HEALTH BEHAVIOR

HEALTH BEHAVIOR
THEORY, RESEARCH, AND PRACTICE

Sixth Edition

EDITED BY

Karen Glanz
University of Pennsylvania
Philadelphia
PA, USA

Barbara K. Rimer
University of North Carolina
Durham
NC, USA

K. Viswanath
Harvard University
Boston
MA, USA

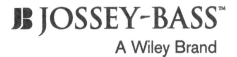
JB JOSSEY-BASS™
A Wiley Brand

Published by John Wiley & Sons, Inc., Hoboken, New Jersey.
Published simultaneously in Canada.

For general information on our other products and services or for technical support, please contact our Customer Care Department within the United States at (800) 762-2974, outside the United States at (317) 572-3993 or fax (317) 572-4002.

Wiley also publishes its books in a variety of electronic formats. Some content that appears in print may not be available in electronic formats. For more information about Wiley products, visit our web site at www.wiley.com.

Library of Congress Cataloging-in-Publication Data applied for:

ISBN 9781394211302 (Hardback)

Cover Design: Wiley
Cover Image: © AniGraphics/Getty Images

Set in 10.5/14pt WarnockPro by Straive, Pondicherry, India

SKY10081176_080624

With warm appreciation to Howard Weitz, who has supported me so steadfastly on this journey and made me laugh when I needed to.

K.G.

With thanks to my husband, Bernard Glassman, whose support has enabled me accomplish more than I could achieve alone, and to all the colleagues who have been there along the way.

B.K.R.

To my parents and their parents who modeled a life of honesty, industry and kindness to their children and grandchildren, and to my teachers and mentors who taught me what pay it forward *means.*

K.V.

CONTENTS

Tables

Figures

The role of behavior in achieving healthy individuals, communities, and populations around the world is becoming ever clearer, and the need to understand behavior and how to enable change ever more urgent. This decade has seen a global pandemic that brought many governments and non-governmental organizations to recognize the vital importance of people's behavior in preventing infection and ameliorating its harms. Key behaviors included social distancing, ensuring ventilation and wearing facemasks in social situations to reduce transmission, being vaccinated to reduce harm, and communicating in ways that engage diverse communities.

Other global existential threats to health include the environmental and biodiversity crises, the dangers of antimicrobial resistance and concerns around cybersecurity and artificial intelligence. These issues and the related behaviors add to the large number that have influenced our health for centuries—for example, tobacco, alcohol, and other drug use; eating and physical activity; adherence to medication and other health interventions; delivery of healthcare; and implementation of evidence-based practice more generally.

In all these global threats, human behavior is at the center of creating and exacerbating them—but also at the heart of reducing or eliminating them.

The harm caused by some behaviors affects not only the well-being of people, their families, and communities, but also people's contribution to society and therefore societal and economic strength. Harms are distributed unequally within and across societies, with those with fewest resources suffering the greatest harm. In recognition of this, in 2023 the World Health Assembly for the first time agreed to a resolution on Behavioral Sciences for Health.

It is in this context that I welcome the 6th edition of *Health Behavior: Theory, Research, and Practice.* The accessible knowledge packed within its pages is foundational for understanding the huge range of behaviors related to health across diverse contexts. This volume also enables the reader to learn about how to apply that understanding to research, public health and clinical practice and policy, communications, education, and training. Each chapter begins with a "vignette" to engage readers' attention, introducing a contemporary problem that can be addressed with relevant theory or evidence.

It reflects advances in the last decade, updating applications and evidence, and two new chapters: Ch 14 on race, health, and health equity; and Ch 22 on social media and health.

The strengths of this outstanding book are many. Here are five that make this a comprehensive and compelling companion for anyone interested in health behavior.

1. It describes **theories of health behavior** and their importance in advancing research and practice in an accessible, compelling way.

Why is theory so important? First, good theories summarize what we know about a field at any point in time, bringing together research findings across diverse domains, populations, and settings. This is essential for accumulating knowledge and advancing the study and application of health behaviors. Second, they outline processes of change, that is how any intervention, policy, or program has an effect on desired outcomes. This enables those designing interventions to target mechanisms that are most likely to bring about change in the behavior of interest. Third, a good theory will also explain variation of effects across contexts, e.g. across populations, settings, and points in time. This is incredibly important as practitioners and policymakers want to be able to ascertain the relevance of research findings conducted in particular contexts for the setting and population they are concerned about. Thus, theories are essential for informing the development of interventions to change behaviors, both because this is likely to lead to more effective interventions, but also because whatever the findings, new knowledge will be generated that can be built on in the future.

2. It demonstrates the **connectedness of theory, research, and practice**.

Just as applying theoretical understanding leads to better policy and practice, feedback from applying theory in practice strengthens understanding. Research is the activity that connects theory and practice. By collecting data in an organized way, research studies can systematically test theoretical propositions and provide evidence to strengthen policy and practice. Well-designed studies can do both of these simultaneously.

3. It recognizes **the importance of context** when considering health behaviors.

Major public health problems can only be successfully addressed by taking into account both local and global contexts, as outlined in Chapter 3 on ecological models. These represent examples of systems thinking and methods which are being increasingly used in considering health behaviors. Systems approaches, including ecological models, can combine population, community, and individual levels in research. They are strengthened by linking the general with the specific in terms of specifying intervention content and mechanisms of action.

The majority of research is conducted in the global North and among relatively advantaged populations, but the majority of health need is in the global South and among disadvantaged communities. This poses the challenge of knowing what evidence can be generalized from research populations to the culturally, socially, and racially diverse populations that health behavior interventions and policies seek to benefit. This edition addresses important issues in the areas of race, health, and health equity in Chapter 14, and of community engagement in Chapter 15.

4. It evaluates **evidence** about the application of theories and models and mechanisms of change.

Over the decade since the 5th edition of *Health Behavior: Theory, Research, and Practice,* there have been significant advances in study designs and methods of data collection. Behavioral interventions can be specified in terms of their component techniques, enabling the evaluation of the effectiveness of particular techniques, along with their links with theoretical processes. The last decade has also seen a digital revolution. Behavior can now be measured directly in real-time, ecologically valid settings, for example via wearables, smartphones, physiological monitors, and environmental sensors. This provides a wealth of data about how behavior changes in response to environmental, physiological, and reported psychological processes. This has huge potential to advance our theories and models about how health behaviors can be changed. Complex data sets require complex analyses; harnessing the power of machine learning and artificial intelligence open up new horizons for the field.

5. It is **accessible and engaging**, aimed at a wide spectrum of readers.

The many groups that this book will interest and inform include health, education, and communication practitioners; intervention developers and policy planners; and researchers seeking to generate the best possible evidence and theoretical understanding. Chapters draw the reader in by beginning with a contemporary problem that can be addressed with the theory or model, followed by critiques and evaluation of evidence. This includes the all-important issue as to how theoretical constructs are conceived in practice and measured. New topics that were not a "thing" 10 years ago are included, for example, social media and health in Chapter 22.

This book will be an invaluable resource for all those wanting an accessible and authoritative source to guide all aspects of the research process from conceptualizing problems in behavioural terms to writing protocols or research reports to synthesize evidence to consult with those wishing to use research findings in their work. The combination of rigorous thinking and methods with practical applications and case studies make this book shine out in an already sunny landscape.

Susan Michie
London, UK
November 2023

Programs to influence health behavior, including health promotion and education programs and interventions, generally are more likely to benefit participants and communities when guided by a theory or theories of health behavior. Theories of health behavior can help program planners consider the sources of influence on particular health behaviors and identify the targets for behavior change and methods for accomplishing these changes. Theories also can inform the evaluation of change efforts by helping planners, evaluators, and others to specify the outcomes to be measured and the timing and methods of study. Although the evidence is not unequivocal, when they are developed and implemented thoughtfully and systematically, theory-driven health promotion and education efforts stand in contrast to programs based primarily on precedent, tradition, intuition, or general principles.

Theory-driven health behavior change interventions and programs require an understanding of the components of health behavior theories and operational or practical forms of the theories. The first edition of this book, published in 1990, was the first text to provide an in-depth analysis of various theories of health behavior relevant to health education in a single volume. It brought together dominant health behavior theories, research based on those theories, and examples of health education practice derived from theory that had been tested through evaluation and research. The second (1996), third (2002), fourth (2008), and fifth (2015) editions of this book updated and improved upon the earlier volumes. People around the world are using this book. It has been translated into multiple languages, including, most recently, Japanese, Korean, and Chinese editions.

We are confident that the sixth edition of *Health Behavior: Theory, Research, and Practice* improves upon on the preceding edition, as each earlier edition has done. The main purpose of the book is the same: to advance the science of understanding health behavior and the practice of health behavior change through the informed application of theories of health behavior. Likewise, this book serves as the definitive text for students, practitioners, and scientists in these areas and education in three ways: by analyzing the key components of health behavior theories, by describing current applications of these theories in selected public health and health promotion programs and interventions, and by identifying important future directions for research and practice in health behavior change.

The sixth edition responds to new developments in health behavior theories and the application of theories in new settings, to new populations, and in new ways. This edition includes an enhanced focus on the application of theories for diverse populations and settings, and there are more chapters written by diverse authors. There is a corresponding integration of issues related to race and ethnicity in multiple chapters and a new chapter (Chapter 14) focused on theories of race and racism. Authors recognize the complexity of race/ethnicity; these are not mere variables. Rather, they are the lenses through which people experience the world. Issues of culture and health inequities are also integrated into many chapters. These issues are of broad and growing importance across many theories and models. We believe that these additions strengthen the book and increase its value for use in settings around the world. The world is more global than ever before, and professionals working on behavior change often will work in multiple countries. We have a heightened commitment to addressing health risks and threats in low- and middle-income countries (LMICs). Thus, more global applications from both developing and developed countries are included.

As new information and communication technologies have opened up an unprecedented range of strategies for health behavior change, this edition integrates expanded coverage of social media and digital health behavior interventions examples throughout the book.

Audiences

This book is written for graduate students, practitioners, and scientists who spend part or all of their time in the broad arenas of health behavior change, public health, health promotion, and health education; the text will assist them both to understand the theories and to apply them in practical settings. Practitioners, as well as students, should find this text a major reference for the development and evaluation of theory-driven health behavior change programs and interventions. Researchers should emerge with a recognition of areas where empirical support is deficient or inconclusive, helping set the research agenda for health behavior going forward.

This book is intended to assist all professionals who value the need to influence health behavior positively. Their fields include health promotion and education, health communication, medicine, nursing, public health, health psychology, behavioral medicine, health communications, nutrition and dietetics, dentistry, pharmacy, social work, exercise science, clinical psychology, and occupational and physical therapy.

Overview of the Book

The chapters, written expressly for this sixth edition, address theories and models of health behavior at the level of the individual, interpersonal, group, organization, and community and approaches that are integrated across multiple levels.

The book is organized into five parts. Part One defines key terms and concepts and introduces ecological models. The next three parts reflect important units of health behavior and education practice: the individual, the interpersonal or group level, and the community or aggregate level. Each of these parts begins with an introductory chapter to orient readers to the next chapters and their interrelationships, and has several chapters. Part Two covers theories of individual health behavior, and its chapters focus on variables *within individuals* that influence their health behavior and response to health promotion and education interventions. Three bodies of theory are reviewed in separate chapters: Health Belief Model; Theory of Reasoned Action/Theory of Planned Behavior/Integrated Behavioral Model and the Reasoned Action Approach, and The Transtheoretical Model. Part Three examines interpersonal theories, which emphasize elements in the *interpersonal* environment that affect individuals' health behavior. Four chapters examine Social Cognitive Theory: social support, social networks; and stress and coping. Part Four covers models for the *community or aggregate level* of change and includes chapters on race, health, and health equity; community engagement; implementation, dissemination, and diffusion of innovations; and media communications. Part Five explores "Using Theory," which presents the key components and applications of overarching planning and process models and integrated models and approaches to health behavior change. It includes chapters on theory-based planning models, behavioral economics, social marketing, and social media (new for this edition).

The major emphasis of this book is on the analysis and application of health behavior theories to public health and health promotion practice. The section introductory chapters in Parts Two, Three, Four and Five introduce the theories in their sections; summarize their potential application to the development of health behavior change interventions; and highlight strengths, weaknesses, gaps and areas for future development and research, and promising strategies. Each core chapter in Parts Two, Three, and Four begins with a discussion of the background of the theory or model and a presentation of the theory; reviews empirical support for it; and concludes with one or two applications.

Chapter authors are established, highly regarded researchers, and practitioners who draw on their experiences in state-of-the-art research to critically analyze and apply the theories to health behavior and education. This text makes otherwise lofty theories accessible and practical, and advances both research and practice in the process.

No single book can be truly comprehensive and still be concise and readable. Decisions about which theories to include were made with both an appreciation of the evolution of the study of health behavior and a vision of its future (see Chapter 2). We emphasize theories and conceptual frameworks that encompass a range from the individual to the societal level. We acknowledge that there is substantial variability in the extent to which various theories and models have been codified, tested, and supported by empirical evidence. Of necessity, some promising emerging theories were not included.

The first five editions of this book grew out of the editors' own experiences, frustrations, and needs as well as their desire to synthesize many literatures and to draw clearly the linkages between theory, research, and practice in health behavior and education. We have sought to show how theory, research, and practice interrelate and to make each accessible and practical. In this sixth edition, we have attempted to respond to changes in the science and practice of public health and health promotion and to update the coverage of these areas in a rapidly evolving field. Substantial efforts have been taken to present findings from health behavior change interventions based on the theories that are described and to illustrate the adaptations needed to successfully reach diverse and unique populations.

Through the preceding five editions, *Health Behavior: Theory, Research and Practice* has become established as a widely used text and reference book.

It is our sincere hope that the sixth edition will continue to be relevant and useful, and to stimulate readers' interest in theory-based health behavior and health education. We aspire to provide readers with the information and skills to ask critical questions, think conceptually, and stretch their thinking beyond using formulaic strategies to improve health. Ultimately, we aim to encourage users to use, test, refine, and even develop theories with the goal of improving health for people around the world and to benefit especially those populations that have suffered disproportionately from the conditions that predispose to poor health.

Acknowledgments

We owe deep gratitude to all the authors whose work is included in this book. They worked diligently with us to produce an integrated volume, and we greatly appreciate their willingness to tailor their contributions to realize the vision of the book. Their collective depth of knowledge and experience across the broad range of theories and topics far exceeds the expertise that the editors can claim.

We acknowledge authors who contributed to the first five editions of this book; although some of them did not write chapters for this edition, their intellectual contributions form an important foundation for this volume.

We pay special tribute to Dr. James Prochaska and Dr. Kay Bartholomew, luminaries in our field whose work appeared in earlier editions of this book who passed away since the last edition was published. Their work is an influential foundation for chapters in this edition that were written by their colleagues.

The editorial team at Wiley provided valuable support to us for development, production, and marketing of this edition. We also are grateful to Terra Ziporyn for her exceptional technical editing support for this edition.

The editors are indebted to their colleagues and students who, over the years, have taught them the importance of both health behavior theories and their cogent and precise representation. They have challenged us to stretch, adapt, and continue to learn through our years of work at the University of Michigan, the University of North Carolina (UNC) at Chapel Hill, the University of Pennsylvania (UPenn), Emory University, Harvard University, the University of Minnesota, Ohio State University, Johns Hopkins University, Temple University, Fox Chase Cancer Center, Duke University, the University of Hawai'i, and the National Cancer Institute (NCI).

We thank Daniel Holman and Alisha Suhag from the University of Sheffield (UK), who collaborated on the umbrella review of theory-behavior change intervention effectiveness that is described in Chapter 2. We also thank members of the Viswanath Lab at Harvard/Dana-Farber and the Center for Health Behavior Research team at Penn, who respectively made it possible for Vish Viswanath and Karen Glanz to focus on the book while they ensured progress on active projects. Further, completion of this manuscript would not have been possible without the dedicated assistance of Lisa Warren and Ellie Bernstein at UNC, and Claudia Caponi at UPenn.

We also express our thanks to our colleagues, staffs, friends, and families, whose patience, good humor, and encouragement sustained us through our work on this book.

January 2024

Karen Glanz
Philadelphia, Pennsylvania

Barbara K. Rimer
Chapel Hill, North Carolina

K. Viswanath
Boston, Massachusetts

ABOUT THE EDITORS

Karen Glanz is George A. Weiss University Professor, Professor in the Perelman School of Medicine and the School of Nursing, and Director of the UPenn Prevention Research Center and the Center for Health Behavior Research at the University of Pennsylvania. She is Program Co-Leader of the Cancer Control Program at the Abramson Cancer Center and has been Director of the Community Engagement and Research (CEAR) Core of the UPenn CTSA since 2011.

Glanz is a senior fellow of the Leonard Davis Institute of Health Economics and the Center for Public Health Initiatives, a distinguished fellow of the Annenberg Public Policy Center, and a fellow of the Penn Institute for Urban Research. She was previously at Emory University (2004–2009), the University of Hawaii (1993–2004), and Temple University (1979–1993). She received her MPH (1977) and PhD (1979) degrees in health behavior and health education from the University of Michigan.

A globally influential public health scholar whose work spans psychology, epidemiology, nutrition, and other disciplines, her research in community and healthcare settings focuses on obesity, physical activity, nutrition, and the built environment; cancer prevention and control; chronic disease management and control; reducing health disparities; and implementation science. Her research and publications about understanding, measuring, and improving healthy food environments, beginning in the 1980s, has been widely recognized and replicated. She served on the NHLBI Advisory Council from 2016 to 2021 and was a member of the US Task Force on Community Preventive Services from 2006 to 2016. Her scholarly contributions consist of more than 550 journal articles and book chapters.

Dr. Glanz has been recognized with local and national awards for her work, including being elected to membership in the National Academy of Medicine in 2013. She was elected to be a fellow of the College of Physicians of Philadelphia, named a fellow of the Society for Behavioral Medicine and received the Elizabeth Fries Health Education Award. She was designated a highly cited author by Clarivate (formerly ISI), in the top 0.5% of authors in her field over a 20-year period, beginning in 2016.

Barbara K. Rimer is Dean Emerita and Alumni Distinguished Professor Emerita of Health Behavior at the University of North Carolina at Chapel Hill Gillings School of Global Public Health. In her 17 years of leading the Gillings School, she was known for her strong commitment to inclusive excellence.

Dr. Rimer received an MPH (1973) from the University of Michigan, with joint majors in health education and medical care organization, and a DrPH (1981) in health education from the Johns Hopkins School of Hygiene and Public Health. Previously, she served as Deputy Director for Population Sciences at UNC Lineberger Comprehensive Cancer Center at UNC-Chapel Hill (2003-2005), and as Director of the Division of Cancer Control and Population Sciences at the National Cancer Institute (part of the National Institutes of Health), from 1997 to 2002.

Dr. Rimer has conducted research in several areas, including informed decision-making, long-term maintenance of behavior changes (such as diet, cancer screening, and tobacco use), interventions to increase adherence to cancer prevention and early detection, dissemination of evidence-based interventions, and use of new technologies for information, support, and behavior change.

Dr. Rimer is the author of over 270 peer-reviewed articles, 55 book chapters, and six books, and serves on several journal editorial boards. She is the recipient of numerous awards and honors; in 2013, she was awarded the American Cancer Society's Medal of Honor for her cancer research, which has guided national research, practice, and policy for more than 20 years. In 2024, she received the Welch-Rose Award from the Association of Schools and Programs of Public Health.

Dr. Rimer was the first woman and behavioral scientist to lead the National Cancer Institute's National Cancer Advisory Board, a presidential appointment. She was elected to the Institute of Medicine (now the National Academy of Medicine) in 2008 and appointed by President Obama to chair the President's Cancer Panel in 2011, for which served as Chair through 2019.

K. Viswanath is Lee Kum Kee Professor of Health Communication in the Department of Social and Behavioral Sciences at the Harvard T. H. Chan School of Public Health (HSPH) and in the McGraw-Patterson Center for Population Sciences at the Dana-Farber Cancer Institute (DFCI). He is also the Director of Lee Kum Sheung Center for Health and Happiness, Harvard Chan, Director of the Center for Translational Communication Science, DFCI, Associate Director for Community Outreach and Engagement, Dana-Farber/Harvard Cancer Center, and Director, Harvard Chan India Research Center.

Dr. Viswanath's work is driven by two fundamental concerns: (i) how to center equity in drawing on translational communication science to promote health and well-being for all population groups and (ii) to involve community-based organizations and stakeholders in promoting social change. His work has documented the relationship between communication inequalities, poverty and health inequalities, and knowledge translation to address health inequalities. He has written more than 320 journal articles, reviews, commentaries, and book chapters and coedited three books and monographs (in addition to co-editing two earlier editions of this book): *Mass Media, Social Control, and Social Change* (Iowa State University Press, 1999), *The Role of Media in Promoting and Reducing Tobacco Use* (National Cancer Institute, 2008), and *A Socioecological Approach to Addressing Tobacco-Related Health Disparities* (National Cancer Institute, 2017). He was the Editor of the Social and Behavioral Research section of the 12-volume *International Encyclopedia of Communication* (Blackwell Publishing, 2008).

He served on and chaired several national committees for the US Government and the National Academy of Sciences, Engineering, and Medicine (NASEM) and currently Chairs the NASEM Consensus Study Committee on Understanding and Addressing Misinformation in Science.

In recognition of his academic and professional achievements, Dr. Viswanath received several awards including the Outstanding Health Communication Scholar Award from the International and National Communication Associations, and the Mayhew Derryberry Award from the American Public Health Association for contributions to health education research and theory. He is an elected fellow of the International Communication Association (2011), the Society for Behavioral Medicine (2008), and the Midwest Association for Public Opinion Research (2006).

Zinzi Bailey is an associate professor in the Department of Epidemiology and Community Health at the University of Minnesota School of Public Health.

Sara G. Balestrieri is the director of research at the National Resident Matching Program.

Mesfin A. Bekalu is a program officer at the National Institute of Mental Health at the National Institutes of Health.

Ganga Bey is an assistant professor in the Department of Epidemiology at Gillings School of Global Public Health at the University of North Carolina at Chapel Hill.

Amy Bleakley is a professor in the Department of Communication at the University of Delaware.

Noel T. Brewer is a professor in the Department of Health Behavior at Gillings School of Global Public Health at the University of North Carolina at Chapel Hill.

Tamara J. Cadet is an associate professor in the School of Social Policy and Practice at the University of Pennsylvania.

Jessica L. Cohen is a Beal associate professor in the Department of Global Health and Population at the Harvard T. H. Chan School of Public Health.

Casey Durand was an assistant professor at the University of Texas Health Science Center at Houston.

Shari Esquenazi-Karonika is a senior program director in the Department of Integrative Health at New York University (NYU) Langone Health.

Kerry E. Evers is the co-president and CEO of Pro-Change Behavior Systems, Inc. in Rhode Island.

María E. Fernández is the vice president of Population Health and Implementation Science and Lorne Bain distinguished professor at the University of Texas Health Science Center at Houston.

Sarah E. Gollust is a professor in the Division of Health Policy and Management at the University of Minnesota School of Public Health.

Deanna M. Hoelscher is John P. McGovern professor in health promotion and the director of the Michael and Susan Dell Center for Healthy Living the University of Texas School of Public Health in Austin.

Julianne Holt-Lunstad is a professor of psychology and neuroscience at Brigham Young University.

Shawnika Hull is an associate professor of communication in the School of Communication and Information at Rutgers University.

Ethan T. Hunt is an assistant professor of health promotion and behavioral sciences at the University of Texas School of Public Health.

Alejandra Jáuregui is the chair of the Department of Physical Activity and Healthy Lifestyles at the Mexican National Institute of Public Health.

Joseph Keawe'aimoku (Keawe) Kaholokula is a professor and chair of the Department of Native Hawaiian Health at the John A. Burns School of Medicine, University of Hawai'i at Mānoa.

Steven H. Kelder is Beth Toby Grossman professor in spirituality and healing and professor of epidemiology, human genetics and environmental sciences at the University of Texas School of Public Health.

Racquel E. Kohler is an assistant professor in the Department of Health Behavior, Society, and Policy at the Rutgers University School of Public Health

Evelyn Kumoji is with the Johns Hopkins Center for Communication Programs.

Dale S. Mantey is an assistant professor of health promotion and behavioral sciences at the University of Texas School of Public Health.

Christine Markham is Alan King professor and chair of the Division of Health Promotion and Behavioral Sciences at the University of Texas School of Public Health.

Patricia Dolan Mullen is a professor of health promotion and behavioral sciences and Distinguished Teaching Professor at the University of Texas School of Public Health.

Rebekah H. Nagler is an associate professor in the Hubbard School of Journalism and Mass Communication at the University of Minnesota.

John G. Oetzel is a professor in the Department of Management Communication in the Waikato Management School at the University of Waikato in New Zealand.

Melissa Peskin is an assistant professor of health promotion and behavioral sciences and epidemiology at the University of Texas School of Public Health.

Sarah E. Piombo is a PhD candidate in the Department of Population and Public Health Sciences at Keck School of Medicine, University of Southern California.

Andrew Scot Proctor is a PhD candidate in social and health psychology at Brigham Young University.

Shoba Ramanadhan is an associate professor of social and behavioral sciences at the Harvard T.H. Chan School of Public Health.

Fred Rariewa is with the sustainability and social enterprise division at the Johns Hopkins Center for Communication Programs.

Serena A. Rodriguez is an assistant professor of health promotion and behavioral sciences at the University of Texas School of Public Health.

Deborah Salvo is an associate professor in the Department of Kinesiology and Health Education in the College of Education at the University of Texas at Austin.

Rachel C. Shelton is an associate professor of sociomedical sciences at the Columbia University Mailman School of Public Health.

Ka'imi A. Sinclair (deceased) was an associate professor in the College of Nursing at Washington State University.

J. Douglas Storey is a professor emeritus and was director for Communication Science and Research at the Center for Communication Programs, in the Johns Hopkins University Bloomberg School of Public Health.

Celette Sugg Skinner is Parkland Community Medicine professor at the University of Texas Southwestern School of Public Health.

Harsha Thirumurthy is a professor in the Department of Medical Ethics and Health Policy at the University of Pennsylvania, Perelman School of Medicine.

Jasmin A. Tiro is a professor in the Department of Public Health Sciences at University of Chicago Medicine.

Ridvan (Riz) Tupai-Firestone is an associate professor and associate dean at the Centre for Public Health Research at Massey University in New Zealand.

Thomas W. Valente is a professor of population and public health sciences at the University of Southern California Keck School of Medicine.

Yunita Wahyuningrum (deceased) was a project director at the Center for Communication Programs at the Johns Hopkins University.

Cheryl L. Woods-Giscombe is Levine Family Distinguished professor in the School of Nursing at the University of North Carolina at Chapel Hill.

ABOUT THE COMPANION WEBSITE

This book is accompanied by a companion website:

www.wiley.com/go/glanz/healthbehavior6e

The website includes:

- Test Bank
- Power Points
- Transition Guide

CHAPTER 1

THE SCOPE OF HEALTH BEHAVIOR

The Editors

In 2020–2022, the world experienced the COVID-19 pandemic, which brought about the most profound changes globally since the influenza pandemic of 1918–1919. The SARS-CoV-2 virus spread across the world. Conservatively, almost 7 million people died, economies sputtered, governments faltered, and inequities were highlighted in searing ways. Quickly, COVID-19, the disease caused by the virus, became one of the world's worst killers in multiple countries, with most of those deaths coming from low- and middle-income countries (LMICs). In tragedy, there also was dramatic progress and innovation as vaccines and treatments for COVID-19 were developed at lightning speed. The pandemic underlined more acutely than any recent event the centrality of health behavior and the threats of health inequities. In the early days of the pandemic (winter/spring 2020), before there were vaccines and treatments, it was necessary to rely on what was learned in 1918 and since—the importance of masks, physical distancing, and good hygiene, such as handwashing. Unfortunately, these proven, common-sense activities became highly politicized. Some countries, such as South Korea, were remarkably successful in applying interventions to prevent sickness and death early in the pandemic, though the country proved vulnerable in its later stages. Other countries had leaders who distrusted science and waited too long to adopt proven interventions. Millions became infected and died as a result, and the economies in these countries were hard-hit. Then, a concerning pattern emerged with the adoption of vaccines: while overall vaccine uptake was relatively high, disadvantaged populations often did not get vaccinated due to mistrust and/or lack of access. COVID also drew attention to an emerging *infodemic*, or spread of information, often false, at a volume and great speed, affecting health behaviors and challenging people's and systems' capacities to cope with the pandemic.

The 2020 pandemic is one of the strongest historical cases of why understanding health behavior and applying science-driven interventions is a matter of life and death. The pandemic also showed that we cannot separate health behaviors from communities and health systems, and that multiple levels of interventions, including policies, are needed to address a deadly viral threat. And it demonstrated that unprepared health systems and communities are not resilient when faced with a pandemic like COVID-19. To prevent future infectious disease outbreaks on a

Health Behavior: Theory, Research, and Practice, Sixth Edition. Edited by Karen Glanz, Barbara K. Rimer, and K. Viswanath.
© 2024 John Wiley & Sons, Inc. Published 2024 by John Wiley & Sons, Inc.
Companion website: www.wiley.com/go/glanz/healthbehavior6e

global scale and improve population health, societal issues, including deeply embedded structural inequities, must be tackled (Lancet Editors, 2020).

There are many other examples to demonstrate why health behavior is so important to health. More than half the top 10 causes of death worldwide are attributed to unhealthy behaviors (World Health Organization, 2023b). 30–50% of cancers are preventable, mostly by behavioral means. With 18 million cancers projected in 2023, changing behavior could save millions of lives globally (Shiels et al., 2023). Infectious and chronic diseases and the factors that drive them—including failure to vaccinate and practice good hygiene, obesity, and physical inactivity, overuse of opioids, and underuse of proven methods to screen and treat diseases when they are early and curable—all contribute to avoidable illness and mortality. Globalization and westernization have accelerated the speed with which diseases of developed countries, such as diabetes and cancers, are increasing in the developing world. Life expectancy is falling for less-educated groups and is eclipsing racial inequities (Case & Deaton, 2021). In many parts of the world, increasing affluence has made automobile accidents a growing threat. There is growing recognition that health behavior changes are needed across the world if population health is to improve.

Where professionals once might have seen their roles as working at a particular level of intervention (such as changing organizational or individual health behaviors) or employing a specific type of behavior change strategy (such as group interventions or individual counseling), evidence shows that multiple kinds of interventions at different levels often are needed to initiate and sustain behavior change effectively. This is true for tobacco use, physical activity, and obesity. During the pandemic, policy interventions were used to mandate masking and provide special funding and services, such as food assistance, for unemployed and low-income families. Community interventions were developed for at-risk groups. Media, pharmacy, and clinical interventions aimed to persuade people to be vaccinated. Environmental approaches, such as wastewater surveillance, were used to understand transmission and provide early warning systems. Any of these alone would have been insufficient to achieve maximal impact. The determinants of health behavior and health are multicomponent and multilevel, and the strategies to improve them are equally complex.

What is Health Behavior?

In the broadest sense, *health behavior* refers to the actions of individuals, groups, and organizations and the determinants, correlates, and consequences of actions, including social change, policy development and implementation, improved coping skills, and enhanced quality of life (Parkerson et al., 1993). This is aligned with the working definition of *health behavior* that Gochman proposed, although his definition emphasized individuals: it includes not only observable, overt actions but also the mental events and feeling states that can be reported and measured. Gochman defined health behavior as "those personal attributes such as beliefs, expectations, motives, values, perceptions, and other cognitive elements; personality characteristics, including affective and emotional states and traits; and overt behavior patterns, actions, and habits that relate to health maintenance, to health restoration, and to health improvement" (Gochman, 1982, 1997).

Gochman's definition is consistent with and embraces the definitions of specific categories of overt health behavior proposed by Kasl and Cobb in their seminal articles. Kasl and Cobb defined three categories of health behavior along a continuum of health and illness: preventive health behavior (primary prevention), illness behavior (disease detection and care-seeking); and sick-role behavior (medical treatment, adherence, and self-care) (Kasl & Cobb, 1966a, b).

Health, Disease, and Health Behavior: Global Needs and Goals

Substantial suffering, premature mortality, and medical costs can be avoided by positive changes in behavior at multiple levels. During the past 30 years, there has been a dramatic increase in public, private, and professional interest and investment in preventing disability and death through changes in lifestyle and increasing participation in screening programs. Much of the interest in disease prevention and early detection was stimulated by the growth of noncommunicable diseases around the world, while injuries and old and emerging infections continue to pose growing threats to health. Risks associated with the highest number of deaths worldwide now include behavioral risk factors such as tobacco use, alcohol use, and dietary risks; child and maternal malnutrition; unhealthy air; and chronic disease risk factors and conditions such as obesity, kidney dysfunction, and elevated blood pressure, blood glucose, and lipids. Leading causes of disability-adjusted life years (DALYs) are heart disease, stroke, diabetes, lung diseases, road injuries, neonatal disorders, and congenital birth defects (Institute for Health Metrics and Evaluation, 2020). Global aging is bringing rapidly escalating healthcare costs and large increases in dementia, currently the seventh highest cause of death, with catastrophic costs (World Health Organization, 2023a).

Country and global population health goals are an essential part of strategies to improve health behavior and health. Landmark reports in Canada and the United States during the 1970s and 1980s heralded the commitment of governments to health education and promotion (Epp, 1986; Lalonde, 1974; U.S. Department of Health, Education, and Welfare, 1979). In the United States, federal initiatives for public health education and monitoring population-wide behavior patterns were spurred by the development of the *Health Objectives for the Nation* (U.S. Department of Health and Human Services, 1980) and their successors that have been released each decade (U.S. Department of Health and Human Services, 2023). International agencies have drawn attention to the global burden of diseases and health inequalities (World Health Organization, 2014) as have the United Nations' Sustainable Development Goals (SDGs), released in 2015 (United Nations, 2023). Several of the SDGs focus specifically on health and health-related behaviors, including zero hunger, clean water and sanitation, climate action, reduced inequalities, and the broad category of good health and well-being (United Nations, 2023). Increased interest in behavioral and social determinants of health behavior change has spawned numerous training programs and public and commercial service programs.

Health Behavior and Health Behavior Change

The Changing Scope of Health Behavior

Since the first edition of this book in 1990, the interconnectedness of the world has become accepted as a fact. If there were doubts, the pandemic cemented this realization. Rapid changes in communication technologies have contributed to making the world a much smaller place and accelerated the pace of sharing information and ideas, with both positive and negative consequences (Galea et al., 2023; Viswanath et al., 2021). As was observed during the pandemic, mis- and disinformation pose major threats to health. We discuss some of these issues later in the book. To the extent that public health is global health, and global health is local, we are committed in this volume to exploring the use of health behavior theories globally and to discussing the potential relevance of what is learned in one setting to other settings. We also recognize that old ideas about global health must change. It is widely recognized that those who seek to change people's health behaviors must work collaboratively with communities to understand the culture and more of those whose behaviors they aim to alter. Lessons may move from the developing to developed world and back in reciprocal ways. As a result, the ways public health graduates will work globally have changed dramatically—from directing those in LMICs to partnering with them, co-learning about the problems, and co-developing solutions. Understanding theory is an important asset in the toolboxes of health professionals.

The science and art of health behavior and health behavior change are eclectic, rapidly evolving, and reflect an amalgamation of approaches, methods, and strategies from social and health sciences. They draw on the theoretical perspectives, research, and practice tools of such diverse disciplines as psychology, sociology, data science, anthropology, communications, nursing, economics, and marketing. Health behavior research and practice also depend on epidemiology, statistics, and medicine. Big data are now a tool for health behavior and other fields. Artificial intelligence and machine learning are emerging as powerful forces and will play even larger roles in intervention development. We should engage with them thoughtfully.

There is also increasing emphasis on an interdisciplinary or even a transdisciplinary focus and the use of team science to solve big, complex problems, such as health inequities, climate threats, obesity, and mental health. Many kinds of health, social service, and social science professionals contribute to and conduct health behavior research and practice. Ultimately, their work is strengthened by collaboration among professionals of different disciplines, each concerned with the behavioral and social intervention process, and contributing unique perspectives.

Evidence-Based Health Behavior for the 21ˢᵗ Century

The evidence base for health behavior change has grown dramatically over the past three decades. Today, there are many tools and strategies accessible from journals, books, and web-based repositories to understand the role that health behavior theories can play in producing effective, sustained behavior changes. Evidence-based groups like the Cochrane Collaboration (Cochrane, 2023) and the CDC's Guide to Community Preventive Services (U.S. DHHS, 2023a, b) offer regular syntheses of behavioral interventions, some of which include theoretical constructs as variables in analyses of effectiveness.

The topics on which health professionals and health behavior experts focus have evolved as health problems have changed around the world. Professionals may counsel people at risk for AIDS about safe sex and medication to prevent HIV infections; help children avoid tobacco, alcohol, and drugs; assist adults to stop smoking; encourage physicians to avoid opioid overprescribing; teach patients to manage and cope with their chronic illnesses; and organize communities and advocate policy changes aimed at fostering health improvement and reducing environmental injustice. Health systems, physicians, and other clinicians increasingly see a role for themselves and their teams to intervene in patients' social determinants (Vanjani et al., 2023). Health professionals also may address environmental concerns, such as safe, accessible water and unhealthy air. Exposure to unhealthy particulates due to climate-related wildfires, and extreme heat, are also medical issues. Where effective strategies to promote healthful behaviors and prevent diseases are available, they should be widely adopted and consistently implemented. A central premise of this book is that public health and medicine are not in opposition. As Kaney (2023) has written, it should not be either/or, it should be both/and.

Health Behavior Change

Positive, informed changes in health behaviors are typically the ultimate aims of health behavior change programs. If behaviors change but health is not improved, it is possible that the theory connecting the behavior to health is wrong or inadequate, or the way behavior was measured is flawed. Efforts to improve environments, policies, and other outcomes should be evaluated for their effects on health behaviors and health. If a policy changes, but does not lead to measurable changes in behavior, it may be either too weak, too shortlived, ineffectively implemented, or only a limited determinant of behavior.

Settings and Audiences for Health Behavior Change

Public health professionals work around the world, in a variety of settings, including schools, worksites, government and nongovernmental organizations (including voluntary health organizations), medical and dental settings, and communities and community organizations. Even professionals not in the health field may influence health behaviors. Applications in the book offer many examples of different settings, health problems, and the role of theory in addressing them. During the past century, and more specifically during the past few decades, the scope and methods of health behavior change strategies have broadened and diversified dramatically. This section briefly reviews the range of settings and audiences for health behavior change today.

Settings: Health behavior interventions can occur almost anywhere. Seven major settings are particularly relevant to contemporary health behavior: schools, communities, worksites, healthcare settings, where people live, where people worship, the consumer marketplace, and the communications environment. Policy interventions may be delivered at the level of governments and other organizations. Examples of types of interventions in these settings are shown in Table 1.1.

Audiences: For health behavior change interventions to be effective, strategies should be designed with an understanding of the recipients, or audiences, their health, cultural context, and social characteristics, and their beliefs, attitudes, values, skills, and past behaviors. These audiences consist of people who may be reached as individuals, in groups, through organizations, as communities or sociopolitical entities, or through some combination of these. They may be health professionals, clients, people at risk for disease, or patients. Table 1.2 describes four dimensions along which the potential audiences can be characterized: social determinants of health (Adler et al., 2016; Centers for Disease Control, 2023; World Health Organization, 2023c), ethnic or racial background, life cycle stage, and disease or at-risk status.

Table 1.1   Settings for Health Behavior Interventions

Settings	Key Types of Interventions
Schools	• Changes in school environment and policies • Capacity-building among school personnel (e.g., teachers) • Inclusion/interventions through existing or new curricula
Worksites	• Workplace conditions that constrain or facilitate worker health behaviors • Total Worker Health: Integration of workplace safety with health promotion • Workplace wellness and well-being programs to change lifestyles
Healthcare Settings	• Programs for high-risk patients and their families and caregivers • In-service training for healthcare providers
Communities	• Community engagement and community mobilization for program design and delivery • Examples of community-based organizations as partners include churches, clubs, recreation centers, and neighborhoods
Consumer Marketplace	• Choice architecture to make the easy choice the healthy choice (Chapter 20) • Counter "commercial determinants" such as promotion of unhealthy lifestyles (e.g., fast food or tobacco) • Use social marketing to encourage healthy lifestyle (Chapter 21)
Communication Environment	• Advances in information and communication technologies and cyber-infrastructure provide opportunities to promote health • Participatory communication technologies such as social media have been successfully used to promote health (Chapter 22) • Mass media campaigns for countering misinformation, defining health, and promoting healthy behaviors (Chapter 17)

Table 1.2   Features of Audiences for Health Behavior Interventions

Audience Characteristics	Examples and Key Considerations
Social Determinants of Health (SDOH) (Adler et al., 2016; WHO, 2023c)	• Nonmedical factors that influence health outcomes; conditions in which people are born, grow, work, live, and age • Wider forces and systems shaping the conditions of daily life • Include income, education, housing, access to health care
Racial and Ethnic Background	• As social constructs, closely aligned with SDOH • Neighborhood racial distribution • Segregation, structural racism • Inequities in morbidity and mortality, often gender-specific
Life-Cycle Stage	• Developmental perspectives help guide intervention design and delivery • Life-course perspective is often aligned with determinants of behaviors, e.g., sense of vulnerability/invulnerability • In the U.S., the aging population, including the very old, is increasing disproportionately
At-Risk and Disease Status	• Risk factors often prompt greater use of health care • Patients' needs vary depending on the nature of their health problems—for example, acute or chronic, disabling or limiting • Self-care strategies can help with disease management and maintaining functional status

Health Behavior Foundations for Theory, Research, and Practice

This chapter has discussed the dynamic nature of health behavior today in the context of emerging patterns of disease and trends in social interaction and communication, health care, health education, and disease prevention in the United States and globally. It has provided definitions of health behavior and described the broad and diverse parameters of this maturing field. Although thousands more studies of health behavior change have been conducted and reported since the last edition of this book, their variable results continue to raise new questions and pose methodological, theoretical, and substantive challenges. The interrelationships and importance of theory, research, and practice are set against a backdrop of the urgent, growing, and complex imperative to improve the health of populations around the world and to do so in a context that recognizes that healthcare services are only some of the forces that influence health status. Today's students, researchers, and practitioners can make a difference in the burden of illness and the potential to develop effective, scalable interventions to improve health.

Observations by McGinnis (1994) are still relevant today: The challenge of understanding and improving health behavior is "one of the most complex tasks yet confronted by science. To competently address that challenge, the . . . research community must simply do more and do it better" in certain key areas of behavioral research. A coordinated and focused effort is essential to resolve many of the most vexing health issues facing our society (Smedley & Syme, 2000). Integration of the best available knowledge from theory, research, and behavior change practice can advance that agenda in the years ahead.

References

Adler, N. E., Cutler, D. M., Fielding, J. E., Galea, S., Glymour, M. M., Koh, H. K., & Satcher, D. (2016). Addressing social determinants of health and health disparities: A vital direction for health and health care. *NAM Perspectives.* Discussion Paper, National Academy of Medicine, Washington, DC. https://doi.org/10.31478/201609t.

Case, A., & Deaton, A. (2021). Life expectancy in adulthood is falling for those without a BA degree, but as educational gaps have widened, racial gaps have narrowed. *Proceedings of the National Academy of Sciences, 118*(11), e2024777118.

Centers for Disease Control and Prevention. (2023). Social determinants of health at CDC. https://www.cdc.gov/about/sdoh/index.html.

Cochrane. (2023). http://www.cochrane.org.

Epp, L. (1986). *Achieving health for all: A framework for health promotion in Canada.* Toronto: Health and Welfare Canada.

Galea, S., Buckley, G. J., & Wojtowicz, A. (Eds.). (2023). *Social media and adolescent health.* Washington, DC: The National Academies Press. https://doi.org/10.17226/27396.

Gochman, D. S. (1982). Labels, systems, and motives: Some perspectives on future research. *Health Education Quarterly, 9,* 167–174.

Gochman, D. S. (1997). Health behavior research: Definitions and diversity. In D. S. Gochman (Ed.), *Handbook of health behavior research I. Personal and social determinants.* New York: Plenum Press.

Institutes for Health Metrics and Evaluation. (2020). The Lancet: Latest global disease estimates reveal perfect storm of rising chronic diseases and public health failures fuelling COVID-19 pandemic. https://www.healthdata.org/news-events/newsroom/news-releases/lancet-latest-global-disease-estimates-reveal-perfect-storm.

Kaney, K. (2023). *Both/and: Public health and medicine together.* Dublin, Ohio: Telemachus Press, LLC.

Kasl, S. V., & Cobb, S. (1966a). Health behavior, illness behavior, and sick-role behavior: I. Health and illness behavior. *Archives of Environmental Health, 12*(2), 246–266.

Kasl, S. V., & Cobb, S. (1966b). Health behavior, illness behavior, and sick-role behavior: II. Sick-role behavior. *Archives of Environmental Health, 12*(4), 531–541.

Lalonde, M. (1974). *A new perspective on the health of Canadians: A working document.* Toronto: Health and Welfare Canada.

Lancet Editors. (2020). Global health: Time for radical change? *Lancet, 396,* 1129.

McGinnis, J. M. (1994). The role of behavioral research in National Health Policy. In S. Blumenthal, K. Matthews, & (Eds.), *New research frontiers in behavioral medicine: Proceedings of the National Conference* (217–222). Bethesda, Md: NIH Health and Behavior Coordinating Committee.

Parkerson, G., Connis, R. T., Broadhead, W. E., Patrick, D. L., Taylor. T. R., & Tse, C. K. (1993). Disease-specific versus generic measurement of health-related quality of life in insulin-dependent diabetic patients. *Medical Care, 31*(7), 629–639.

Shiels, M. S., Lipkowitz, S., Campos, N. G., Schiffman, M., Schiller, J. T., Freedman, N. D., & Berrington de González, A. (2023). Opportunities for achieving the Cancer Moonshot goal of a 50% reduction in cancer mortality by 2047. *Cancer Discovery, 13,* 1084–1099.

Smedley, B. D., & Syme, S. L. (Eds.). (2000). *Promoting health: Intervention strategies from social and behavioral research.* Washington, DC: National Academy Press.

United Nations, Department of Economic and Social Affairs. (2023). U.N. Sustainable development goals: The 17 goals. https://sdgs.un.org/goals.

U. S. Department of Health and Human Services. (1980). *Promoting health and preventing disease: Health objectives for the nation.* Washington, DC: U.S. Government Printing Office.

U.S. Department of Health and Human Services. (2023a). Healthy People 2030: Building a healthier future for all. https://health.gov/healthypeople.

U.S. Department of Health and Human Services. (2023b). The community guide. http://www.thecommunityguide.org/.

U. S. Department of Health, Education, and Welfare. (1979). *Healthy people: The Surgeon General's report on health promotion and disease prevention*. Public Health Service Publication No. 79-55071. Washington, DC: U.S. Government Printing Office.

Vanjani, R., Reddy, N., Giron, N., Bai, E., Martino, S., Smith, M., Harrington-Steppen, S., & Trimbur, M. C. (2023). The social determinants of health—Moving beyond screen-and-refer to intervention. *New England Journal of Medicine, 389*, 569–573.

Viswanath, K., McCloud, R. F., & Bekalu, M. A. (2021). Communication, health, and equity: structural influences. In T. L. Thompson & N. G. Harrington. (Eds.), *The Routledge handbook of health communication* (pp. 426–440). Routledge.

World Health Organization. (2014). Global burden of disease. https://www.who.int/healthinfo/global_burden_disease/gbd/en/.

World Health Organization. (2023a). Dementia. https://www.who.int/news-room/fact-sheets/detail/dementia.

World Health Organization. (2023b). Global health estimates: Life expectancy and leading causes of death and disability. https://www.who.int/data/gho/data/themes/mortality-and-global-health-estimates.

World Health Organization. (2023c). Social determinants of health. https://www.who.int/health-topics/social-determinants-of-health#tab=tab_1.

CHAPTER 2

THEORY, RESEARCH, AND PRACTICE IN HEALTH BEHAVIOR

The Editors

Theory, Research, and Practice: Interrelationships

In the period around 320–380 BCE, the Greek philosopher Aristotle distinguished between *theoria* and *praxis*. *Theoria* signifies those sciences and activities concerned with knowing for its own sake, while *praxis* corresponds to action or doing. This contrast between theory and practice (Bernstein, 1971) permeates Western philosophical and scientific thought from Aristotle to Karl Marx (major work around 1867) and on to John Dewey (groundbreaking essays early 1900s) and other contemporary 20th-century philosophers. Theory and practice often were regarded as irreconcilable opposites. Within academic departments, there is often a hierarchical split between those who conduct theoretical work and those who pursue practice. Dewey attempted to resolve the dichotomy by focusing on similarities and continuities between theoretical and practical judgments and inquiries. Dewey described empirical investigation, that is, research, as the bridge between theory and practice and the testing of theory in action.

The editors of this book follow Dewey's tradition and focus on the similarities and continuities of theory and practice rather than on differences. Theory, research, and practice are a continuum along which the skilled professional should move with ease. Not only are they related but they are each essential to understanding health behavior and health behavior change. The best theory is informed by practice; the strongest practice should be grounded in theory. There is too little of both in health behavior. As Green (2006) wrote compellingly, there is a need for more practice-based evidence. Researchers and practitioners may differ in their priorities, but the relationship between research and its application can and should move in both directions. The world needs more "reflective practitioners," who can ensure that theories and practice build on each other (Schön, 1983).

Among the most important challenges is to understand health behavior and to transform knowledge about behavior into effective strategies for health enhancement. Research in health behavior will be judged by its contributions to improving the health of populations. The authors of this book examine theories in terms of their application. By including an explanation of theories and their applications in each chapter, we aim to dispel the dichotomy between theory and practice.

Health Behavior: Theory, Research, and Practice, Sixth Edition. Edited by Karen Glanz,
Barbara K. Rimer, and K. Viswanath.
© 2024 John Wiley & Sons, Inc. Published 2024 by John Wiley & Sons, Inc.
Companion website: www.wiley.com/go/glanz/healthbehavior6e

Relationships between theory, research, and practice are not simple or linear. The larger picture of health improvement and disease reduction is a cycle of interacting types of endeavors, including fundamental or basic research (research into determinants and development of methods), intervention research (research aimed at change), surveillance research (tracking population-wide trends, including maintenance of behavior changes), and application and program delivery, including what will be discussed later in this book as implementation (Hiatt & Rimer, 1999). At the heart of this cycle is knowledge synthesis. Regularly updated critical appraisals of the available literature are central to identifying interventions that should be disseminated and implemented to reduce the burden of disease (Rimer et al., 2001; Tricco et al., 2011). The use of evidence-based health behavior interventions is essential to improving population health at scale.

This sixth edition of *Health Behavior: Theory, Research and Practice* aims to help healthcare providers, public health professionals, and behavior change experts and educators—whatever their backgrounds or disciplines—understand some of the most important theoretical underpinnings of health behaviors and use theory to inform research and practice. Editors of this volume believe that "there is nothing so useful as a good theory" (Lewin, 1935). Each chapter demonstrates the practical value of theory, summarizes what was learned through conceptually sound research and practice, and draws linkages between theory, research, and practice. Chapter authors, writing based on their own impressive experiences, aim to provide readers with real-world cases in which a specific theory was used to understand and/or change behaviors.

Professionals charged with responsibility for improving health behavior are generally interventionists. They are action-oriented. They use their knowledge to design and implement programs to improve health. Design of interventions that yield desirable changes can be improved when it is done with an understanding of behavior change theories and an ability to use them skillfully in research and practice (Glanz & Bishop, 2010). Most public health educators, managers, and behavior change clinicians work in resource-constrained settings. This makes it essential that they reach evidence-based judgments about the choice of interventions, to achieve efficiency and effectiveness. There may be no second chances to reach a critical target audience. It may be about life and death.

A synthesis of theory, research, and practice will advance what is known about health behavior (Michie et al., 2013). The professional who understands theory and research can comprehend the "why," and design and craft well-tailored interventions. In health behavior, the circumstances include the nature of the target audience, setting, resources, goals, and constraints (Bartholomew et al., 2006). As Chapter 19 shows, there are good planning models to help professionals and communities decide on which problems and variables to focus on and help them understand key elements of the background situation.

The health professional in a community clinic who understands how to use the Transtheoretical Model or Social Cognitive Theory (SCT) may design better interventions to help patients lose weight or stop smoking. The community health educator who understands principles of social marketing and media communication can make better use of relevant tools than one who does not. The nurse, who recognizes that observational learning is important to how people learn, as postulated in SCT, may do a better job of teaching people with diabetes how to administer their injections. A working knowledge of community organizations can help the educator identify and mobilize key individuals and groups to develop or maintain a health promotion program. A physician who understands interpersonal influence can communicate more effectively with patients. The health psychologist who understands the Transtheoretical Model of change will know how to design better smoking cessation and exercise interventions and how to tailor them to the needs of patients.

What is Theory?

A theory is a set of interrelated concepts, definitions, and propositions that present a *systematic* view of events or situations by specifying relations among variables, to *explain* and *predict* the events or situations. The notion of *generality*, or broad application, is important, as is *testability* (van Ryn & Heaney, 1992). Theories are *abstract*: they do not have a specified content or topic area. Like an empty coffee cup, they have a shape and boundaries but nothing concrete inside. They only come alive in public health and health behavior when they are filled with practical topics, goals, and problems.

A formal theory—more an ideal than a reality—is a completely closed deductive system of propositions that identifies the interrelationships among concepts and is a systematic view of the phenomena (Blalock, 1969; Kerlinger, 1986). There is no such system in the social sciences or health promotion and education; it can only be approximated

Table 2.1   Definitions of Theory

Definition	Source
A set of interrelated constructs (concepts), definitions, and propositions that present a systematic view of phenomena by specifying relations among variables, with the purpose of explaining and predicting phenomena	Kerlinger (1986), p. 9
A systematic explanation for the observed facts and laws that relate to a particular aspect of life	Babbie (1989), p. 46
Knowledge writ large in the form of generalized abstractions applicable to a wide range of experiences	McGuire (1983), p. 2
A set of relatively abstract and general statements which collectively purport to explain some aspect of the empirical world	Chafetz (1978), p. 2
An abstract, symbolic representation of what is conceived to be reality—a set of abstract statements designed to "fit" some portion of the real world	Zimbardo et al. (1977), p. 53

(Blalock, 1969). Theory has been defined in a variety of ways, each consistent with Kerlinger's definition. Table 2.1 summarizes several definitions of theory. These definitions, put forth in the 1970s and 1980s, have stood the test of time.

Theories are useful during the stages of planning, implementing, and evaluating interventions. Program planners can use theories to shape the pursuit of answers to *why? what? how?* Theories can be used to guide the search for *why* people are not following public health and medical advice or not caring for themselves in healthy ways. They can help pinpoint *what* one needs to know before developing and organizing an intervention program. They can provide an insight into *how* to shape program strategies to reach people and organizations and make an impact on them. They also identify *what* should be monitored, measured, and/or compared in a program evaluation (Glanz et al., 1996, 2002).

Thus, theories and models *explain* behaviors and suggest ways to achieve behavior *change*. Explanatory theories, often called a *theory of the problem*, help describe and identify why a problem exists. These theories also predict behaviors under defined conditions. They guide the search for modifiable factors like knowledge, attitudes, self-efficacy, social support, lack of resources, and so on. Change theories, or *theories of action*, guide the development of interventions. They also form the basis for evaluation, pushing evaluators to make explicit their assumptions about how a program should work. Implementation theories are change theories that link theory specifically to a given problem, audience, and context (Institute of Medicine, 2002; see Chapter 16). Theories of the problem and theories of action often have different foci but are complementary.

Even though various theoretical models of health behavior may reflect the same general ideas, each theory employs a specific vocabulary to articulate the factors that define it. The *why* explains the processes by which changes occur in target variables. Theories vary in the extent to which they have been conceptually developed and empirically tested, and even the extent to which they can be proven.

As we discuss later in this chapter, many new theories and models have been and continue to be proposed in health behavior (Michie et al., 2014). The proliferation of theories in health behavior poses a challenge: when do we accept a theory as truly advancing understanding of a phenomenon? Sometimes, what appears to be a new theory is merely old wine in new bottles. An established theory should reflect a body of research testing it and supporting it by multiple scientists beyond the original developer(s). A new theory can be considered acceptable if it explains everything that the prior theories explain, provides explanation for phenomena that could *not* be explained by prior theories, and identifies conditions under which the theory could be falsified (Lakatos & Musgrave, 1970).

Concepts, Constructs, and Variables

Concepts are the major components of a theory; they are its building blocks or primary elements. Concepts can vary in the extent to which they have meaning and can be understood outside the context of a specific theory. When concepts are developed or adopted for use in a particular theory, they are called *constructs* (Kerlinger, 1986). The term *subjective normative belief* is an example of a construct within Ajzen and Fishbein's (1980) Theory of Reasoned Action (Chapter 6); the specific construct has a precise definition in the context of that theory. Another example of a construct is *perceived susceptibility* in the Health Belief Model (Chapter 5).

Variables are the empirical counterparts or operational forms of constructs. They specify how a construct is to be measured in a specific situation. *Variables* should be matched to *constructs* when identifying what should be assessed in the evaluation of a theory-driven program.

Principles

Theories go beyond principles. Principles are general guidelines for action, often articulated as assumptions. They are broad and nonspecific. Principles may be based on precedent, history, *or* on research. At their best, principles are based on accumulated research. In their best form, principles are the basis for hypotheses and serve as informed hunches about how or what we should do to obtain a desired outcome in a population. Principles should not be so broad that they invite multiple interpretations and are therefore unreliable. Nor should they be ambiguous so that they can be all things to all people.

Models

Health behavior and guiding concepts for influencing it are far too complex to be explained by a single, unified theory. *Models* draw on multiple theories to understand a specific problem in a particular setting or context. Several models that support program planning processes are widely used in health promotion and education: Green and Kreuter's PRECEDE-PROCEED model (2005; see Chapter 19), social marketing (see Chapter 21), and ecological models (McLeroy et al., 1988; see Chapter 3).

Paradigms for Theory and Research in Health Behavior

A paradigm is a basic schema that organizes our broadly based view of something (Babbie, 1989). Paradigms are widely recognized scientific achievements that, for a time, provide model problem-solving approaches to a community of practitioners and scientists. They include theory, application, and instrumentation, and comprise models that represent coherent traditions of scientific research (Kuhn, 1962). Paradigms gain status because they are more successful than their competitors at solving pressing problems (Kuhn, 1962) but they also can impede scientific progress by protecting inconsistent findings until a crisis point is reached; these crisis points lead to scientific revolutions.

Paradigms create boundaries within which the search for answers occurs. They do not answer specific questions, but they direct the search for answers (Babbie, 1989). Paradigms circumscribe or delimit what is important to examine in a given field of inquiry. The collective judgments of scientists define the dominant paradigm that constitutes the body of science (Wilson, 1952).

In the science of health behavior (and in this text), the dominant paradigm that supports the largest body of theory and research is that of *logical positivism* or *logical empiricism.* This basic view, developed in the Vienna Circle from 1924 to 1936, has two central features: (1) an emphasis on the use of induction, or sensory experience, feelings, and personal judgments as the source of knowledge; and (2) the view that deduction is the standard for verification or confirmation of theory so that theory must be tested through empirical methods and systematic observation of phenomena (Runes, 1984). Logical empiricism reconciles the deductive and inductive extremes; it prescribes that researchers begin inquiries with a hypothesis deduced from a theory and then test it, subjecting it to the jeopardy of disconfirmation through empirical tests (McGuire, 1983).

An alternative worldview that is also important in health behavior relies more heavily on induction and is often identified as a predominantly constructivist paradigm. This perspective argues that the organization and explanation of events should be revealed through a process of discovery rather than organized into prescribed conceptual categories before a study begins. In this paradigm, data collection methods, such as standardized questionnaires and predetermined response categories, have a limited place. Ethnography, phenomenology, and grounded theory are examples of approaches using a constructivist paradigm (Kendler, 2005; Strauss, 1987). It has become increasingly common in the field for work to originate within a constructivist paradigm and shift toward a focus on answering specific research questions using methodologies from the logical positivist paradigm. The use of mixed methods that include both qualitative and quantitative measures has gained traction in health behavior, psychological research, and other social sciences (Cacioppo et al., 2004; Creswell, 2013). However, without quantitative data, a theory is unlikely to be widely accepted because it will lack sufficient data for verification.

Ultimately, those who study and practice in fields that involve health behavior generally are concerned with approaches to solving social problems, and, in many cases, addressing some of the most significant threats and problems facing the world today. They are grappling with fundamental challenges of behavior change in the health and social domains. Considerable scholarly and practitioner efforts have been devoted to developing techniques that change behavior. Although these grew out of a desire to produce a better world, techniques that "push" people to change were experienced by many as manipulative, reducing freedom of choice, and sustaining a balance of power in favor of the "change agent" (Kipnis, 1994). A paradigm shift occurred, and many techniques for promoting individual behavior change (for example, social support, empowerment, personal growth) shifted focus to *reducing obstacles to change* and promoting informed decision making, rather than pushing people to change. This is also consistent with global efforts to empower people in low- or middle-income countries (LMICs), among other areas, to change rather than direct change. Another example of this shift is the growing prominence of community engagement and community-based participatory research in public health sciences (Chapter 15).

New paradigms for understanding, studying, and applying knowledge about human behavior continue to arise and may be influential in the future of health behavior research and practice. More than 20 years ago, the Institute of Medicine's Committee on Capitalizing on Social Science and Behavioral Research to Improve the Public's Health recommended that "interventions on social and behavioral factors should link multiple levels of influence" rather than focusing on a single or limited number of health determinants (Smedley & Syme, 2000, p. 7). Today, this recommendation is echoed as health educators and social scientists struggle with some of the most challenging health behavior issues, such as climate change, communicable diseases, tobacco control, and obesity prevention, at a time when ecological models begin to be more clearly articulated and studied (Chapter 3).

Trends in Use of Health Behavior Theories and Models

Theories that gain recognition in a discipline shape the field, help define the scope of practice, and influence training and socialization of its professionals. No single theory or conceptual framework dominates research or practice for understanding and changing health behavior. Instead, there are many theories.

Most Often Used Theories: 1986–2022

In making decisions about which theories to include in this book, we reviewed available reviews, texts, and highly cited publications. We first examined previously published reviews of health behavior theory use from the first five editions of this book (Glanz et al., 1990, 1996, 2002, 2008, 2015). We also assessed theories covered in other books on health behavior theory (DiClemente et al., 2019; Edberg, 2018; Hayden, 2019; Michie et al., 2014; Sharma, 2017; Simons-Morton et al., 2012).

Next, we reviewed highly cited articles that reviewed and described dominant health behavior theories (Davis et al., 2015; Glanz & Bishop, 2010; Glanz & Rimer, 2021; Holman et al., 2018; Michie & Prestwich, 2010; Painter et al., 2008; Prestwich et al. 2014; Webb et al., 2010). The most highly cited papers emerged clearly from a Google Scholar search, with numbers of citations in the hundreds (Michie & Prestwich, 2010, n = 908; Painter et al., 2008, n = 801; Prestwich et al., 2014, n = 624) to thousands (Davis et al., 2015, n = 1431; Glanz & Bishop, 2010, n = 2773).

Historical Reviews and Trends

Table 2.2 summarizes the most frequently used theories across six reviews from 1986 to the present. Synthesis of the various reviews and books leads to the conclusion that indeed, across more than four decades, only *a small number of theories and models have persisted and have been widely used and/or informed numerous other theories*. Those theories are the same ones that were identified in reviews conducted for the previous editions of this book: Health Belief Model, SCT (and Social Learning Theory, its predecessor), Theory of Planned Behavior (and Theory of Reasoned Action, its predecessor), social support, Diffusion of Innovations, and the Social Ecological Model. Most books also included the PRECEDE-PROCEED Model and Intervention Mapping as leading planning and implementation models.

An important issue in examining use of theories and models for health behavior change *is the level at which they seek to understand and/or influence behavior and its determinants*. Golden and Earp's review of 157 intervention articles published between 1989 and 2008 found that, across all settings, theories, topics, and time periods, the intervention strategies and targets for change were most likely to be at the individual and interpersonal levels, and less often at the

Table 2.2   Trends in Use of Health Behavior Theories and Models

Period of Review and Source	Most-Used Theories/Models/Frameworks
1986–1988 Glanz et al. (1990)	• Health Belief Model • Social Learning Theory • Theory of Reasoned Action
1992–1994 Glanz et al. (1996)	• Health Belief Model • Social Cognitive Theory • Theory of Reasoned Action/Theory of Planned Behavior • The Transtheoretical Model/Stages of Change • Community organization • Social marketing • Social support/social networks
1999–2000 Glanz et al. (2002)	• Health Belief Model • Social Cognitive Theory • Theory of Reasoned Action and Theory of Planned Behavior • The Transtheoretical Model/Stages of Change • Community organization • Social support and social networks • Ecological models/social ecology • Diffusion of Innovations • Patient-provider communication • Stress and coping
2000–2005 Painter et al. (2008)	• Health Belief Model • Social Cognitive Theory • The Transtheoretical Model/Stages of Change
2012–2014 Golden & Earp (2012) Tabak et al. (2012) Michie et al. (2014)	• Health Belief Model • Social Cognitive Theory (and Social Learning Theory, its predecessor) • Theory of Planned Behavior (and Theory of Reasoned Action, its predecessor), • Diffusion of Innovations • Social Ecological Model • Social support
2012–2019 Theories covered in five theory books and reviews: Simons-Morton et al. (2012) Davis et al. (2015) Sharma (2017) Edberg (2018) Hayden (2019) DiClemente et al. (2019)	• Health Belief Model (HBM) • Social Cognitive Theory • Theory of Planned Behavior (TPB)/Theory of Reasoned Action/Integrated Model of Behavior • The Transtheoretical Model/Stages of Change (TTM) • Social Ecological Model • Diffusion of Innovations

institutional, community, and policy levels (Golden & Earp, 2012). Similar findings emerged from a review by Holman et al. (2018), that social context was less emphasized. In contrast, Tabak et al. (2012) found that most models that they identified for dissemination and implementation research were distributed across all levels of the Social Ecological Model. Notably, the Tabak review examined inherently multilevel issues (dissemination and implementation) across a wide range of sources. These contrasting findings suggest that review articles can be drivers of theory use as well as reflect those that are most used in different categories of health behavior research (e.g., individual-focused, and organization- and policy-focused).

Are Interventions More Effective If They Are Based on Theory?

The empirical question of whether intervention strategies are more effective when grounded in theory has been examined in many systematic reviews and meta-analyses on various behavioral topics. We recently conducted an umbrella review of evidence about patterns and effects of using theory in health behavior intervention research (Glanz et al., 2024, forthcoming). The review, the most comprehensive to date, addresses the overarching question: Are behavioral interventions more effective if they are explicitly theory-based?

We assessed English-language review articles published between 2010 and 2022 to analyze whether the use of behavioral science theories is associated with more effective behavior change intervention strategies and programs. Reviews had to include an analysis of behavior change, a health outcome with established association with behavior (e.g., weight loss, diabetes control), or mental health as an outcome. The type of behavior addressed was not prespecified or limited. Analysis of the theory-effectiveness association could be quantitative, qualitative, or a combination of both methods.

The analysis included 6 umbrella reviews and 132 additional systematic reviews, meta-analyses, and narrative reviews. The umbrella reviews yielded mixed results, with positive short-term effects when theory was used (Fiedler et al., 2020; Olanrewaju et al., 2016), lack of greater effectiveness for theory-based interventions (Dalgetty et al., 2019), and a limited role for theories across reviews for some behavioral outcomes (French et al., 2017; Safron et al., 2011; Weston et al., 2020). The 132 review articles also concluded that the use of theory had varied effects: positive or mostly positive in 37% of reviews; certain theories were more effective than others in 16.7%; inconclusive or mixed reviews in 35.5%; and no association or negative effects in 10.9% of the reviews.

The sum of these findings provides substantial support for use of theory as a foundation for health behavior interventions but by no means an overwhelming endorsement of theory-based strategies. How do we reconcile the mixed findings about value of health behavior theory? First, the most common classification of studies in the review articles was "yes/no" regarding the use of theory and "which theory or theories" were applied. Fifty-six reviews used a taxonomy or established system for classifying behavior change techniques and theoretical constructs such as Michie and others' Behavior Change Techniques (Abraham & Michie, 2008), Theory Domain Framework (Cane et al., 2012), CALO-RE taxonomy (Michie et al., 2011), and levels of theory use (Painter et al., 2008); however, these taxonomies were often not used fully due to incomplete information available in the published studies.

Second, the ways that theories were applied to interventions varied widely, both in terms of the level of detail described in primary research publications and in the number of constructs used to design and implement interventions. Use of theory is more complicated than a check-off box. None of the reviews could assess the complexity of theory use because the data in most papers are insufficient. Thus, a simple yes/no conclusion about the utility of health behavior theory may be less meaningful than studies that enable us to discern what works for whom, and under what circumstances (Atkins et al., 2017; Sheeran et al., 2017).

The body of evidence we reviewed does not justify an unequivocal endorsement for use of theory in health behavior interventions. Clearer descriptions of how theory is used and measured are needed. At the same time, the overall weight of evidence from research and practice in public health and preventive medicine is sufficient to recommend that researchers and program planners familiarize themselves with a range of health behavior theories and apply them critically in a variety of settings.

Selection of Theories for this Book

Selection of theories and models for inclusion in the sixth edition of *Health Behavior: Theory, Research and Practice* was based on the published information summarized above, including an updated synthesis of reviews of theory use in the health behavior literature. Each of the most often cited theories and models is the focus of chapters in this volume. They were selected to provide readers with a range of theories representing different units of intervention (for example, individuals, groups, and communities). They also were chosen because they represent, as in the case of SCT, the Transtheoretical Model, and Health Belief Model, dominant theories of health behavior and health behavior change. Others, like social marketing, Intervention Mapping and the PRECEDE/PROCEED Model, and community organization, were selected for their practical value in applying theoretical formulations in a way that has demonstrated usefulness to professionals concerned with health behavior change.

Selection of theories also reflects some difficult editorial decisions. Three criteria helped define selection of material. First, we determined that to be included, a theory must meet basic standards of adequacy for research and practice, thus having the potential for effective use by health behavior practitioners. Second, there must be evidence that the theory is used in *current* health behavior research. (That is why, for example, we include Health Belief Model rather than Lewin's Field Theory.) The third criterion is that there must be at least promising, if not substantial, empirical evidence supporting the theory's validity in predicting or changing health behaviors. This does not preclude the possibility of mixed findings and critiques of the evidence, which we believe are important to bring to light.

In later sections of the book, a purpose/theme or focus rather than theory is the identifying title for a chapter—as in the case of Chapter 12 on stress, which describes different theories of stress and how stress affects health behavior and health. Chapter 14 on Race, Health, and Health Equity introduces racism-related theories and constructs and illustrates how they can be integrated with other widely used health behavior models.

Chapter 15 on Improving Health Through Community Engagement is named for the approach to intervention strategies rather than for the convergent theoretical bases that form the foundation for community organization work. Chapters in Part Five present Intervention Mapping and the PRECEDE-PROCEED Model for program planning, social marketing, behavioral economics, and social media, each of which draws on multiple theories to understand health behavior and assist in development of effective intervention programs and strategies.

We recognize the lack of consensus regarding the definition and classification of theories and have taken a liberal, ecumenical stance toward theory. The lowest common denominator of the theoretical models herein might be that they are all *conceptual or theoretical frameworks, models,* or broadly conceived perspectives used to organize ideas. Nevertheless, we have not abandoned the term *theory* because it accurately describes the spirit of this book and describes the goal to be attained for developing frameworks and tools for refining health education research and practice.

Fitting a Theory or Theories to Research and Practice: Building Bridges and Forging Links

Effective health behavior change depends on marshaling the most appropriate theory *and* practice strategies for a given situation. Different theories are best suited to different units of practice, such as individuals, groups, and organizations. When one is attempting to overcome women's personal barriers to obtaining mammograms, Health Belief Model may be useful. The Transtheoretical Model may be especially useful for smoking cessation interventions. When trying to change physicians' mammography practices by instituting reminder systems, dissemination and implementation science approaches are more suitable. At the same time, physicians might use The Transtheoretical Model to inform their discussions with individual patients about getting a first mammogram or annual screening. The choice of a suitable theory or theories should begin with identifying the problem, goal, and units of practice (Sussman, 2001; van Ryn & Heaney, 1992), *not* with selecting a theoretical framework because it is intriguing, familiar, or in vogue. As Green and Kreuter (2005) have argued, one should start with a logical model of the problem and work backward to identify potential solutions.

The adequacy of a theory most often is assessed with three criteria: (1) its *logic*, or *internal consistency* in not yielding mutually contradictory derivations, (2) extent to which it is *parsimonious*, or broadly relevant while using a manageable number of concepts, and (3) its *plausibility* in fitting with prevailing theories in the field (McGuire, 1983).

Theories also are judged in the context of activities of practitioners and researchers. Practitioners may apply the pragmatic criterion of *usefulness* to a theory and thus would be concerned with its consistency to everyday observations. Researchers make scientific judgments of a theory's *ecological validity*, or the extent to which it conforms to observable reality when empirically tested (McGuire, 1983). We should test theories iteratively in the field and in more controlled settings. When we do so, theory, research, and practice begin to converge.

One of the most frequent questions students around the world ask is, "*What theory should I use?*" It is an important question whose answer is found not just in the readings contained in this book but also in the experiences and judgments that equip readers to apply what is learned here: *theory into practice and research.* We hope that *Health Behavior: Theory, Research and Practice* will provide and strengthen that foundation for readers.

Science is, by definition, cumulative, with paradigm shifts that come more rarely as a result of crises when current theories fail to explain some phenomena (Kuhn, 1962). The same applies to the science base that supports long-standing and innovative health behavior interventions. More research is needed at all points along the research continuum—more basic research to develop and test theories, more intervention research to develop and test evidence-based interventions, more implementation science research and practice to understand and apply the processes of implementation, and more concerted attention to dissemination of evidence-based interventions (Institute of Medicine, 2002; Rimer et al., 2001; Rohrbach et al., 2006; Weinstein, 2007).

Health behavior research and practice communities are sorely in need of more rigor and precision in theory development and testing—in measures, assessment of mediating variables, and in specification of theoretical elements (Rejeski et al., 2000). Theory provides the conceptual underpinnings for well-crafted research and informed practice. "The scientist values research by the size of its contribution to that huge, logically articulated structure of ideas which is already, though not half-built, the most glorious accomplishment of mankind" (Medawar, 1967).

In this book, we aim to demystify theory and communicate theory and theoretically inspired research alongside their implications for practice. We encourage informed criticism of theories. The ultimate test of these ideas and this information rests on their use over time, critical assessment, refinement, and application. The process does not end with publication of a particular study. The goal of theory, for a small number of people, may be proof of the theory. But for most readers of this book, it will be improved health. Theory, then, is a tool to improve health outcomes. Thus, we should think about theory *and* practice, not theory *or* practice. Green said it well: The translational gap between research and practice has long been discussed, often as a one-way street—get practitioners to recognize and utilize the research that is being conducted. While important, equally important is the reverse—integrating practice-based evidence and context into the research conducted (Green, 2006). We need a bridge between the two, not a pipeline. Achieving this vision will require social support, supportive environments, and periodic reinforcement. The beneficiaries will be practitioners, researchers, and participants in formal health behavior change programs—and ultimately, improved public health.

Limitations of this Book

No text can be all-inclusive nor can it meet the needs of all potential audiences. This book is not a how-to guide or manual for program planning and development in health education and health behavior. Other books in health behavior, nursing, medicine, psychology, and nutrition serve that purpose, and readers should seek out key sources in each discipline for more on the "nuts and bolts" of practice. This volume will be most useful when it is included as part of a problem-oriented learning program, whether in a formal professional education setting or through continuing education venues.

Readers should emerge from reading this edition with a critical appraisal of theory and with the curiosity to pursue not only the theories presented in this book but other promising theories as well. This book is a starting point, not the end. Theories—and conceptual frameworks—can be and *are* useful because they enrich, inform, and complement the practical technologies of health promotion and education. Thus, the readers of this book should "pass with relief from the tossing sea of Cause and Theory to the firm ground of Result and Fact" (Churchill, 1898). As the ocean meets the shore, we hope you will find that theory, research, and practice can converge in a single landscape of improved health for all.

References

Abraham, C., & Michie, S. (2008). A taxonomy of behavior change techniques used in interventions. *Health Psychology, 27*(3), 379–387.

Ajzen, I., & Fishbein, M. (1980). *Understanding attitudes and predicting social behavior.* Englewood Cliffs, NJ: Prentice Hall.

Atkins, L., Francis, J., Islam, R., O'Connor, D., Patey, A., Ivers, N., Foy, R., Duncan, E. M., Colquhoun, H., Grimshaw, J. M., Lawton, R., & Michie, S. (2017). A guide to using the Theoretical Domains Framework of behaviour change to investigate implementation problems. *Implementation Science, 12*(1), 1–18.

Babbie, E. (1989). *The practice of social research* (5th ed.). Belmont, CA: Wadsworth.

Bartholomew, L. K., Parcel, G. S., Kok, G., & Gottlieb, N. H. (2006). *Planning health promotion programs: An intervention mapping approach.* San Francisco: Jossey-Bass.

Bernstein, R. (1971). *Praxis and action.* Philadelphia: University of Pennsylvania Press.

Blalock, H. M., Jr. (1969). *Theory construction, from verbal to mathematical constructions.* Englewood Cliffs, NJ: Prentice Hall.

Cacioppo, J. T., Semin, G. R., & Berntson, G. G. (2004). Realism, instrumentalism, and scientific symbiosis: Psychological theory as a search for truth and the discovery of solutions. *American Psychologist, 59*(4), 214–223.

Cane, J., O'Connor, D., & Michie, S. (2012). Validation of the theoretical domains framework for use in behaviour change and implementation research. *Implementation Science, 7*, 37. https://doi:10.1186/1748-5908-7-37.

Chafetz, J. (1978). *A primer on the construction of theories in sociology.* Itasca, IL: Peacock.

Churchill, W. (1898). *The Malakand field force.* London: Longmans Green.

Creswell, J. W. (2013). *Research design: Qualitative, quantitative, and mixed methods approaches.* Los Angeles: Sage Publications.

Dalgetty, R., Miller, C. B., & Dombrowski, S. U. (2019). Examining the theory-effectiveness hypothesis: A systematic review of systematic reviews. *British Journal of Health Psychology, 24*(2), 334–356.

Davis, R., Campbell, R., Hildon, Z., Hobbs, L, Michie S. (2015). Theories of behaviour and behaviour change across the social and behavioural sciences: A scoping review. *Health Psychology Review, 9*(3), 323–344.

DiClemente, R., Salazar, L., & Crosby, R. (2019). *Health behavior theory for public health* (2nd ed.). Burlington, MA: Jones & Bartlett.

Edberg, M. (2018). *Essentials of health behavior: Social and behavioral theory in public health* (3rd ed.). Burlington, MA: Jones & Bartlett.

Fiedler, J., Eckert, T., Wunsch, K., & Woll, A. (2020). Key facets to build up eHealth and mHealth interventions to enhance physical activity, sedentary behavior and nutrition in healthy subjects—an umbrella review. *BMC Public Health, 20*(1), 1605.

French, D. P., Cameron, E., Benton, J. S., Deaton, C., & Harvie, M. (2017). Can communicating personalised disease risk promote healthy behaviour change? A systematic review of systematic reviews. *Annals of Behavioral Medicine, 51*(5), 718–729.

Glanz, K., & Bishop, D. (2010). The role of behavioral science theory in development and implementation of public health interventions. *Annual Review of Public Health, 31*, 399–418.

Glanz, K., Holman, D., & Suhag, A. (2024) [Forthcoming]. Association of health behavior theory use and intervention effectiveness: An umbrella review.

Glanz, K., Lewis, F. M., & Rimer, B. K. (Eds.). (1990). *Health behavior and health education: Theory, research, and practice.* San Francisco: Jossey-Bass.

Glanz, K., Lewis, F. M., & Rimer, B. K. (Eds.). (1996). *Health behavior and health education: Theory, research, and practice* (2nd ed.). San Francisco: Jossey-Bass.

Glanz, K., & Rimer, B. K. (2021). Health behavior theories. In M. L. Boulton (Ed.), *Maxcy-Rosenau-Last public health and preventive medicine* (16th ed., pp. 452–457). Chicago: McGraw-Hill.

Glanz, K., Rimer, B. K., & Lewis, F. M. (Eds.). (2002). *Health behavior and health education: Theory, research, and practice.* (3rd ed.). San Francisco: Jossey-Bass.

Glanz, K., Rimer, B. K., & Viswanath, V (Eds.). (2008). *Health behavior and health education: Theory, research, and practice* (4th ed.). San Francisco: Jossey-Bass, Inc.

Glanz, K., Rimer, B. K., & Viswanath, V. (Eds.). (2015). *Health behavior: Theory, research, and practice* (5th ed.). San Francisco: Jossey-Bass, Inc./Wiley.

Golden, S., & Earp, J. A. (2012). Social ecological approaches to individuals and their contexts: Twenty years of health education and behavior interventions. *Health Education and Behavior, 39*(3), 364–372.

Green, L. W. (2006). Public health asks of systems science: To advance our evidence-based practice, can you help us get more practice-based evidence? *American Journal of Public Health, 96*(3), 406–409.

Green, L. W., & Kreuter, M. W. (2005). *Health promotion planning: An educational and ecological approach* (4th ed.). New York: McGraw-Hill.

Hayden. J. (2019). *Introduction to health behavior theory* (3rd ed.). Burlington, MA: Jones & Bartlett.

Hiatt, R. A., & Rimer, B. K. (1999). A new strategy for cancer control research. *Cancer Epidemiology, Biomarkers and Prevention, 8*(11), 957–964.

Holman, D., Lynch, R., & Reeves A. (2018). How do health behaviour interventions take account of social context? A literature trend and co-citation analysis. *Health, 22*(4) 389–410.

Institute of Medicine, Committee on Communication for Behavior Change in the 21st Century: Improving the Health of Diverse Populations. (2002). *Speaking of health: Assessing health communication strategies for diverse populations.* Washington, DC: National Academies Press.

Kendler, H. H. (2005). Psychology and phenomenology: A clarification. *American Psychologist, 60*, 318–324.

Kerlinger, F. N. (1986). *Foundations of behavioral research* (3rd ed.). New York: Holt, Rinehart & Winston.

Kipnis, D. (1994). Accounting for the use of behavior technologies in social psychology. *American Psychologist, 49*(3), 165–172.

Kuhn, T. S. (1962). *The structure of scientific revolutions.* Chicago: University of Chicago Press.

Lakatos, I., & Musgrave, A. (Eds.). (1970). *Criticism and the growth of knowledge.* Cambridge: Cambridge University Press.

Lewin, K. (1935). *A dynamic theory of personality.* New York: McGraw Hill.

McGuire, W. J. (1983). A contextualist theory of knowledge: Its implications for innovation and reform in psychological research. *Advances in Experimental Social Psychology, 16,* 1–47.

McLeroy, K. R., Bibeau, D., Steckler, A., & Glanz, K. (1988). An ecological perspective on health promotion programs. *Health Education Quarterly, 15,* 351–377.

Medawar, P. B. (1967). *The art of the soluble.* New York: Methuen.

Michie, S., Ashford, S., Sniehotta, F.F., Dombrowski, S. U., Bishop, A., & French, D. P. (2011). A refined taxonomy of behaviour change techniques to help people change their physical activity and healthy eating behaviours: The CALO-RE taxonomy. *Psychology & Health, 26*(11), 1479–1498.

Michie, S., Prestwich, A. (2010). Are interventions theory-based? Development of a theory coding scheme. *Health Psychology, 29,* 1–8.

Michie, S., West, R., Campbell, R., Brown, J., & Gainforth, H. (2014). *ABC of theories of behavioural change.* Great Britain: Silverback Publishing.

Michie, S., West, R., & Spring, B. (2013). Moving from theory to practice and back in social and health psychology. *Health Psychology, 32*(5), 581–585.

Olanrewaju, O., Kelly, S., Cowan, A., Brayne, C., & Lafortune, L. (2016). Physical activity in community dwelling older people: A systematic review of reviews of interventions and context. *PLoS One, 11*(12), e0168614.

Painter, J. E., Borba, C.P., Hynes, M., Mays, D., & Glanz, K. (2008). The use of theory in health behavior research from 2000 to 2005: A systematic review. *Annals of Behavioral Medicine, 35*(3), 358–362.

Prestwich, A., Sniehotta, F. F., Whittington, C., Dombrowski, S. U., Rogers, L., & Michie, S. (2014). Does theory influence the effectiveness of health behavior interventions? Meta-analysis. *Health Psychology, 33*(5), 465–474.

Rejeski, W. J., Brawley, L. R., McAuley, E., & Rapp, S. (2000). An examination of theory and behavior change in randomized clinical trials. *Controlled Clinical Trials, 21*(Suppl. 5), 164S–170S.

Rimer, B. K., Glanz, K., & Rasband, G. (2001). Searching for evidence about health education and health behavior interventions. *Health Education and Behavior, 28*(2), 231–248.

Rohrbach, L. A., Grana, R., Sussman, S., & Valente, T. W. (2006). Type II translation: Transporting prevention interventions from research to real-world settings. *Evaluation & the Health Professions, 29*(3), 302–333.

Runes, D. (1984). *Dictionary of philosophy.* Totawa, N.J.: Rowman and Allanheld.

Safron, M., Cislak, A., Gaspar, T., & Luszczynska, A. (2011). Effects of school-based interventions targeting obesity-related behaviors and body weight change: a systematic umbrella review. *Behavioral Medicine, 37*(1), 15–25.

Schön, D. (1983). *The reflective practitioner. How professionals think in action.* London: Temple Smith.

Sharma, M. (2017). *Theoretical foundations of health education and health promotion* (3rd ed.). Burlington, MA: Jones & Bartlett, 2017.

Sheeran, P., Klein, W. M. P., & Rothman, A. J. (2017). Health behavior change: Moving from observation to intervention. *Annual Review of Psychology, 68,* 573–600.

Simons-Morton, B., McLeroy, K., & Wendel, M. (2012). *Behavior theory in health promotion practice and research.* Burlington, MA: Jones & Bartlett.

Smedley, B. D., & Syme, S. L (Eds.). (2000). *Promoting health: Intervention strategies from social and behavioral research.* Washington, DC: National Academy Press.

Strauss, A. L. (1987). *Qualitative analysis for social scientists.* Cambridge, England: Cambridge University Press.

Sussman, S. (Ed.). (2001). *Handbook of program development for health behavior research and practice.* Thousand Oaks, CA: Sage Publications.

Tabak, R. G., Khoong, E. C., Chambers, D. A., & Brownson, R. C. (2012). Bridging research and practice: Models for dissemination and implementation research. *American Journal of Preventive Medicine, 43*(3), 337–350.

Tricco, A. C., Tetzlaff, J., & Moher, D. (2011). The art and science of knowledge synthesis. *Journal of Clinical Epidemiology, 64*(1), 11–20.

van Ryn, M., & Heaney, C. A. (1992). What's the use of theory? *Health Education Quarterly*, *19*(3), 315–330.

Webb, T. L., Sniehotta, F. F., & Michie, S. (2010). Using theories of behaviour change to inform interventions for addictive behaviours. *Addiction*, *105*(11), 1879–1892.

Weinstein, N. D. (2007). Misleading tests of health behavior theories. *Annals of Behavioral Medicine*, *33*(1), 1–10.

Weston, D., Ip, A., & Amlôt, R. (2020). Examining the application of behaviour change theories in the context of infectious disease outbreaks and emergency response: A review of reviews. *BMC Public Health*, *20*(1), 1483.

Wilson, E. B. (1952). *An introduction to scientific research*. New York: McGraw-Hill.

Zimbardo, P. G., Ebbesen, E. B., & Maslach, C. (1977). *Influencing attitudes and changing behavior* (2nd ed.). Reading, MA: Addison-Wesley.

CHAPTER 3

ECOLOGICAL MODELS OF HEALTH BEHAVIOR

Deborah Salvo
Casey Durand
Alejandra Jáuregui

KEY POINTS

- Ecological models offer a broad framework for understanding the totality of influences on health behavior.

- Ecological models posit that health behaviors are influenced by factors at multiple levels, from the individual to the interpersonal, and to the environmental, policy, and planetary scales.

- Ecological models are flexible and can be adapted to explain the multilevel influences of different health behaviors, in varying populations, and across different settings.

- Ecological models can guide the selection of study design, measures, analytic techniques, and intervention strategies and can inform data analysis and interpretation of findings for single- or multilevel interventions.

- Ecological models are a helpful framework in advocating for multilevel, systems-oriented solutions to major public health problems across local and global contexts.

- An important limitation of ecological models is that they do not provide specificity to explain behavioral mechanisms and pathways, and empirical evidence testing of ecological models has been mostly through observational research.

- The emerging integration of salient planetary health issues (especially climate change) and complex systems methods (simulations) with ecological models, and the use of natural experiments to test multilevel interventions, provide viable options to expand the evidence on the utility of ecological models.

Vignette

A Day in the Life of Sophie and Sofia

Sophie and Sofia have never met but have many things in common. They are both 26-year-old, working-class, single women living in big, bustling cities: Sophie in Houston, United States and Sofia in Mexico City, Mexico. Both are relatively healthy and work in an office. The vignettes below describe their daily routines.

Sophie

Sophie's alarm clock goes off at 7 a.m. She lives in a single-family home in East Houston, with two roommates. The home is not too big but is on a quiet street and has a small yard where her dog can play. Upon waking, Sophie lets her dog into the yard and has a quick bite and some coffee while getting ready for work. Because it would take her over one hour to walk to the nearest light-rail stop that can get her to her job downtown, and most streets in her area do not have sidewalks or shade, using public transit is not feasible. A few years ago, she saved enough money to buy a used but reliable car that gets her everywhere.

Sophie leaves her home no later than 7:50 a.m. since traffic can be bad in Houston, and it takes her about one hour to get to work, which starts at 9 a.m. Once she finds a good parking spot, she walks about five minutes to reach the entrance of her building and takes the elevator up to the 12th floor where her cubicle is located. She spends her day on her computer, taking video conference calls and a few in-person meetings on the same floor. Her floor does not have a kitchen. So, when it's time for lunch, she warms up her food from home in the microwave oven on the 10th floor. She usually takes the elevator to the 10th floor, but if it is taking too long, she walks down the hall and takes the stairs two floors down. She usually eats lunch in the common dining area with other administrative assistants who work there too. On busy workdays, she brings her warm dish back to her cubicle and eats while catching up on email.

Work usually ends by 5:30 p.m. The drive back home is about an hour long, due to traffic. Once home, she takes her dog out on a long walk, which usually involves a stop at the nearby neighborhood park that has a nice off-leash area where her dog loves to run, and where Sophie enjoys the fresh air. About 45–60 minutes later, they

Health Behavior: Theory, Research, and Practice, Sixth Edition. Edited by Karen Glanz, Barbara K. Rimer, and K. Viswanath.
© 2024 John Wiley & Sons, Inc. Published 2024 by John Wiley & Sons, Inc.
Companion website: www.wiley.com/go/glanz/healthbehavior6e

come back home, and Sophie prepares dinner. Depending on the day of the week, she eats with her roommates, or alone while watching her favorite Netflix show. After dinner, she catches up on chores or calls her parents, who live in Arizona. Later in the evening, at around 9:30 p.m., she takes her dog on a quick 10-minute stroll and calls it a night.

Sometimes, Sophie feels lonely and wishes she lived closer to family, but she has already invested in her career in Houston and would find it hard to start over in a different place.

Sofia

Sofia's alarm clock goes off at 5:30 a.m. She lives in Northeastern Mexico City with her parents and three siblings—in the same home where they all grew up, which is in the neighborhood where her entire extended family has always lived. Her job starts at 8 a.m. and is in a central business district. Sofia takes a quick shower, and leaves no later than 6 a.m. after her mom routinely reminds her to be careful to avoid certain routes that are known to be unsafe for women walking alone when it is still dark outside.

Sofia walks about 15 minutes to a busy intersection located along the path of the "feeder bus system" (small buses that make frequent stops anywhere along their route, connecting riders to more structured mass transit systems in the city). Conveniently, a *tamales* and *atole* (a hot sweet beverage) stall is located there. So, she buys breakfast while waiting for the bus. About five minutes later, Sofia is on the bus, which at this hour is still quite empty, although it soon fills up with people of all ages (including many children with their parents heading to school). Forty-five minutes later, she gets off and walks about 10 minutes to reach a Metro (subway) station. Fortunately, virtually all roads in Mexico City have sidewalks (although some are full of cracks or are very narrow), but at least they keep people separated from traffic— this is nice in a city where about 2/3 of all daily trips are not done by car! Once at the Metro station, she waits less than six minutes to board a train. She must be very careful at this point, as the trains are crowded, and sometimes, the front wagons, which are officially reserved for women and children (as a safe environment), are already full at this hour. Pickpocketing and sexual harassment are, unfortunately, very common in crowded city trains and buses. About 20 minutes later, Sofia gets off at a station in the business district where she works.

Now, there is an *EcoBici* station right outside of the Metro stop. *EcoBici* is an inexpensive, city-run bicycle-sharing program. Sofia became an *EcoBici* user when she realized how convenient it was in helping her travel the last portion of her commute, with a short, 10-minute bike ride. The business district where she works has invested a lot in building protected bicycle lanes, so she feels safe. There is an *EcoBici* docking station less than a three-minute walk from her work, so it is perfect!

Once she gets to work, at around 7:45–8 a.m., she takes the stairs to the third floor, and greets her co-workers, who are all close friends after more than three years on the job together. They are all preparing a warm pot of coffee to kick off the workday. She then gets to her workstation, answers emails, and works the phone all morning. At around noon, the administrative staff, including Sofia, usually take a quick coffee break while walking around the block, or head to a nearby public square, to get some fresh air and stretch their legs. Later, at about 2 p.m., they all walk together to one of the many *fondas* (affordable, prix-fix local diners offering home-cooked, three-course menus) in the area. There, they eat lunch together (lunch in Mexico happens at around this time and is the main meal of the day).

At about 7 p.m., Sofia leaves her office and starts heading back home. She gets home between 8:30 and 9 p.m., and helps her mother and siblings prepare dinner. Her father arrives shortly after, and they all eat together. At around 10:30 p.m., she goes to bed.

Sometimes, Sofia wishes she could afford a car to avoid the long commute via multimodal public transit. She even considers moving closer to work. However, living near her work would be very expensive, and she would miss her family. Also, buying and maintaining a car is very expensive in Mexico City. She would like to have a dog one day, too, but worries about not having enough time to take care of one during the week.

Contextual Differences and Health

The stories of Sophie and Sofia help underscore *contextual differences* across settings (Houston, Texas, United States, and Mexico City, Mexico), operating at *multiple ecological levels*, including family life, social norms, work-life culture, and built environments. Although at first glance, Sophie and Sofia may appear to be similar *individuals*, their day-to-day routines tell a different story about their *interpersonal* (e.g., family), *organizational* (e.g., worksite), *social* (e.g., crime in their neighborhood), and *built* (e.g., transit infrastructure) *environments*. These different environments help explain some of the differences between them in physical activity, sleep, mental health, and overall quality of life.

Ecological Models of Health Behavior: Introduction

Ecological models offer a framework for understanding the totality of the influences on health behavior (Bronfenbrenner, 1989). Ecological models recognize that health behaviors are complex processes that rarely can be linked to a single defining influence. They also recognize that influences on behavior can vary considerably from behavior to behavior. Broadly, ecological models organize influences from those internal to an individual to those that are most external: intrapersonal, interpersonal, community/societal, and environmental factors can all have an impact on the behavior in question (Richard et al., 2011). While there is general agreement on the basic structure of ecological models, scholars have proposed different versions of this structure that differ in some key constructs, and in their level of detail.

Ecological models do not make assertions regarding specific elements within each level, nor the directionality among the levels. They also do not always specify how to measure elements at each level nor how to conduct multilevel analyses. These features introduce key aspects of ecological models: they are much more general and flexible than what we traditionally think of as fully articulated theories of health behavior.

History

Ecological models are based on a rich conceptual tradition in the behavioral and social sciences. There has been a progression from the early concept that only *perceptions* of environments were important (Lewin & Cartwright, 1951) to an emphasis on the direct effects of environments on behaviors (Barker, 1968). Categories and hierarchies of behavioral influences have been described in numerous ways, including Bronfenbrenner's micro-, meso-, and exo-environment approaches and McLeroy and colleagues' five sources of influence: intrapersonal, interpersonal, institutional, community, and policy (Bronfenbrenner, 1989; McLeroy et al., 1988). Earlier models were developed to apply broadly across behaviors, but more recent models are designed for specific health behaviors (Cohen et al., 2000; Ginja et al., 2018; Glanz et al., 2005; Glass & McAtee, 2006; Richard et al., 2011; Sazzad et al., 2020; Story et al., 2008; Wold & Mittelmark, 2018).

Given the initial emphasis on schools, workplaces, and other levels of social organization, ecological models are also commonly referred to as "socio-ecological models" or "social-ecological models." In this chapter, we adopt the simpler, yet broader, term of "ecological models," recognizing that the totality of influences on health behaviors is the result of multiple factors, including social factors as well as environmental and policy factors such as the physical availability and proximity of parks, supermarkets, hospitals, bicycle lanes, and levels of air pollution and heat in an area.

Key Components of Ecological Models

Ecological models do not propose a specific set of constructs, with hypothesized directional relationships among those constructs. For this reason, we refer to ecological *models* or *frameworks*, rather than ecological *theories*. Ecological models are centered on a hierarchical organization of broad influences on behavior (see Figure 3.1). These levels, as they are typically called, of the ecological model, broadly include the following:

Intrapersonal: Characteristics of individuals, including biological factors and psychological factors such as self-efficacy, attitudes, knowledge, personal history, and experience.

Interpersonal: Relationships and interactions among individuals and the people around them. These factors may include social norms among individuals who directly interact, such as relatives, coworkers, and friends, parent-child communications, and peer modeling.

Community/Societal: Factors that operate at a larger scale. That is, factors that affect entire organizations (e.g., schools, workplaces), neighborhoods, cities, and states. Can include the built environment (e.g., transportation infrastructure, walkability, accessibility to jobs, housing density, housing quality, access to parks and recreational spaces). May also include broad cultural norms and values, and the degree to which organizations (schools, workplaces, places of worship, and other institutions) act as social forces.

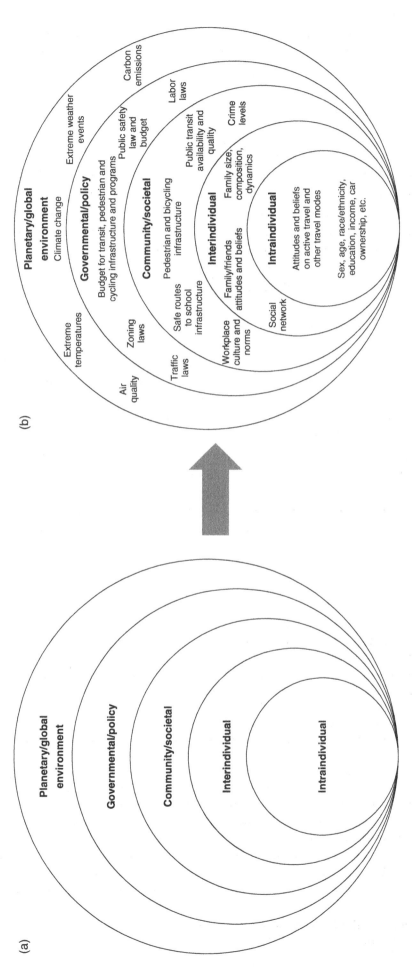

Figure 3.1 Ecological Models of Health Behavior: General and Behavior Specific Models. (a) A General Representation of Ecological Models of Health Behavior; (b) An Ecological Model of the Totality of Influences on Active Travel Behaviors (Walking, Cycling, and Public Transit Use)

Policy: Includes policies and laws established by governmental and nongovernmental entities (such as worksite policies) that are directly or indirectly related to health behavior of an individual or businesses required to adhere to them. In some cases, policies or laws directly influence community-level factors such as walkability and prices or accessibility of healthful products.

Planetary: Often referred to as the "global environment," characteristics of natural ecosystems, weather, climate, geology, etc. (Santos et al., 2021).

Note that we have included an additional, distal level to this version of the Ecological Model focused on planetary factors. There is growing evidence of the multiple influences that things like the weather and climate (including climate change and its determinants, like carbon emissions) can have on health behaviors and outcomes (Marinova & Bogueva, 2019; Santos et al., 2021; Sorensen et al., 2018). For example, extreme weather events resulting from climate change can lead to food shortages, which, in turn, can have an impact on food insecurity and food-purchasing and consumption behaviors (Leisner, 2020). Also, the term "environment" can be used in different ways to describe different levels of ecological models. For instance, many researchers define the built *environment* of neighborhoods or cities as a specific level of interest (Mahmoudi & Zhang, 2020), which is usually best fitting under the broader umbrella of community/societal level factors, while we describe global *environmental* or planetary factors as a more distal level of influence. An implicit underpinning of the idea of including the "planetary level" is that human behavior over time has contributed to many important changes in the natural environment.

Table 3.1 provides definitions of key concepts for understanding ecological models. Scholars have chosen various terms to name the levels of the ecological model; these names may or may not be identical to our chosen terminology for this chapter. However, they are usually consistent. Possible differences across versions of the ecological model should, however, be seen as a feature of ecological models. This is an example of their flexibility and adaptability to the specific circumstances of settings and health behaviors.

Although the term *hierarchical* is used above to describe the organization of the ecological model, ecological models do not assert that any level is more or less important in terms of its potential influence on the behavior at hand. Rather, the term *hierarchical* is in reference to how proximal or distant the given factor is to the individual level. Importantly, not only do ecological models posit that factors at higher levels affect the behavior of individuals, but they also assume that the components of the higher levels of the model (e.g., policies of an organization, state or country; or

Table 3.1   Ecological Models: Key concepts

Concept	Definition
Influence on health behaviors	Ecological models recognize that health behaviors are complex processes and rarely are the result of a single defining influence, but rather, are the consequence of multiple influencing factors.
Hierarchical levels of influence	Ecological models organize the influences of health behavior "hierarchically," from those most internal to an individual to those most external: intrapersonal, interpersonal, community/societal, policy, and planetary. The term "hierarchical" does not imply that one level is more important than another one, but rather, denotes proximity or distance to the individual.
Interactions across levels of influence	The influences of health behaviors interact across levels; they "work together" in influencing the given health behavior of interest. Therefore, the effectiveness of strategies targeting one level of the ecological model on a given health behavior may vary depending on other factors at other levels of the ecological model.
Reciprocal determinism	Ecological models recognize the bidirectional influence of the higher levels of influence (community/societal, governmental/policy and planetary factors) on the health behavior of individuals, and the effects of actions of individuals and groups on the outer rings of the ecological model. Ecological models recognize that people can affect social, physical, and natural environments and policies, and vice versa.
Behavior-specific ecological models	Ecological models are most useful to guide research and interventions when they are adapted to specific health behaviors, as societal, environmental and policy drivers tend to be behavior-specific.
Context-specific ecological models	Many times, the cultural, economic, environmental, and planetary factors that influence the same health behavior vary substantially by context. An illustration of this is the different food and policy environments that align with people's diets across continents such as the United States and Africa.
Single-level interventions	Interventions that target only one level, whichever it may be (intrapersonal, interpersonal, community/societal, policy, or planetary).
Multilevel interventions	Multilevel interventions aim to affect factors at multiple levels of influence. The ecological model proposes that these should logically have a stronger effect on health behavior than those operating at a single level.

the social and physical assets of a neighborhood) can be changed by groups of individuals, and often, by their collective health behaviors. This bidirectional interdependence is referred to as reciprocal determinism, a concept that is well known to many readers from its use in Social Cognitive Theory (see Chapter 9).

Also inherent to the idea of ecological models is that these models are not merely convenient ways of organizing discrete influences on behavior. Rather, ecological models assume that, for virtually any health behavior, there will be interactions among the various levels. That is, the effects of factors within a certain level do not operate on health behavior in isolation; instead, they influence each other, and together, they influence the health behavior at hand (Van Dyck et al., 2014). The interactive nature of influences from multiple levels highlights the insufficiency of merely knowing a health behavior is influenced by factors at multiple levels: rather, interventions must be designed to account for these factors.

Ecological Models in Practice

Like other theories and frameworks of health behavior, ecological models generally are used in one of two ways: (1) to explain the antecedents—that is, the determinants, or the causes or etiology—of a health behavior; or, (2) as a framework to guide the design of health promotion interventions targeting multiple levels of influence on health behaviors (*multilevel interventions*). Using ecological models to guide the design of multilevel interventions typically assumes that the antecedents have already been identified. That is, it would be unwise to use the ecological model to inform multilevel intervention development if an analysis to understand the specific elements of the different levels that influence particular health behaviors has not already been conducted. (see Chapter 19, Theory-Based Planning Models, for in-depth treatment of this idea.)

Ecological Models for Explaining Antecedents of Health Behaviors

There are several ways to move from the general framework provided by an ecological model to a behavior-specific one (see Figure 3.1). First, virtually any of the theories presented in this book can be incorporated into an ecological model. Suppose, for example, that a team of researchers wants to develop a version of the ecological model specific to teenage smoking. Evidence shows that the Theory of Planned Behavior (TPB and the Reasoned Action Approach, see Chapter 6) is useful for understanding teenage smoking. So the investigators decide to use TPB in its entirety to fill in the intrapersonal and interpersonal levels of the model (see also Chapter 11, Social Networks). For the remaining levels, there is epidemiological evidence that may help explain societal and community-level factors that influence teenage smoking (Calo & Krasny, 2013). Most health behaviors have sufficient evidence at this point to begin to flesh out the higher levels of an ecological model.

An important caveat to the approach outlined above is that where behavior-specific ecological models are created based on existing research measuring single-level influences on behavior, they do not stand alone as tests of the model in its entirety, that is, at all levels. This is a crucial information gap because for most health behaviors, we lack data to examine the combined or interactive effects of factors at all levels. Simultaneously testing the interactive impact of all factors at all levels on a given health behavior is challenging. Nonetheless, there are good examples of how evidence of the ecological influences of a given health behavior has been generated via independent yet interconnected studies. Perhaps, the best example is tobacco control research. Studies have been conducted assessing different levels (or combinations of levels) and with varying study designs that have informed the next steps for research at other levels (US National Cancer Institute, 2017).

Ecological Models for Informing Multilevel Interventions

As with explanatory research, it is possible to synthesize existing intervention studies with an ecological framework to inform future multilevel intervention work. Historically, most health behavior interventions focused on a single level of the ecological model, with earlier work most often centered on individual and interpersonal strategies for behavior change. Since 2006, however, researchers have increasingly invoked ecological models that emphasize environmental change such as the built environment or public policy (Holman et al., 2018). This is evidence of the robust influence of ecological models for designing and implementing strategies to improve health behaviors in populations. Further, since 2006, we have witnessed a rapid increase in multilevel intervention studies (Holman et al., 2018). Some of the most visible examples come from tobacco control, nutrition, and physical activity research.

It can be challenging to implement multilevel interventions. Sallis (2018) recently addressed this issue. He noted that although groups of individuals can affect the higher levels of the ecological model (environments, policies), and that scientific evidence can and often does play a role in shaping these changes, when it comes to single research projects, investigators may lack direct control over these types of factors. For example, it is not realistic to design and implement a built environment or state policy intervention as part of a short-term funded research project in the same controlled fashion that is possible for an interpersonal intervention, with a randomized controlled study design. This is because the unit of randomization and intervention would be neighborhoods or cities. Because this is financially and/or practically impossible, interventionists interested in empirically testing the effect of factors at the higher levels of the ecological model on health behaviors often use "windows of opportunity," and study large-scale environmental and policy using designs called "natural experiments." Examples of this type of study include a natural experiment to evaluate a new light rail system in Seattle (Saelens et al., 2022) and studies of state and local restaurant menu labeling policies (VanEpps et al., 2016). Because these policy and built environment intervention strategies target individuals both directly and indirectly via changes in the food and transportation environments, they make it possible to conduct opportunistic multilevel intervention trials.

All this is not to say that there are no good examples of investigator-led multilevel interventions. For example, a recent study by Glanz and colleagues demonstrated that interpersonal educational strategies combined with modifications to the built environment in public swimming pools (physical prompts and signage, sunscreen stations, and increased shading structures) were successful in improving skin cancer preventive environments and behaviors (Glanz et al., 2015). Branas and colleagues conducted a randomized trial of the greening of vacant lots in Philadelphia in partnership with the City and a nonprofit community group, and found reductions in crime, increased perceptions of safety and improved quality of life in neighborhoods where blighted land was remediated (Branas et al., 2018).

There are other examples of successful investigator-led multilevel interventions that do not rely on natural experiments. However, most focus on relatively proximal levels of influence on the individual (interpersonal strategies plus organizational setting policy and asset changes; versus changing the urban landscape of entire cities or passing laws at the municipal, state or national levels) (Parkinson et al., 2022; Stotz et al., 2021). Successfully designing and implementing investigator-driven multilevel interventions typically requires a long-term commitment and strong engagement with community or organizational partnerships (schools, churches, swimming pools, workplaces, urban planners, healthcare organizations, and nongovernmental organizations).

Ecological Models for Informing Measurement

Another use of ecological models, relevant for both antecedent and intervention work, is to guide decisions about what should be measured in a research study or program evaluation (Elder et al., 2007; Ogilvie et al., 2011). For example, a researcher might be designing a worksite intervention to promote physical activity. The intervention will target the built and social environments by providing new designated spaces for organized, instructor-led exercise classes. It will also target the individual level through email prompts and goal-setting tools. Other factors at various levels, like the out-of-work social network of employees, their home neighborhood environment, or broader city policies, will not be targeted by the intervention. However, the investigators know that these factors can influence physical activity behaviors and thus decide to measure them so they can adjust their analyses accordingly (remove the influence of these variables as potential confounders, so the unbiased effect of the intervention can be assessed). In some cases, they may even want to determine whether some of these factors occurring at other levels of the ecological model affect the success of their intervention strategies. For example, the research team may be interested in finding out if their intervention works better for women versus men, younger versus older employees, or for those living further versus nearer to work.

Applications

Application 1: Using Ecological Models to Conduct Natural Experiments of Large-scale Changes to Urban Travel Infrastructure Across Different Global Settings

In this section, we outline two examples of how ecological frameworks helped guide the evaluation of major urban travel infrastructure changes in Houston, United States and Mexico City, Mexico, and their impact on active travel behaviors.

Although urban design, planning, and transport play an important role for health behaviors (Boulange et al., 2017; Bull et al., 2010; Frank et al., 2016; Sallis et al., 2016), there is a lack of data from controlled, prospective studies quantifying the impact of urban modifications (e.g., adding more parks to a city) on health. Conducting built environment and urban policy interventions is something that is generally out of the control of researchers, leaving traditional randomized controlled trials as a virtually impossible option. Nonetheless, naturally occurring changes in a city's built environment offer researchers the opportunity to assess their impact, by treating these infrastructure changes as *natural experiments* (Craig et al., 2012; Huang et al., 2017; Leatherdale, 2019; Ogilvie et al., 2020). This includes large infrastructure projects funded by governments and/or private investment, which ultimately modify the urban landscape of the city: more and/or better sidewalks, bicycle lanes, transit stations or entirely new transit systems, and public open spaces.

Ecological models offer a helpful framework for assessing the impact of natural experiments on health behaviors. Despite their cost and scale, if unaccompanied by complementary strategies like a broad communications campaign, or financial incentives for individuals working in certain locations or residing in certain areas to use the new infrastructure, urban infrastructure modifications are essentially single-level interventions (built environment). However, when assessing the impact of natural experiments, ecological models can be used as an organizing framework, to account for elements at the same level or at different levels that can influence study outcomes. Indeed, given that natural experiments are in essence *quasi-experimental studies*, with lack of random assignment to the intervention versus comparison arms, it is essential to account for any known confounder, at any level of the ecological model (Leatherdale, 2019). Hence, ecological models can help investigators make decisions about the design, selection of measures, power calculations, and analytical approaches within the context of complex natural experiments. In this section, we outline two examples on how ecological frameworks helped guide the evaluation of major urban travel infrastructure changes in Houston, the United States and Mexico City, Mexico, and their impact on active travel behaviors (see Figure 3.1b).

Houston and Mexico City are both large, dynamic cities, but also face pressing challenges, including rapid population growth, traffic congestion, air pollution, and high levels of obesity and known comorbidities amongst their populations (Tamayo-Ortiz et al., 2021; Zhang, 2018). However, while Houston has invested heavily in highway and toll-way projects (car-centric infrastructure), Mexico City has a widespread public transit system, including one of the largest subway systems in the world, bus rapid transit, and several types of "feeder buses" (informal transit options). In recent years, both cities have undergone major investments in transformative infrastructure that could potentially increase active travel. In December 2013, Houston began major expansions to its light-rail system across the city, connecting many low-income, predominantly minority neighborhoods, to the downtown business core of the city, through 15 miles of new lines including 24 new stations (Gates & United States Department of Transportation, 2013). On the other hand, since 2018, Mexico City began a massive expansion plan of its bicycling infrastructure plan, including expanding the geographic reach of its already large public bicycle-sharing program (*EcoBici*), and the addition of over 50 km of protected bicycle lanes throughout the city, with emphasis in low-income areas (Mexico City Government, 2018).

Given these major infrastructure investments and expansion plans, research teams in the United States and Mexico secured funds for conducting rigorous, longitudinal assessments of the impacts of these *natural experiments* on active travel outcomes (transit use in Houston and bicycle ridership in Mexico City). While these two studies were conducted independently of each other, they share many commonalities worth highlighting, as they are a direct result of the investigators' use of ecological models for guiding study design, implementation, and analytical decisions. For instance, in addition to assessing the exposures (light-rail access in Houston, and bicycle-infrastructure access in Mexico City) and outcomes of interest (physical activity as a result of increased transit use and bicycle ridership, respectively), both studies relied on a wide array of instruments to collect data on individual (e.g., sociodemographics, attitudes, and perceptions on active travel), interpersonal (family size, social support for active travel), and community-level factors (perceived and objective measures of the social and built environment of neighborhoods) (Durand et al., 2016; Jáuregui et al., 2020). Both research teams used objective measures to quantify their outcome of interest (accelerometers, GPS monitors), and relied on validated questionnaires, environmental audits, and Geographic Information Systems for assessing the exposure to the natural experiment, and multiple other factors at varying levels of the ecological model.

These studies used sample size calculations and analytical approaches that accounted for the clustered nature of data. Similar statistical approaches, consistent with concepts articulated in ecological models, were used in both studies to determine whether any of the individual, societal, or environmental factors interacted with the new urban infrastructure to differentially affect study outcomes.

Application 2: Using Ecological Models as a Framework to Assess the Bidirectional Relationship of Health Behavior, Human Health, and Planetary Health

Planetary health is a newer field that focuses on understanding the relationships between humans and the conditions of the planet Earth (Horton & Lo, 2015). The planetary health approach recognizes that for humans to lead healthy lives, we must achieve and sustain a healthy planet (with all of its natural systems at balance, and with threats like climate change being mitigated). Hence, planetary health is explicit about the bidirectional nature of human and environmental interactions—in full alignment with the ecological model framework and its embrace of the concept of reciprocal determinism. That is, the health status of our planet (e.g., how frequently do extreme weather events occur?) exerts an influence on our health behaviors, which naturally occur at the individual level. Conversely, the collective behaviors of individuals impact the health of the planet. For example, if most residents of a city choose to drive, even for short-distance trips, this could ensue a series of consequences at the planetary level (bad local air quality due to high traffic and congestion, and ultimately, increased carbon emissions—the main contributor to global warming and climate change).

Although traditionally, ecological models have been used almost exclusively to explain the upstream influences of individual-level health behaviors (i.e., in a unidirectional fashion), there is no reason why they cannot or should not be used to understand the influence of collective behaviors of individuals on societal and environmental/planetary outcomes. That is, an ecological framework, as applied to planetary health, can and should consider that factors occurring within and beyond the individual level can simultaneously be "exposures" (causes) and "outcomes" (effects) of interest. This is arguably a more realistic representation of the world.

In 2021, Salvo and colleagues published their findings of a study using an *agent-based model* to test the effect of major urban infrastructure changes (built environment interventions) on both health-related (physical activity behaviors) and planetary outcomes (local air quality, carbon emissions). Agent-based modeling is a method that uses real-world data to simulate a given environment (e.g., a real-world city), its inhabitants (referred to as "agents" in the simulation), and their interactions—based on known ecological determinants of health behavior (Auchincloss & Diez Roux, 2008). When based on solid empirical evidence and properly calibrated (the process of comparing the way in which agents of a simulated city behave, relative to real residents of the real-world city under current, known conditions), agent-based modeling can be a powerful tool to test the impact of the higher levels of the ecological model on multiple outcomes at once. Simulation-based approaches, such as agent-based modeling, provide an alternative and complementary approach to traditional empirical (data-based) methods for testing the effects of complex, multilevel interventions.

In their work, Salvo and colleagues designed three simulated cities representing general city typologies in low-, middle-, and high-income countries. Notably, the type of high-income city that they simulated was meant to represent a sprawling, car-dependent North American city, rather than a walkable, transit-oriented European city. After carefully calibrating their model for the three city types, they simulated the following built-environment interventions: (a) large expansion in coverage and near-complete reduction in inequities in access to high-quality, frequently running public transit across the city; (b) large expansion in coverage and near-complete reduction in inequities in access to pedestrian (sidewalk, walking paths) and bicycling infrastructure (protected bicycle lanes and paths);

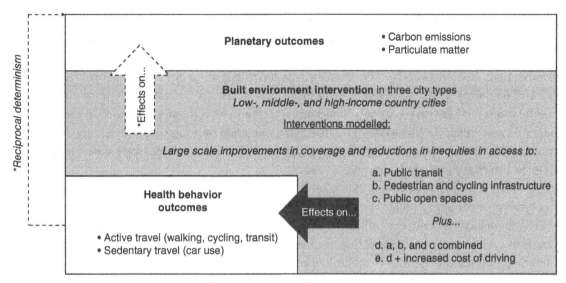

Figure 3.2 Reciprocal Determinism in Ecological Models: Example of the Impact of Built Environment Interventions on Health Behavior and Planetary Outcomes, Based on a Modeling Study by Salvo et al. (2021)

(c) large expansion in coverage and near-complete reduction in inequities in access to parks and other public open spaces; (d) scenarios a-c combined; (e) scenario d, plus an increases cost of driving (via car ownership taxes, gas taxes, and parking restrictions). Outcomes included: proportion of trips in each city done by active travel (walking, cycling), public transit (known to be connected to more walking trips than driving), and car (sedentary travel); proportion of the population engaging regularly in recreational physical activity; air quality (measured by particulate matter); and carbon emissions (main contributor to climate change). Figure 3.2 shows the ecological relationships that this study explored, highlighting the fact that it tested the reciprocal determinism principle of ecological models by assessing the effect of population shifts in health-related behaviors (sedentary versus active travel modes) on planetary outcomes.

Findings revealed that context matters: scenario d (all built environment strategies combined) worked the best for low- and middle-income country cities, simultaneously yielding significant increases in active travel, recreational physical activity, and reductions in particulate matter and carbon emissions. However, in sprawling, high-income country cities, it was necessary to include bold complementary strategies that increase the cost of driving, alongside all other built-environment changes, to observe health behavior and planetary benefits.

This study, and others using similar methodologies (Kaplan et al., 2017), demonstrate the utility of complex systems-science methods for testing the ecological model across varying settings, and of exploring outcomes at different levels (i.e., reciprocal determinism principle). More importantly, these types of studies provide important evidence in support of the major built-environment and economic-policy changes needed across the world to improve the health of humans and of the planet.

Discussion

To date, ecological models have mostly been used conceptually for explaining the totality of influence of health behaviors, and to determine what needs to be measured or accounted for when designing observational, program evaluation, or intervention studies. A common criticism of ecological models is that despite their excellent face validity, they remain "too general" and are perceived as being "hard to test" through traditional empirical approaches. Another consistent critique is that while it is often safe to assume that there are multiple levels of influence on health behavior, most health behavior interventions to date focus on the more proximal levels—the individual (interpersonal and community levels)—versus the more distal ones (policy and planetary levels) (Parkinson et al., 2022). The still-limited work on multilevel interventions that include strategies across all or most levels of influence likely has several causes. Simply determining the specific influences on which to intervene at each level is challenging, while multilevel interventions are more complex, and may require more expertise and resources for implementation and evaluation.

Although individual researchers and interventionists may have little or no direct control over factors at the societal, environmental, and planetary levels, the evidence produced by research is critical to advocate effectively for health-promoting modifications to these very systems. Tobacco research and its influence on policy in the United States, and the work by nutrition researchers in Mexico to evaluate sugar-sweetened beverage tax policies, are both excellent examples of how science based on ecological models has influenced policies and large-scale environmental changes for improving public health (Batis et al., 2016; Warner & Tam, 2012).

Some studies have tested interventions that target only one level of the ecological model—with those at the community/societal, governmental/policy, or planetary level more likely to be explicitly identified as informed by ecological models. Ecological models can still be useful for guiding this work. A single-level intervention could be acceptable if existing evidence has established, that, for this specific behavior, that level exerts an outsized influence on behavioral outcomes, and that the optimal use of limited resources is to focus on a single level. One classic public health example is fluoridated water (Newbrun, 1989). While the occurrence of dental caries is influenced by factors across multiple levels, fluoridating the public water supply, an upstream, single-level environmental intervention, is a simple, cost-effective approach with major impact. This is not to say, however, that fluoridated water minimizes *all* risk of dental caries, and that a multilevel intervention would not be preferable. Indeed, recent evidence points to significant increases in dental caries incidence among children globally (Bagramian et al., 2009), which further emphasizes that multilevel approaches are necessary for better controlling the issue. It should also be noted that examples like the case of water fluoridation and dental caries are increasingly rare, and hence, for most health behaviors, a multilevel approach is usually preferable.

Another instance for which single-level interventions may be useful is as part of a larger effort to flesh out the behavior-specific ecological model, and to help establish credible evidence on the causal link between factors at a given level of the ecological model on the behavior *while accounting for the influence of factors at other levels.* When there is consistent etiologic evidence for a problem at multiple levels, it is increasingly important for intervention work to focus on more than one level.

There are some comprehensive analyses that attempt to quantify the relative influence of different levels, and of different factors within each level, on health behaviors. There are many good examples of this type of work in the food environment and obesity-behavior literature (Cobb et al., 2015). One example is the comprehensive analysis by Ohri-Vachaspati et al. (2015), who combined individual respondent survey data with neighborhood environment data to understand the relative contributions of factors from different levels of the ecological model to understand childhood obesity. These levels included child, parent, household and neighborhood characteristics, parental perceptions of the neighborhood environment, and measured presence of food and physical activity facilities. The investigators found that the strongest contributors were parental characteristics (such as education and body mass index) and parental perceptions of the neighborhood environment (such as safety from crime and traffic, availability of fruits and vegetables, and condition of sidewalks). This type of research can help indicate where to prioritize intervention efforts to reduce childhood obesity. On the basis of this analysis, a future multilevel intervention might target certain important changeable factors, including increasing the availability of fruits and vegetables at nearby stores and quantity and quality of spaces for physical activity, as well as parental perceptions of those facilities. Parental perceptions might be targeted either directly, such as by individually directed interventions to address concerns around safety, or indirectly, through further environmental interventions, such as sidewalk reconstruction, crosswalk painting, and the like.

Other important factors to consider when thinking about which levels to prioritize for intervention are the expected effect sizes for proximal versus distal influences, and the need (or desire) to achieve individual- versus population-level impact. It is reasonable to expect interventions targeting intrapersonal or interpersonal factors (proximal influences) to generally result in larger effect sizes for behavior change in individuals than those operating at higher levels of the ecological model (distal influences). However, the reach, long-term maintenance, and scalability potential of these strategies may be limited. So, if the goal is to find solutions to address a large-scale, public health problem such as the obesity epidemic in the United States or Mexico, one might argue that targeting the most upstream-level factors (policies, environments) that promote unhealthy eating and sedentary lifestyles may be the most effective approach. Previous sections of this chapter have discussed the complexities entailed by this type of intervention, occurring at the outermost rings of ecological models. Still, let us assume that all of those challenges have been overcome and that we have successfully implemented a policy-level intervention involving a junk food and soda tax in a large city to reduce caloric intake and unhealthy eating. Under this scenario, it would be reasonable to expect that the individual-level effect size of this type of policy intervention (say on the average reduction in caloric intake per person) would be low. However, from a public health standpoint, achieving small health behavioral improvements among a large proportion of the population may be preferable to achieving larger changes among only a few people (Letson et al., 2016). Obviously, the ideal scenario would be to implement effective, complementary, and coordinated strategies targeting multiple levels of the ecological model. However, this is not always feasible in real life and in the short term. Hence, the thresholds for what we consider effective may need to be adapted to reasonable expectations depending on the level(s) targeted by health behavior interventions.

Finally, other emerging considerations with respect to the use of ecological models for identifying strategies to improve health behaviors involve the need to develop *globally and locally varying ecological models*. It is not enough to recognize that the ecological model for one health behavior will operate differently for another health behavior. For example, it is possible that the ecological model for gun violence in the United States includes very different factors or elements at all levels when compared to the ecological model for gun violence in Australia, as each country has different policies and social norms around gun ownership. The same could be said about any health behavior. In fact, new evidence even suggests that the factors populating each level of the ecological model for a given health behavior can vary across neighborhoods within a single city (Feuillet et al., 2015). More research exploring the global and local variations of ecological models for "the same health behavior" is needed, as this type of work is not just interesting, but most importantly, can help us design and implement more effective health behavior change strategies for specific settings, contexts, and population groups.

Summary

Ecological models provide a framework for understanding the totality of influence of health behaviors, and how people interact with their broader contexts. Ecological models emphasize the influence that levels beyond the individual can exert on health behaviors, including the interpersonal, societal or community, policy, and planetary levels. Further, ecological models posit that factors at these levels interact with each other when influencing health behaviors. A key advantage of ecological models is their flexibility, allowing for tailoring the ecological framework to any health behavior and/or setting or population group of interest. Additionally, behavior change theories can be integrated or embedded within an ecological framework and used to design multilevel interventions. Ecological models are also useful for designing and implementing observational and evaluation studies, as they can help investigators identify which factors must be measured across multiple levels. Although there are logistical challenges for implementing multilevel behavior change interventions, this chapter included examples of successful multilevel interventions and of creative solutions for overcoming these challenges, including natural experiments. When informed by high-quality empirical studies, complex systems models—which use sophisticated simulation-based techniques to test the effects that major societal, policy, and environmental changes could have on human and planetary health outcomes—provide a novel approach for examining the potential impacts of multilevel interventions. Furthermore, regardless of the availability of empirical evidence demonstrating the utility of ecological models, their face validity is excellent, and their premise is simple: if we create environments that are conducive to healthy choices, entire populations, and perhaps even our planet, will benefit. Also, the effectiveness and long-term maintenance of behavioral interventions targeting more proximal levels to individuals could be optimized.

Acknowledgments

The authors would like to acknowledge Drs. James F. Sallis and Neville Owen, authors of previous versions of this chapter that appeared in earlier editions of this book. Most of the text used in the first paragraph of the "History" section of our chapter is borrowed from their work.

References

Auchincloss, A. H., & Diez Roux, A. V. (2008). A new tool for epidemiology: The usefulness of dynamic-agent models in understanding place effects on health. *American Journal of Epidemiology*, *168*(1), 1–8.

Bagramian, R. A., Garcia-Godoy, F., & Volpe, A. R. (2009). The global increase in dental caries. A pending public health crisis. *American Journal of Dentistry*, *22*(1), 3–8.

Batis, C., Rivera, J. A., Popkin, B. M., & Taillie, L. S. (2016). First-year evaluation of Mexico's tax on nonessential energy-dense foods: An observational study. *PLoS Medicine*, *13*(7), e1002057.

Boulange, C., Gunn, L., Giles-Corti, B., Mavoa, S., Pettit, C., & Badland, H. (2017). Examining associations between urban design attributes and transport mode choice for walking, cycling, public transport and private motor vehicle trips. *Journal of Transport & Health*, *6*, 155–166.

Branas, C., South, E., Kondo, M., Hohl, B., Bourgois, P., Wiebe, D., & MacDonald, J. (2018). Citywide cluster randomized trial to restore blighted vacant land and its effects on violence, crime, and fear. *Proceedings of the National Academy of Sciences*, 115, 2946–2951.

Bronfenbrenner, U. (1989). Ecological systems theory. In R. Vasta (Ed.), *Annals of child development* (vol. 6, pp. 187–249). London: Jessica Kingsley Publishers.

Bull, F. C., Gauvin, L., Bauman, A., Shilton, T., Kohl, H. W., & Salmon, A. (2010). The Toronto charter for physical activity: A global call for action. *Journal of Physical Activity and Health*, *7*(4), 421–422.

Calo, W. A., & Krasny, S. (2013). Environmental determinants of smoking behaviors: The role of policy and environmental interventions in preventing smoking initiation and supporting cessation. *Current Cardiovascular Risk Reports*, *7*(6), 446–452.

Cobb, L. K., Appel, L. J., Franco, M., Jones-Smith, J. C., Nur, A., & Anderson, C. A. (2015). The relationship of the local food environment with obesity: A systematic review of methods, study quality, and results. *Obesity*, *23*(7), 1331–1344.

Cohen, D. A., Scribner, R. A., & Farley, T. A. (2000). A structural model of health behavior: A pragmatic approach to explain and influence health behaviors at the population level. *Preventive Medicine*, *30*(2), 146–154. https://doi.org/10.1006/pmed.1999.0609

Craig, P., Cooper, C., Gunnell, D., Haw, S., Lawson, K., Macintyre, S., Ogilvie, D., Petticrew, M., Reeves, B., & Sutton, M. (2012). Using natural experiments to evaluate population health interventions: New Medical Research Council guidance. *Journal of Epidemiology and Community Health*, *66*(12), 1182–1186.

Durand, C. P., Oluyomi, A. O., Gabriel, K. P., Salvo, D., Sener, I. N., Hoelscher, D. M., Knell, G., Tang, X., Porter, A. K., & Robertson, M. C. (2016). The effect of light rail transit on physical activity: Design and methods of the travel-related activity in neighborhoods study. *Frontiers in Public Health*, *4*, 103.

Elder, J. P., Lytle, L., Sallis, J. F., Young, D. R., Steckler, A., Simons-Morton, D., Stone, E., Jobe, J. B., Stevens, J., & Lohman, T. (2007). A description of the social–ecological framework used in the trial of activity for adolescent girls (TAAG). *Health Education Research*, *22*(2), 155–165.

Feuillet, T., Charreire, H., Menai, M., Salze, P., Simon, C., Dugas, J., Hercberg, S., Andreeva, V. A., Enaux, C., & Weber, C. (2015). Spatial heterogeneity of the relationships between environmental characteristics and active commuting: Towards a locally varying social ecological model. *International Journal of Health Geographics*, *14*(1), 1–14.

Frank, L., Giles-Corti, B., & Ewing, R. (2016). The influence of the built environment on transport and health. *Journal of Transport and Health*, *3*(4), 423–425.

Gates, A., & United States Department of Transportation. (2013). *U.S. Department of Transportation celebrates opening of new light rail line, expanding transit options in Houston region*. Federal Transit Administration. https://www.transit.dot.gov/about/news/us-department-transportation-celebrates-opening-new-light-rail-line-expanding-transit

Ginja, S., Arnott, B., Namdeo, A., & McColl, E. (2018). Understanding active school travel through the Behavioural Ecological Model. *Health Psychology Review*, *12*(1), 58–74. https://doi.org/10.1080/17437199.2017.1400394

Glanz, K., Escoffery, C., Elliott, T., & Nehl, E. J. (2015). Randomized trial of two dissemination strategies for a skin cancer prevention program in aquatic settings. *American Journal of Public Health*, *105*(7), 1415–1423.

Glanz, K., Sallis, J. F., Saelens, B. E., & Frank, L. D. (2005). Healthy nutrition environments: concepts and measures. *American Journal of Health Promotion*, *19*(5), 330–333, ii. https://doi.org/10.4278/0890-1171-19.5.330

Glass, T. A., & McAtee, M. J. (2006). Behavioral science at the crossroads in public health: Extending horizons, envisioning the future. *Social Science & Medicine*, *62*(7), 1650–1671.

Holman, D., Lynch, R., & Reeves, A. (2018). How do health behaviour interventions take account of social context? A literature trend and co-citation analysis. *Health*, *22*(4), 389–410.

Horton, R., & Lo, S. (2015). Planetary health: A new science for exceptional action. *The Lancet*, *386*(10007), 1921–1922.

Huang, R., Moudon, A. V., Zhou, C., Stewart, O. T., & Saelens, B. E. (2017). Light rail leads to more walking around station areas. *Journal of Transport & Health*, 6, 201–208.

Jáuregui, A., Salvo, D., Medina, C., Unar, M., Barrientos, T., Barquera, S., Velázquez, D., & Reséndiz, E. (2020). Effects of improved bicycling infrastructure developed in response to COVID-19: A natural experiment in Mexico City (The SALURBAL Study). LAC-Urban Health (Urban Health Network for Latin America and the Caribbean). Drexel Urban Health Collaborative. https://drexel.edu/lac/data-evidence/policy-evaluations/effect-of-a-public-bicycle-sharing-program-on-urban-health-in-mexico-city/

Kaplan, G. A., Roux, A. V. D., Simon, C. P., & Galea, S. (2017). *Growing inequality: Bridging complex systems, population health, and health disparities.* Washington, DC: Westphalia Press.

Leatherdale, S. T. (2019). Natural experiment methodology for research: A review of how different methods can support real-world research. *International Journal of Social Research Methodology*, 22(1), 19–35.

Leisner, C. P. (2020). Climate change impacts on food security-focus on perennial cropping systems and nutritional value. *Plant Science*, 293, 110412.

Letson, G. W., French, J., Ricketts, S., Trierweiler, K., Juhl, A., Gujral, I., Archer, L., & McGregor, J. A. (2016). Utility of population attributable fraction assessment in guiding interventions to reduce low birthweight in the high-altitude state of Colorado. *Maternal and Child Health Journal*, 20(12), 2457–2464.

Mahmoudi, J., & Zhang, L. (2020). Impact of the built environment measured at multiple levels on nonmotorized travel behavior: An ecological approach to a Florida case study. *Sustainability*, 12(21), 8837.

Marinova, D., & Bogueva, D. (2019). Planetary health and reduction in meat consumption. *Sustainable Earth*, 2(1), 1–12.

McLeroy, K. R., Bibeau, D., Steckler, A., & Glanz, K. (1988). An ecological perspective on health promotion programs. *Health Education Quarterly*, 15(4), 351–377. https://doi.org/10.1177/109019818801500401

Mexico City Government. (2018). *Plan Bici CDMX.* Banco Interamericano de Desarrollo, Universidad Nacional Autónoma de México.

Newbrun, E. (1989). Effectiveness of water fluoridation. *Journal of Public Health Dentistry*, 49(5), 279–289.

Ogilvie, D., Adams, J., Bauman, A., Gregg, E. W., Panter, J., Siegel, K. R., Wareham, N. J., & White, M. (2020). Using natural experimental studies to guide public health action: Turning the evidence-based medicine paradigm on its head. *Journal of Epidemiology and Community Health*, 74(2), 203–208.

Ogilvie, D., Bull, F., Powell, J., Cooper, A. R., Brand, C., Mutrie, N., Preston, J., Rutter, H., & iConnect Consortium. (2011). An applied ecological framework for evaluating infrastructure to promote walking and cycling: The iConnect study. *American Journal of Public Health*, 101(3), 473–481.

Ohri-Vachaspati, P., DeLia, D., DeWeese, R. S., Crespo, N. C., Todd, M., & Yedidia, M. J. (2015). The relative contribution of layers of the Social Ecological Model to childhood obesity. *Public Health Nutrition*, 18(11), 2055–2066.

Parkinson, R., Jessiman-Perreault, G., Frenette, N., & Allen Scott, L. K. (2022). Exploring multilevel workplace tobacco control interventions: A scoping review. *Workplace Health & Safety*, 70(8), 368–382.

Richard, L., Gauvin, L., & Raine, K. (2011). Ecological models revisited: their uses and evolution in health promotion over two decades. *Annual Review of Public Health*, 32, 307–326. https://doi.org/10.1146/annurev-publhealth-031210-101141

Sallis, J. F. (2018). Needs and challenges related to multilevel interventions: Physical activity examples. *Health Education & Behavior*, 45(5), 661–667.

Sallis, J. F., Cerin, E., Conway, T. L., Adams, M. A., Frank, L. D., Pratt, M., Salvo, D., Schipperijn, J., Smith, G., & Cain, K. L. (2016). Physical activity in relation to urban environments in 14 cities worldwide: A cross-sectional study. *The Lancet*, 387(10034), 2207–2217.

Santos, O., Virgolino, A., Carneiro, A. V., & de Matos, M. G. (2021). Health Behavior and Planetary Health. *European Psychologist*, 26(3), 212–218.

Sazzad, H. M. S., McCredie, L., Treloar, C., Lloyd, A. R., & Lafferty, L. (2020). Violence and hepatitis C transmission in prison—A modified social ecological model. *PLoS One*, 15(12), e0243106. https://doi.org/10.1371/journal.pone.0243106

Sorensen, C., Murray, V., Lemery, J., & Balbus, J. (2018). Climate change and women's health: Impacts and policy directions. *PLoS Medicine*, 15(7), e1002603.

Story, M., Kaphingst, K. M., Robinson-O'Brien, R., & Glanz, K. (2008). Creating healthy food and eating environments: Policy and environmental approaches. *Annual Review of Public Health*, 29, 253–272. https://doi.org/10.1146/annurev.publhealth.29.020907.090926

Stotz, S. A., McNealy, K., Begay, R. L., DeSanto, K., Manson, S. M., & Moore, K. R. (2021). Multi-level diabetes prevention and treatment interventions for native people in the USA and Canada: A scoping review. *Current Diabetes Reports*, 21(11), 1–17.

Tamayo-Ortiz, M., Téllez-Rojo, M. M., Rothenberg, S. J., Gutiérrez-Avila, I., Just, A. C., Kloog, I., Texcalac-Sangrador, J. L., Romero-Martinez, M., Bautista-Arredondo, L. F., & Schwartz, J. (2021). Exposure to PM2. 5 and obesity prevalence in the Greater Mexico City area. *International Journal of Environmental Research and Public Health, 18*(5), 2301.

US National Cancer Institute. (2017). A socioecological approach to addressing tobacco-related health disparities. *National Cancer Institute Tobacco Control Monograph 22*. NIH Publication No. 17-CA-8035A.

Van Dyck, D., Cerin, E., Conway, T. L., De Bourdeaudhuij, I., Owen, N., Kerr, J., Cardon, G., & Sallis, J. F. (2014). Interacting psychosocial and environmental correlates of leisure-time physical activity: A three-country study. *Health Psychology, 33*(7), 699–709. https://doi.org/10.1037/a0033516

Warner, K. E., & Tam, J. (2012). The impact of tobacco control research on policy: 20 years of progress. *Tobacco Control, 21*(2), 103–109.

Wold, B., & Mittelmark, M. B. (2018). Health-promotion research over three decades: The social-ecological model and challenges in implementation of interventions. *Scandinavian Journal of Public Health, 46*(20_suppl), 20–26.

Zhang, X. (2018). *Traffic, air pollution, built environment and obesity in Greater Houston*. Publication Number AAI10789762. Houston: The University of Texas School of Public Health. https://digitalcommons.library.tmc.edu/dissertations/AAI10789762

Salvo, D., Garcia, L., Reis, R. S., Stankov, I., Goel, R., Schipperijn, J., Hallal, P. C., Ding, D., & Pratt, M. (2021). Physical activity promotion and the United Nations sustainable development goals: building synergies to maximize impact. *Journal of Physical Activity and Health, 18*(10), 1163–1180.

Barker, R. G. (1968). *Ecological psychology*. Stanford, CA: Stanford University Press.

Lewin, K., & Cartwright, D. (1951). *Field theory in social science*. New York: Harper.

VanEpps EM, Roberto CA, Park S, Economs CD, & Bleich SN (2016). Restaurant menu labeling policy: review of evidence and controversies. *Current Obesity Reports*, 5: 72–80.

Saelens BE, Hurvitz PM, Zhou C, Colburn T, Marchese A, & Moudon AV (2022). Impact of a light rail transit line on physical activity: Findings from the longitudinal Travel Assessment and Community (TRAC) study. *Journal of Transport & Health*, 27: 101527.

MODELS OF INDIVIDUAL HEALTH BEHAVIOR

CHAPTER 4

INTRODUCTION TO HEALTH BEHAVIOR THEORIES THAT FOCUS ON INDIVIDUALS

Noel T. Brewer
Barbara K. Rimer

This section of *Health Behavior: Theory, Research and Practice* covers three health behavior theories centered on individuals. They are the Health Belief Model (HBM); Reasoned Action Approach (RAA) models (Theory of Reasoned Action [TRA], Theory of Planned Behavior [TPB], Integrative Behavioral Model [IBM], and Reasoned Action Approach [RAA]); and The Transtheoretical Model (TTM). These theories were developed and refined over the past 40–70 years, and thousands of studies have shown their value in improving how researchers and practitioners think about public health, conceptualize public health problems, and design, implement, and evaluate behavior change interventions. This pre-eminence makes understanding these theories a basic and required tool for those working on health behavior. Examples in the chapters show the theories' importance for understanding well-characterized health behaviors and newly emergent threats like COVID-19.

Health Belief Model (HBM)

HBM has intuitive logic and clear central tenets, with defined ways to measure them (Chapter 5). The first study that used HBM addressed the very practical question: "Why did some people not get tuberculosis screening when it was available to them?"

Expectancy and value are central to HBM. The theory posits that people will engage in a health behavior when they believe that doing so can reduce a threat that is likely (expectancy) and would have severe consequences (value). HBM suggests that a health behavior is also more likely when people expect it to have more benefits and fewer barriers. The intuition behind expectancy and value also animates several other health behavior theories, most notably, RAA models (Weinstein, 1993).

Another core construct of HBM—cues to action—may be as varied as medical symptoms, a doctor's recommendation, reminders from a health plan, a poster near the checkout counter in a pharmacy, or a media campaign. The construct of cues to action is unusual among health behavior theories in providing a specific place for the effect of health symptoms in motivating behavior.

Health Behavior: Theory, Research, and Practice, Sixth Edition. Edited by Karen Glanz, Barbara K. Rimer, and K. Viswanath.
© 2024 John Wiley & Sons, Inc. Published 2024 by John Wiley & Sons, Inc.
Companion website: www.wiley.com/go/glanz/healthbehavior6e

Self-efficacy, originally part of Social Cognitive Theory, proposed as an addition after HBM was formulated, is not derived directly from an expectancy-value approach. Substantial research has shown that self-efficacy is a strong predictor of many health behaviors (see Chapter 9 on Social Cognitive Theory), and researchers made a logical case for incorporating it into HBM (Rosenstock et al., 1988). However, we have not found systematic reviews that examined the predictive utility of adding self-efficacy to HBM.

HBM is parsimonious, requiring as few as six questions to assess key constructs. It is a proven way to identify correlates of health behavior that may be important in behavior changes and is useful for informing intervention design and evaluation. The theory is especially well-suited to understanding preventive behaviors for infectious diseases and screening for a range of diseases. Studies have shown the utility of HBM in understanding uptake of many health behaviors beyond screening and vaccination.

Reasoned Action Approach Models

RAA models focus on behaviors that involve planning or deliberation. The Theory of Reasoned Action (TRA), the first iteration of the theories, aimed to explain health and non-health outcomes, including organ donation and voting (Chapter 6). Later theories—the Theory of Planned Behavior (TPB), Integrative Behavioral Model (IBM), and Reasoned Action Approach (RAA)—retained this general focus but added some new dimensions. These theories are notable for the way they built upon one another in a sequential fashion (Yzer, 2017), well-supported by data from laboratory experiments and health behavior interventions (Sheeran et al., 2016).

An important feature of RAA is the centrality of behavioral intentions. Positive attitudes toward a health behavior, social norms favoring the behavior, and perceived behavioral control all strengthen behavioral intentions, which then activate health behavior. Longitudinal, observational studies have found strong intention-behavior associations (Sheeran, 2002), while experiments show small-to-moderate effect sizes (Webb and Sheeran, 2006). Intentions can be an important step along the pathway to behavior change. However, because intentions may not translate directly into behavior changes, they are not an adequate proxy for behavior change, especially in large behavior change trials (Sheeran and Webb, 2016).

People must be able to perform a health behavior for intentions to translate into action. Thus, RAA developers (Fishbein and Ajzen, 2010) added the construct of actual control as moderating intention-behavior relationships. Actual control recognizes the importance of the environment, defined broadly, and a person's skills for performing a particular behavior.

RAA models prescribe a systematic method to identify issues most important to specific contexts and to individuals' decisions about performing specific behaviors. These methods require detailed preliminary work, elicitation methods, to assess the populations of interest and contexts under study. While potentially time-consuming, the methods are especially important when studying new topic areas and different cultures.

The Transtheoretical Model (TTM)

TTM evolved from theories of psychoanalysis to consolidate many varied approaches and understand how people change health behaviors, such as smoking (Chapter 7). The creators examined what self-changers did, and how people changed in formal programs. TTM became a widely used theory of health behavior, and informed the understanding of many health behaviors, across prevention, screening, and treatment.

TTM posits that people are in different stages of readiness to make health behavior changes, starting in precontemplation and progressing toward action and maintenance. Prior to development of TTM, a common assumption was that everyone was ready for action even though many people were not even contemplating behavior change. According to TTM, people are more likely to change when they receive interventions appropriate to their stage in the behavior change process.

One of the greatest values of TTM may be in encouraging researchers and practitioners to think about interventions from the recipient's perspective. Why might they not be ready to quit? What are the benefits they derive from smoking? What are the perceived benefits of quitting? What are the downsides of quitting? TTM looks at how people weigh these pros or cons, called decisional balance.

Processes of change, a diverse set of activities that people naturally engage in as part of behavior change, such as consciousness-raising, seeking support, and substituting healthier options, are a strength of TTM. Data about processes of change can provide insights for intervention development. As Chapter 7 notes, the processes warrant as much or more attention than stages of change but often are ignored by those creating and evaluating interventions. Finally, the theory includes people's beliefs that they can perform the health behavior successfully, also called self-efficacy.

Interventions that leverage constructs from TTM, such as matching by stage of change, should be more effective than those not doing so. A systematic review of 33 randomized trials found improved physical activity behaviors from TTM-based interventions that delivered stage-matched interventions or selected people based on their stage, but the interventions were equally effective when they did not match interventions or participants by stage (Romain et al., 2018). Interventions were more impactful when based on some constructs in the theory (interventions that were tailored on more theoretical constructs or that emphasized self-efficacy), but not when based on other constructs (decisional balance, temptation, or processes of change). The findings suggest that stage matching may not be necessary. One interpretation is that even people in the same stage might have very different beliefs (Sussman et al., 2022).

Stages of change may have substantially practical value in interventions. A recent systematic review of 51 studies examined physical activity interventions for cancer survivors (Sheeran et al., 2023). Two intervention techniques (barrier identification and tailoring intervention on motivational readiness) were associated with the adoption of physical activity, but they did not also promote maintenance or the continued practice of new behaviors. Two intervention techniques (providing general encouragement and safety information) were associated with less adoption and maintenance. Only use of supervised exercise sessions was associated with greater adoption and maintenance. Findings show the potential importance of distinguishing among stages of change as targets of intervention.

Similarities and Differences in the Theories' Constructions

Theories in this section have some marked similarities, and all of them include some focus on motivation, attitudes, and self-efficacy. Motivation is central to all three theories but appears in different forms. RAA posits that behavior change for deliberative health behaviors occurs through behavioral intentions. Attitudes, norms, and perceived behavioral control also operate through intentions in RAA. In contrast, TTM views behavior change as a series of stages through which people progress—beginning in precontemplation and moving toward action and maintenance. While HBM does not explicitly include a variable for motivation, it is implicit in the theory.

The three theories in this section all include attitudes toward health behavior. Because many important attitudes *are* changeable, they are ideal targets for intervention. In HBM, perceived benefits of engaging in health behavior are a predictor of behavior, and RAA includes attitudes and an antecedent to behavioral intentions and behavior. TTM focuses on decisional balance of pros and cons (positive and negative attitudes toward the behavior). The three theories all include self-efficacy, though RAA calls it perceived behavioral control.

The three health behavior theories also have important differences. They conceptualize risk appraisals in different ways. HBM includes perceived vulnerability (feeling susceptible) and perceived severity (how bad that harm is). Some views of HBM, for example, in this book, interpret the theory's original proposal of perceived vulnerability as being about perceived likelihood (chances of being harmed).

Social norms are another area where the theories diverge. HBM and TTM do not include social norms per se, although processes of change in TTM include social processes. RAA specifies injunctive norms (what a person thinks others want them to do), which are measured as the multiplication of powerful others wanting the respondent to perform the behavior and motivation to comply. In the last iteration of RAA, the authors dropped multiplication and focused on awareness of the norm, based on data showing that motivation to comply did not add predictive power (Fishbein and Ajzen, 2010). This evolution is an example of how RAA models have changed over time.

Finally, theories of health behavior that focus on individuals generally incorporate race, ethnicity, and other demographic characteristics as distal influences, peripheral to more central psychological constructs, such as attitudes. Theorists of race and racialization have challenged this approach, quite appropriately, by placing race as central to people's lived experiences, where they first experience the world through the lens of race (see Chapter 14). One potential approach is to blend individual-level theories with other theories built explicitly to address race and racism. New insights from such synthesis may include explaining greater variance in health behavior, designing more effective interventions, and better understanding intersectionality of race with other constructs and experiences. Additional research is needed to quantify these potential impacts.

Other Considerations

The rise of theories in this section over more than 50 years, and their integration into research and practice, have advanced understanding about how to improve health behaviors. These individual-level health behavior theories have strengths as psychological theories of what is on people's minds that might affect their behaviors. However, no theories are panaceas for all health behavior problems or foundations for easy solutions to create behavior change. Forces external to the person, including social processes and environmental contexts, can exert powerful influences on health behavior that must also be considered (see Chapter 3). Other parts of the book address some of these forces beyond individuals.

Particular problems and contexts may require new and expanded ways of thinking that transcend individual theories. Some researchers use elements of individual-level theories (such as risk perceptions and attitudes) and pair them with constructs from other theories (such as the experience of racism or neighborhood characteristics). Individual theories can serve as building blocks. This type of approach is encouraged through systematic planning models such as PRECEDE-PROCEED and Intervention Mapping (Chapter 19), using multiple theories and multi-level approaches.

Conclusion

Theories of health behavior that focus on individuals are widely used and valuable tools for public health practitioners, researchers, and policymakers. They offer generally agreed upon descriptions of how people think and feel, and how those thoughts and feelings influence health behavior. While theories that are good predictors and intervention foundations in some health behavior contexts may fall short in others (Brewer et al., 2019), the theories in this section provide an important starting point for understanding health behaviors.

It is critical to consider the larger context of health behavior, including environment, broadly defined, in efforts to improve population health (Hagger and Weed, 2019). That means going beyond some variables in individual-level theories of health behavior. Additional constructs, such as implementation intentions, may be important in directing a focus on performance of desired behaviors (Gollwitzer and Sheeran, 2006). Implementation intentions involve making plans that are specific to external events or contexts, for example, how to avoid smoking while socializing with friends who smoke.

More attention also should be given to understanding what kinds of behaviors different theories are best suited to address. Theories of the individual should give more consideration to race and racism and to biologic and regulatory systems that may affect the gap between what people want to do and are able to do (Rejeski and Fanning, 2019). Later sections of this book provide more detail on strategies, such as incentives, race, and racism, and structured approaches for developing theory-based interventions.

Part 2 of this book includes individual-level theories that are well-established and have benefited from recent refinements. Development of health behavior theories is an evolutionary process. We urge careful attention to research design and measurement in studies that aim to explain how variables in the theories contribute to explaining behaviors and other outcomes.

References

Brewer, N. T., Parada Jr, H., Hall, M. G., Boynton, M. H., Noar, S. M., & Ribisl, K. M. (2019). Understanding why pictorial cigarette pack warnings increase quit attempts. *Annals of Behavioral Medicine, 53*(3), 232–243.

Fishbein, M., & Ajzen, I. (2010). *Predicting and changing behavior: The reasoned action approach.* New York, NY: Psychology Press.

Gollwitzer, P. M., & Sheeran, P. (2006). Implementation intentions and goal achievement: A meta-analysis of effects and processes. *Advances in Experimental Social Psychology, 38,* 69–119.

Hagger, M. S., & Weed, M. Debate: Do interventions based on behavioral theory work in the real world? *International Journal of Behavioral Nutrition and Physical Activity,* 2019, *16*(36), 1–10.

Rejeski, W. J., & Fanning, J. (2019). Models and theories of health behavior and clinical interventions in aging: A contemporary, integrative approach. *Clinical Interventions in Aging, 14*, 1007–1019.

Romain, A. J., Bortolon, C., Gourlan, M., Carayol, M., Decker, E., Lareyre. O., Ninot, G., Boiche, J., & Bernard, P. (2018). Matched or nonmatched interventions based on the transtheoretical model to promote physical activity. A meta-analysis of randomized controlled trials. *Journal of Sport and Health Science, 7*(1), 50–57.

Rosenstock, I. M., Strecher, V. J., & Becker, M. H. (1988). Social learning theory and the health belief model. *Health Education and Behavior, 15*, 175–188.

Sheeran, P. (2002). Intention-behavior relations: A conceptual and empirical review. *European Review of Social Psychology, 12*(1), 1–36.

Sheeran, P., Maki, A., Montanaro, E., Avishai-Yitshak A., Bryan, A., Klein, W. M. P., Miles, E., & Rothman, A. J. (2016). The impact of changing attitudes, norms, and self-efficacy on health-related intentions and behavior: A meta-analysis. *Health Psychology, 35*(11), 1178–1188.

Sheeran, P., & Webb, T. L. (2016). The intention–behavior gap. *Social and Personality Psychology Compass, 10*(9), 503–518.

Sheeran, P., Wright, C. E., Listrom, O., Klein, W. M. P., & Rothman, A. J. (2023). Which intervention strategies promote the adoption and maintenance of physical activity? Evidence from behavioral trials with cancer survivors. *Annals of Behavioral Medicine, 57*(9), 708–721.

Sussman, S. Y., Ayala, N., Pokhrel, P., & Herzog, T. A. (2022). Reflections on the continued popularity of The Transtheoretical Model. *Health Behavior Research, 5*(3), 2.

Webb, T. L., & Sheeran, P. (2006). Does changing behavioral intentions engender behavior change? A meta-analysis of the experimental evidence. *Psychological Bulletin, 132*, 249–268.

Weinstein, N. D. (1993). Testing four competing theories of health-protective behavior. *Health Psychology, 12*(4), 324–333.

Yzer, M. (2017). Reasoned action as an approach to understanding and predicting health, essage outcomes. In R. Parrott (Ed.), *Encyclopedia of health and risk message design and processing* (pp. 1–21). Oxford University Press.

CHAPTER 5

THE HEALTH BELIEF MODEL

Celette Sugg Skinner
Jasmin A. Tiro
Serena A. Rodriguez

KEY POINTS

This chapter will:

- Suggest health problems that can be addressed by the Health Belief Model (HBM).

- Introduce the HBM's historical development, key components, supporting evidence, and how its constructs are measured and used in interventions.

- Present applications of the HBM to perceptions of diabetes risk and receipt of COVID-19 vaccination.

Vignette: "I Thought This Wouldn't Be a Problem Once We Had a Vaccine"

The development of effective vaccines has allowed us to address some of the most serious health threats to humans and animals alike. To health professionals and many others, receiving a shot might appear to be a fairly straightforward and discrete behavior, particularly in comparison to more difficult behavior changes, such as weight loss and stopping smoking, that require repeated actions to achieve and maintain desired outcomes. However, vaccines' potential for prevention has not always translated into swift or sustained acceptance. Adoption by US adolescents of the first and only cancer-prevention HPV vaccine—first introduced in 2006 and requiring two doses for full coverage—was only 75% for initial vaccination by 2020, with only 58.6% of adolescents fully up-to-date in that year (Pingali et al., 2021). As of September 2022, when COVID-19 had taken the lives of over a million people in the United States and 6.5 million worldwide, only 67% of people eligible in the United States and 61% of the world population had received the first two recommended doses of the vaccine (Mathieu et al., 2022). Health behavior theory can help us understand what's going on here by elucidating key factors that influence whether people take recommended actions to protect their health.

We may feel just as frustrated today explaining these behaviors as the developers of the first widely used health behavior theory—the Health Belief Model (HBM)—back in the 1950s. In those years, tuberculosis (TB) was still a major health threat in the United States. Toward the goal of reducing morbidity and mortality, the US Public Health Service rolled out a program for neighborhood-based screening via mobile vans. The plan was innovative, and the potential benefits seemed obvious. But even when vans were deployed into people's neighborhoods, many fewer people than expected came to be screened. That put millions of people at risk for contracting TB—a highly contagious and potentially deadly and debilitating disease.

Health Behavior: Theory, Research, and Practice, Sixth Edition. Edited by Karen Glanz, Barbara K. Rimer, and K. Viswanath.
© 2024 John Wiley & Sons, Inc. Published 2024 by John Wiley & Sons, Inc.
Companion website: www.wiley.com/go/glanz/healthbehavior6e

The Public Health Service, wisely, realized a need to involve behavioral scientists who could help to explain the complex decisions influencing adoption of TB screening and, ultimately, other health-related behaviors. Thus was born the field of modern health behavior theory, and its first product was the HBM (Hochbaum, 1958).

Introduction

The HBM remains one of the most widely used conceptual frameworks in health behavior research and practice. Over the decades, it has been expanded, compared, and contrasted to other theories and frameworks, and used to inform behavior-change interventions—both alone and in combination with other theories.

In this chapter, we review the HBM's historical development, core constructs, hypotheses, and relationships of constructs to each other and to specific health behaviors, as well as the empirical evidence supporting it. Of the many health behaviors to which researchers have applied the HBM, we provide examples relevant to diabetes risk and COVID-19 mitigation measures, using the first example to focus on how the constructs of this model are measured, and the second on how they can be used in interventions to change health behavior.

Origins of the Health Belief Model

The HBM was originally developed by Dr. Godfrey Hochbaum, a social psychologist who immigrated to the United States from Austria following World War II, and his colleagues at the US Public Health Service to explain the widespread failure of people to participate in programs to prevent and detect disease (Hochbaum, 1958; Rosenstock, 1960). It was then extended to study people's behavioral responses to opportunities for early detection of potentially curable diseases, and their response to illnesses, with particular focus on adherence to medical regimens (Becker, 1974; Kirscht, 1974). HBM constructs were built on tenets of *Cognitive Theory* briefly discussed below.

During the first half of the 20th century, social psychologists had developed two major approaches for explaining behavior: *Stimulus-Response (S-R) Theory* (Watson, 1925) and *Cognitive Theory* (Lewin, 1951). S-R Theory posited that events (termed *reinforcements*) affect physiological drives that, in turn, activate behavior. American psychologist B. F. Skinner (1938) hypothesized that behavior is determined by its consequences, or reinforcements, and that the mere temporal association between a behavior and a reward or punishment immediately following that behavior was sufficient to increase the probability that the behavior would be repeated or avoided. According to S-R Theory, behavior is automatic and does not require mental processes, such as *reasoning* or *thinking*. Researchers now regard behavior as more complicated in most cases.

Conversely, cognitive theorists argued that reinforcements operated by influencing expectations rather than by influencing behavior directly. Mental processes—thinking, reasoning, hypothesizing, or expecting—are critical components of cognitive theories, which are often termed *value-expectancy* models because they propose that behavior is a function of the degree to which individuals value an outcome of a specific behavior and their assessment of the probability, or *expectation*, that a particular action will achieve that outcome (Lewin et al., 1944). For health-related behaviors, the *value* is avoiding illnesses and staying or getting well. The *expectation* is that a specific health action may prevent (or ameliorate) an illness or condition for which people believe they may be at risk.

Key Components of the HBM

Findings from Hochbaum's initial study of participation in TB screening were striking (Hochbaum, 1958). Among individuals who believed that they were more susceptible to TB, and who believed that early detection offered benefits, 82% had at least one voluntary chest X-ray. In contrast, only 21% of those who perceived lower personal susceptibility and benefits obtained X-rays. Some recent studies have found more modest associations between perceived susceptibility and health behavior.

In addition to TB screening, the HBM can be applied to many other health behaviors (such as medication adherence) with potential to reduce risk of developing a health condition and/or the effects of an existing disease or condition. As Charles Abraham and Paschal Sheeran explain, the cognitive theorists who developed and refined this model did not ignore social factors that influence health behaviors. They understood that demographic and socioeconomic factors were associated with both preventive behaviors and accessing health services. However, because their goal was to develop a framework that could be used to influence behavior change, they focused on specifying a set of "common-sense beliefs" that might be modified via health education interventions (Abraham & Sheeran, 2015). In our 21st-century conceptualization of multi-level determinants of both health and health behaviors, the HBM should be understood as primarily applicable to individual-level factors. However, it can be combined with constructs from other theories that operate at different levels. Other chapters in this book address some of those theories.

The HBM contains several primary components (or *constructs*) associated with whether and why people act to prevent, detect, or control illness condition. The model's overall premise is that people are likely to engage in health behavior if they believe:

1. They are at risk for (or susceptible to) a condition.

2. The condition could have potentially serious or severe consequences.

3. A course of action (behavior) available to them could reduce their susceptibility to and/or the severity of the condition.

4. There are benefits to taking action.

5. The perceived barriers (or costs) would not be strong enough to prevent action.

Other internal or external experiences ("cues") may also prompt action, either working through or outside of these beliefs.

The more precise definitions of these HBM constructs are summarized below:

Perceived Susceptibility is a belief about the likelihood of developing a disease or condition. For instance, people must believe they are at risk of getting colon cancer or breast cancer before they are willing to get screened for these cancers. Those being asked to take statins to prevent heart disease and stroke must believe they are at risk of these serious health problems if their high cholesterol is not managed.

Perceived Severity is a belief about the seriousness of contracting a condition or of leaving it untreated, including health consequences (e.g., death, disability, and pain) and social consequences (e.g., ability to work, maintain relationships, or feeling stigmatized).

Perceived Threat is sometimes described as the construct formed by the combination of susceptibility and severity.

Perceived Benefits are beliefs about positive effects or advantages of a recommended action to reduce threat of a disease, health condition, or its consequences. Other nonhealth-related benefits might be tangible ("I'll save money by quitting smoking") or social {"I'll feel better about myself if I follow my doctor's recommendation" or "my family member concerned about my cancer risk will be satisfied if I have a colonoscopy").

Perceived Barriers are possible negative consequences associated with an action. They may impede initial action or subsequent repeat of the behavior, and may be tangible ("If I quit, I'll be ridiculed by my still-smoking friends") or psychological ("trying to quit might cause me anxiety").

Cues to Action. In 1958, Hochbaum originally proposed that perceived susceptibility and perceived benefits were relevant only if activated by other factors that he termed "cues" to instigate action (Hochbaum, 1958). These cues could be internal (such as noticing a symptom that increased perceived threat), or external (such as media publicity; receiving a recommendation from a doctor, a free sample, or an individualized reminder from a health center; or even learning about a friend's diagnosis).

In the 1990s, Victor Strecher, Victoria Champion, and Irwin Rosenstock suggested that cues operate mainly as perceived threats, such as a painful sunburn increasing perceived risk of skin cancer and prompting people to add sunscreen to their shopping list (Strecher et al., 1997). However, Hochbaum (1958) also suggested scenarios through which the cue directly prompts behaviors without operating through beliefs. His often-used classroom example was a point-of-purchase display at the drugstore counter that prompts a person to add a tube of sunscreen to the cart even if her perceptions do not change: she already believes in the benefits of sunscreen but would have left the store without it were it not for the prompt and easy access at the cash register. This construct of a cue resembles more recent suggestions by behavioral economists that a simple "nudge" may prompt a person to change behavior (Thaler & Sunstein, 2009) (Also see Chapter 20).

Efficacy Expectations. Years after the HBM was developed, Albert Bandura (2005) introduced the constructs of self-efficacy and outcome efficacy expectations in his Social Cognitive Theory, postulating that behavior is guided by cognitive and affective (emotional) factors as well as biological and external events (see Chapter 9). Outcome efficacy—beliefs about the extent to which a particular behavior will lead to a certain outcome (Bandura, 1997, 1999)—resembles the HBM construct of perceived benefits. The construct of self-efficacy—the conviction that one can successfully execute a behavior—was not clearly represented by an HBM construct (although lack of self-efficacy was sometimes noted as a barrier to taking action) (Mahoney et al., 1995). In 1988, Rosenstock and colleagues suggested that self-efficacy be added to the HBM as a separate construct (Rosenstock et al., 1988).

Other Variables. An early assumption of the HBM was that demographic, structural, and psychosocial factors may affect beliefs and indirectly influence health behaviors. For example, sociodemographic factors, such as educational attainment, can indirectly influence behaviors by altering perceptions of susceptibility, severity, benefits, and barriers (Rosenstock, 1974; Salloway et al., 1978). However, the model does not specify *how* such factors operate or interact with other constructs. This remains a major gap in the HBM.

Operationalization of the HBM (Critical Assumptions and Hypotheses)

Figure 5.1 depicts components of the HBM, with arrows indicating pathways through which the model's constructs are linked to each other and to health behaviors. As shown, sociodemographic variables, such as age, sex/gender, race/ethnicity, education, income, and insurance status, may moderate relationships between health beliefs and health behaviors. For example, because cancer is more prevalent among older people, a person's age may moderate the relationship between perceived threat and cancer screening behavior such that older individuals believe themselves to be at a greater risk for cancer and rate cancer as a more severe disease than younger adults. Gender may moderate the effects

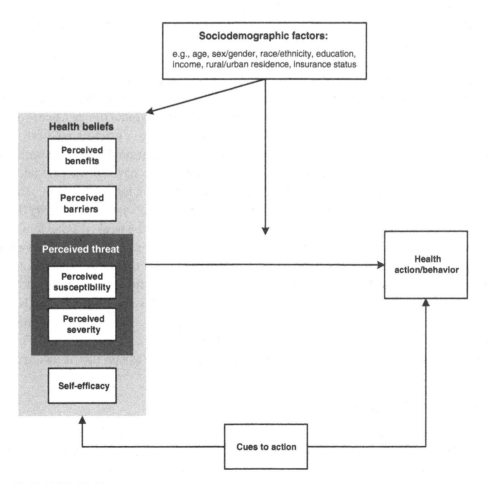

Figure 5.1 Components of the Health Belief Model

of perceived susceptibility and benefits regarding HPV vaccination because more attention has been drawn to the link between HPV infection and cervical cancer than to anal, penile, and oropharyngeal cancers. In addition, cues to action may affect health behaviors either directly or indirectly through their influence on health beliefs.

The HBM clearly specifies that health beliefs collectively affect behaviors, but it does not delineate precise combinations, weights, and relationships among variables (Abraham & Sheeran, 2015). This ambiguity has led to variations in how the HBM is applied in research. For example, while many studies have evaluated the direct path between beliefs and a given health behavior, others have tested constructs by using mathematical combinations that were not part of the model's original specification.

In the 1970s, Marshall Becker and Lois Maiman (1975) evaluated whether barriers should be subtracted from benefits. Conceptually, they argued that a kind of unconscious cost-benefit analysis occurs wherein individuals weigh the behavior's expected benefits against perceived barriers: "It could help me," the person might think, "but it may be expensive, painful, unpopular, unpleasant, or inconvenient." This combination of benefits and barriers is similar to the *Transtheoretical Model*'s later proposition that people weigh pros and cons of a given behavior against each other to form a single decisional balance score (see Chapter 7). However, Neil Weinstein (1988) later argued that benefits and barriers are qualitatively different and should be treated as distinct constructs with the potential to be linked to other HBM constructs and behavior through different pathways. Weinstein's position has been borne out in the HBM context through psychometric testing of barrier and benefit scales, showing that they act as separate factors influencing behavior (Tiro et al., 2005). Studies using structural equation modeling to test multiple pathways have also shown that perceived benefits and barriers have independent associations with behavior (Gerend & Shepherd, 2012; Murphy, et al., 2013). The HBM was developed long before these statistical models were available to conduct such analyses.

Empirical Evidence Supporting the HBM

Over the years, critical reviews of the HBM's predictive validity have combined or analyzed results from many studies to assess its performance. Generally, the model's constructs have been found consistently to predict health behaviors (Carpenter, 2010; Harrison et al., 1992; Janz & Becker, 1984; Jones et al., 2014; Zimmerman & Vernberg, 1994). Researchers' interest in the relative predictive value of individual HBM constructs has waxed and waned over time.

Studies that have assessed individual contributions of various constructs have found that the construct *perceived barriers* seem to be the most powerful single predictor of behavior (Carpenter, 2010; Harrison et al., 1992), followed by *perceived benefits*, with the magnitude of effect higher for prevention and risk-reduction behaviors (such as vaccination, child safety restraints) than for treatment behaviors (such as adherence to a drug or medical regimen). *Perceived susceptibility* was found to follow the same pattern as *benefits*, being a stronger predictor of preventive health behaviors (Janz & Becker, 1984), some of which are one-time or periodic actions, like having a vaccine (although the need for multiple vaccine doses for HPV and COVID-19 adds complexity) or screening test, rather than behaviors like smoking cessation or physical activity, that must be practiced daily. In some meta-analyses, *perceived severity* (Harrison et al., 1992; Janz & Becker 1984) and *perceived susceptibility* (Carpenter, 2010) have been the weakest behavioral predictors.

In the 1990s, some researchers (such as Lewis, 1994) suggested that susceptibility and severity should be combined additively or multiplicatively to create the overarching construct of perceived threat (threat = susceptibility + [susceptibility × severity]). Others suggested that low variance in perceived severity for some health conditions—such as the almost universal perception that lung cancer is very severe—empirically leads to small effect sizes (Harrison et al., 1992). No reviews have evaluated the contribution of cues to action due, in part, to the fact that few studies have explained whether or how cues were measured or used for interventions (Abraham & Sheeran, 2015). Finally, no systematic reviews have evaluated whether the addition of self-efficacy increases the HBM's predictive validity.

Measurement of HBM Constructs

One of the most important limitations in both observational and intervention research using the HBM has been variability in measurement of its central constructs (Carpenter, 2010; Harrison et al., 1992; Janz & Becker, 1984). If researchers do not measure people's HBM-related perceptions consistently, they will be unable to understand the extent to which those perceptions are related to health behaviors and whether interventions are effective in changing these perceptions.

Several important principles should thus be used to guide HBM measurement. First, construct definitions should be consistent with the HBM as originally conceptualized. Measures also should be specific to the behavior being addressed (e.g., barriers to mammography may be quite different from barriers to colonoscopy) and relevant to the population among whom they will be used (e.g., groups with lower versus higher health literacy may respond differently to certain measures). Further, to ensure content validity of each HBM construct, it is important to measure the full range of factors that may influence behaviors, especially where the constructs are inherently complex. For example, measuring a single barrier to a health behavior would be insufficient if a person perceived multiple barriers to a health behavior. Formative research can identify factors perceived as particular benefits, barriers, and susceptibility beliefs for particular health behaviors, among particular populations, and in particular settings. Once identified, these beliefs may be incorporated into scales that include multiple items for each construct (King et al., 2012; Rawl et al., 2000, 2001; Russell, et al., 2003; Vernon et al., 1997).

Applications of the Health Belief Model

In this section, we discuss how the HBM has been applied to research related to two very different health behaviors. First, we examine how perceived risk for diabetes has been measured, realizing that those who do not perceive they are at risk will see no reason to engage in risk-reducing behaviors. Next, we discuss how HBM constructs have been employed in studies of COVID-19 vaccinations.

HBM and Diabetes Risk

Type 2 diabetes is a chronic condition characterized by high blood sugar, occurring when the pancreas cannot effectively use the hormone insulin that regulates blood sugar levels. Resulting complications include hypoglycemia, kidney disease, nerve damage, poor circulation, heart disease, and vision problems. Globally, type 2 diabetes ranks among the top ten leading causes of death. Screening individuals at high risk for developing diabetes (including those who are overweight/obese and/or have a family history of the disease); detecting diabetes at an early stage; and connecting the newly diagnosed to treatment can reduce diabetes-related morbidity and mortality (Herman et al., 2015; US Preventive Services Task Force, 2021). However, many people at high risk for developing type 2 diabetes—and even many people who already have the condition—are unaware of their status. In the United States, more than 20% of individuals with diabetes remain undiagnosed (Centers for Disease Control and Prevention, 2022).

Multiple studies have used the HBM to examine beliefs and attitudes, such as perceived susceptibility, among *undiagnosed* individuals. These studies are important to determine if these perceptions influence individual decisions to participate in screening for diabetes and in risk-lowering lifestyle interventions, such as diet and physical activity programs (Esquives et al., 2021). For example, Dorman and colleagues sought to assess perceived susceptibility in individuals without a diagnosis of diabetes (Dorman et al., 2012). Researchers employed a single-item measure: "Compared to most people your age and sex, what would you say your chances are for developing diabetes?" among three groups with increasingly elevated risk: (1) no family history of diabetes risk factors (e.g., diabetes, coronary heart disease, and stroke); (2) family history of diabetes alone; and (3) family history of multiple risk factors. Perceived susceptibility varied among the three groups, and there was a stronger association with risk factors as they increased from none to diabetes alone, to multiple risk factors. However, most people within each group perceived themselves as being at or below "average risk." Therefore, despite differences in actual risk factors, most participants with elevated risk of developing diabetes due to familial history still perceived themselves at a risk level that, according to the HBM, would not induce behavior change.

In 2023, Serena Rodriguez and colleagues published a systematic review of studies assessing perceived susceptibility of developing diabetes among people without a diagnosis (Rodriguez et al., 2022). They found multiple ways in which the construct had been measured in different studies: (1) multi-item scales with composite scores; (2) multiple items with no composite score; and (3) a single item. An example of a multi-item scale includes the Perception of Risk Factors for Type 2 Diabetes (PRF-T2DM) scale that sums the score of six questions about personal and behavioral risk factors (e.g., "What is the effect of your exercise habits on your risk for type 2 diabetes?") and six questions about environmental risk factors (Sousa et al., 2010). In contrast, the Risk Perception Survey for Developing Diabetes (RPS-DD) is a multi-item measure that assesses different aspects of perceived susceptibility—internal and external control, worry, and optimistic bias—but does not create a composite score (Walker et al., 2003).

Even among studies using a single item to measure perceived susceptibility, Rodriguez et al. (2022) found a variety of ways to operationalize it. As noted above, Dorman et al. (2012) item asked a respondent to compare their own susceptibility to others using a Likert scale ranging from less to more likely (Ranby et al., 2010). Other researchers ask about absolute perceived susceptibility—perception of one's own risk without comparison (Ranby et al., 2010). Response options for these items often use numerical scales such as "on a scale from 0 to 100, how likely are you to develop diabetes at some point in your life?" Interpreting numerical responses to absolute perceived susceptibility questions can be challenging (Dillard et al., 2012).

Overall, variations in the operationalization of perceived susceptibility make it difficult to summarize the direction and magnitude of association across studies. Increasing use of reliable and validated scales such as the PRF-T2DM (Rodriguez et al., 2022), can help researchers synthesize findings across studies by helping to make researchers more confident in their measurement of constructs and to guide manipulations of perceived susceptibility to, in turn, influence health-promoting behaviors such as diabetes screening or treatment. Finally, high-quality measurement of perceived susceptibility can help enable researchers to determine whether interventions, such as lifestyle interventions to increase physical activity or change diet, are effective in changing behavior because they first influence this hypothesized intermediate variable.

HBM and COVID-19 Vaccination

With the onset of the COVID-19 pandemic in 2020, the HBM would have been a useful way for researchers to examine response to vaccination. In fact, there has been a general increase in the application of HBM constructs to various health behaviors since 2000 by researchers working in international settings. A Medline search of peer-reviewed articles from 2001 to 2021 with "Health Belief Model" as a search term identified more than 2,000 articles with over 600 published in a language other than English, an international journal, or conducted outside the United States. In addition, several studies have found significant associations between HBM constructs and vaccination for infectious diseases that have pandemic potential, including swine flu, H1N1, SARS, and MERS (Bish et al., 2011).

To better understand the application of HBM to COVID-19 vaccination, we conducted a systematic Medline search that identified 109 articles, published in English from January 2020 to December 2021, that applied the HBM to COVID-19 behaviors. Here, we focus on the 29 studies that measured COVID-19 vaccination or vaccination intentions. As described below, this approach allowed us to: (1) describe quality and completeness of measuring HBM constructs; (2) summarize patterns of association between HBM constructs and a COVID-19 vaccine outcome (either actual behavior or vaccination intention); and (3) describe whether constructs from other health behavior theories were integrated into the multivariate models examining correlations between these constructs and vaccination.

Most of the studies (21 of 29) were conducted in non-US settings during 2020 (before vaccines became available to the public) and measured the five main HBM constructs: susceptibility, severity, benefits, barriers, and cues to action. Self-efficacy was rarely measured (Table 5.1). Studies found strong, consistent support for perceived benefits being positively associated and perceived barriers negatively associated with vaccination intentions. For perceived susceptibility, severity, and cues to action, findings were mixed; some showed statistically significant positive associations and others found no association (Table 5.1). Measurement of cues to action varied greatly across studies. Some only defined cues as recommendations from healthcare providers, the government, and family/friends, whereas others acknowledged that reminders in one's environment could include personal or family experiences of COVID-19 disease and exposure to information via various media channels or public education campaigns. Such variability in operational definitions for HBM constructs continues to weaken our ability to draw conclusions of what might be driving differences in findings.

A few of these recent studies employing the HBM found that susceptibility and severity may conceptually combine to denote an individual's perceived threat, but only one study (Zampetakis & Melas, 2021) sought to test this through a factorial survey experiment; this approach highlighted interactions between HBM constructs, associating an interaction between high perceived susceptibility and severity with positive intentions to be vaccinated. The lack of significant main effects more generally may suggest that susceptibility and severity are more distal predictors of vaccination

Table 5.1 Summary of Patterns of Association for Health Belief Model Constructs and COVID-19 Vaccine Intentions or Uptake[a]

HBM Construct	N Studies	Associations: N Studies	Studies
Perceived Susceptibility/Risk	22	Positive: 12 Negative: 0 No significant association: 9 Mixed: 1 Not measured: 1	Positive: Ahmed et al. (2021), Banik et al. (2021), Chen et al. (2021), Guillon and Kergall (2021), Hossain et al. (2021), Lopez-Cepero et al. (2021), Tao et al. (2021), Toth-Manikowski et al. (2022), Tsutsui et al. (2021), Wijesinghe et al. (2021), Wong et al. (2020), Zampetakis and Melas (2021) No significant association: Al-Metwali et al. (2021), Berg and Lin (2021), Chu and Liu (2021), Jiang et al. (2021), Mir et al. (2021), Shmueli (2021), Wong et al. (2020), Yu et al. (2021) Mixed: Lin et al. (2020) Not measured: Al-Hasan et al. (2021)
Perceived Severity	21	Positive: 11 Negative: 0 No significant association: 9 Mixed: 1 Not measured: 2	Positive: Al-Hasan et al. (2021), Hossain et al. (2021), Lopez-Cepero et al. (2021), Shmueli (2021), Toth-Manikowski et al. (2022), Tsutsui et al. (2021), Wong et al. (2020), Wong et al. (2021), Ye et al. (2021), Yu et al. (2021), Zampetakis and Melas (2021) No significant association: Ahmed et al. (2021), Al-Metwali et al. (2021), Banik et al. (2021), Berg and Lin (2021), Chen et al. (2021), Chu and Liu (2021), Jiang et al. (2021), Tao et al. (2021), Wijesinghe et al. (2021) Mixed: Lin et al. (2020) Not measured: Guillon and Kergall (2021), Mir et al. (2021)
Perceived Benefits	22	Positive: 21 Negative: 0 No significant association: 1 Mixed: 0 Not measured: 1	Positive: Ahmed et al. (2021), Al-Hasan et al. (2021), Al-Metwali et al. (2021), Banik et al. (2021), Chen et al. (2021), Chu and Liu (2021), Guillon and Kergall (2021), Hossain et al. (2021), Jiang et al. (2021), Lin et al. (2020), Lopez-Cepero et al. (2021), Mir et al. (2021), Shmueli (2021), Tao et al. (2021), Toth-Manikowski et al. (2022), Wijesinghe et al. (2021), Wong et al. (2020, 2021), Ye et al. (2021), Yu et al. (2021), Zampetakis and Melas (2021) No significant association: Berg and Lin (2021) Not measured: Tsutsui et al. (2021)
Perceived Barriers	20	Positive: 0 Negative: 18 No significant association: 2 Mixed: 0 Not measured: 3	Positive: Ahmed et al. (2021), Al-Hasan et al. (2021), Al-Metwali et al. (2021), Banik et al. (2021), Berg and Lin (2021), Chen et al. (2021), Chu and Liu (2021), Guillon and Kergall (2021), Hossain et al. (2021), Jiang et al. (2021), Lin et al. (2020), Lopez-Cepero et al. (2021), Tao et al. (2021), Toth-Manikowski et al. (2022), Wong et al. (2020), Wong et al. (2021), Ye et al. (2021), Zampetakis and Melas (2021) No significant association: Shmueli (2021), Yu et al. (2021) Not measured: Mir et al. (2021), Tsutsui et al. (2021), Wijesinghe et al. (2021)
Cues to Action	17	Positive: 12 Negative: 0 No significant association: 4 Mixed: 1 Not measured: 6	Positive: Al-Hasan et al. (2021), Al-Metwali et al. (2021), Chen et al. (2021), Jiang et al. (2021), Lin et al. (2020), Lopez-Cepero et al. (2021), Shmueli (2021), Tao et al. (2021), Toth-Manikowski et al. (2022), Wong et al. (2020, 2021), Yu et al. (2021) No significant association: Banik et al. (2021), Berg and Lin (2021), Guillon and Kergall (2021), Hossain et al. (2021) Mixed: Ahmed et al. (2021) Not measured: Chu and Liu (2021), Mir et al. (2021), Tsutsui et al. (2021), Wijesinghe et al. (2021), Ye et al. (2021), Zampetakis and Melas (2021)
Self-Efficacy	3	Positive: 2 Negative: 0 No significant association: 1 Mixed: 0 Not measured: 20	Positive: Chen et al. (2021), Yu et al. (2021) No significant association: Chu and Liu (2021) Not measured: Ahmed et al. (2021), Al-Hasan et al. (2021), Al-Metwali et al. (2021), Banik et al. (2021), Berg and Lin (2021), Guillon and Kergall (2021), Hossain et al. (2021), Jiang et al. (2021), Lopez-Cepero et al. (2021), Mir et al. (2021), Tao et al. (2021), Toth-Manikowski et al. (2022), Tsutsui et al. (2021), Wijesinghe et al. (2021), Ye et al. (2021)

[a] Review of the full text from the 29 articles revealed reasons to exclude: two studies used nontraditional measures of HBM constructs (Kalam et al. 2021; Mercadante & Law, 2021), two studies did not quantitatively examine associations between HBM constructs and the target health behavior: vaccination or vaccination intention (Marquez et al., 2021; Williams et al. 2021), one study analyzed qualitative interviews (Walker et al., 2021), and one study had difficult-to-interpret multivariate models (Cerda & Garcia, 2021). As a result of these exclusions, the table summarizes patterns of associations for measured HBM constructs for the remaining 23 studies.

Some studies included each survey item measuring the particular HBM construct in the multivariate model instead of an aggregate scale score. Thus, it was possible for a construct to have a positive, negative, and no association when looking across the set of survey items.

acceptance (Brewer et al., 2017; Carpenter, 2010). Almost all the studies in our narrative review were cross-sectional, which precludes discussion of how health beliefs, vaccination intentions, and vaccination behaviors evolved as information and misinformation about COVID-19 and the vaccines were disseminated. Longitudinal studies and experiments are critical to better understand mechanisms of influence among the HBM constructs, intention, and actual behavior.

Twelve studies integrated constructs from another theory along with the HBM, with Theory of Planned Behavior (TPB, Chapter 6) being the predominant addition. Studies that examined both HBM and TPB constructs did not address the conceptual overlap between perceived benefits and barriers and attitude towards the behavior, nor did they consider overlap of cues to action and subjective norms. More rigorous conceptualization and competitive testing of these two theories may be helpful in understanding their unique or overlapping contributions to understanding behavior. In addition, future work might include studies, not considered in our review, that examined HBM constructs, such as perceived susceptibility, but did not specify that this construct came from the HBM (Viswanath et al., 2021).

Discussion and Summary

In this chapter, we described origins of the HBM, reviewed and defined its key components and hypothesized relationships, summarized critical reviews, and provided examples of applications—most recently in the study of COVID-19-related behaviors. The model, which has been used for more than 60 years to predict health-related behaviors and inform development of behavior-change interventions, is still being used in health behavior research today. The model's intuitive concepts have made its modifiable beliefs popular for designing interventions (e.g., messages to strengthen perception of benefits and weaken perceived barriers). As the chapter describes, this approach has been exceptionally popular in global studies.

However, we still know relatively little about relationships among HBM constructs, such as whether they all directly predict behavior or whether some beliefs have indirect effects or mediate relationships to behaviors. Notable exceptions are studies by Gerend and Shepherd (2012), comparing the value of HBM and the TPB in predicting HPV vaccine uptake, and Murphy et al. (2013), comparing the value of HBM and Theory of Reasoned Action in evaluating mammography behavior. In addition, few researchers have investigated factors that moderate HBM constructs' effects on behaviors (Li et al. 2003). Another persistent limitation is that the way HBM constructs are measured and addressed varies widely. However, as shown during the COVID-19 pandemic, the HBM is alive and well—informing assessment of health beliefs and interventions to change those perceptions and, ultimately, behaviors. As with all models, a good measurement of the constructs and effective intervention components addressing them will continue to be important as we use the HBM to influence behavior change.

References

Abraham, C., & Sheeran, P. (2015). The health belief model. In M. Conner & P. Norman (Eds.), *Predicting health behaviour: Research and practice with social cognition models* (3rd ed., pp. 30–69). Maidenhead: Open University Press.

Ahmed, T. F., Ahmed, A., Ahmed, S., & Ahmed, H. U. (2021). Understanding COVID-19 vaccine acceptance in Pakistan: An echo of previous immunizations or prospect of change? *Expert Review of Vaccines, 20*(9), 1185–1193.

Al-Hasan, A., Khuntia, J., & Yim, D. (2021). Does seeing what others do through social media influence vaccine uptake and help in the herd immunity through vaccination? A cross-sectional analysis. *Frontiers in Public Health, 9*, 715931.

Al-Metwali, B. Z., Al-Jumaili, A. A., Al-Alag, Z. A., & Sorofman, B. (2021). Exploring the acceptance of COVID-19 vaccine among healthcare workers and general population using health belief model. *Journal of Evaluation in Clinical Practice, 27*(5), 1112–1122.

Bandura, A. (1997). *Self-efficacy: The exercise of control.* New York: Freeman.

Bandura, A. (1999). *Social learning theory.* Engelwood Cliffs, NJ: Prentice Hall.

Bandura, A. (2005). The primacy of self-regulation in health promotion. *Applied Psychology. An International Review, 54*(2), 245–254.

Banik, R., Islam, M. S., Pranta, M. U. R., Rahman, Q. M., Rahman, M., Pardhan, S., Driscoll, R., Hossain, S., & Sikder, M. T. (2021). Understanding the determinants of COVID-19 vaccination intention and willingness to pay: findings from a population-based survey in Bangladesh. *BMC Infectious Diseases, 21*(1), 892.

Becker, M. H. (1974). The health belief model and sick role behavior. *Health Education Monographs, 2*, 409–419.

Becker, M. H., & Maiman, L. A. (1975). Sociobehavioral determinants of compliance with health and medical care recommendations. *Medical Care, 13*(1), 10–24.

Berg, M. B., & Lin, L. (2021). Predictors of COVID-19 vaccine intentions in the United States: The role of psychosocial health constructs and demographic factors. *Translational Behavioral Medicine, 11*(9), 1782–1788.

Bish, A., Yardley, L., Nicoll, A., & Michie, S. (2011). Factors associated with uptake of vaccination against pandemic influenza: A systematic review. *Vaccine, 29*(38), 6472–6484.

Brewer, N. T., Chapman, G. B., Rothman, A. J., Leask, J., & Kempe, A. (2017). Increasing vaccination: Putting psychological science into action. *Psychological Science in the Public Interest, 18*(3), 149–207.

Carpenter, C. J. (2010). A meta-analysis of the effectiveness of health belief model variables in predicting behavior. *Health Communication, 25*(8), 661–669.

Centers for Disease Control and Prevention. (2022). *Prevalence of both diagnosed and undiagnosed diabetes.* U.S. Department of Health and Human Services. https://www.cdc.gov/diabetes/data/statistics-report/diagnosed-undiagnosed-diabetes.html

Cerda, A. A., & Garcia, L. Y. (2021). Hesitation and refusal factors in individuals' decision-making processes regarding a coronavirus disease 2019 vaccination. *Frontiers in Public Health, 9*, 626852.

Chen, H., Li, X., Gao, J., Liu, X., Mao, Y., Wang, R., Zheng, P., Xiao, Q., Jia, Y., Fu, H., & Dai, J. (2021). Health Belief Model perspective on the control of COVID-19 vaccine hesitancy and the promotion of vaccination in China: Web-based cross-sectional study. *Journal of Medical Internet Research, 23*(9), e29329.

Chu, H., & Liu, S. (2021). Integrating health behavior theories to predict American's intention to receive a COVID-19 vaccine. *Patient Education and Counseling, 104*(8), 1878–1886.

Dillard, A. J., Ferrer, R. A., Ubel, P. A., & Fagerlin, A. (2012). Risk perception measures' associations with behavior intentions, affect, and cognition following colon cancer screening messages. *Health Psychology, 31*(1), 106–113.

Dorman, J. S., Valdez, R., Liu, T., Wang, C., Rubinstein, W. S., O'Neill, S. M., Acheson, L. S., Ruffin, M. T., & Khoury, M. J. (2012). Health beliefs among individuals at increased familial risk for type 2 diabetes: Implications for prevention. *Diabetes Research and Clinical Practice, 96*(2), 156–162.

Esquives, B. N., Ramos, K. Q., Stoutenberg, M. (2021). Exploring strategies to engage Hispanic patients in screening for a diabetes prevention program at a local community health center. *Journal of Health Care for the Poor and Underserved, 32*(1), 487–505.

Gerend, M. A., & Shepherd, J. E. (2012). Predicting human papillomavirus vaccine uptake in young adult women: Comparing the health belief model and theory of planned behavior. *Annals of Behavioral Medicine, 44*(2), 171–180.

Guillon, M., & Kergall, P. (2021). Factors associated with COVID-19 vaccination intentions and attitudes in France. *Public Health, 198*, 200–207.

Harrison, J. A., Mullen, P. D., & Green, L. W. (1992). A meta-analysis of studies of the health belief model with adults. *Health Education Research, 7*(1), 107–116.

Herman, W. H., Ye, W., Griffin, S. J., Simmons, R. K., Davies, M. J., Khunti, K., Rutten, G. E. H. M., Sandbaek, A., Lauritzen, T., Borch-Johnsen, K., Brown, M.B., & Wareham, N. J. (2015). Early detection and treatment of type 2 diabetes reduce cardiovascular morbidity and mortality: A simulation of the results of the Anglo-Danish-Dutch Study of Intensive Treatment in People With Screen-Detected Diabetes in Primary Care (ADDITION-Europe). *Diabetes Care, 38*(8), 17449–55.

Hochbaum, G. M. (1958). *Public participation in medical screening programs: A socio-psychological study*: US Department of Health, Education, and Welfare (No. 572). US Department of Health, Education, and Welfare. Public Health Service, Bureau of State Services, Division of Special Health Services, Tuberculosis Program.

Hossain, M. B., Alam, M. Z., Islam, M. S., Sultan, S., Faysal, M. M., Rima, S., Hossain, M.A., & Mamun, A. A. (2021). Health Belief Model, Theory of Planned Behavior, or psychological antecedents: What predicts COVID-19 vaccine hesitancy better among the Bangladeshi adults? *Frontiers in Public Health, 9*, 711066.

Janz, N. K., & Becker, M. H. (1984). The health belief model: A decade later. *Health Education Quarterly, 11*(1), 1–47.

Jiang, T., Zhou, X., Wang, H., Dong, S., Wang, M., Akezhuoli, H., & Zhu, H. (2021). COVID-19 vaccination intention and influencing factors among different occupational risk groups: A cross-sectional study. *Human Vaccines & Immunotherapeutics, 17*(10), 3433–3440.

Jones, C. J., Smith, H., & Llewellyn, C. (2014). Evaluating the effectiveness of health belief model interventions in improving adherence: A systematic review. *Health Psychology Review, 8*(3), 253–269.

Kalam, M. A., Davis, T. P., Jr., Shano, S., Uddin, M. N., Islam, M. A., Kanwagi, R., Islam, A., Hassan, M. M., & Larson, H. J. (2021). Exploring the behavioral determinants of COVID-19 vaccine acceptance among an urban population in Bangladesh: Implications for behavior change interventions. *PLoS One, 16*(8), e0256496.

King, R. B., Champion, V. L., Chen, D., Gittler, M. S., Heinemann, A. W., Bode, R. K., & Semik, P. (2012). Development of a measure of skin care belief scales for persons with spinal cord injury. *Archives of Physical Medicine and Rehabilitation*, *93*(10), 1814–1821.

Kirscht, J. P. (1974). The health belief model and illness behavior. *Health Education Monographs*, *2*(4), 387–408.

Lewin, K. (1951). The nature of field theory. In M. H. Marx (Ed.), *Psychological theory: Contemporary readings*. New York: Macmillan.

Lewin, K., Dembo, T., Festinger, L., & Sears, P. S. (1944). Level of aspiration. In J. Hunt (Ed.), *Personality and the behavior disorders* (pp. 333–378). Somerset, NJ: Ronald Press.

Lewis, K. S. (1994). An examination of the health belief model when applied to diabetes mellitus. [Unpublished doctoral dissertation]. University of Sheffield.

Li, C., Unger, J. B., Schuster, D., Rohrbach, L. A., Howard-Pitney, B., & Norman, G. (2003). Youths' exposure to environmental tobacco smoke (ETS): Associations with health beliefs and social pressure. *Addictive Behaviors*, *28*(1), 39–53.

Lin, Y., Hu, Z., Zhao, Q., Alias, H., Danaee, M., & Wong, L. P. (2020). Understanding COVID-19 vaccine demand and hesitancy: A nationwide online survey in China. *PLoS Neglected Tropical Diseases*, *14*(12), e0008961.

Lopez-Cepero, A., Cameron, S., Negron, L. E., Colon-Lopez, V., Colon-Ramos, U., Mattei, J., Fernández-Repollet, E., & Perez, C. M. (2021). Uncertainty and unwillingness to receive a COVID-19 vaccine in adults residing in Puerto Rico: Assessment of perceptions, attitudes, and behaviors. *Human Vaccines & Immunotherapeutics*, *17*(10), 3441–3449.

Mahoney, C. A., Thombs, D. L., & Ford, O. J. (1995). Health belief and self efficacy models: Their utility in explaining college student condom use. *AIDS Education and Prevention*, *7*, 32–49.

Marquez, R. R., Gosnell, E. S., Thikkurissy, S., Schwartz, S. B., & Cully, J. L. (2021). Caregiver acceptance of an anticipated COVID-19 vaccination. *Journal of the American Dental Association*, *152*(9), 730–739.

Mathieu, E., Ritchie, H., Rodés-Guirao, L., Appel, C., Gavrilov, D., Giattino, C., Hasell, J., Macdonald, B., Dattani, S., Beltekian, D., Ortiz-Ospina, E., & Roser, M. (2022). Coronavirus Pandemic (COVID-19). https:/ourworldindata.org/coronavirus

Mercadante, A. R., & Law, A. V. (2021). Will they, or won't they? Examining patients' vaccine intention for flu and COVID-19 using the Health Belief Model. *Research in Social and Administrative Pharmacy*, *17*(9), 1596–1605.

Mir, H. H., Parveen, S., Mullick, N. H., & Nabi, S. (2021). Using structural equation modeling to predict Indian people's attitudes and intentions towards COVID-19 vaccination. *Diabetes & Metabolic Syndrome*, *15*(3), 1017–1022.

Murphy, C. C., Vernon, S. W., Diamond, P. M., & Tiro, J. A. (2013). Competitive testing of health behavior theories: How do benefits, barriers, subjective norm, and intention influence mammography behavior? *Annals of Behavioral Medicine*, *47*(1), 120–129.

Pingali, C., Yankey, D., Elam-Evans, L. D., Markowitz, L. E., Williams, C. L., Fredua, B., McNamara, L. E., Stokley, S., & Singleton, J. A. (2021). National, regional, state, and selected local area vaccination coverage among adolescents aged 13-17 years - United States, 2020. *MMWR. Morbidity and Mortality Weekly Report*, *70*(35), 1183–1190.

Ranby, K. W., Aiken, L. S., Gerend, M. A., & Erchull, M. J. (2010). Perceived susceptibility measures are not interchangeable: Absolute, direct comparative, and indirect comparative risk. *Health Psychology*, *29*(1), 20–28.

Rawl, S., Champion, V., Menon, U., Loehrer, P. J., Vance, G. H., & Skinner, C. S. (2001). Validation of scales to measure benefits of and barriers to colorectal cancer screening. *Journal of Psychosocial Oncology*, *19*(3-4), 47–63.

Rawl, S. M., Menon, U., Champion, V. L., Foster, J. L., & Skinner, C. S. (2000). Colorectal cancer screening beliefs. Focus groups with first-degree relatives. *Cancer Practice*, *8*(1), 32–37.

Rodriguez, S. A., Tiro, J. A., Baldwin, A. S., Hamilton-Bevil, H., & Bowen, M. (2022). Measurement of perceived risk of developing diabetes mellitus: A systematic literature review. (2023). *Journal of General Internal Medicine*, *38*, 1928–1954.

Rosenstock, I. M. (1960). What research in motivation suggests for public health. *American Journal of Public Health and the Nations Health*, *50*, 295–302.

Rosenstock, I. M. (1974). Historical origins of the health belief model. *Health Education Monographs*, *2*, 1–8.

Rosenstock, I. M., Strecher, V. J., & Becker, M. H. (1988). Social learning theory and the health belief model. *Health Education Quarterly*, *15*(2), 175–183.

Russell, K. M., Champion, V. L., & Perkins, S. M. (2003). Development of cultural belief scales for mammography screening. *Oncology Nursing Forum*, *30*(4), 633–640.

Salloway, J. C., Pletcher, W. R., & Collins, J. J. (1978). Sociological and social-psychological models of compliance with prescribed regimen: In search of synthesis. *Sociological Symposium*, 23, 100–121.

Shmueli, L. (2021). Predicting intention to receive COVID-19 vaccine among the general population using the health belief model and the theory of planned behavior model. *BMC Public Health*, *21*(1), 804.

Skinner, B. F. (1938). *The behavior of organisms*. Engelwood Cliffs, NJ: Appleton-Century-Crofts.

Sousa, V. D., Ryan-Wenger, N. A., Driessnack, M., & Jaber, A. A. F. (2010). Factorial structure of the perception of risk factors for type 2 diabetes scale: Exploratory and confirmatory factor analyses. *Journal of Evaluation in Clinical Practice, 16*(6), 1096–1102.

Strecher, V. J., Champion, V. L., & Rosenstock, I. M. (1997). The health belief model and health behavior. In D. S. Goschman (Ed.), *Handbook of Health Behavior Research* (vol. 1, pp. 71–91). New York: Plenum Press.

Tao, L., Wang, R., Han, N., Liu, J., Yuan, C., Deng, L., Han, C., Sun, F., Lius, M., & Liu, J. (2021). Acceptance of a COVID-19 vaccine and associated factors among pregnant women in China: A multi-center cross-sectional study based on health belief model. *Human Vaccines & Immunotherapeutics, 17*(8), 2378–2388.

Thaler, R. H., & Sunstein, C. R. (2009). *Nudge: Improving decisions about health, wealth, and happiness*. New York: Penguin Books.

Tiro, J. A., Diamond, P. M., Perz, C. A., Fernandez, M., Rakowski, W., DiClemente, C. C., & Vernon, S. W. (2005). Validation of scales measuring attitudes and norms related to mammography screening in women veterans. *Health Psychology, 24*(6), 555.

Toth-Manikowski, S. M., Swirsky, E. S., Gandhi, R., & Piscitello, G. (2022). COVID-19 vaccination hesitancy among health care workers, communication, and policy-making. *American Journal of Infection Control, 50*(1), 20–25.

Tsutsui, Y., Shahrabani, S., Yamamura, E., Hayashi, R., Kohsaka, Y., & Ohtake, F. (2021). The willingness to pay for a hypothetical vaccine for the coronavirus disease 2019 (COVID-19). *International Journal of Environmental Research & Public Health, 18*(23), 26.

U.S. Preventive Services Task Force. (2021). Prediabetes and type 2 diabetes: Screening. https://www.uspreventiveservicestaskforce.org/uspstf/recommendation/screening-for-prediabetes-and-type-2-diabetes

Vernon, S. W., Myers, R. E., & Tilley, B. C. (1997). Development and validation of an instrument to measure factors related to colorectal cancer screening adherence. *Cancer Epidemiology, Biomarkers & Prevention, 6*(10), 825–832.

Viswanath, K., Bekalu, M., Dhawan, D., Pinnamaneni, R., Lang, J., McCloud, R. (2021). Individual and social determinants of COVID-19 vaccine uptake. *BMC Public Health, 21*(1), 818.

Walker, E. A., Mertz, C. K., Kalten, M. R., & Flynn, J. (2003). Risk perception for developing diabetes: Comparative risk judgments of physicians. *Diabetes Care, 26*(9), 2543–2548.

Walker, K. K., Head, K. J., Owens, H., & Zimet, G. D. (2021). A qualitative study exploring the relationship between mothers' vaccine hesitancy and health beliefs with COVID-19 vaccination intention and prevention during the early pandemic months. *Human Vaccines & Immunotherapeutics, 17*(10), 3355–3364.

Watson, J. B. (1925). *Behaviorism*. New York: Norton.

Weinstein, N. D. (1988). The precaution adoption process. *Health Psychology, 7*(4), 355–386.

Wijesinghe, M. S. D., Weerasinghe, W., Gunawardana, I., Perera, S. N. S., & Karunapema, R. P. P. (2021). Acceptance of COVID-19 vaccine in Sri Lanka: Applying the health belief model to an online survey. *Asia-Pacific Journal of Public Health, 33*(5), 598–602.

Williams, L. B., Fernander, A. F., Azam, T., Gomez, M. L., Kang, J., Moody, C. L., Bowman, H., & Schoenberg, N. E. (2021). COVID-19 and the impact on rural and black church congregants: Results of the C-M-C project. *Research in Nursing & Health, 44*(5), 767–775.

Wong, L. P., Alias, H., Wong, P. F., Lee, H. Y., & AbuBakar, S. (2020). The use of the health belief model to assess predictors of intent to receive the COVID-19 vaccine and willingness to pay. *Human Vaccines & Immunotherapeutics, 16*(9), 2204–2214.

Wong, M. C. S., Wong, E. L. Y., Huang, J., Cheung, A. W. L., Law, K., Chong, M. K. C., Chan, P. K. S. (2021). Acceptance of the COVID-19 vaccine based on the health belief model: A population-based survey in Hong Kong. *Vaccine, 39*(7), 1148–1156.

Ye, W., Li, Q., & Yu, S. (2021). Persuasive effects of message framing and narrative format on promoting COVID-19 vaccination: A study on Chinese college students. *International Journal of Environmental Research & Public Health, 18*(18), 08.

Yu, Y., Lau, J. T. F., She, R., Chen, X., Li, L., Li, L., & Chen, X. (2021). Prevalence and associated factors of intention of COVID-19 vaccination among healthcare workers in China: Application of the health belief model. *Human Vaccines & Immunotherapeutics, 17*(9), 2894–2902.

Zampetakis, L. A., & Melas, C. (2021). The health belief model predicts vaccination intentions against COVID-19: A survey experiment approach. *Applied Psychology. Health and Well-Being, 13*(2), 469–484.

Zimmerman, R. S., & Vernberg, D. (1994). Models of preventive health behavior: Comparison, critique, and meta-analysis. *Advances in Medical Sociology, 4*, 45–67.

CHAPTER 6

THEORY OF REASONED ACTION, THEORY OF PLANNED BEHAVIOR, INTEGRATIVE BEHAVIORAL MODEL, AND REASONED ACTION APPROACH

Amy Bleakley
Shawnika Hull

KEY POINTS

This chapter will:

- Describe assumptions and main constructs of Theory of Reasoned Action (TRA), Theory of Planned Behavior (TPB), Integrative Model of Behavioral Prediction (IM), and Reasoned Action Approach (RAA).

- Explain research methods, measurements, and analyses used with these reasoned action theories.

- Demonstrate how reasoned action theories were used to (1) understand intention to use pre-exposure for prophylaxis (PrEP) to prevent HIV infections; and (2) identify salient constructs and beliefs for message design regarding enrollment in a brain health registry for Alzheimer's-related research.

- Present commonly cited critiques of the reasoned action theories and future directions.

Vignette

> The last five years of her life, she probably did not know who I was. It's . . . I got emotional about it. Because just about everyone in my mother's family has experienced dementia and Alzheimer's.
>
> —Kay's story (National Institute on Aging, 2019)

Alzheimer's disease (AD) is a family disease not because of its hereditary component but due to the emotional and other challenges families face watching a loved one's cognitive decline. Having a family history of AD is one reason people may participate in AD research. Unfortunately, there are not nearly enough volunteers, especially from historically underrepresented groups who are at higher risk of developing AD. For example, Black adults are twice as likely to have AD compared to their non-Hispanic white counterparts; Hispanic adults are 1.5 times as likely. Research to develop improved prevention, treatment, and care for AD is advancing, but it could be accelerated by having more diverse study participants. Diversifying prevention and clinical trial participation in medical research is a priority, with both scientific and ethical justification. Efforts to recruit participants should be based on an understanding of different beliefs and motivations that can inform recruitment efforts and promote enrollment. Researchers and practitioners can use health behavior theories for that purpose. They offer a framework to identify individual-level determinants specific to specific groups—such as specific racial or ethnic groups, genders, or political identifications—that may predict and explain participation. More importantly, they provide a structure to identify salient group-specific modifiable beliefs that can be used to design effective messaging about participating in AD research and build an evidence base to advance the science of recruitment. The theories described in this chapter—Theory of Reasoned Action (TRA), Theory of Planned Behavior (TPB), Integrative Model of Behavioral Prediction (IM), and Reasoned Action Approach (RAA)—offer frameworks that can help understand and address challenges like this.

Health Behavior: Theory, Research, and Practice, Sixth Edition. Edited by Karen Glanz, Barbara K. Rimer, and K. Viswanath.
© 2024 John Wiley & Sons, Inc. Published 2024 by John Wiley & Sons, Inc.
Companion website: www.wiley.com/go/glanz/healthbehavior6e

Introduction and History

One measure of a theory's contribution is the degree to which subsequent theorizing and research are informed by its key constructs and applications. By that standard, Theory of Reasoned Action (Fishbein & Ajzen,1975), Theory of Planned Behavior (Ajzen, 1985, 1991), Integrative Model of Behavioral Prediction (Fishbein, 2000), and the most recent iteration, and Reasoned Action Approach (Fishbein & Ajzen, 2010) are some of the most influential psychosocial theories of individual behavioral prediction and explanation. Since the TRA was first introduced almost 50 years ago, the theoretical approach continued to evolve and expand into TPB, Integrative Model of Behavioral Prediction (IM), and, finally, Reasoned Action Approach (RAA). As articulated by Marco Yzer, "The different formulations build on one another in a developmental fashion and reflect improvements—in conceptualization and measurement of the theory's key constructs for the purpose of improving the precision with which behavior can be explained" (Yzer, 2017, p. 2). The popularity of these *reasoned action theories* is tied to their theoretical robustness, parsimonious conceptualization of the factors that contribute to behavior, meticulous attention to measuring those constructs, and utility for guiding intervention development and evaluation. *The main proposition in all formulations is that intention is the best predictor of one's behavior, and that intentions are formed by some combination of attitudes, norms, and control or efficacy.* We define these constructs in more detail below, but first offer a brief history of the evolution of this framework. At times, we refer to "reasoned action framework" or "the framework" to represent the set of these theories which share common propositions and constructs (Figure 6.1).

Evolution of Reasoned Action Theories from TRA to RAA

Figure 6.1 shows a graphical depiction of the TRA and TPB—and Table 6.1 highlights the differences in the four versions since the inception of TRA. The TRA was formulated to address the weakness of general attitudes in the prediction of behavior. In TRA, the most powerful predictor of behavior is intention to perform a behavior. Intentions are a function of attitudes and social norms regarding the behavior. Generally, attitudes are a disposition or tendency to evaluate a psychological object, such as a behavior, as favorable or unfavorable. Social norms, however, refer to the acceptability of a behavior by a group (or society in general). In TRA, social norms are referred to as subjective norms. These subjective norms are injunctive, which are perceptions concerning whether important people in an individual's life think they should or should not perform the behavior (approval). TPB was developed to extend the utility of TRA, with addition of the perceived behavioral control (PBC) construct to account for agency, or the capacity to influence one's own thoughts and behaviors. In TPB, PBC was added as a distinct predictor of intention that can exert a direct

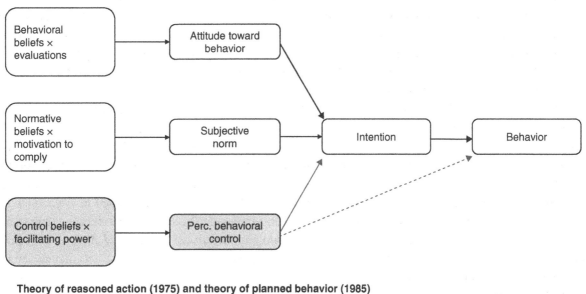

Theory of reasoned action (1975) and theory of planned behavior (1985)

Shaded areas/constructs and paths were added to TPB

Figure 6.1 Visual Depictions of TRA and TPB

Table 6.1   Constructs and Pathways for TRA, TPB, IM, and RAA

Theory	Predictors of Direct Determinants	Predictors of Intention	Predictors of Behavior
Theory of Reasoned Action			
	Behavioral beliefs × Evaluation →	Attitude →	Intention
	Normative beliefs × Motivation to comply →	Subjective norm →	
Theory of Planned Behavior			
	Behavioral beliefs × Evaluation →	Attitude →	Intention
	Normative beliefs × Motivation to comply →	Subjective norm →	**PBC**
	Control beliefs × facilitating power →	**Perceived Behavioral Control →**	
Integrative Model of Behavioral Prediction			
	Behavioral beliefs × Evaluation →	Attitude →	Intention
	Normative beliefs × Motivation to comply →	Normative Pressure (Injunctive and Descriptive) →	**Skills, Abilities**[a]
	Efficacy beliefs →	**Self-efficacy →**	**Environmental constraints**[a]
Reasoned Action Approach			
	Behavioral beliefs × Evaluation →	Attitude (Instrumental and Experiential) →	Intention
	Normative beliefs × Motivation to comply →	Normative Pressure (Injunctive and Descriptive) →	**Actual control**[a]
	Control beliefs × facilitating? Power →	Perceived Behavioral Control (**Autonomy and Capacity**) →	

[a] Moderators of the intention-behavior relationship.

influence on behavior as well, unlike attitudes and perceived norms which are thought to operate through their effects on intention.

Other behavioral theories commonly used in the context of public health and public health communication when TPB was developed had considerable overlap. These theories, including Health Belief Model (Janz & Becker, 1984) (Chapter 5), Social Cognitive Theory (Bandura, 1986) (Chapter 9), and Theory of Subjective Culture and Interpersonal Relations (Triandis, 1977), share assumptions of reasoned action and also focus on outcome expectations, norms and efficacy. To examine this overlap, the National Institutes of Mental Health convened a small group of prominent behavioral theorists in 1991, including Drs. Martin Fishbein, Albert Bandura, Marshall Becker, Harry Triandis, and Frederick Kanfer, for a workshop to reach consensus around which variables are the most important determinants of behavior. Though the workshop did not result in consensus, there was general agreement on eight propositions relevant to the process of behavior change involving assertions about the importance of (1) positive behavioral intentions, (2) prohibitive environmental constraints, (3) requisite skills and abilities, (4) positive attitudes toward the behavior, (5) supportive social norms, (6) perceived self-efficacy to perform the behavior, (7) consistency with one's self-image, and (8) positive emotional reactions to behavioral performance (Fishbein et al., 2001). Fishbein further refined these propositions when he introduced Integrative Model of Behavioral Change and Prediction, or IM (Fishbein, 2000), also referred to as the *Integrated* Behavioral Model (Montano & Kasprzyk, 2015) or the *Integrative* Model of Behavioral Prediction (IM).

IM was a step forward in the reasoned action lineage, as it began to account more comprehensively for the complex ways perceptions of social pressure shape intention formation by including a descriptive normative component (Cialdini et al., 1990; Fishbein, 2000). In IM, descriptive norms are incorporated into the normative pressure construct along with injunctive norms. The IM also reconfigures the constructs introduced earlier, such that consistency with self-image and emotions are considered outcome expectations and background factors, respectively. Finally, IM includes self-efficacy rather than PBC.

In 2010, Fishbein and Ajzen published *Predicting and Changing Behavior: A Reasoned Action Approach*, which presents the latest iteration in this set of theories—RAA (Figure 6.2). The most significant distinction between RAA and previous versions is its emphasis on the dual aspects of attitudes, norms, and control. Attitudes are conceptualized as experiential and instrumental. Normative pressure, as in IM, includes an injunctive and descriptive component. And the PBC construct, which is treated synonymously with self-efficacy, is based on autonomy and capacity. RAA also diverges from IM by conceptualizing skills and environmental constraints as a single construct: *actual control*. Actual

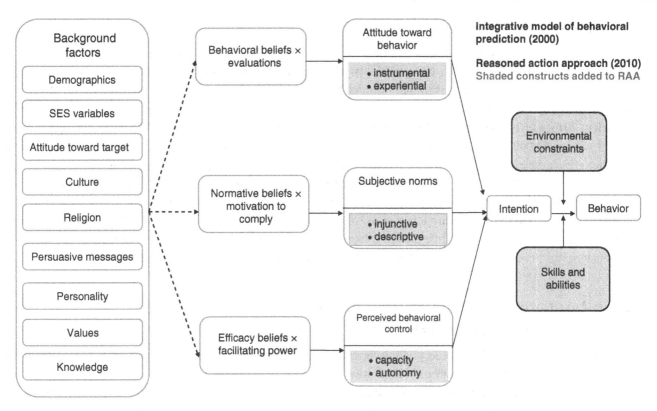

Figure 6.2 Visual Depictions of IM and RAA

control over a behavior is proposed to moderate the intention-behavior relationship and shapes perceptions of behavioral control. As in earlier models, perceptions of behavioral control moderate the intention-behavior relationship when actual control is not measured or accounted for in the model.

Key Constructs

In TRA, TPB, IM, and RAA, the most powerful determinant of behavioral performance is intention to enact the behavior. Performing the behavior is most likely if individuals have the necessary skills and/or abilities, believe they can perform the target behavior, and if environmental constraints are not prohibitive. Depending on the theoretical iteration, intention formation is determined by attitudes, social norms, and PBC. Generally, attitudes refer to the perceived favorability or unfavorability of a behavior. Perceived norms (also, normative pressure) are of two types. *Injunctive norms* are perceptions about whether the behavior is approved by people who are important to an individual, and *descriptive norms* are whether these important others themselves perform the behavior. PBC refers to perceptions about one's capability to accomplish the behavior, even in the context of important barriers (self-efficacy), and about having the autonomy to do so.

Each of these determinants is a function of corresponding underlying beliefs, which have an *expectancy-value form* (Ajzen & Fishbein, 2000). That is, attitudes (favorability) are determined by experiential (having to do with affective or emotional responses) and instrumental (having to do cognitive responses about outcomes) beliefs weighted by the valence of the outcome. For example, to the extent that someone feels that exercising to sweat for at least 30 minutes/day, 5 days/week leads to primarily positive outcomes (e.g., increased energy, increased self-confidence, better health outcomes), she would demonstrate a more positive attitude toward exercising. If she associates exercising primarily with negative outcomes (e.g., soreness, discomfort, embarrassment), she would have a more negative attitude toward the behavior. This formulation of attitudes accounts for the fact that two individuals might hold the same belief (that exercising to sweat for at least 30 minutes/day, 5 days/week results in weight loss), but that belief may contribute differently to attitudes, depending on the evaluation of the outcome as desirable or undesirable. Similarly, normative pressure is determined by normative beliefs; beliefs about whether specific important others (normative or social referents) approve of the behavior weighted by the motivation to comply with the referent. PBC is determined by *control beliefs*: perceptions of one's ability to overcome specific barriers to behavioral performance.

Which Theory Should be Used?

With each iteration in this set of theories, construct measurement and conceptualizations became more refined, and predictive validity improved. However, the availability of multiple versions may raise questions about which version should be used for a new purpose. For example, although IM and RAA are more recent, TPB is more frequently referred to in the scientific literature, even in recent publications. In an informal search on Google Scholar since the last edition of this book in 2015, approximately 408,000 results were returned from a search simply for "theory of planned behavior" compared to about 64,000 results for "reasoned action approach." Decisions about which model to use involve several considerations, including the empirical question(s) being asked, context of use (e.g., for intervention development versus explanation), and measures available. The process for identifying beliefs may also vary depending on available resources. For example, the measurement development process, including elicitation research, can be labor-intensive and costly. When resources are limited, some researchers may use alternative strategies to identify salient beliefs, including literature review and secondary data analysis. While the latest iteration of the model may offer a more complete understanding of various behaviors and maximize explained variance (McEachan et al., 2016), earlier versions still are valuable.

Common Assumptions of TRA, TPB, IM, and RAA

Reasoned is Not Necessarily Rational

The use of the word "reasoned" may lead to a misconception about these theories. Critics sometimes assume that the intention formation process is "rational" or "deliberative" (Ajzen, 2011; Reyna & Farley, 2006). However, here, the word "reasoned" reflects how intention formation is predicted by development of attitudes, norms, and control beliefs in a consistent way, but not necessarily through a process that is unbiased or logical. In other words, these theories assume nothing about how attitudes are cognitively constructed. In addition, these theories recognize that individuals' underlying beliefs may be "irrational" and may not be grounded in objective reality, yet, still be predictive of behavior.

Behavioral Specificity and Compatibility

According to this reasoned action framework, the target behavior must be defined at "various levels of generality or specificity" based on the four *TACT components: target, action, context, and time (TACT)*. RAA posits that changing any aspect of the formulation results in a different behavior (Fishbein & Ajzen, 2010, p. 30). For example, suppose we are interested in the goal of women asking health providers about pre-exposure prophylaxis (PrEP, an HIV prevention medication). The action is "asking about PrEP," the target is the "health care provider," the context might be "during your check-up" or "at your local clinic," and the time "in the next 30 days" or "the next time you go to your provider." A behavior defined only by action and time, for example, is the most general application of the components but is often appropriate for some behaviors in which the target and context are not applicable.

A common mistake is confusing goals, behavioral categories, and behaviors. For example, "losing weight" is not a behavior; it is a goal. Behaviors needed to achieve this goal might be a range of actions, such as avoiding sugary drinks, walking to work, increasing exercising, or bariatric surgery. A behavior in the avoiding sugary drink category would be "eliminating sugary drinks at mealtimes every day for the next six weeks." The general principle is that a target behavior should be specifically defined using TACT so there is a clear understanding of what is being predicted or explained, but not so detailed that the behavior is impractical or of little interest.

Related to defining the target behavior is the concept of compatibility. Compatibility refers to measuring intention and behavior at the same level of TACT specificity (Ajzen & Fishbein, 1980; Fishbein & Ajzen, 2010). Compatibility extends to measures for attitudes, norms, and control as well. That is, they should all refer to the same definition of the target behavior. A lack of compatibility attenuates the relationships among intention, its determinants, and the target behavior.

Volitional Control

Volitional control refers to the actual (not perceived) ability of an individual to act on their intention to perform a behavior. In TRA, behavioral intention is determined based only on attitudes and norms because it was presumed that agency was high, and the target behavior was volitional. In response to criticisms about this assumption, PBC was added to TRA, creating TPB, to account for behaviors in which volitional control is low, or may be perceived as low. Studies have shown that PBC explains more variance in behavior beyond that explained by intention when perceived control is low; its contribution to behavioral prediction is limited in other instances when perceived control is higher (Fishbein & Ajzen, 2010). In RAA, PBC moderates the relationship between intention and behavior, as does actual control. Although some behaviors may occur involuntarily, those behaviors were not meant to be explained by the theory, as they are "outside of awareness."

Theoretical Sufficiency

In the context of the reasoned action framework, theoretical sufficiency is the notion that performance of the target behavior is predicted directly by intention to perform the behavior and, sometimes, actual behavioral control; and behavioral intention is predicted solely by attitude, normative pressure, and control factors. The effect of additional variables (demographics, media exposure, personality traits) on intention and behavior is *mediated* through these attitudinal, normative pressure, and control factors. In instances where sufficiency may not occur or intention is a poor predictor of behavior, measurement error (e.g., poor reliability) or a lack of compatibility among measures are often to blame (Ajzen, 2020).

Measurement of TRA, TPB, IM, and RAA Constructs

In the formative stages of program or intervention development, application of reasoned action theories can help identify important pathways to behavioral intention as well as the specific beliefs within those pathways that are relevant for intention formation (Cappella et al., 2001). This is a common theme across these theories and can guide identification of intervention and communication strategies that address the salient pathways and beliefs. In evaluation stages, the theories are also useful for guiding analyses to explain intervention and program effects (Yzer, 2017). This is possible, in part, because processes for measuring the theoretical constructs in RAA are well-prescribed (Bleakley & Hennessy, 2012; Fishbein & Ajzen, 2010; Hennessy et al., 2012). Table 6.2 includes the direct and indirect measures for each model component, their definition, and examples of commonly used wording. The measures fall into two categories: *direct* and *indirect*. *Direct measures* are those of attitudes, perceived norms, and PBC, the three primary or proximal determinants of intention (these may also be referred to as *global or universal measures*). The wording of these items does not vary across different target behaviors. *Indirect measures* are those assessing the underlying beliefs: wording of these items is specific to each target behavior. Usually, direct and indirect items are measured on a 5-point or 7-point scale, although scoring may vary from either 1 to 7 or –3 to 3. Composite measures of the beliefs for each proximal determinant should correlate with that determinant.

Intention. Measures of behavioral intention represent an individual's readiness to perform the behavior, which includes aspects of willingness and expectation. Various wording is used in intention items, which can be framed as statements such as "I will [*perform the behavior*]," "I intend to [*perform the behavior*]," "I plan to [*perform the behavior*]," or questions such as "How likely are you to [*perform the behavior*]?" Responses are typically on a seven-point scale with response options based on a Likert index (Likert, 1932). Thus, respondents indicate their level of agreement with statements ranging from "strongly disagree" to "strongly agree" on a 7-point or 5-point scale.

Attitudes are specific to the behavior of interest and reflect the extent to which an object or behavior is evaluated favorably or unfavorably. They are determined by salient *behavioral beliefs* weighted by evaluations of the attribute or outcome. These beliefs focus on expectations about the likely outcomes of performing (or not performing) the target behavior. The more one believes that the behavior will lead to positive consequences and prevent negative ones, the more favorable the attitude toward the behavior.

Attitudes are measured using a series of semantic differential items that use pairs relevant to a particular behavior and ask respondents to rate each item using a scale with opposite adjectives at each end (such as easy-hard, ugly-beautiful, safe-dangerous). The series of items should result in a unidimensional scale that evaluates the object or behavior according to positive and negative valence. However, attitude items may be classified into two factors: experiential (e.g., unpleasant-pleasant) and instrumental (e.g., harmful-beneficial) evaluations. Some commonly used pairs for the semantic differential items include good-bad, unpleasant-pleasant, foolish-wise, and harmful-beneficial. Other adjectives can also be added as additional items that are relevant to the target behavior of interest.

Table 6.2 RAA Construct Definitions, Measures, and Example Wording

Construct	Definition	Measure	Item Wording Examples
Attitude		5- or 7- point scale	
Direct measures		Semantic differentials	
Experiential attitude	Overall evaluation of the positive or negative experiences of engaging the behavior	E.g., pleasant/ unpleasant; enjoyable/ unenjoyable	[*Performing the behavior*] is. . . Please rate whether [*performing the behavior*] would be . . .
Instrumental attitude	Overall evaluation of positive or negative consequences of performing the behavior	E.g., good/bad; wise/foolish	[*Performing the behavior*] is. . . Please rate whether [*performing the behavior*] would be. . .
Indirect measures		Likert	
Behavioral beliefs	Belief that behavioral performance is associated with certain attributes or outcomes	Extremely unlikely to extremely likely	How likely do you think each of the following are? If I were to [*perform the behavior*], it would. . . If you were to [*perform the behavior*], it would. . .
Evaluation	Value attached to a behavioral outcome or attribute	Bad to good	[*Behavioral outcome mentioned in belief*] would be a bad/good result of [*performing the behavior*]?
Perceived norm			
Direct measures		Likert	
Injunctive norm	Belief about whether most people important to individual approves or disapproves of the behavior	Think I should not/Think I should Strongly disapprove/strongly approve	Most people important to me think I should/should not [*perform the behavior*] or would approve/disapprove of me [*performing the behavior*]. Most people who are important to me want me to [*perform the behavior*].
Descriptive norm	Belief about whether most people perform the behavior	"Most people like me will not" to "Most people like me will"	How many people like you will [*perform the behavior*]?
Indirect measures		Likert	
Injunctive belief	Belief about whether each referent approves or disapproves of the behavior	SD/SA	[*Referent*] thinks that I should [*perform the behavior*].
Motivation to comply	Motivation to do what each referent thinks	SD/SA	In general, I want to do what my [*referent*] wants me to do.
Descriptive belief	Belief about whether each referent performs the behavior	SD/SA None, a few, some, a lot, all[a]	My [*referent group*] [*performs the behavior*]. About how many of the following people or groups do you think would [*perform the behavior*]?
Perceived behavioral control			
Direct measures		Likert	
Capacity	Belief about ability to perform the behavior and the perceived ease or difficulty of performing the behavior	SD/SA "Certain I could *not*" to "certain I could"	I am confident/I am certain that I can [*perform the behavior*]. If you really wanted to, how certain are you that you could [*perform the behavior*]?
Autonomy	Belief about the degree of control over performing the behavior	"Not at all up to me" to "Completely up to me" SD/SA	It is not at all up to me/completely up to me whether I [*perform the behavior*]. I have complete control over [*performing the behavior*].
Indirect measures		Likert	
Control beliefs	Belief about factors that can impede or facilitate performing the behavior	"Certain I could *not*" to "Certain I could for overall behavior" (Self-efficacy) SD/SA Overall behavior (Control) SD/SA	The following are some situations in which certain people might find it hard to [*perform the behavior*]. How certain are you that you could [*perform the behavior*] even if [*barriers or facilitators present*]? I will have [*the control factor*].
Power of control	Belief in the factor's power to facilitate or impede behavioral performance	Difficult to easy	[*The factor*] would make [*performing the behavior*] . . .
Intention	Perceived readiness of performing the behavior	Extremely unlikely to extremely likely	How likely are you to [*behavior*]. . .? I intend to [*perform the behavior*].

[a] Not Likert scale; SD/SA = Strongly disagree to strongly agree.

Perceived norms, or perceived social pressure, refers to perceptions about what others think and do with regard to performing the behavior, reflecting the contribution of both injunctive and descriptive normative influences. Normative pressure is determined by underlying *normative beliefs* that refer (1) to whether important referents approve or disapprove of performing the behavior, weighted by their motivation to comply with the referents (i.e., injunctive norms), and (2) beliefs about whether similar others are performing or not performing the behavior (i.e., descriptive norms).

Direct measures of norms capture the injunctive and descriptive components of normative pressure. The injunctive norm item deals with approval or disapproval from "important people in your life," whereas the descriptive normative item(s) refers to perceptions about whether others, and what percentage of others like the individual are performing the behavior.

PBC is based on beliefs about capacity to perform the behavior in the presence of barriers and the autonomy to do so. *Control beliefs* emphasize the ability to perform the behavior and the perceived ease or difficulty of doing so, as well as the degree of control over performing the behavior. PBC is often used as a proxy for actual control when contextual factors, skills, and abilities are not measured. *Self-efficacy* (Bandura, 1986) is another way to describe beliefs about capabilities and is conceptually indistinguishable from PBC (Fishbein & Ajzen, 2010), although it has distinct measures. *Efficacy beliefs* are based on perceptions about factors that can impede or facilitate performing the behavior.

Direct measures of PBC reflect perceived capabilities to perform the behavior. Aspects of autonomy and capacity are captured in a combination of items that ask about the extent to which behavioral performance is up to an individual and/or under their control. Self-efficacy measures are also used to measure PBC, and are often used to operationalize autonomy (McEachan et al., 2016).

Constructing Indirect Measures Using Elicitation Research

Direct measures in RAA generally are standardized across behaviors, but underlying beliefs for each of the corresponding constructs should be specific to the target behavior. *Elicitation research* should be conducted to identify which beliefs are important to the population of interest for a particular behavior (Erbe et al., 2020; Vézina-Im et al., 2021). Elicitation research is crucial to determine salient beliefs that are potentially modifiable and can be incorporated into persuasive health messaging (Yzer, 2012) and intervention design. When new elicitation research is not feasible (it can be labor-intensive and costly), scientific literature and other studies of the same behavior in the same or similar populations can be used to generate a list of beliefs that will likely be relevant.

An elicitation study can be conducted using focus groups or interviews, although interviews are preferred because they involve open-ended discussion and center participants' perspectives to identify relevant beliefs. To elicit underlying behavioral beliefs, individuals are asked about "good things" (advantages) and "bad things" (disadvantages) that would happen if they were to perform the behavior. For normative beliefs, important referents who might approve or disapprove of performing the behavior are listed (e.g., spouse/partner, family doctor). Referents for descriptive norms are elicited by asking about groups performing the behavior and/or groups that might be relied upon by the individual in figuring out whether s/he will perform the behavior. *Barriers* ("what makes it hard") to performing the behavior and *facilitators* ("what makes it easy") often are elicited to represent control beliefs.

Behavioral beliefs are measured through extent of agreement with statements about the consequences of performing a behavior. Beliefs incorporate the same aspects of the behavior mentioned in measures of the proximal determinant and intention (TACT). Each belief/consequence/expectation is then *evaluated* as being a good thing or a bad thing, also on a 5- to 7-point scale. Evaluation and beliefs item scores are then multiplied. Often, evaluation of a particular expectation is straightforward—some consequences are inherently negative (e.g., getting lung cancer from smoking) or positive (e.g., feeling less stressed after exercise), and a separate evaluation item is not necessary. Others may require a more formal evaluation. For example, adolescents' evaluation of "losing their virginity" because of having sex could be perceived by some as good and by others as negative. The product terms can be summed to create a composite measure of beliefs.

Normative beliefs. Injunctive normative beliefs assess the extent to which each identified social referent (ideally elicited as "important" approves or disapproves of the individual performing the behavior). *Motivation to comply* with each of the referents is assessed using a unipolar scale and multiplied by the normative belief. Although motivation to comply appears in RAA, it rarely is used. Empirical evidence has not supported its contribution to the prediction of injunctive norms (Fishbein & Ajzen, 2010). Descriptive normative belief items ask about perceptions of whether specific referents are performing the behavior.

Control beliefs. These are items to assess perceived presence of barriers and facilitators and the extent to which they impede or foster the behavior. More specifically, control beliefs comprise two measures for each control factor (barrier or facilitator): (1) assessments of the *belief strength* regarding the presence of specific control factors and the *power of (specific) control* factors to facilitate or impede behavioral performance.

Analyzing TPB, TRA, IM, and RAA Data

Causal pathways in the RAA are the starting points for statistical analysis. The various ways the RAA frameworks are analyzed are related directly to two main uses of the model: to explain and predict behavior and to identify salient underlying beliefs as a basis for intervention development. A multiple regression model with direct measures predicting intention will identify which factors predict a particular behavior.

However, often the effects of various background or precursor variables on a behavior are the focus of empirical studies. In each version of reasoned action, effects of all precursor variables on intention and behavior are mediated through attitudes, norms, and control (Hennessy et al., 2010; Lee et al., 2018), although in Figure 6.2, they are only pictured for IM and RAA.

It is always an empirical question whether a particular variable will be related to any of the underlying beliefs or direct determinants, and which precursors to include in a model varies according to the population and behavior of interest. Background variables are not limited to individual-level characteristics and may also include social or structural variables (such as density of health care providers in a community). In instances when precursors are included in the model, *path analysis*, which is a regression-based approach that allows one to assess the effects of a system of variables, is used to estimate mediated effects from the precursor to the observed determinants and then on to intention. Advanced statistical techniques, such as structural equation modeling, also can be appropriate (Hennessy et al., 2012).

Ideally, component items for the higher-order constructs (injunctive and descriptive norms; autonomy and capacity) should be combined into a single measure. However, they can be separate and entered individually into regression models. One important reason to keep component measures separate is that they can be used individually if there is interest in exploring the underlying beliefs, or if they are not well-correlated.

Because underlying beliefs specific to a target behavior are often modifiable, they may be incorporated into messaging and other behavior-change interventions. They can also be used to divide a population according to a particular characteristic (Slater, 1996): In analyses using the reasoned action framework, the audience is segmented by their behavioral intention into intenders and nonintenders (Fishbein & Yzer, 2003). Several data points on the belief level may be used together to inform selection of salient beliefs. These may include: correlation of the belief with intention, mean difference in the beliefs between intenders and nonintenders, and the percent of agreement with the belief within intenders and nonintenders (for examples see Bleakley et al., 2018; Hornik et al., 2019).

Supporting Evidence

The RAA and its various iterations have been used widely in developing and evaluating a diverse range of behavioral and public health communication interventions. As a result, many meta-analyses show support for the theories applied to a range of behaviors, including: condom use (TRA, TPB; Albarracin et al., 2001), alcohol consumption (TPB; Cooke et al., 2016), exercise (TRA, TPB; Hagger et al., 2002), sun protection (TPB; Starfelt Sutton & White, 2016), smoking (TPB; Topa & Moriano, 2010), vaccine hesitancy (TRA, TPB, RAA; Xiao & Wong, 2020), and dietary choices (TPB; McDermott et al., 2015).

Other meta-analytic studies that pool research reports across behavioral domains also have shown support for reasoned action-hypothesized relationships (e.g., TPB Godin & Kok, 1996; Hagger et al., 2018). McEachan et al. (2011) conducted a meta-analysis of 237 prospective tests of the TPB. They found that the TPB constructs account for a considerable amount of variance in behavioral outcomes (19%) and intentions (44%) and the intention-behavior correlation was .43, which indicates a moderate relationship. Some argue that intention does not always translate into behavior. In a later meta-analysis, McEachan et al. (2016) demonstrated significant prospective intention-behavior relationships and showed that the components of the RAA were associated with behavioral intentions. Experiential and instrumental attitudes, descriptive and injunctive norms, and capacity, but not autonomy, were significant predictors of intentions, and these variables explained more than half of the variance in intentions (59%). In turn, intention and capacity but not autonomy, significantly predicted behavior, explaining almost one-third of the variance in behavior (31%). These analyses provide strong support for RAA but also raise important unanswered questions about the autonomy dimension of the PBC construct.

Applications

Case 1: Analyzing Background Variables in the Context of PrEP for HIV

This section offers an example to demonstrate how to identify the ways sociodemographic and other background characteristics exert their influence on behavioral intentions by shaping determinants of intention. The analysis is based on data collected from women in the District of Columbia, one of the 48 US counties with the highest HIV incidence (HHS, 2019), to understand why women do or do not plan to use PrEP (Hull et al., 2022). PrEP is a pill that is highly effective in preventing HIV infection when taken daily and is recommended for people without HIV who are at risk of being exposed to HIV through sex or injection drug use. PrEP is underutilized by women generally and particularly by Black women relative to the number of HIV infections diagnosed in these groups (Siegler et al., 2018). Because of low rates of PrEP uptake, this study sought to understand Black women's perspectives about PrEP and psychosocial factors most relevant to their intentions to use PrEP to inform the development of communication efforts to increase its use. The data were used to identify how potentially relevant background variables—age, a history of injection substance use, and the proportion of casual (as opposed to committed) sex partners—affect attitudes, norms, and perceived control to ultimately shape women's intentions to use PrEP.

The study was conducted in community (rented private office space in the community) and clinic settings. Recruitment methods included approaching women in the waiting room of the women's health clinic to invite them to be screened, outreach by community-based partners, and distributing flyers and palm cards. Cisgender women (or women who identified socially as female) who met study criteria based on an eligibility screening survey were invited to participate ($n = 398$). Eligibility criteria included being sexually active, HIV negative, age 20–49 and potentially eligible for PrEP due to residence in high prevalence area and the presence of any HIV risk factor (having an HIV-positive sex partner, a recent sexually transmitted infection, participation in sex work, inconsistent condom use).

The survey assessed risk perceptions, knowledge of PrEP, demographic and background characteristics, HIV risk and prevention behaviors, and reasoned action theoretical constructs (behavioral intention, attitudes, injunctive and descriptive norms, PBC). The target behavior was "My using PrEP daily for HIV prevention in the next 12 months." Attitudes were assessed with a semantic differential item: "Overall, would you say that using PrEP daily to prevent HIV is a good or a bad thing?" In addition, 5-point Likert scales were used to measure injunctive norms ("Thinking about the people who are important to you, would they support or not support your using PrEP for HIV prevention in the next 12 months?"), descriptive norms ("Thinking about people who are similar to you, how likely would they be to use PrEP for HIV prevention in the next 12-months."), and PBC (i.e., "If I really wanted to, I could use PrEP daily for HIV prevention,"). All items were coded such that higher scores represented more positive attitudes, more normative support, and higher PBC. Age was assessed continuously; injection drug use was a dichotomous assessment of participants' lifetime history of "inject[ing] any drug other than those prescribed to you." Sexual partnerships were assessed by asking: "Of the men you had sex with in the past 12 months, how many were casual sex partners?" (Responses: none, a few, some, most, all).

The statistical analysis tested mediation of the relationship between the background variables and intentions to use PrEP, through the proximal determinants. A path analysis was conducted with age, substance use history, and number of partners as the independent variables, behavioral intention as the dependent variable and attitudes, descriptive and injunctive norms, and PBC as parallel mediators. Injunctive and descriptive norms were kept separate in this analysis, because they were correlated at.23. As shown in Figure 6.3, attitudes, descriptive norms, and PBC were significantly associated with intentions at the $p<.05$ level, but the injunctive normative path was not significant.

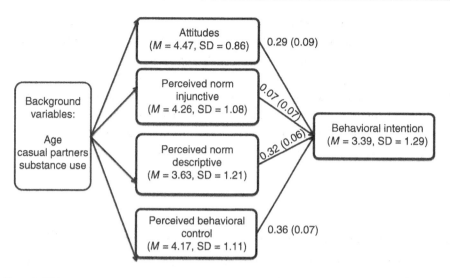

Notes: Coefficients are unstandardized b (SE); *p < 0.05. Age-> descriptive norms (b = 0.10, SE = 0.04: indirect effect
(b = 0.06, SE = 0.02)); Casual partners-> PBC (b = −0.09, SE = 0.04; indirect effect (b = −0.06, SE = 0.03));

Figure 6.3 Conceptual Model with RAA and Precursor for Intention to Use PrEP (Case Study 1)

Figure 6.3 shows statistically significant paths for background variables to the determinants. Age was associated positively with descriptive norms, and the relationship between age and behavioral intentions worked (in part) through descriptive norms, as mediation was significant. That is, older women anticipated to a greater extent that their peers would utilize PrEP to prevent HIV infection, relative to younger women, and this belief shaped intentions. In addition, those with more casual partnerships reported lower PBC for using PrEP daily. Further, having more casual partnerships was associated with lower intentions to use PrEP, and this relationship is explained in part by lower PBC to utilize PrEP. Evidence suggests that women perceive PrEP to be a tool primarily for those in serodiscordant relationships, in which one of the partners is known to be living with HIV (Bond & Gunn, 2016). We anticipate that those with more casual partnerships may have low certainty about their HIV risk exposure and may have less confidence in their ability to adhere to such a tool, which has uncomfortable side-effects and required a daily pill at the time the research was conducted.

History of injection-drug use was not associated significantly with attitudes, norms, or self-efficacy in this context; however, substance use may be related to other important background variables. For example, Roth and her colleagues (Roth et al., 2015) reported that, among a sample of individuals who inject drugs, PrEP awareness was associated positively with use of syringe-exchange programs, STI testing, and drug treatment. Injection-drug use may shape and constrain individuals' abilities to enact intentions, thereby moderating the intention-behavior relationship.

Considering persistent inequities in HIV infection, and disparately low utilization of PrEP among women, raising awareness of this HIV prevention option among women who may benefit from using it is an important step toward ending the epidemic. Findings from analyses like those reported here are being used to inform communication strategies to increase the use of PrEP. For example, given that older women in this sample were more likely to perceive their peers would use PrEP, strategies that cultivate positive descriptive norms and/or that rely on important normative referents to convey information may be particularly promising strategies for communicating effectively about PrEP. These results also suggest that efforts to build actual and perceived efficacy may be an important component of communication strategies that are designed to reach women in casual sexual relationships who may be eligible for PrEP.

Case 2: Using the RAA to Increase Recruitment into Alzheimer's Disease Research Registries

The advancement of medical science depends on rigorous and representative trials to test new preventive therapies and treatments for diseases. Such trials require participation from people who are affected or are at-risk and who come from diverse groups—including people of different race/ethnic groups. Health behavior theories can help understand and address the behaviors and intentions of individuals and groups participating in clinical trials. Black and Hispanic participation in registries and clinical trials related to AD is quite low (Langbaum et al., 2019; Manly & Glymour, 2021; Weiner et al., 2018). However, under-representation of traditionally marginalized groups in clinical trials is not unique to AD trials. Nonwhite racial and ethnic groups report lower rates of participation in clinical trials across a range of diseases (Coakley et al., 2012).

Although there are structural barriers such as access and system-level barriers such as inclusion criteria that may reduce Black and Hispanic participant enrollment, individual-level factors and decision-making are also consequential. This second case demonstrates how the RAA can be used to determine whether the determinants of behavioral intention vary for different subgroups based on race and ethnicity, sex, and/or any number of possible individual or structural characteristics.

The StepUp (Study to Expand registry Participation of Underrepresented Populations) is designed to increase enrollment of cognitively healthy older adults and to advance recruitment science. StepUp is aimed at increasing participation of groups that are underrepresented in AD-focused participant registries for AD prevention trials. Examples of these registries include the Alzheimer's Prevention Registry (APR), the Alzheimer's Association's TrialMatch, the Brain Health Registry, and APR's GeneMatch Program.

The message-design process began with formative research that included elicitation interviews with 60 white, Black, and Hispanic older adults ages 49–80 years old, from the Philadelphia, PA area. Phone interviews were conducted in spring and summer 2020 by two experienced interviewers and were about 30 minutes long. The goal of elicitation interviews was to identify attitudinal, normative, and control beliefs among the target audience that were associated with registry enrollment and could serve as a basis for subsequent quantitative research. Findings from the elicitation study (Bleakley et al., 2022) were incorporated into a nationally representative survey about one year later. RAA data on the target behavior of "signing up for a brain health research registry" were collected through an online survey using a probability-based sample of adults ages 49–80 years old ($n = 1,501$) with oversamples of Black ($n = 334$) and Hispanic ($n = 309$) adults. Direct measures and underlying beliefs were used to measure all three determinants of intention. Table 6.3 provides descriptive statistics on the RAA direct measures for the three racial and ethnic subgroups of women.

Regression analysis of proximal determinants on intention was conducted within subgroups of interest—white women (for comparison; $n = 415$), Black women ($n = 194$), and Hispanic women ($n = 134$). In these analyses, the control and efficacy items (used to measure autonomy and capacity) were correlated with one another at $r = 0.44$, and the injunctive and descriptive norms were correlated at $r = 0.55$, and so they were each entered separately into the models. Attitudes were related significantly to intentions for all subgroups of women at the $p < 0.01$ level (see Table 6.4 for all regression coefficients), and the association between intention and descriptive norms was also significant ($p < 0.05$) for all three groups. Capacity was related uniquely to intention for Black women. These findings emphasize the importance of assessing specific groups within the target audience: different determinants are relevant for different groups. This has implications for interventions, such as health messaging, in which persuasive efforts are focused on specific beliefs about the salient determinants. Here, there are clear similarities and differences in important constructs for intention formation. This type of analysis could be conducted with an intersectional lens, which attends to the ways power and privilege are conveyed differently for people at different intersectional locations to examine the "dynamics of differences and sameness" (Cho et al., 2013, p. 787). For example, one might examine regional differences or differences between socioeconomic categories within groups of racially similar women.

Having identified salient global constructs, our next step was to conduct a belief-level analysis that offered more specific information on potentially modifiable underlying beliefs for each group. Although attitudes are important for all groups of women, the beliefs that underlie those attitudes may be very different. Using an audience segmentation approach in which respondents were categorized into intenders and nonintenders, we examined relevant beliefs for each subgroup. For the purposes of an illustrative example, Table 6.4 includes only select behavioral beliefs.

Beliefs are ordered by correlations of intention and each belief for Black women, from strongest to weakest. Highlighted cells represent beliefs identified as most salient for each group. Some beliefs about joining a registry, such as "help to advance science, "and "help people like you in the future" would be candidates for inclusion in a message aimed at women in general, although "helping others like me" is stronger for Black and Hispanic women, who are the actual groups targeted for enrollment. "Improve one's community trust in medical research" also is more salient for Black and Hispanic women. Segmentation reveals numerous beliefs that, if bolstered, could lead to increased intentions for this behavior. The combination of these statistics helps researchers, practitioners, and clinicians make assessments

Table 6.3 Measures and Descriptive Statistics for RAA Proximal Determinants of Enrolling in a Brain Health Registry, by Racial and Ethnic Subgroups

Construct	Items Range of Scores from −3 to 3	Black Women n = 194	White Women n = 415	Hispanic Women n = 134
Outcome		Mean (SD)	Mean (SD)	Mean (SD)
Intention	How likely are you to sign up for a brain health registry in the next 30 days? Extremely unlikely/extremely likely	−0.49 (1.84)	−0.32 (1.74)	−0.43 (1.79)
% Intenders		36.6%	34%	31.3%
Proximal determinants				
Attitudes Alpha=0.93	Signing up for a brain health registry in the next 30 days would be... Bad/good, Unpleasant/pleasant, Harmful/beneficial Selfish/altruistic, Unnecessary/necessary, Foolish/wise	Mean (SD) 0.65 (1.27) b(SE) **0.63 (0.10)**	Mean (SD) 0.57 (1.19) b(SE) **0.60 (0.08)**	Mean (SD) 0.47 (1.33) b(SE) **0.42 (0.13)**
Perceived norms				
Injunctive norm	Do you think most people who are important to you think that you should or should not sign up for a brain health registry in the next 30 days? Should not/should	Mean (SD) −0.12 (1.38) b(SE) 0.09 (0.09)	Mean (SD) 0.13 (1.28) b(SE) 0.06 (0.07)	Mean (SD) −0.15 (1.50) b(SE) 0.11 (0.11)
Descriptive norm	Will most people like you sign up for a brain health registry in the next 30 days? Will not/will	Mean (SD) −0.40 (1.63) b(SE) **0.21 (0.08)**	Mean (SD) −0.30 (1.53) b(SE) **0.24 (0.06)**	Mean (SD) −0.09 (1.58) b(SE) **0.23 (0.09)**
Perceived behavioral control				
Autonomy	It is completely up to me whether I sign up for a brain health registry in the next 30 days. Strongly disagree/ Strongly agree	Mean (SD) 1.86 (1.74) b(SE) −0.00 (0.06)	Mean (SD) 2.23 (1.28) b(SE) −0.11 (0.07)	Mean (SD) 1.74 (1.73) b(SE) 0.002 (0.08)
Capacity	If I really wanted to, I am certain that I could sign up for a brain health registry in the next 30 days. Strongly disagree/ Strongly agree	Mean (SD) 0.84 (1.68) b(SE) 0.09 (0.06)	Mean (SD) 1.09 (1.44) b(SE) 0.23 (0.08)	Mean (SD) 0.63 (1.82) b(SE) 0.13 (0.09)

Notes: Scores were coded −3–3. Unstandardized regression coefficients (b) and standard errors (SE) in regression model on intention with all six determinants included. Bolded, italicized coefficients are statistically significant at least at the $p < 0.05$ level.

Table 6.4 Audience Segmentation Analysis for Women: Enrolling in Brain Health Registries for Alzheimer's Research

	Black Women (n = 194)			White Women (n = 415)			Hispanic Women (n = 134)		
	r with intention	Mean difference	% Likely difference	r with intention	Mean difference	% Likely difference	r with intention	Mean difference	% Likely difference
Behavioral beliefs									
Help people like you in the future[a,c]	0.42	1.09	27.4	0.34	0.64	14.6	0.42	1.17	30.5
Help to advance science[a–c]	0.35	0.79	26.7	0.35	0.62	17.5	0.35	0.94	23.7
Help others in the future[b]	0.35	0.73	15.2	0.41	0.76	20.1	0.35	0.80	17.3
Be a novel experience[a,b]	0.30	0.77	29.0	0.31	0.62	15.7	0.32	0.51, ns	8.8, ns
Improve your community's trust in medical research[a,c]	0.27	0.73	23.8	0.21	0.38	15.1	0.32	0.85	21.9
Make others think of you as a role model	0.11, ns	0.38, ns	11.5, ns	0.16	0.25, ns	5.3, ns	0.17, ns	0.36, ns	11.9, ns
Compromise your privacy[b]	−0.25	−0.83	19.0	−0.34	−0.76	15.0	−0.20	−0.71	20.2

Notes: Differences were calculated from intender-nonintenders.
[a] Black women.
[b] white women.
[c] Hispanic women.
Mean and likely differences are statistically significant at $p < 0.05$ unless otherwise noted. Shaded cells represent beliefs identified as most salient for each group.

about which beliefs are most salient and promising for intervention. For each belief, the larger the difference between intenders and nonintenders, the more room there is to move individuals; conversely, if the belief is not correlated with intention or attitude, it would not be a good candidate. This example highlights the versatility of the RAA, and all its predecessors, to find both similar and different points of potential intervention to encourage behavior change among various groups and demonstrates the necessity of moving beyond a one-size-fits-all approach as it applies to understanding underlying behavioral determinants.

Critiques

While the models described in this chapter have been used widely over several decades, critics (Amaro & Raj, 2000; Sniehotta et al., 2014; Trafimow, 2015; Ogden, 2003) have raised issues that warrant consideration. Some of the most common critiques include that it is difficult to falsify, too parsimonious or simplified, and it inappropriately asserts theoretical sufficiency. For a review of more critiques, see Hagger (2019).

Falsifiability. Ogden (2003) argued that models are not falsifiable on the grounds that when data from a study ostensibly provide disconfirmation, the results could be explained as conceptually consistent with theoretical assumptions or as the result of methodological shortcomings. In their response to these and other critiques, proponents have countered that it is indeed plausible to disconfirm the theories, as would be the case if none of the theoretical predictors was significantly associated with behavior (Ajzen, 2015; Ajzen & Fishbein, 2004; Ogden, 2003). Ajzen (2020) also points out that the models hypothesize various "mediation and moderation processes," grounded in its sufficiency claims, that can also be disproven.

Parsimony. Other critics argue that this reasoned action framework is too parsimonious because it oversimplifies factors shaping behavior and excludes important variables (Sniehotta et al., 2014). For example, emotions, including anticipated affect (Conner et al., 2013) and behavioral consistency with self-identity (Armitage & Conner, 1999) have received considerable empirical attention, leading researchers to advocate including these factors in the reasoned action framework. s As noted earlier, this framework does not preclude adding predictor variables that are not redundant with the original constructs and that consistently add additional variance across a range of behaviors (Ajzen, 2020). Further, the reasoned action theory predicts considerable variance in intentions and behaviors across a wide array of behavioral domains with relatively few predictors.

Theoretical sufficiency. The sufficiency principle in a reasoned action context also has been challenged (Sniehotta et al., 2014), particularly with the inclusion of past behavior in the prediction of intention and/or behavior. According to the theories, the effect of past behavior on intention should be mediated through attitudes, norms, and intentions. There is empirical evidence, however, that demonstrates that adding past behavior to the prediction of intention as well as behavior can increase the variance explained in those outcomes (Albarracin et al., 2001; Hagger et al., 2018; Rise et al., 2010). The causal mechanism through which past behavior influences intention remains unclear.

Future Directions

As models of individual decision-making, TRA, TPB, IM, and RAA consistently are invoked in developing individual-level interventions and in explaining the psychosocial mechanisms of behavioral performance. Scholars have noted that these models rarely have been applied to understand social and structural factors that shape behavior, particularly in the context of underserved groups where a social-structural approach could produce the most relative impact (Sniehotta et al., 2014). However, factors like these, which are external to the individual, can be incorporated and these models accommodate such factors in two ways. First, social and structural factors could/should be treated as precursors that shape intentions indirectly through their direct effect on perceptions of behavioral control. Additionally, structural and social barriers may represent environmental constraints that reduce an individual's *actual control* to perform the behavior. Actual control and PBC (Hagger et al., 2022) not only moderate the intention-behavior relationship but can also precipitate a feedback loop that affects underlying beliefs of any of the proximal determinants. Though the importance of actual control is highlighted in RAA, few studies assess actual control. Methodological advances in measurement of social-structural factors in health behaviors, such as spatial stigma (Smiley et al., 2020; Taggart et al., 2022), police-based discrimination (English et al., 2017) and structural racism (Doshi et al., 2020), facilitate more accurate modeling of this important set of factors in behavior. Conceptual and empirical integration of reasoned action constructs within social-ecological models of communication (Goulbourne & Yanovitzky, 2021; Young & Bleakley, 2020) and behavior (Bronfenbrenner, 1992) is also fertile ground for future scholarship.

Summary

TRA (1975), TPB (1985, 1991), IM (2000), and RAA (2010), together, offer behavioral researchers and practitioners a comprehensive framework of psychosocial factors to understand decision-making across a wide range of behavioral domains and populations. The explanatory power of the models, validated in thousands of studies, the intuitive appeal of their constructs, explicit causal specifications, and standardized measurement protocols help account for its popularity, and numerous promising areas of future research and application remain to be explored, including expanded efforts to more accurately model the social and structural factors that shape health behaviors.

References

Ajzen, I. (1985). From intentions to actions: A theory of planned behavior In J. Kuhl, J. Beckmann (Eds.), *Action control* (pp. 11–39). SSSP Springer Series in Social Psychology. https://doi.org/10.1007/978-3-642-69746-3_2

Ajzen, I. (1991). The theory of planned behavior. *Organizational Behavior and Human Decision Processes, 50*(2), 179–211.

Ajzen, I. (2011). The theory of planned behaviour: Reactions and reflections. *Psychology & Health, 26*(9), 1113–1127).

Ajzen, I. (2015). The theory of planned behaviour is alive and well, and not ready to retire: A commentary on Sniehotta, Presseau, and Araújo-Soares. *Health Psychology Review, 9*(2), 131–137.

Ajzen, I. (2020). The theory of planned behavior: Frequently asked questions. *Human Behavior and Emerging Technologies, 2*(4), 314–324.

Ajzen, I., & Fishbein, M. (1980). *Understanding attitudes and predicting social behavior*. Prentice-Hall.

Ajzen, I., & Fishbein, M. (2000). Attitudes and the attitude-behavior relation: Reasoned and automatic processes. *European Review of Social Psychology, 11*, 1–33.

Ajzen, I., & Fishbein, M. (2004). Questions raised by a reasoned action approach: Comment on Ogden (2003). *Health Psychology, 23*(4), 431–434.

Albarracin, D., Johnson, B. T., Fishbein, M., & Muellerleile, P. A. (2001). Theories of reasoned action and planned behavior as models of condom use: A meta-analysis. *Psychological Bulletin, 127*(1), 142.

Amaro, H., & Raj, A. (2000). On the margin: Power and women's HIV risk reduction strategies. *Sex Roles, 42*(7), 723–749.

Armitage, C. J., & Conner, M. (1999). Distinguishing perceptions of control from self-efficacy: Predicting consumption of a low-fat diet using the theory of planned behavior. *Journal of Applied Social Psychology, 29*(1), 72–90.

Bandura, A. (1986). *Social foundations of thought and action: A social cognitive theory*. Prentice-Hall, Inc.

Bleakley, A., & Hennessy, M. (2012). The quantitative analysis of reasoned action theory. *The Annals of the American Academy of Political and Social Science, 640*(1), 28–41.

Bleakley, A., Jordan, A., Ellithorpe, M. E., Lazovich, D., Grossman, S., & Glanz, K. (2018). A national survey of young women's beliefs about quitting indoor tanning: Implications for health communication messages. *Translational Behavioral Medicine, 8*(6), 898–906.

Bond, K. T., & Gunn, A. J. (2016). Perceived advantages and disadvantages of using pre-exposure prophylaxis (PrEP) among sexually active black women: An exploratory study. *Journal of Black Sexuality and Relationships, 3*(1), 1.

Bronfenbrenner, U. (1992). Ecological systems theory. In R. Vasta (Ed.), *Six theories of child development: Revised formulations and current issues* (pp. 187–249). Jessica Kingsley Publishers.

Cappella, J. N., Fishbein, M., Hornik, R., Ahern, R. K., & Sayeed, S. (2001). Using theory to select messages in antidrug media campaigns. In R. E. Rice & C. K. Atkin (Eds.), *Public communication campaigns* (3rd ed., pp. 214–230). Sage Publications, Inc.

Cho, S., Crenshaw, K. W., & McCall, L. (2013). Toward a field of intersectionality studies: Theory, applications, and praxis. *Signs: Journal of Women in Culture and Society, 38*(4), 785–810.

Cialdini, R. B., Reno, R. R., & Kallgren, C. A. (1990). A focus theory of normative conduct: Recycling the concept of norms to reduce littering in public places. *Journal of Personality and Social Psychology, 58*(6), 1015.

Coakley, M., Fadiran, E. O., Parrish, L. J., Griffith, R. A., Weiss, E., & Carter, C. (2012). Dialogues on diversifying clinical trials: Successful strategies for engaging women and minorities in clinical trials. *Journal of Women's Health, 21*(7), 713–716.

Conner, M., Godin, G., Sheeran, P., & Germain, M. (2013). Some feelings are more important: Cognitive attitudes, affective attitudes, anticipated affect, and blood donation. *Health Psychology*, *32*(3), 264.

Cooke, R., Dahdah, M., Norman, P., & French, D. P. (2016). How well does the theory of planned behaviour predict alcohol consumption? A systematic review and meta-analysis. *Health Psychology Review*, *10*(2), 148–167.

Department of Health & Human Services. (2019). What is ending the HIV epidemic in the U.S.? https://www.hiv.gov/federal-response/ending-the-hiv-epidemic/overview

Doshi, R. K., Bowleg, L., & Blankenship, K. M. (2020). Tying structural racism to HIV viral suppression. *Clinical Infectious Diseases*, *72*(10), e646–e648.

English, D., Bowleg, L., del Río-González, A. M., Tschann, J. M., Agans, R. P., & Malebranche, D. J. (2017). Measuring Black men's police-based discrimination experiences: Development and validation of the Police and Law Enforcement (PLE) Scale. *Cultural Diversity and Ethnic Minority Psychology*, *23*(2), 185.

Erbe, R. G., Middlestadt, S. E., Lohrmann, D. K., & Beckmeyer, J. J. (2020). A salient belief elicitation examining adolescents' meditation beliefs using the reasoned action approach. *Health Promotion Practice*, *21*(4), 633–641.

Fishbein, M. (2000). The role of theory in HIV prevention. *AIDS Care*, *12*(3), 273–278.

Fishbein, M., & Ajzen, I. (2010). *Predicting and changing behavior: The reasoned action approach*. Psychology Press, Taylor & Francis Group.

Fishbein, M., & Yzer, M. C. (2003). Using theory to design effective health behavior interventions. *Communication Theory*, *13*(2), 164–183. https://doi.org/10.1111/j.1468-2885.2003.tb00287.x

Fishbein, M., Triandis, H., Kanfer, F., Becker, M., Middlestadt, S., & Eichler, A. (2001). Factors influencing behavior and behavior change. In A. Baum, T. Reveson, & J. Singer (Eds.), *Handbook of health psychology* (vol. 3, pp. 3–17). Lawrence Erlbaum Associates.

Godin, G., & Kok, G. (1996). The theory of planned behavior: A review of its applications to health-related behaviors. *American Journal of Health Promotion*, *11*(2), 87–98.

Goulbourne, T., & Yanovitzky, I. (2021). The communication infrastructure as a social determinant of health: Implications for health policymaking and practice. *The Milbank Quarterly*, *99*(1), 24–40.

Hagger, M. S. (2019). The reasoned action approach and the theories of reasoned action and planned behavior. In D. S. Dunn (Ed.), *Oxford bibliographies in psychology*. Oxford University Press.

Hagger, M., Chatzisarantis, N., & Biddle, S. (2002). A meta-analytic review of the theories of reasoned action and planned behavior in physical activity: Predictive validity and the contribution of additional variables. *Journal of Sport & Exercise Psychology*, *24*(1), 3–32.

Hagger, M. S., Polet, J., & Lintunen, T. (2018). The reasoned action approach applied to health behavior: Role of past behavior and tests of some key moderators using meta-analytic structural equation modeling. *Social Science & Medicine*, *213*, 85–94.

Hagger, M. S., Cheung, M. W-L., Ajzen, I., & Hamilton, K. (2022). Perceived behavioral control moderating effects in the theory of planned behavior: A meta-analysis. *Health Psychology*, *41*(2), 155–167.

Hennessy, M., Bleakley, A., Fishbein, M., Brown, L., DiClemente, R., Romer, D., Valois, R., Vanable, P., Carey, M., & Salazar, L. (2010). Differentiating between precursor and control variables when analyzing reasoned action theories. *AIDS and Behavior*, *14*(1), 225–236. http://dx.doi.org/10.1007/s10461-009-9560-z

Hennessy, M., Bleakley, A., & Fishbein, M. (2012). Measurement models for reasoned action theory. *The Annals of the American Academy of Political and Social Science*, *640*(1), 42–57.

Hornik, R. C., Volinsky, A. C., Mannis, S., Gibson, L. A., Brennan, E., Lee, S. J., & Tan, A. S. (2019). Validating the Hornik & Woolf approach to choosing media campaign themes: Do promising beliefs predict behavior change in a longitudinal study? *Communication Methods and Measures*, *13*(1), 60–68.

Hull, S. J., Duan, X., Brant, A. R., Ye, P. P., Lotke, P., Huang, J. C., Coleman, M. E., Nalls, P., & Scott, R. K. (2022). Understanding psychosocial determinants of PrEP uptake among cisgender women experiencing heightened HIV risk: Implications for multi-level communication intervention. *Health Communication*, *18*, 1–12. https://doi.org/10.1080/10410236.2022.2145781

Janz, N. K., & Becker, M. H. (1984). The health belief model: A decade later. *Health Education Quarterly*, *11*(1), 1–47.

Langbaum, J. B., Karlawish, J., Roberts, J. S., Wood, E. M., Bradbury, A., High, N., Walsh, T. L., Gordon, D., Aggarwal, R., & Davis, P. (2019). GeneMatch: A novel recruitment registry using at-home APOE genotyping to enhance referrals to Alzheimer's prevention studies. *Alzheimer's & Dementia*, *15*(4), 515–524.

Lee, C. G., Middlestadt, S. E., Seo, D.-C., Lin, H.-C., Macy, J. T., & Park, S. (2018). Incorporating environmental variables as precursor background variables of the Theory of Planned Behavior to predict quitting-related intentions: A comparative study between adult and young adult smokers. *Archives of Public Health*, *76*(1), 66. https://doi.org/10.1186/s13690-018-0311-3

Likert, R. (1932). A technique for the measurement of attitudes. *Archives of Psychology, 140*, 5–55.

Manly, J. J., & Glymour, M. M. (2021). What the aducanumab approval reveals about Alzheimer disease research. *JAMA Neurology, 78*(11), 1305–1306.

McDermott, M. S., Oliver, M., Simnadis, T., Beck, E., Coltman, T., Iverson, D., Caputi, P., & Sharma, R. (2015). The theory of planned behaviour and dietary patterns: A systematic review and meta-analysis. *Preventive Medicine, 81*, 150–156.

McEachan, R. R., Conner, M., Taylor, N. J., & Lawton, R. J. (2011). Prospective prediction of health-related behaviours with the theory of planned behaviour: A meta-analysis. *Health Psychology Review, 5*(2), 97–144.

McEachan, R. R., Taylor, N., Harrison, R., Lawton, R., Gardner, P., & Conner, M. (2016). Meta-analysis of the Reasoned Action Approach (RAA) to understanding health behaviors. *Annals of Behavioral Medicine, 50*(4), 592–612.

Montano, D. E., & Kasprzyk, D. (2015). Theory of reasoned action, theory of planned behavior, and the integrated behavioral model. *Health Behavior: Theory, Research and Practice, 70*(4), 231.

National Institute on Aging. (2019). Why I Participate in Alzheimer's Research—Kay's Story. https://www.youtube.com/watch?v=0A0RZAw2N9c

Ogden, J. (2003). Some problems with social cognition models: A pragmatic and conceptual analysis. *Health Psychology, 22*(4), 424.

Reyna, V., & Farley, F. (2006). Risk and rationality in adolescent decision making. *Psychological Science in the Public Interest, 7*(1), 1–44.

Rise, J., Sheeran, P., & Hukkelberg, S. (2010). The role of self-identity in the Theory of Planned Behavior: A meta-analysis. *Journal of Applied Social Psychology, 40*(5), 1085–1105.

Roth, A. M., Armenta, R. A., Wagner, K. D., Roesch, S. C., Bluthenthal, R. N., Cuevas-Mota, J., & Garfein, R. S. (2015). Patterns of drug use, risky behavior, and health status among persons who inject drugs living in San Diego, California: A latent class analysis. *Substance Use & Misuse, 50*(2), 205–214.

Siegler, A. J., Mouhanna, F., Giler, R. M., Weiss, K., Pembleton, E., Guest, J., Jones, J., Castel, A., Yeung, H., & Kramer, M. (2018). The prevalence of PrEP use and the PrEP-to-need ratio in the fourth quarter of 2017, United States. *Annals of Epidemiology, 28*(12), 841–849. https://doi.org/10.1016/j.annepidem.2018.06.005

Slater, M. D. (1996). Theory and method in health audience segmentation. *Journal of Health Communication, 1*(3), 267–284.

Smiley, S. L., Milburn, N. G., Nyhan, K., & Taggart, T. (2020). A systematic review of recent methodological approaches for using ecological momentary assessment to examine outcomes in US based HIV research. *Current HIV/AIDS Reports, 17*(4), 333–342.

Sniehotta, F. F., Presseau, J., & Araújo-Soares, V. (2014). Time to retire the theory of planned behaviour. *Health Psychology Review, 8*(1), 1–7.

Starfelt Sutton, L. C., & White, K. M. (2016). Predicting sun-protective intentions and behaviours using the theory of planned behaviour: A systematic review and meta-analysis. *Psychology & Health, 31*(11), 1272–1292.

Taggart, T., Rendina, J., Boone, C., Burns, P., Carter, J., English, D., Hull, S., Massie, J., Mbaba, M., Mena, L., del Río-González, A., Shalhav, O., Talan, A., Wolfer, C., & Bowleg, L. (2022). Stigmatizing spaces and places as axes of intersectional stigma among sexual minority men in HIV prevention research. *American Journal of Public Health 112*(S4), S371–S373.

Topa, G., & Moriano, J. A. (2010). Theory of planned behavior and smoking: Meta-analysis and SEM model. *Substance Abuse and Rehabilitation, 1*, 23–33. https://doi.org/10.2147/SAR.S15168

Trafimow, D. (2015). On retiring the TRA/TPB without retiring the lessons learned: A commentary on Sniehotta, Presseau and Araújo-Soares. *Health Psychology Review, 9*(2), 168–171.

Triandis, H. C. (1977). Subjective culture and interpersonal relations across cultures. *Annals of the New York Academy of Sciences, 285*(1), 418–434.

Vézina-Im, L.-A., Beaulieu, D., Thompson, D., Nicklas, T. A., & Baranowski, T. (2021). Beliefs of women of childbearing age on healthy sleep habits: A reasoned actionapproach elicitation study. *Women & Health, 61*(8), 751–762.

Weiner, M. W., Nosheny, R., Camacho, M., Truran-Sacrey, D., Mackin, R. S., Flenniken, D., Ulbricht, A., Insel, P., Finley, S., & Fockler, J. (2018). The brain health registry: An internet-based platform for recruitment, assessment, and longitudinal monitoring of participants for neuroscience studies. *Alzheimer's & Dementia, 14*(8), 1063–1076.

Xiao, X., & Wong, R. M. (2020). Vaccine hesitancy and perceived behavioral control: A meta-analysis. *Vaccine, 38*(33), 5131–5138.

Young, D. G., & Bleakley, A. (2020). Ideological health spirals: An integrated political and health communication approach to COVID interventions. *International Journal of Communication, 14*, 17.

Yzer, M. (2012). The integrative model of behavioral prediction as a tool for designing health messages. In H. Cho (Ed.), *Designing messages for health communication campaigns: Theory and practice* (pp. 21–40). Sage.

Yzer, M. (2017). Reasoned action as an approach to understanding and predicting health message outcomes In R. Parrott (Ed.), *Encyclopedia of health and risk message design and processing* (pp. 1–21). Oxford University Press. https://doi.org/10.1093/acrefore/9780190228613.013.255

CHAPTER 7

THE TRANSTHEORETICAL MODEL AND STAGES OF CHANGE

Kerry E. Evers
Sara G. Balestrieri

Vignette

At 24 years old, Brenda had a car accident on her way to the grocery store, leading to several doctor visits. One of these doctors prescribed her opioid pain medication. Brenda does not recall being warned about the risks of using prescription opioids or the potential for misuse. She was in significant pain, and the medication provided relief. After filling her prescription, Brenda increased her dosage one day and continued to do so, deviating from the prescribed instructions. She began seeing multiple doctors to obtain more pills and eventually resorted to buying them in her community. This isolation left her suffering and pushed aside her friends and family.

During her annual check-up, Brenda's physician inquired about her medication use, leading Brenda to disclose her misuse. The doctor gave her a referral to a treatment program and stressed the importance of seeking help urgently. Brenda, feeling defensive, discarded the referral, believing that the doctors had prescribed the medication for her pain, and she was not ready to stop using it.

Several months later, after her pill use intensified due to another car accident with her child, Brenda spoke with another medical professional. This provider, rather than pressuring her to quit immediately, empathized with Brenda and discussed the potential benefits of seeking treatment. Brenda, still hesitant but more open, agreed to continue the discussion and explore treatment options. The new provider acknowledged that seeking help to quit using the painkillers might not be easy and could take a series of steps or stages.

An estimated 21.7 million (8.1%) Americans aged 12 and older need treatment for substance use disorders (SUDs), but only 10–11% of those requiring treatment receive it (Center for Behavioral Health Statistics and Quality, 2016). The gap between those who need treatment and those who receive it has led to associated annual economic costs of $193 billion for illicit substance use (National Drug Intelligence Center, 2011), $78.5 billion for prescription opioid misuse (Florence et al., 2016), and $249 billion for excessive alcohol use (Sacks et al., 2015), due to lost productivity, health care costs, and criminal justice costs. These statistics are

The authors dedicate this chapter to the memory of James O. Prochaska, Ph.D., our dear teacher, mentor, colleague, and friend, who will forever inspire us.

KEY POINTS

This chapter will:

- Explain stages of change and the other core Transtheoretical Model (TTM) constructs.

- Explore empirical support for and challenges to TTM.

- Illustrate how the utility of TTM continues to be extended to increasingly diverse populations, settings, and target behaviors.

publicized widely and discussed in the media. So why do so few people seek and receive treatment if there are a variety of treatment options (Cherpitel & Ye, 2008)? Part of the answer lies within patients' readiness to receive treatment and to stop using their substance of choice. The availability of, and resources to pursue treatment will be moot for patients who are not ready to receive this treatment. Additionally, patients who are not ready for treatment probably will not benefit from traditional action-oriented communications, referrals, and pressure from society, friends, and family.

The literature suggests that one approach to filling the gap between secondary and tertiary prevention is screening and referral by physicians, as an estimated two-thirds of individuals with addictions see primary care or urgent care providers every six months (Bowman et al., 2013). Screening, Brief Intervention, and Referral to Treatment (SBIRT) was designed to facilitate referrals to specialty care for patients who need it (Ghitza & Tai, 2014). Given their reach, primary care providers are in a unique position to identify patients who have a SUD and to provide referrals. However, as with other efforts, there are many barriers to primary care providers providing SBIRT, one being a lack of and resistance to using messaging tailored to a patient's readiness to engage in cessation and treatment. When health professionals use communication techniques tailored to an individual's readiness, patient resistance and noncompliance are more likely to be reduced (Prochaska, 2004). It is important for health promotion, medical, and public health providers to understand how to tailor communications to an individual's readiness to engage in the behavior if they are to maximize the impact they can have, given other barriers to change that may exist, such as lack of access to care.

Overview

Significance

The Transtheoretical Model (TTM) conceptualizes the process of intentional behavior change and provides a framework for behavior change communications and interventions. The TTM includes and integrates key constructs from other theories into a comprehensive theory of change that provides a framework for matching interventions to an individual's readiness along a continuum of change. TTM can be applied to a variety of behaviors, populations, and settings—hence, the name Transtheoretical. While often referred to as the "stages of change model," this term can be misleading as the stages of change are only one aspect of the complete model.

Since it was first introduced in the late 1970s (Prochaska & Norcross, 1979), researchers across the world have expanded, validated, applied, and challenged core constructs of TTM (Imeri et al., 2022; Mastellos et al., 2014; Prochaska et al., 2008; Sussman et al., 2022). Originally developed to address smoking cessation, the TTM has been tested and applied to a broad range of health and social behaviors, including alcohol and substance abuse, COVID-19 vaccinations, financial well-being, resilience, anxiety disorders, bullying, delinquency, depression, overall well-being, weight management, high-fat diets, HIV/AIDS prevention, mammography and other cancer screening, medication compliance, domestic violence, unplanned pregnancy prevention, sedentary lifestyles, sun exposure, and physicians practicing preventive medicine (Hall & Rossi, 2008; Hashemzadeh et al., 2019). However, to conceptualize the importance of using a theoretical model when approaching change management, it is helpful to use a specific public health concern for context.

Background

Historically, behavior change was viewed as a specific moment in time, either all or nothing. Someone either adopts a new behavior, or they do not. They stop harmful behaviors, or they do not. After an intervention, individuals who took actions leading to positive outcomes were considered successes, while those who did not were considered to have failed. When the majority of individuals in programs "fail," as they often do, it can be demoralizing for researchers, clinicians, public health providers, and patients (Hartmann-Boyce et al., 2021; Wewers et al., 2003). However, this is based upon the belief that change only happens at one particular moment. This is where TTM comes into play.

The TTM emerged from a comparative analysis of 25 leading theories of psychotherapy in an effort to integrate a field that had fragmented into more than 300 theories (Prochaska & Norcross, 1979, 2018). Those theories had much more to say about *why* people change than about *how* they change. They were really theories of behavior, such as theories of personality and psychopathology, rather than theories of behavior *change*.

Early research identified 10 processes of change that described the key ways in which people changed their behaviors. These included consciousness raising from the Freudian tradition (Freud, 1959), contingency management from B. F. Skinner (Skinner, 1966), and forming helping relationships from Carl Rogers' work (Rogers, 1951). Further research included an analysis of self-changers compared to those in professional treatment. An integrative model of change should reflect *how* people change on their own and with professional guidance. A study by DiClemente and Prochaska (1982) assessed the frequency of use of each of the 10 processes of change previously identified (DiClemente & Prochaska, 1982) and found that participants used different processes of change at different times in their smoking cessation journeys. Upon further investigation, it was determined that their behavior change processes unfolded through a series of stages with different change processes used at different stages (Prochaska & DiClemente, 1983). This was the first exploration and definition of the TTM of Behavior Change.

Key Components

The TTM is, by definition, an integrative theoretical framework that encompasses many other models and theories by differentially promoting the use of a wide range of behavior change techniques and intervention strategies based on an individual participant's readiness to change. It is built on the premise that, depending upon where an individual is in their readiness to change behavior, different communication and behavior change techniques are effective or ineffective. By helping people move through the readiness to change continuum, their chances of taking successful action are improved. Therefore, the goal of any intervention or communication is to move someone at least one stage of change forward and then adjust the technique being used appropriately. The TTM provides the "map" of what processes and principles of behavior change, including those highlighted in other theories, should be used at each point in time of the behavior change journey.

Stages of Change

Stage of change is an index of a person's readiness to act on a particular behavior that describes readiness to change as a continuum that includes five stages: (1) Precontemplation stage—not ready; (2) Contemplation—thinking about it; (3) Preparation—getting ready; (4) Action—taken recent action; and (5) Maintenance—taken action that began more than six months ago. It also offers guidelines around when a person intends to act. Because of the strong evidence base, stage of change also can be used to predict who will change successfully. For example, if we tell a smoker to quit smoking when they are not ready to quit, they are unlikely to succeed. In that case, we have ignored the person's stage of change and only provided them with a one-size-fits-all direction. The same applies to other behaviors.

Stages of change are dynamic and change over time. People will progress, and they will relapse—it is all part of the process. However, because we can measure it, we can tailor communications and interventions to match an individual's stage. Also, movement through the stages is not a linear process. Individuals do not always complete one stage of change before moving to the next stage. Knowing an individual's stage of change provides the central organizing construct to apply the rest of the constructs within TTM to communications.

Once we know an individual's stage of change for a particular behavior, we can begin to shape communications and interventions accordingly and meet the person where they are. Stage of change describes where an individual is for a specific behavior. In fact, they are probably in different stages for different behaviors. For example, a person may be ready to act on eating healthy but have no intention to start exercising.

Note the phrase "ready to take action" or act, rather than "ready to change." It is another important distinction. Change happens across *all* stages. Taking action is when a person reaches the point when they go from engaging in the negative behavior, such as smoking, to no longer engaging in the behavior. Or, when they begin engaging in a healthy behavior at an established criterion, such as eating five servings of fruits and vegetables a day. The first step in determining the stage of change for a behavior is to define what the criterion is for taking action. In the example of smoking, this means the day an individual quits.

Precontemplation is the stage in which an individual has no intention to act on the specific behavior in the future. The person may be uninformed, underinformed, unwilling, or too discouraged to take action to change that specific behavior. They underestimate the pros of changing and overestimate the cons. Although they may wish to change, they are not intending to do so in the foreseeable future. Someone in Precontemplation can be resistant to recognizing or modifying the behavior and may minimize the underlying associated negative behavior. These individuals may be demoralized and defensive concerning the behavior, especially when they are pressured to act. They are least likely to believe that they can change and expect little support for their efforts. This may be due to being unsuccessful in previous efforts to change and/or previous experience with traditional health programs not being well matched to their needs. However, by using appropriate processes and principles of change in communications and interventions, they can engage in the behavior change process. The goal is to help these individuals move at least one stage forward, and not simply to take action.

An individual in the *Contemplation* stage for a behavior is thinking about taking action but not in the near future, typically within the next six months. They perceive almost equal pros and cons about the behavior and are ambivalent about acting. Ambivalence can keep them in this stage for years. While they are more likely to acknowledge that they should change and less resistant than when in Precontemplation, they are not ready for traditional action-oriented programs that expect participants to take immediate action. If someone in contemplation of a behavior is pushed into such programs, they are unlikely to succeed.

In the *Preparation* stage, an individual intends to act soon, usually measured as within the next month. Typically, they have taken some steps toward positive behavior in the past year. They have a plan of action and may have set a date for it, for example, they may have signed up for a program or made an appointment. These individuals will welcome assistance and guidance and are those for whom traditional health promotion and public health programs were designed.

People in the *Action* stage have made specific overt modifications to their behaviors within the past six months. Taking action is when a person reaches the point when they go from engaging in the negative behavior, such as smoking or drug use, to no longer engaging in the behavior, or when they begin engaging in a behavior at an established criterion for a healthful behavior, such as eating five servings of fruits and vegetables a day or meeting the national recommendations for physical activity. Individuals in action for a behavior may experience strong urges to slip back into old behavior patterns during times of distress or when they encounter obstacles to a positive behavior change. Relapse to an earlier stage is common, especially among those who have unrealistic goals or who were not adequately prepared.

Individuals in the *Maintenance* stage for a behavior took action more than six months ago. These individuals experience fewer temptations to slip back into old behaviors, and they are more confident than when they were in the Action stage. However, they are still at risk for relapse during times of distress. Maintenance is a dynamic. not static, stage. For many people, staying in maintenance can be a lifelong challenge, especially for addictive behaviors.

While stage of change is a central organizing construct and perhaps the most well-known part of the TTM, the full TTM includes three other key constructs which are outlined below. Stage of change is a construct, not a theory. A theory requires systematic relationships between a set of constructs, and a formal theory ideally specifies these as mathematical relationships.

Historical TTM Constructs

Additional TTM constructs that are considered central to change include: (1) decisional balance—the pros and cons of changing (Janis & Mann, 1977); (2) self-efficacy—confidence to make and sustain the change in difficult situations (Bandura, 1977); and (3) processes of change—10 cognitive, affective, and behavioral activities that facilitate progress through the stages (DiClemente & Prochaska, 1982; Prochaska, 1984). More than 40 years of research on the TTM have identified particular principles and strategies that work best in each stage to facilitate progress towards eventual action and maintenance—for example, that the pros of changing go up, and the cons go down as people progress through the stages (Hall & Rossi, 2008); self-efficacy increases in the later stages (Henry et al., 2006; Hoving, 2006; Prochaska, 2013); people in the early stages rely more on cognitive and affective processes of change; and people in the later stages rely more on behavioral processes (Henry et al., 2006; Prochaska & Norcross, 2001).

Decisional balance reflects an individual's weighing of the pros and cons of changing. Initially, the TTM relied on the Janis and Mann (1977) model of decision-making that included four categories of pros (instrumental gains for self and others and approval from self and others) and four categories of cons (instrumental costs to self and others and disapproval from self and others). Over many studies, a simpler two-factor structure was developed: pros and cons of changing.

Self-efficacy is the situation-specific confidence to take and sustain action and to overcome the temptation to relapse. This construct was integrated into the TTM from Bandura's (1977) Social Cognitive Theory (see Chapter 9). As mentioned previously, the *processes of change* originally were derived from leading theories of psychotherapy and counseling (Prochaska & Norcross, 1979). Table 7.1 describes the core constructs of the TTM, as well as the 10 processes that have received the most empirical support in research to date and a technique for applying each process.

Table 7.1 Transtheoretical Model Constructs

Constructs	Description
Stages of Change	
Precontemplation	Not ready. No plan to take action in the next six months
Contemplation	Getting ready. Individuals in this stage are more likely to recognize the pros (benefits) of changing. However, they continue to overestimate the cons (costs) of changing and therefore are ambivalent and not ready to take action
Preparation	Ready. Individuals in this stage have decided to make a behavior change in the near future and have already begun to take small steps toward that goal
Action	Doing it. Took action less than six months ago
Maintenance	Keeping it up. Took action six or more months ago
Processes of Change	Covert and overt activities used to progress through stages
Consciousness Raising	Finding and learning new facts, ideas, and tips that support the healthy behavior change, e.g., nutrition education.
Dramatic Relief	Experiencing the negative emotions (e.g., fear, anxiety, worry) that go along with unhealthy behaviors or the positive emotions (e.g., inspiration) that go along with success in changing, e.g., testimonials
Self-Reevaluation	Realizing that the behavior change can enhance one's identity, e.g., values clarification
Environmental Reevaluation	Realizing the negative impact of the unhealthy behavior or the positive impact of the healthy behavior on one's social and physical environment, e.g., empathy training
Self-Liberation	Believing in one's ability to change and making commitments based on those beliefs
Helping Relationships	Seeking and using social support for the healthy behavior change, e.g., a positive social network
Social Liberation	Realizing that social norms and environments are changing to support the healthy behavior change, e.g., easy access to walking paths
Counterconditioning	Substituting healthier thoughts and behaviors for unhealthy behaviors
Stimulus Control	Modifying one's environment to facilitate the healthy behavior and to reduce cues to engage in the unhealthy behavior e.g., remove all ashtrays from the house and car
Reinforcement Management	Increasing the intrinsic and extrinsic rewards for the positive behavior change and decreasing the rewards for the unhealthy behavior, e.g., incentives
Decisional Balance	
Pros	Benefits of changing
Cons	Costs of changing
Self-Efficacy	
Confidence	Confidence that one can engage in the healthy behavior across different challenging situations
Temptation	Temptation to engage in the unhealthy behavior across different challenging situations

Critical Assumptions

There are several critical assumptions about the nature of behavior change and how population health interventions can best facilitate such changes upon which the TTM is based. The first is that behavior change is a process that unfolds over time through a sequence of stages that are both stable and open to change. Second, programs, interventions, and initiatives should emphasize specific principles and processes of change at specific stages for individuals to make forward progress through the stages. Finally, most at-risk populations are not prepared for action and will not be well-served by traditional programs that emphasize action. Setting realistic goals, such as progressing to the next stage of change, facilitates the change process and eventual progression to action.

Empirical Evidence

Stage Distribution

To match the needs of individuals in entire populations, it is important to know population stage distributions for specific high-risk behaviors (Norcross et al., 2011). A series of studies (e.g., Wewers et al., 2003) demonstrated that fewer than 20% of US smokers were preparing to quit using tobacco. About 40% of smokers were in Contemplation, and another 40% were in Precontemplation. In countries without a long history of tobacco control campaigns, stage distributions were quite different. In Germany, about 70% of smokers were in Precontemplation, and about 10% of smokers were in Preparation (Etter et al., 1997); in China, more than 70% were in Precontemplation, and about 5% in Preparation (Yang, 2001). In a sample of just under 20,000 members of a Health Maintenance Organization (HMO) across 10 health risk behaviors, only a small minority were ready for action and the majority were in Precontemplation for many of the behaviors. This pattern has also been found in other studies (Etter et al., 1997; Nigg et al., 1999; Wewers et al., 2003).

Pros and Cons Structure and Integration with Stages of Change across 12 Behaviors

Across studies of 12 behaviors (smoking cessation, quitting cocaine, weight control, dietary fat reduction, safer sex, condom use, exercise acquisition, sunscreen use, radon testing, delinquency reduction, mammography screening, and physicians practicing preventive medicine), a two-factor structure of pros and cons was remarkably stable (Prochaska et al., 1994). For all 12 studies, cons of changing were higher than pros for people in Precontemplation, and pros increased from Precontemplation to Contemplation. For all twelve behaviors, from Contemplation to Action, the cons of changing were lower in Action than Contemplation. In 11 studies, pros were higher than cons for people in Action. These relationships suggest that to progress from Precontemplation to Contemplation, Action, and subsequent stages, the pros of changing the behavior should increase. To progress from Contemplation, cons should decrease. To move to Action, ratings for pros should be higher than ratings for cons.

Most theories have not derived mathematical principles for integrating theoretical variables, in part, because few behavior-change theories have generated such principles. In fact, most have not even developed constructs that are subject to such mathematical principles. Across the 12 studies, however, mathematical relationships between pros and cons of changing and progress across the stages were found (Prochaska et al., 1994): The Strong Principle and The Weak Principle.

The Strong Principle is PC → A ≅ 1 SD ↑ PROS. Progress from Precontemplation to Action involves about one standard deviation (SD) increase in the pros of changing. A 1 SD increase is a substantial increase. Predicting the magnitude of this principle across a much broader range of behaviors and across diverse populations is much more challenging, given the error variance that can be generated by so much heterogeneity. Nevertheless, in a meta-analysis of 48 behaviors and 120 data sets from 10 countries, it was predicted that the pros of changing would increase by 1 SD. The Strong Principle was confirmed to the second decimal with the increase being 1.00 SD (Hall & Rossi, 2008).

The Weak Principle is PC → A ≅ 0.5 SD ↓ CONS. Progress from Precontemplation to Action involves ~0.5 SD decrease in the cons of changing. Evidence from the Hall and Rossi meta-analysis for the Weak Principle was not as precise: 0.56 SD (Hall & Rossi, 2008). Nevertheless, data on 48 behaviors from 120 datasets were integrated into a single graph that supported these two mathematical principles (Hall & Rossi, 2008).

The practical implications of these principles are that the pros of changing must increase about twice as much as cons decrease for a person to move from one stage to another. Perhaps twice as much emphasis should be placed on raising benefits as on reducing costs or barriers to enacting recommended behaviors. For example, if an individual in Precontemplation for physical activity can only list 5 pros of exercise, then, being too busy will be a big barrier to change. But if program participants accept that there can be more than 60 benefits of physical activity most days of the week, being too busy may become a smaller barrier.

Processes of Change across Behaviors

Building TTM based on 10 processes originally identified by theorists with sometimes incompatible assumptions about humans and their behaviors (such as Freud, Carl Rogers, and B.F. Skinner) has been a tough test that TTM has passed only partially. The assumption is that people can apply a common set of change processes across a broad range of behaviors. The higher-order measurement structure of the processes (experiential and behavioral) has been replicated across problem behaviors better than the individual processes (Rossi, 1992). Typically, support has been found for the set of 10 processes across behaviors, including smoking, diet, cocaine use, exercise, condom use, and sun exposure. But the measurement structure of processes has not been as consistent as the mathematical relationships between stages and pros and cons of changing. In some studies, fewer processes are found. Occasionally, evidence for one or two additional processes is found. It is also possible that, for some behaviors or some people, fewer change processes may be used. With regular but infrequent behavior like yearly mammograms, fewer processes may be required to progress to long-term Maintenance (Rakowski et al., 1998).

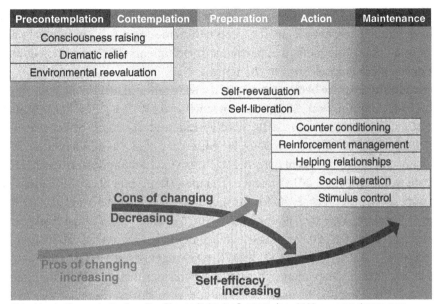

Note. Used with permission from Pro-Change Behavior Systems, Inc., 2023, www.prochange.com

Figure 7.1 Processes of Change that Mediate Progression Between the Stages of Change

The discovery of systematic relationships between stages and processes is reflected in the empirical integration shown in Figure 7.1. (Prochaska & DiClemente, 1983; Prochaska et al., 1992). This integration suggests that, in early stages, people rely upon cognitive, affective, and evaluative processes. In action-oriented stages, people draw more on commitments, conditioning, reinforcement, environmental controls, and support for progressing toward Maintenance. The relationships between stage of change and these behavior change constructs provide an evidence-based framework for delivering tailored feedback that is more likely to be remembered (Brug et al., 1999; Kreuter et al., 1999), to be considered personally relevant and credible (Johnson et al., 2006; Kreuter et al., 1999; Prochaska et al., 2001), and to change behavior. Meta-analyses found that health interventions tailored to Stage of Change produced significantly greater effects than those not tailored to stage (Krebs et al., 2010; Noar et al., 2007; Norcross et al., 2011). The TTM has also been used as a robust conceptual and empirical foundation that informs digital interventions that have been effective in promoting behavior change in hundreds of behavior change domains, including stress management (Evers et al., 2006), depression prevention (Levesque et al., 2011), chronic disease management, and shared decision making (Cummins et al., 2004). It influences program design (i.e., assessments, decision rules, content, embedded program features, user interface, frequency of interaction) as well as engagement and re-engagement messaging. Initial engagement messages, for example, must resonate with end users at all levels of readiness to engage with the program. This ensures a true population approach that engages all individuals, not just those ready to change.

The relationships of processes of change to the stages of change have important practical implications. To help people progress from Precontemplation to Contemplation, processes like consciousness-raising and dramatic relief should be used. Encouraging use of processes, such as reinforcement management and stimulus control, in Precontemplation would be a theoretical, empirical, and practical mistake. But for people in Action, such strategies would reflect optimal matching.

As with the structure of processes, relationships between the processes and stages have not been as consistent as relationships between stages and pros and cons of changing. While part of the problem may be due to the greater complexity of integrating 10 processes across 5 stages, processes of change need more basic research and may be more specific to each problem behavior.

Applied Studies

Since health behavior change theories should be the basis for applied science, it is not enough to apply tests of generalization, integration, and prediction. Theory-driven interventions should pass stringent tests to demonstrate that they can produce important impacts across a variety of problem behaviors, populations, and treatments. Across a diverse body of applied TTM studies, several trends are clear. The most common applications—TTM-based, computerized, tailored interventions and digital therapeutics—match intervention messages to an individual's needs across TTM constructs, based on information about the individual participants or patients. For example, people in Precontemplation could receive feedback designed to increase pros of changing.

TTM-based intervention studies have been conducted on a wide range of health behavior topics, including smoking cessation (Barnett et al., 2014; Cummins et al., 2004; Hashemzadeh et al., 2019; J. J. Prochaska et al., 2014; Ravi et al., 2021; Rios et al., 2019); diet (Carvalho de Menezes, 2016; Hashemzadeh et al., 2019; Nakabayashi et al., 2020); exercise (Carvalho de Menezes, 2016; Hashemzadeh et al., 2019; Jiménez-Zazo et al., 2020; Kleis et al., 2021; Nunes et al., 2017; Rhodes et al., 2021; Romain et al., 2018); stress management (Evers et al., 2006), substance use (Freyer-Adam et al., 2022; Hashemzadeh et al., 2019; Mauriello et al., 2011); cancer screening (Dsouza et al., 2021; Salinas-Martínez et al., 2018); participating in community service (Fenn et al., 2022); advanced care planning (Levoy et al., 2019); chronic disease management (Selçuk-Tosun & Zincir, 2019; Tseng et al., 2017; Winter et al., 2016); mental health (Hoy et al., 2016; Krebs et al., 2010; Levesque et al., 2011; Li et al., 2020); weight management (de Freitas et al., 2020; Johnson et al., 2008); medication adherence (Imeri et al., 2022; Patton et al., 2017); pain management (Hashemzadeh et al., 2019; Johnson et al., 2017; Kamioka et al., 2022); sleep management (Hashemzadeh et al., 2019), and safer sex (Hashemzadeh et al., 2019). TTM also has been applied in many settings and with diverse populations, including worksites (e.g., Sanaeinasab et al., 2018), primary care (e.g., Hollis et al., 2005), communities (e.g., de Freitas et al., 2020), those in treatment for substance use (J. J. Prochaska et al., 2004), faith-based organizations (e.g., Vincent-Doe et al., 2022) and schools (e.g., Evers et al., 2012). While many of these applications have been effective, some have not (e.g., Aveyard et al., 1999).

Two reviews of commonly used theories of behavior change across a broad range of behaviors—a meta-analysis of tailored print communications (Noar et al., 2007) and of web-delivered tailored health behavior change interventions (Lustria et al., 2013)—found that TTM was the most commonly used theory of behavior change for the applications studied. For print communications, significantly greater effect sizes were found when tailored communications included the following TTM constructs: stages of change, pros and cons of changing, self-efficacy, and processes of change. In contrast, interventions that included the non-TTM construct of perceived susceptibility had significantly worse outcomes. In that analysis, which included articles published through 2005, tailoring on non-TTM constructs like social norms and behavioral intentions did not produce significantly greater effect sizes.

While each TTM construct (stage, pros and cons, self-efficacy, and processes) produced greater effect sizes when included in tailored communications, what happens when only some constructs were used? Spencer, Pagell, Hallion, and Adams (Spencer et al., 2002) systematically reviewed 23 interventions that used one or more TTM variables for smoking cessation. Most studies used just stage; of these, only about 40% produced significant effects. Five used stage and pros and cons or self-efficacy; 60% had significant effects. Another five used all TTM variables; 80% found significant effects. This analysis raises the important dissemination question of what it means for practice and applied research to be theory-driven. Most studies were construct-driven (for example, using only the stage of change construct) rather than theory-driven. Future research and more recent reviews/meta-analyses should determine whether interventions are most effective when a full set of constructs from a theory, like TTM, is applied or whether there is an optimal number of theoretical variables that can produce the same effect sizes. They also should consider the incremental cost of adding more variables. Determining the right balance of variables and point of diminishing returns are important future considerations.

Applications of TTM

Application 1: SBIRT for Substance Use Disorders

As described at the beginning of the chapter, there is a major gap in the identification and successful treatment of SUDs in the United States. While Screening Brief Intervention and Referral to Treatment (SBIRT) has demonstrated some success when delivered in clinical settings, many barriers can prevent it from being applied, resulting in SBIRT only being administered to a fraction of patients, or not being delivered at all. Even when SBIRT *is* delivered, there is an additional concern that it is not taking into account the readiness to quit or patterns of use for each individual patient and is instead taking a "one-size-fits-all" approach. As several research syntheses have found with other behaviors, the more tailored an intervention is to an individual's readiness to change, the greater its efficacy (Krebs et al., 2010; Noar et al., 2007; Norcross et al., 2011).

Connect2BWell, a mobile device-optimized, online SBIRT program was developed to address these concerns. This program was designed to be integrated into clinical workflow in a variety of clinical settings, removing much of the burden for SBIRT delivery from clinical staff. Leveraging this mobile-optimized, online delivery platform allows the administration of SBIRT to be much more flexible: patients with upcoming appointments can even engage with the program before going to the clinic. This streamlines the process and allows clinic staff to focus their efforts on delivering additional intervention and referring to treatment for those patients with the riskiest patterns of substance use. The integrative program allows patients to interact over any internet-enabled device, a clinician-facing view of the program, and communication directly with the electronic health record (EHR). *Connect2BWell*'s integration into EHRs allows for the direct transmission of patient results between the program and the EHR, informing clinicians when a patient has screened positive for an SUD and providing clinicians with details of a patient's pattern of use. Not only are these results available to view in the EHR but they also can be viewed in an interactive, clinician dashboard aimed at facilitating discussions regarding substance use between a patient and a member of their care team.

In addition to these important technological innovations aimed at improving the delivery of SBIRT, another critical component of *Connect2BWell* is the use of the TTM to inform the development of all intervention content, communications, and referral to treatment. Approaching intervention development using this TTM-based lens facilitates the tailoring that *Connect2BWell* provides. When patients first enter the program, they are screened for SUDs using the Alcohol, Smoking and Substance Involvement Test (ASSIST). The ASSIST is a widely used, validated measure for identifying substance-specific levels of risk (low, moderate, high) and provides substance involvement scores for tobacco, alcohol, cannabis, cocaine, stimulants, inhalants, sedatives, hallucinogens, and opioids. Based on a series of decision rules built into the program, the highest-risk substance is determined and used as the focus for the brief intervention piece of the program. Based upon the ASSIST and other information regarding their use, a specific program track is identified for each patient. The program includes five tracks, each defined by a different target behavior: (1) quitting, (2) limiting use of alcohol to low-risk drinking guidelines, (3) quitting drinking with the guidance of a medical professional, (4) limiting use of a prescription drug to as prescribed by a health care provider, and (5) limiting medical marijuana to medically advised use. Once a track has been determined, the patient is assessed for their readiness to engage in their relevant target behavior (stage of change). From this point forward, stage of change is used to tailor their intervention experience and dictates other TTM-based principles on which interventions are tailored. The online intervention experience is also complemented by behavior and stage-matched text messages, which are sent to patients every one to three days when they are in-between intervention sessions.

Once a patient completes the online intervention portion of *Connect2BWell*, the data are shared with their care team via the EHR and the clinician dashboard. A member of the care team then reaches out to the patient to schedule a "face-to-face" (either in-clinic or via a telehealth platform) intervention session. The care team member uses the program's clinician dashboard to facilitate this discussion, reflecting on patterns of use and other information the patient provided in their online session. The clinician dashboard also provides a message field that allows the clinician to send messages directly to patients. Another key feature of the dashboard is the Action Plan, which allows clinicians to choose from a list of pre-determined action steps that are populated based on the patient's target behavior and stage of change. Clinicians and patients work together to determine which action steps are best suited for particular patients. Once the Action Plan is created, it is available to patients through their patient homepages. Patients can view their assigned action steps on their homepage and mark steps as "done" as they are completed. As action steps are marked as complete by the user, the clinician dashboard updates in real-time to reflect these completions. The homepage also features a list of behavior and stage-matched activities for each patient to complete.

All aspects of *Connect2BWell* are built around a TTM framework. All patient communications, either from the online program or from the clinician who uses the clinical dashboard to guide their interactions, are tailored to the patient's specific behavioral risk and stage of change. All action planning, goal setting, and referrals to treatment take into account the patient's stage of change and make appropriate recommendations based upon their readiness. In addition, stage information is transmitted to the EHR so that all clinical staff interacting with the individual around this behavior have additional knowledge as to the patient's behavior change journey. While the final data from a randomized controlled trial evaluating the efficacy of *Connect2BWell* in a large Federally Qualified Health Center

(FQHC) are not yet available, data from a pilot of the program demonstrated high levels of acceptability with participants' average ratings above a 4 out of 5 on all acceptability measures and clinicians also averaging above a 4 out of 5 on all but one of the acceptability questions regarding their use of the clinician dashboard (Evers, 2019). The clinical trial has retention rates of over 70% across nine months, indicating a high level of engagement with the program.

Application 2: Advance Care Planning

The TTM can be applied in novel ways. One recent example of this is a TTM-based intervention for engaging people in advance care planning activities (Fried et al., 2016, 2021). Advance care planning activities allow individuals to prepare for potential healthcare decisions ahead of time and communicate their preferences with loved ones and healthcare providers (Advance Care Planning, n.d.). While there has been an increase in advance care planning over time, only about one-third of adults in the United States have completed an advance directive, a living document allowing an individual to record their healthcare decision preferences and update them over time as their situation changes. Some interventions have been effective in increasing advanced care plan use, but they have limitations (MacKenzie et al., 2018). Facilitator-led interventions typically demonstrate the strongest effects, but they are resource-intensive and may not be scalable. Self-administered tools are more widely available, but these interventions are less efficacious than those with face-to-face guidance and often require access to the Internet. There is a need to bridge the gap between these two types of interventions for advanced care planning and develop a solution that is widely accessible but also offers high levels of efficacy to individuals.

One program that has addressed this gap, STAMP (Sharing and Talking about my Preferences), was developed with a firm theoretical grounding in the TTM. This program was organized around readiness to participate in four key advance care planning behaviors: completion of a living will, formal assignment of a healthcare proxy, identifying a trusted person and communicating with this person about views on quality versus quantity of life, and ensuring that written documents are in the medical record. Intervention feedback was tailored for each user based on three TTM constructs: (1) stages of change for these four key behaviors, (2) decisional balance, and (3) values/beliefs. For example, for those who were in the early stages of change on a given behavior, intervention feedback focused on changing attitudes and addressing barriers, while feedback for those in the later stages provided specific actions the individual(s) could perform. Those engaging with STAMP can complete their assessments either online or over the phone, assuring that those without a device or internet access are not denied support. Based on these assessment answers, STAMP generates an individual-tailored feedback report, which is then shared with the participant.

STAMP has shown efficacy in a cluster randomized controlled trial conducted in primary care and specialty practices (Fried et al., 2021). Randomization occurred at the practice level to avoid contamination, and sites were randomized in matched pairs based on a series of practice and patient characteristics. Patients who were age 55 or older and presented for in-person visits at any study site were considered for inclusion. There were also many exclusion criteria, including the visit being an urgent care encounter, severe hearing or vision loss, moderate-to-severe cognitive impairment, inability to complete informed consent, a primary language other than English, and having already completed advance care planning. Participants in practices randomly assigned to receive STAMP received the computer-tailored intervention, while those receiving care at control sites were engaged in usual care. All participants received assessments either online or over the phone (based on participant preference) at baseline and after two, four, and six months. The primary outcome of interest was the self-reported completion of all four advance care planning behaviors at the six-month follow-up.

A total of 909 participants completed baseline sessions, including 455 intervention and 454 usual care participants. At the six-month follow-up, 91% of intervention participants and 95% of those assigned to usual care completed their final assessments. Using intent-to-treat analyses, the predicted probability of completing all four advance care planning activities was greater for intervention participants (14.1%, 95% CI 11.0–17.2%) than for those in usual care (8.2%, 95% CI 4.9–11.4%). Results for the four individual behaviors mirrored these overall results, such that for all four behaviors, intervention participants had a higher predicted probability for completing the behavior than those receiving usual care (Fried et al., 2021).

Not only does the conceptualization of the STAMP program overcome known barriers to engaging individuals in advance care planning activities, but it is clear that it is also effective in practice. The creation of a computerized tailored intervention using the TTM addresses both the concern of scalability posed by facilitator-led applications as well as the lack of individualization and efficacy of previous computerized programs (Fried et al., 2016). The application of the TTM to the development and implementation of STAMP demonstrates the flexibility of the model and should encourage us to think creatively about new ways to apply this evidence-based model.

Limitations

Several commentaries, studies, and evaluations have challenged the applicability and/or utility of the TTM. One criticism is that stage of change is not the most appropriate predictor of long-term outcomes. Several studies have been conducted to examine, within the TTM, which variables predict long-term outcomes across multiple behaviors (Blissmer et al., 2010; Redding et al., 2011). Some researchers have emphasized that severity, or level of addiction, is a more important predictor of long-term outcomes than stage of change (Abrams et al., 2000; Farkas et al., 1996); indeed, severity has been confirmed as an important variable in addition to stage. However, the second important variable is a stage in which participants in Preparation at baseline have better 24-month outcomes for smoking, diet, and sun exposure than those in Contemplation, and those in Contemplation do better than those in Precontemplation (Blissmer et al., 2010; Redding et al., 2011). The third variable is treatment in which participants in treatment do better at 24 months than those randomly assigned to control groups for smoking, diet, and sun exposure. The fourth and final variable is an effort effect, in which participants in both treatment and control groups who progressed to Action and Maintenance at 24 months were making better efforts with TTM variables like pros and cons, self-efficacy, and processes at baseline. There were no consistent demographic effects across the three behaviors. What these and other similar results indicate is that either-or thinking (such as either severity or stage) is not as helpful as an approach that seeks to identify the most important effects, whether they are based on TTM or an addiction or severity model.

Another frequent criticism of the TTM is the categorization of the stages of change. O'Keefe (2016) raises the concern that classification criteria into stages may seem artificial or vary between studies and across behaviors. A review of the literature may seem to show that this is true, but discrepancies are often due to misinterpretation of the stage definitions or a lack of fidelity in the application of the theory. In addition, the TTM has been widely used in studies of diverse behaviors and populations including low-income individuals, nurses, pregnant women, adolescents, children, elderly, employees, primary care patients, and those receiving in-patient treatment (see Hashemzadeh et al., 2019; Jiménez-Zazo et al., 2020; Kleis et al., 2021; Nunes et al., 2017 for examples), and researchers have adapted the definitions based upon their knowledge of specific behaviors. O'Keefe (2016) also raises the concern that the stages may not be mutually exclusive categories and that a continuum may be better suited for understanding behaviors than discrete stages. However, in all early publications on the topic of the stages of change, they were in fact described as a continuum.

Some researchers have explored alternative ways of formulating stages or have attempted to develop more parsimonious theories that use fewer constructs (Abrams et al., 2000; Herzog et al., 1999, 2000). Other research has found that change processes and other TTM variables predict stage progress (for example, DiClemente et al., 1991; Dijkstra et al., 2006; Evans et al., 2000; Prochaska et al., 1985, 2004, 2008; Sun, et al., 2007; Velicer et al., 2007). Evans et al. (2000) explained some of the inconsistencies in previous research by demonstrating better predictions over 6 months versus 12 months, and better predictions using all 10 processes of change instead of a subset.

Although TTM has been applied across at least 48 behaviors and populations from many countries, limitations of its application have been identified. To date, population trials based on TTM have not produced significant effects in preventing substance abuse among children (see, for example, Aveyard et al., 1999; Hollis et al., 2005). For example, in 2000, Peterson et al. (2000) commented that most school-based smoking prevention trials failed and suggested that the field should move beyond social influence models but raised the question of whether this was due to methodological issues or actual failure of the interventions. Indeed, individually focused prevention trials are challenging across theories. Further, after the Master Tobacco Settlement in 1998, and with the increase in policies restricting tobacco sales to minors, it became increasingly difficult to find intervention effects due to the overall reduction in adolescent use of combustible tobacco products.

It might be concluded that TTM does not apply very well to children and adolescents. There is a basic question regarding the age at which intentional behavior change begins. Applied studies of bullying prevention in elementary, middle, and high schools produced significant results (Prochaska et al., 2007). Similarly, early intervention with adolescent smokers using TTM-tailored treatments produced significant abstinence rates at 24 months that were almost identical to rates with treated adult smokers (Hollis et al., 2005). This was also true for TTM-tailored interventions targeting sun-protective behaviors in adolescents (Norman et al., 2007). Because there has been much more research done applying the TTM to reducing risks than to preventing risks, conclusions about intervention effects related to life stage may be confused with questions of reduction versus prevention of risks.

Given the global application of TTM, it will be important to determine in which cultures TTM can be applied effectively and in which cultures it may require major adaptations or if other theoretical frameworks may be a better fit. In a meta-analysis of the relationships between stages and pros and cons of changing in studies conducted in 10 countries, there was no significant effect by country (Hall & Rossi, 2008). However, the studies included were only in 10 of the many countries in the world, and mainly in industrialized higher-income nations.

Future Research

While many efficacy studies and implementation trials support the use of the TTM, much still needs to be done to advance understanding about the processes of behavior change, effective interventions to achieve population impact and other issues related to the TTM, specifically, and behavior change research more generally. Basic research should be done with other theoretical variables, such as processes of resistance, well-being, and problem severity, to determine if such variables relate systematically to the stages and predict progress across specific stages.

More research is also needed on the structure and integration of processes and stages of change across a broad range of behaviors, such as acquisition behaviors, like exercise, and cessation behaviors, like smoking cessation (Rosen, 2000). It is important to examine what modifications are needed for specific types of behaviors, such as fewer processes perhaps for infrequent behaviors, like mammography screening, or behaviors that may relapse less often, such as sunscreen use.

Since tailored communications have been found to be the most promising interventions for applying TTM to date, more research is needed to compare the cost-effectiveness and impacts of alternative technologies. As technologies evolve, it will be important to evaluate the best modalities to increase engagement and retention in programs. The costs of personnel and technology required for developing tailored interventions have dropped dramatically over the past two decades. One promising approach is to add tailored texting to best-practice internet-based computer-tailored interventions and digital therapeutics. In one study, this enhancement produced an improvement in cigarette abstinence of 11 percentage points (44% versus 33%) (Evers et al., in press). In addition, the use of computerized, tailored interventions and digital therapeutics based upon the TTM should be applied in multi-level interventions, such as biological (e.g., pharmacological adjuncts), community, and social (e.g., policy) level interventions.

While the application of the TTM to diverse populations and evaluation of the effectiveness of TTM-tailored interventions minority populations has been promising (for examples see Albright et al., 2005; Benitez et al., 2017; Gazabon et al., 2007; Paxton et al., 2008; J. M. Prochaska, 2007), more research should be done to compare alternative communication modalities for engaging such populations. It is possible that alternative intervention modalities—such as mobile applications, conversational agents (Martinengo et al., 2022), text messaging, neighborhood or church leaders, gaming (Mulchandani et al., 2022), or community programs—may empower diverse populations to engage with and increase the impact of health-enhancing programs.

Changing multiple behaviors creates special challenges, including the demands placed on participants and providers. Alternative strategies beyond the sequential (one at a time) and simultaneous (each treated intensely at the same time) should be assessed. Integrative approaches are promising. With bullying prevention, multiple behaviors (for example, hitting, stealing, ostracizing, mean gossiping and labeling, damaging personal belongings) and multiple roles (bully, victim, and passive bystander) require attention. The available classroom intervention time may be as little as 30 minutes. If behavior change is construct-driven (for example, by stage or self-efficacy), what is a higher-order construct that is common to the behaviors that could be used as an integrative factor for the focus of an intervention? In one case, that concept was "relating with respect." Significant and important improvements across roles and behaviors have been found with elementary, middle, and high school students (Prochaska et al., 2007). Effective applications may be limited more by our creativity and resources for testing than by the ability of the theory to drive significant research and effective interventions.

The TTM is dynamic and open to modifications and enhancements as more students, scientists, and practitioners apply the TTM to a growing number of theoretical issues, diverse behaviors, and at-risk populations.

Summary

This chapter described the core constructs of TTM and how these constructs can be integrated across the stages of change. Empirical support for basic constructs of TTM and for applied research was presented, along with conceptual and empirical challenges from critics. Applications of TTM-tailored interventions with diverse populations and behaviors were explored with an example of programs developed for SBIRT within primary care practices for individuals with SUDs and for advanced care planning. These examples illustrate the range of behaviors and populations to which the TTM has been successfully applied, and how programs can be successfully designed using a TTM approach. A major theme is that programmatically building and applying core constructs of TTM at the individual level can lead to high-impact programs for enhancing health at the population level.

References

Abrams, D. B., Herzog, T. A., Emmons, K. M., & Linnan, L. (2000). Stages of change versus addiction: A replication and extension. *Nicotine & Tobacco Research, 2*(3), 223–229. https://doi.org/10.1080/14622200050147484

Advance care planning: Health care directives. (n.d.). National Institute on Aging. https://www.nia.nih.gov/health/advance-care-planning-health-care-directives

Albright, C. L., Pruitt, L., Castro, C., Gonzalez, A., Woo, S., & King, A. C. (2005). Modifying physical activity in a multiethnic sample of low-income women: One-year results from the IMPACT (Increasing Motivation for Physical ACTivity) project. *Annals of Behavioral Medicine: A Publication of the Society of Behavioral Medicine, 30*(3), 191–200. https://doi.org/10.1207/s15324796abm3003_3

Aveyard, P., Cheng, K. K., Almond, J., Sherratt, E., Lancashire, R., Lawrence, T., Griffin, C., & Evans, O. (1999). Cluster randomised controlled trial of expert system based on the transtheoretical ("stages of change") model for smoking prevention and cessation in schoolsBMJ *[British Medical Journal], 319*(7215), 948–953. https://www.ncbi.nlm.nih.gov/pmc/articles/PMC28247/

Bandura, A. (1977). Self-efficacy: Toward a unifying theory of behavioral change. *Psychological Review, 84*(2), 191. http://psycnet.apa.org/journals/rev/84/2/191/

Barnett, N. P., Ott, M. Q., Rogers, M. L., Loxley, M., Linkletter, C., & Clark, M. A. (2014). Peer associations for substance use and exercise in a college student social network. *Health Psychology, 33*(10), 1134.

Benitez, T. J., Tasevska, N., Coe, K., & Keller, C. (2017). Cultural relevance of the transtheoretical model in physical activity promotion: Mexican-American women's use of the Processes of Change. *Journal of Health Disparities Research and Practice, 10*(1), 2. https://digitalscholarship.unlv.edu/jhdrp/vol10/iss1/2

Blissmer, B., Prochaska, J. O., Velicer, W. F., Redding, C. A., Rossi, J. S., Greene, G. W., Paiva, A., & Robbins, M. (2010). Common factors predicting long-term changes in multiple health behaviors. *Journal of Health Psychology, 15*(2), 205–214. https://doi.org/10.1177/1359105309345555

Bowman, S., Eiserman, J., Beletsky, L., Stancliff, S., & Bruce, R. D. (2013). Reducing the health consequences of opioid addiction in primary care. *The American Journal of Medicine, 126*(7), 565–571. https://doi.org/10.1016/j.amjmed.2012.11.031

Brug, J., Steenhuis, I., Van Assema, P., Glanz, K., & Vries, H. (1999). Computer-tailored nutrition education: Differences between two interventions. *Health Education Research, 14*(2), 249–256.

Carvalho de Menezes, M. (2016). Interventions directed at eating habits and physical activity using the transtheoretical model: A systematic review. *Nutrición Hospitalaria, 33*(5), 1194–1204. https://doi.org/10.20960/nh.586

Center for Behavioral Health Statistics and Quality. (2016). Key substance use and mental health indicators in the United States: Results from the 2015 National Survey on Drug Use and Health. HHS Publication No. SMA 16-4984, NSDUH Series H-51). http://www.samhsa.gov/data/

Cherpitel, C. J., & Ye, Y. (2008). Drug use and problem drinking associated with primary care and emergency room utilization in the US general population: Data from the 2005 National Alcohol Survey. *Drug and Alcohol Dependence, 97*(3), 226–230. https://doi.org/10.1016/j.drugalcdep.2008.03.033

Cummins, C. O., Evers, K. E., Johnson, J. L., Paiva, A., Prochaska, J. O., & Prochaska, J. M. (2004). Assessing stage of change and informed decision making for internet participation in health promotion and disease management. *Managed Care Interface, 17*(8), 27–32.

DiClemente, C. C., & Prochaska, J. O. (1982). Self-change and therapy change of smoking behavior: A comparison of processes of change in cessation and maintenance. *Addictive Behaviors, 7*(2), 133–142.

Dijkstra, A., Conijm, B., & DeVries, H. A. (2006). A match-mismatch test of a stage model of behaviour change in tobacco smoking. *Addiction, 101*(7), 1035–1043.

Dsouza, J. P., Van den Broucke, S., Pattanshetty, S., & Dhoore, W. (2021). The application of health behavior theories to promote cervical cancer screening uptake. *Public Health Nursing, 38*(6), 1039–1079. https://doi.org/10.1111/phn.12944

Etter, J.-F., Perneger, T. V., & Ronchi, A. (1997). Distributions of smokers by stage: International comparison and association with smoking prevalence. *Preventive Medicine, 26*(4), 580–585. https://doi.org/10.1006/pmed.1997.0179

Evans, J. L., Regan, R. M., Maddock, J. E., Fava, J. L., Velicer, W. F., Rossi, J. S., & Prochaska, J. O. (2000). What predicts stage of change for smoking cessation? *Annals of Behavioral Medicine, 22*(S173). Poster presented at the Twenty-first Annual Scientific Sessions of the Society of Behavioral Medicine, Nashville, TN.

Evers, K. E. (2019). *Stage-based mobile intervention for substance use disorders in primary care: Implementation and cluster-randomized trial* (Grant Proposal R44 DA044840). Pro-Change Behavior Systems, Inc. https://reporter.nih.gov/search/VAM4Q4rUcUC0IeB6NwyKWA/project-details/10173734#similar-Projects

Evers, K. E., Prochaska, J. O., Johnson, J. L., Mauriello, L. M., Padula, J. A., & Prochaska, J. M. (2006). A randomized clinical trial of a population- and transtheoretical model-based stress-management intervention. *Health Psychology, 25*(4), 521–529. https://doi.org/10.1037/0278-6133.25.4.521

Evers, K. E., Paiva, A. L., Johnson, J. L., Cummins, C. O., Prochaska, J. O., Prochaska, J. M., Padula, J., & Gökbayrak, N. S. (2012). Results of a transtheoretical model-based alcohol, tobacco and other drug intervention in middle schools. *Addictive Behaviors, 37*(9), 1009–1018. https://doi.org/10.1016/j.addbeh.2012.04.008

Farkas, A. J., Pierce, J. P., Zhu, S.-H., Rosbrook, B., Gilpin, E. A., Berry, C., & Kaplan, R. M. (1996). Addiction versus stages of change models in predicting smoking cessation. *Addiction, 91*(9), 1271–1280. https://doi.org/10.1046/j.1360-0443.1996.91912713.x

Fenn, N., Reyes, C., Monahan, K., & Robbins, M. L. (2022). How ready are young adults to participate in community service? An application of the transtheoretical model of behavior change. *American Journal of Health Promotion, 36*(1), 64–72. https://doi.org/10.1177/08901171211034742

Florence, C. S., Zhou, C., Luo, F., & Xu, L. (2016). The economic burden of prescription opioid overdose, abuse, and dependence in the United States, 2013. *Medical Care, 54*(10), 901–906. https://doi.org/10.1097/MLR.0000000000000625

de Freitas, P. P., de Menezes, M. C., dos Santos, L. C., Pimenta, A. M., Ferreira, A. V. M., & Lopes, A. C. S. (2020). The transtheoretical model is an effective weight management intervention: A randomized controlled trial. *BMC Public Health, 20*(1), 652. https://doi.org/10.1186/s12889-020-08796-1

Freud, S. (1959). *Inhibitions, symptoms and anxiety* (Standard ed., vol. 20). Hogarth Press.

Freyer-Adam, J., Baumann, S., Bischof, G., Staudt, A., Goeze, C., Gaertner, B., & John, U. (2022). Social equity in the efficacy of computer-based and in-person brief alcohol interventions among general hospital patients with at-risk alcohol use: A randomized controlled trial. *JMIR Mental Health, 9*, e31712.

Fried, T. R., Redding, C. A., Robbins, M. L., Paiva, A. L., O'Leary, J. R., & Iannone, L. (2016). Development of personalized health messages to promote engagement in advance care planning. *Journal of the American Geriatrics Society, 64*(2), 359–364. https://doi.org/10.1111/jgs.13934

Fried, T. R., Paiva, A. L., Redding, C. A., Iannone, L., O'Leary, J. R., Zenoni, M., Risi, M. M., Mejnartowicz, S., & Rossi, J. S. (2021). Effect of the STAMP (Sharing and Talking About My Preferences) intervention on completing multiple advance care planning activities in ambulatory care: A cluster randomized controlled trial. *Annals of Internal Medicine, 174*(11), 1519–1527. https://doi.org/10.7326/M21-1007

Gazabon, S. A., Morokoff, P. J., Harlow, L. L., Ward, R. M., & Quina, K. (2007). Applying the transtheoretical model to ethnically diverse women at risk for HIV. *Health Education & Behavior, 34*(2), 297–314. https://doi.org/10.1177/1090198105285328

Ghitza, U. E., & Tai, B. (2014). Challenges and opportunities for integrating preventive substance-use-care services in primary care through the Affordable Care Act. *Journal of Health Care for the Poor and Underserved, 25*(1A), 36–45. https://doi.org/10.1353/hpu.2014.0067

Hall, K. L., & Rossi, J. S. (2008). Meta-analytic examination of the strong and weak principles across 48 health behaviors. *Preventive Medicine, 46*(3), 266–274. https://doi.org/10.1016/j.ypmed.2007.11.006

Hartmann-Boyce, J., Livingstone-Banks, J., Ordóñez-Mena, J. M., Fanshawe, T. R., Lindson, N., Freeman, S. C., Sutton, A. J., Theodoulou, A., & Aveyard, P. (2021). Behavioural interventions for smoking cessation: An overview and network meta-analysis. *Cochrane Database of Systematic Reviews, 1*. https://doi.org/10.1002/14651858.CD013229.pub2

Hashemzadeh, M., Rahimi, A., Zare-Farashbandi, F., Alavi-Naeini, A. M., & Daei, A. (2019). Transtheoretical model of health behavioral change: A systematic review. *Iranian Journal of Nursing and Midwifery Research, 24*(2), 83. https://doi.org/10.4103/ijnmr.IJNMR_94_17

Henry, H., Reimer, K., Smith, C., & Reicks, M. (2006). Associations of decisional balance, processes of change, and self-efficacy with stages of change for increased fruit and vegetable intake among low-income, African-American mothers. *Journal of the American Dietetic Association*, *106*(6), 841–849. https://doi.org/10.1016/j.jada.2006.03.012

Herzog, T. A., Abrams, D. B., Emmons, K. M., Linnan, L. A., & Shadel, W. G. (1999). Do processes of change predict smoking stage movements? A prospective analysis of the transtheoretical model. *Health Psychology*, *18*(4), 369. https://doi.org/10.1037/0278-6133.18.4.369

Herzog, T. A., Abrams, D. B., Emmons, K. M., & Linnan, L. (2000). Predicting increases in readiness to quit smoking: A prospective analysis using the contemplation ladder. *Psychology & Health*, *15*(3), 369–381. https://doi.org/10.1080/08870440008401999

Hollis, J. F., Polen, M. R., Whitlock, E. P., Lichtenstein, E., Mullooly, J. P., Velicer, W. F., & Redding, C. A. (2005). Teen reach: Outcomes from a randomized, controlled trial of a tobacco reduction program for teens seen in primary medical care. *Pediatrics*, *115*(4), 981–989. https://doi.org/10.1542/peds.2004-0981

Hoving, E. (2006). Smoking and the O pattern; Predictors of transitions through the stages of change. *Health Education Research*, *21*(3), 305–314. https://doi.org/10.1093/her/cyl033

Hoy, J., Natarajan, A., & Petra, M. M. (2016). Motivational interviewing and the transtheoretical model of change: Under-explored resources for suicide intervention. *Community Mental Health Journal*, *52*(5), 559–567. https://doi.org/10.1007/s10597-016-9997-2

Imeri, H., Toth, J., Arnold, A., & Barnard, M. (2022). Use of the transtheoretical model in medication adherence: A systematic review. *Research in Social and Administrative Pharmacy*, *18*(5), 2778–2785. https://doi.org/10.1016/j.sapharm.2021.07.008

Janis, I. L., & Mann, L. (1977). *Decision making: A psychological analysis of conflict, choice, and commitment*. Free Press.

Jiménez-Zazo, F., Romero-Blanco, C., Castro-Lemus, N., Dorado-Suárez, A., & Aznar, S. (2020). Transtheoretical model for physical activity in older adults: Systematic review. *International Journal of Environmental Research and Public Health*, *17*(24), 9262. https://doi.org/10.3390/ijerph17249262

Johnson, S. S., Driskell, M.-M., Johnson, J. L., Dyment, S. J., Prochaska, J. O., Prochaska, J. M., & Bourne, L. (2006). Transtheoretical model intervention for adherence to lipid-lowering drugs. *Disease Management: DM*, *9*(2), 102–114. https://doi.org/10.1089/dis.2006.9.102

Johnson, S. S., Paiva, A. L., Cummins, C. O., Johnson, J. L., Dyment, S. J., Wright, J. A., Prochaska, J. O., Prochaska, J. M., & Sherman, K. (2008). Transtheoretical model-based multiple behavior intervention for weight management: Effectiveness on a population basis. *Preventive Medicine*, *46*(3), 238–246. https://doi.org/10.1016/j.ypmed.2007.09.010

Johnson, S. S., Levesque, D. A., Broderick, L. E., Bailey, D. G., & Kerns, R. D. (2017). Pain self-management for veterans: Development and pilot test of a stage-based mobile-optimized intervention. *JMIR Medical Informatics*, *5*(4), e40. https://doi.org/10.2196/medinform.7117

Kamioka, H., Okuizumi, H., Handa, S., Kitayuguchi, J., & Machida, R. (2022). Effect of non-surgical interventions on pain relief and symptom improvement in farmers with diseases of the musculoskeletal system or connective tissue: An exploratory systematic review based on randomized controlled trials. *Journal of Rural Medicine*, *17*(1), 1–13. https://doi.org/10.2185/jrm.2021-038

Kleis, R. R., Hoch, M. C., Hogg-Graham, R., & Hoch, J. M. (2021). The effectiveness of the transtheoretical model to improve physical activity in healthy adults: A systematic review. *Journal of Physical Activity and Health*, *18*(1), 94–108. https://doi.org/10.1123/jpah.2020-0334

Krebs, P., Prochaska, J. O., & Rossi, J. S. (2010). A meta-analysis of computer-tailored interventions for health behavior change. *Preventive Medicine*, *51*(3–4), 214–221. https://doi.org/10.1016/j.ypmed.2010.06.004

Kreuter, M. W., Strecher, V. J., & Glassman, B. (1999). One size does not fit all: The case for tailoring print materials. *Annals of Behavioral Medicine*, *21*(4), 276–283.

Levesque, D. A., Van Marter, D. F., Schneider, R. J., Bauer, M. R., Goldberg, D. N., Prochaska, J. O., & Prochaska, J. M. (2011). Randomized trial of a computer-tailored intervention for patients with depression. *American Journal of Health Promotion: AJHP*, *26*(2), 77–89. https://doi.org/10.4278/ajhp.090123-QUAN-27

Levoy, K., Salani, D. A., & Buck, H. (2019). A systematic review and gap analysis of advance care planning intervention components and outcomes among cancer patients using the transtheoretical model of health behavior change. *Journal of Pain and Symptom Management*, *57*(1), 118–139.e6. https://doi.org/10.1016/j.jpainsymman.2018.10.502

Li, X., Yang, S., Wang, Y., Yang, B., & Zhang, J. (2020). Effects of a transtheoretical model—based intervention and motivational interviewing on the management of depression in hospitalized patients with coronary heart disease: A randomized controlled trial. *BMC Public Health*, *20*(1), 420. https://doi.org/10.1186/s12889-020-08568-x

Lustria, M. L. A., Noar, S. M., Cortese, J., Van Stee, S. K., Glueckauf, R. L., & Lee, J. (2013). A meta-analysis of web-delivered tailored health behavior change interventions. *Journal of Health Communication*, *18*(9), 1039–1069. https://doi.org/10.1080/10810730.2013.768727

MacKenzie, M. A., Smith-Howell, E., Bomba, P. A., & Meghani, S. H. (2018). Respecting choices and related models of advance care planning: A systematic review of published evidence. *American Journal of Hospice & Palliative Medicine, 35*(6), 897–907. https://doi.org/10.1177/1049909117745789

Martinengo, L., Jabir, A. I., Goh, W. W. T., Lo, N. Y. W., Ho, M.-H. R., Kowatsch, T., Atun, R., Michie, S., & Tudor Car, L. (2022). Conversational agents in health care: Scoping review of their behavior change techniques and underpinning theory. *Journal of Medical Internet Research, 24*(10), e39243. https://doi.org/10.2196/39243

Mastellos, N., Gunn, L. H., Felix, L. M., Car, J., & Majeed, A. (2014). Transtheoretical model stages of change for dietary and physical exercise modification in weight loss management for overweight and obese adults. *Cochrane Database of Systematic Reviews, 2014*(2), CD008066. https://doi.org/10.1002/14651858.CD008066.pub3

Mauriello, L. M., Gökbayrak, N. S., Van Marter, D. F., Paiva, A. L., & Prochaska, J. M. (2011). An Internet-based computer-tailored intervention to promote responsible drinking: Findings from a pilot test with employed adults. *Alcoholism Treatment Quarterly, 30*(1), 91–108. https://doi.org/10.1080/07347324.2012.635528

Mulchandani, D., Alslaity, A., & Orji, R. (2022). Exploring the effectiveness of persuasive games for disease prevention and awareness and the impact of tailoring to the stages of change. *Human Computer Interaction*, 1–36. https://doi.org/10.1080/07370024.2022.2057858

Nakabayashi, J., Melo, G. R., & Toral, N. (2020). Transtheoretical model-based nutritional interventions in adolescents: A systematic review. *BMC Public Health, 20*(1), 1543. https://doi.org/10.1186/s12889-020-09643-z

National Drug Intelligence Center. (2011). *National Threat Assessment: The economic impact of illicit drug use on American society.* Department of Justice.

Nigg, C. R., Burbank, P. M., Padula, C., Dufresne, R., Rossi, J. S., Velicer, W. F., Laforge, R. G., & Prochaska, J. O. (1999). Stages of change across ten health risk behaviors for older adults. *The Gerontologist, 39*(4), 473–482. https://doi.org/10.1093/geront/39.4.473

Noar, S. M., Benac, C. N., & Harris, M. S. (2007). Does tailoring matter? Meta-analytic review of tailored print health behavior change interventions. *Psychological Bulletin, 133*(4), 673–693. https://doi.org/10.1037/0033-2909.133.4.673

Norcross, J. C., Krebs, P. M., & Prochaska, J. O. (2011). Stages of change. *Journal of Clinical Psychology, 67*(2), 143–154. https://doi.org/10.1002/jclp.20758

Norman, G. J., Adams, M. A., Calfas, K. J., Covin, J., Sallis, J. F., Rossi, J. S., Redding, C. A., Cella, J., & Patrick, K. (2007). A randomized trial of a multicomponent intervention for adolescent sun protection behaviors. *Archives of Pediatrics & Adolescent Medicine, 161*(2), 146–152. https://doi.org/10.1001/archpedi.161.2.146

Nunes, H. E. G., Silva, D. A. S., & Gonçalves, E. C. de A. (2017). Prevalence and factors associated with stages of behavior change for physical activity in adolescents: A systematic review. *World Journal of Pediatrics, 13*(3), 202–209. https://doi.org/10.1007/s12519-017-0027-4

O'Keefe, D. J. (2016). *Persuasion: Theory and research* 3rd ed. SAGE.

Patton, D. E., Hughes, C. M., Cadogan, C. A., & Ryan, C. A. (2017). Theory-based interventions to improve medication adherence in older adults prescribed polypharmacy: A systematic review. *Drugs & Aging, 34*(2), 97–113. https://doi.org/10.1007/s40266-016-0426-6

Paxton, R. J., Nigg, C. R., Motl, R. W., McGee, K., McCurdy, D., Matthai, C. H., & Dishman, R. K. (2008). Are constructs of the Transtheoretical model for physical activity measured equivalently between sexes, age groups, and ethnicities? *Annals of Behavioral Medicine, 35*(3), 308–318. https://doi.org/10.1007/s12160-008-9035-x

Peterson, A. V., Kealey, K., Mann, S., Marek, P., & Sarason, I. (2000). Hutchinson smoking prevention project: Long-term randomized trial in school-based tobacco use prevention—results on smoking. *Journal of the National Cancer Institute, 92*(24), 1979–1991. https://doi.org/10.1093/jnci/92.24.1979

Prochaska, J. O. (1984). *Systems of psychotherapy: A transtheoretical analysis.* Oxford University Press.

Prochaska, J. O. (2004). Population treatment for addictions. *Current Directions in Psychological Science, 13*(6), 242–246. https://doi.org/10.1111/j.0963-7214.2004.00317.x

Prochaska, J. M. (2007). The Transtheoretical model applied to the community and the workplace. *Journal of Health Psychology, 12*(1), 198–200. https://doi.org/10.1177/1359105307071754

Prochaska, J. O. (2013). Transtheoretical model of behavior change. In M. D. Gellman & J. R. Turner (Eds.), *Encyclopedia of behavioral medicine* (pp. 1997–2000). Springer. http://link.springer.com/10.1007/978-1-4419-1005-9_70

Prochaska, J. O., & DiClemente, C. C. (1983). Stages and processes of self-change of smoking: Toward an integrative model of change. *Journal of Consulting and Clinical Psychology, 51*(3), 390–395. https://doi.org/10.1037/0022-006X.51.3.390

Prochaska, J. O., & Norcross, J. C. (1979). *Systems of psychotherapy: A transtheoretical analysis.* Oxford University Press.

Prochaska, J. O., & Norcross, J. C. (2001). Stages of change. *Psychotherapy: Theory, Research, Practice, Training, 38*(4), 443–448. https://doi.org/10.1037/0033-3204.38.4.443

Prochaska, J. O., & Norcross, J. C. (2018). *Systems of psychotherapy: A transtheoretical Analysis*. Oxford University Press.

Prochaska, J. O., DiClemente, C. C., Velicer, W. F., Ginpil, S., & Norcross, J. C. (1985). Predicting change in smoking status for self-changers. *Addictive Behaviors, 10*(4), 395–406.

Prochaska, J. O., DiClemente, C. C., & Norcross, J. C. (1992). In search of how people change. Applications to addictive behaviors. *The American Psychologist, 47*(9), 1102–1114. https://doi.org/10.1037//0003-066x.47.9.1102

Prochaska, J. O., Velicer, W. F., Rossi, J. S., Goldstein, M. G., Marcus, B. H., Rakowski, W., Fiore, C., Harlow, L. L., Redding, C. A., Rosenbloom, D., & Rossi, S. R. (1994). Stages of change and decisional balance for 12 problem behaviors. *Health Psychology, 13*(1), 39. http://psycnet.apa.org/journals/hea/13/1/39/

Prochaska, J. O., Velicer, W. F., Fava, J. L., Ruggiero, L., Laforge, R. G., Rossi, J. S., Johnson, S. S., & Lee, P. A. (2001). Counselor and stimulus control enhancements of a stage-matched expert system intervention for smokers in a managed care setting. *Preventive Medicine, 32*(1), 23–32. http://www.sciencedirect.com/science/article/pii/S0091743500907679

Prochaska, J. J., Delucchi, K., & Hall, S. M. (2004). A meta-analysis of smoking cessation interventions with individuals in substance abuse treatment or recovery. *Journal of Consulting and Clinical Psychology, 72*(6), 1144–1156. https://doi.org/10.1037/0022-006X.72.6.1144

Prochaska, J. O., Evers, K. E., Prochaska, J. M., Van Marter, D., & Johnson, J. L. (2007). Efficacy and effectiveness trials: Examples from smoking cessation and bullying prevention. *Journal of Health Psychology, 12*(1), 170–178. https://doi.org/10.1177/1359105307071751

Prochaska, J. O., Wright, J. A., & Velicer, W. F. (2008). Evaluating theories of health behavior change: A hierarchy of criteria applied to the transtheoretical model. *Applied Psychology. An International Review, 57*(4), 561–588. https://doi.org/10.1111/j.1464-0597.2008.00345.x

Prochaska, J. J., Hall, S. E., Delucchi, K., & Hall, S. M. (2014). Efficacy of initiating tobacco dependence treatment in inpatient psychiatry: A randomized controlled trial. *American Journal of Public Health, 104*(8), 1557–1565. https://doi.org/10.2105/AJPH.2013.301403

Rakowski, W., Ehrich, B., Goldstein, M. G., Rimer, B. K., Pearlman, D. N., Clark, M. A., Velicer, W. F., & Woolverton, H. (1998). Increasing mammography among women aged 40–74 by use of a stage-matched, tailored intervention. *Preventive Medicine, 27*(5), 748–756. https://doi.org/10.1006/pmed.1998.0354

Ravi, K., Indrapriyadharshini, K., & Madankumar, P. (2021). Application of health behavioral models in smoking cessation—a systematic review. *Indian Journal of Public Health, 65*(2), 103. https://doi.org/10.4103/ijph.IJPH_1351_20

Redding, C. A., Prochaska, J. O., Paiva, A., Rossi, J. S., Velicer, W., Blissmer, B. J., Greene, G. W., Robbins, M. L., & Sun, X. (2011). Baseline stage, severity, and effort effects differentiate stable smokers from maintainers and relapsers. *Substance Use & Misuse, 46*(13), 1664–1674. https://doi.org/10.3109/10826084.2011.565853

Rhodes, R. E., Boudreau, P., Josefsson, K. W., & Ivarsson, A. (2021). Mediators of physical activity behaviour change interventions among adults: A systematic review and meta-analysis. *Health Psychology Review, 15*(2), 272–286. https://doi.org/10.1080/17437199.2019.1706614

Rios, L. E., Herval, Á. M., Ferreira, R. C., & Freire, M. do C. M. (2019). Prevalences of stages of change for smoking cessation in adolescents and associated factors: Systematic review and meta-analysis. *Journal of Adolescent Health, 64*(2), 149–157. https://doi.org/10.1016/j.jadohealth.2018.09.005

Rogers, Carl R. (1951). Client-centered therapy. *Journal of Clinical Psychology, 7*(3), 294–295. https://doi.org/10.1002/1097-4679(195107)7:3<294::AID-JCLP2270070325>3.0.CO;2-O

Romain, A. J., Bortolon, C., Gourlan, M., Carayol, M., Decker, E., Lareyre, O., Ninot, G., Boiché, J., & Bernard, P. (2018). Matched or nonmatched interventions based on the transtheoretical model to promote physical activity. A meta-analysis of randomized controlled trials. *Journal of Sport and Health Science, 7*(1), 50–57. https://doi.org/10.1016/j.jshs.2016.10.007

Rosen, C. S. (2000). Is the sequencing of change processes by stage consistent across health problems? A meta-analysis *Health Psychology, 19*(6), 593–604.

Rossi, J. S. (1992). *Common processes of change across nine problem behaviors*. Paper presented at the 100th meeting of the American Psychological Association, Washington, D. C.

Sacks, J. J., Gonzales, K. R., Bouchery, E. E., Tomedi, L. E., & Brewer, R. D. (2015). 2010 National and state costs of excessive alcohol consumption. *American Journal of Preventive Medicine, 49*(5), e73–e79. https://doi.org/10.1016/j.amepre.2015.05.031

Salinas-Martínez, A. M., Castañeda-Vásquez, D. E., García-Morales, N. G., Oliva-Sosa, N. E., de-la-Garza-Salinas, L. H., Núñez-Rocha, G. M., & Ramírez-Aranda, J. M. (2018). Stages of change for mammography among Mexican women and a decisional balance comparison across countries. *Journal of Cancer Education*, *33*(6), 1230–1238. https://doi.org/10.1007/s13187-017-1236-1

Sanaeinasab, H., Saffari, M., Valipour, F., Alipour, H. R., Sepandi, M., Al Zaben, F., & Koenig, H. G. (2018). The effectiveness of a model-based health education intervention to improve ergonomic posture in office computer workers: A randomized controlled trial. *International Archives of Occupational and Environmental Health*, *91*(8), 951–962. https://doi.org/10.1007/s00420-018-1336-1

Selçuk-Tosun, A., & Zincir, H. (2019). The effect of a transtheoretical model–based motivational interview on self-efficacy, metabolic control, and health behaviour in adults with type 2 diabetes mellitus: A randomized controlled trial. *International Journal of Nursing Practice*, *25*(4), e12742. https://doi.org/10.1111/ijn.12742

Skinner, B. F. (1966). Contingencies of reinforcement in the design of a culture. *Behavioral Science*, *11*(3), 159–166. https://doi.org/10.1002/bs.3830110302

Spencer, L., Pagell, F., Hallion, M. E., & Adams, T. B. (2002). Applying the transtheoretical model to tobacco cessation and prevention: A review of literature. *American Journal of Health Promotion*, *17*(1), 7–71. https://doi.org/10.4278/0890-1171-17.1.7

Sun, X., Prochaska, J. O., Velicer, W. F., & Laforge, R. G. (2007). Transtheoretical principles and processes for quitting smoking: A 24-month comparison of a representative sample of quitters, relapsers and non-quitters. *Addictive Behaviors*, *32*(12), 2707–2726.

Sussman, S. Y., Ayala, N., Pokhrel, P., & Herzog, T. A. (2022). Reflections on the continued popularity of the transtheoretical model. *Health Behavior Research*, *5*(3). 2. https://doi.org/10.4148/2572-1836.1128

Tseng, H.-M., Liao, S.-F., Wen, Y.-P., & Chuang, Y.-J. (2017). Stages of change concept of the transtheoretical model for healthy eating links health literacy and diabetes knowledge to glycemic control in people with type 2 diabetes. *Primary Care Diabetes*, *11*(1), 29–36. https://doi.org/10.1016/j.pcd.2016.08.005

Velicer, W. F., Redding, C. A., Sun, X., & Prochaska, J. O. (2007). Demographic variables, smoking variables, and outcome across five studies. *Health Psychology*, *26*(3), 278–287.

Vincent-Doe, A., Sneed, R., Jordan, T., Key, K., Bailey, R. S., Jefferson, B. B., Sanders, R. P. E., Brewer, A., Scott, J. B., Calvin, K., Summers, M., Farmer, B., & Johnson-Lawrence, V. (2022). Exploring the readiness of African-American churches to engage in a community-engaged blood pressure reduction research study: Lessons learned from the church challenge. *Journal of Community Engagement and Scholarship*, *14*(2), 10.

Wewers, M. E., Stillman, F. A., Hartman, A. M., & Shopland, D. R. (2003). Distribution of daily smokers by Stage of Change: Current population survey results. *Preventive Medicine*, *36*(6), 710–720. https://doi.org/10.1016/S0091-7435(03)00044-6

Winter, S. J., Sheats, J. L., & King, A. C. (2016). The use of behavior change techniques and theory in technologies for cardiovascular disease prevention and treatment in adults: A comprehensive review. *Progress in Cardiovascular Diseases*, *58*(6), 605–612. https://doi.org/10.1016/j.pcad.2016.02.005

Yang, G. (2001). Smoking cessation in China: Findings from the 1996 national prevalence survey. *Tobacco Control*, *10*(2), 170–174. https://doi.org/10.1136/tc.10.2.170

PART THREE

MODELS OF INTERPERSONAL HEALTH BEHAVIOR

CHAPTER 8

INTRODUCTION TO MODELS OF INTERPERSONAL INFLUENCES ON HEALTH BEHAVIOR

Racquel E. Kohler
K. Viswanath

Humans are social beings, and the power of social connections to influence health is one of the most pervasive, consistent findings in the public health and social science literature. There have been myriad and divergent changes in our social fabric over the last two decades. Almost a quarter-century ago, in his book *Bowling Alone*, political scientist Robert Putnam (2000) documented how participation in many traditional social groups and structures (such as bowling leagues, religious organizations, and parent/teacher associations) has been diminishing. The US Surgeon General drew attention to the diminishing social connections as the reason for the loneliness "epidemic" and issued an Advisory and guidance to promote social connections (Office of Surgeon General, 2023). The importance of interpersonal connections is further amplified by an exponential growth in social media and virtual communications as important ways for people to connect, with an estimated 4.7 billion users worldwide (Data Reportal, 2023; Pew Research Center, 2021). Social media use has been blamed for both promoting and diminishing social connections, with mixed evidence (See Chapter 22).

The mechanisms that link individuals' social contexts with health effects revolve around two important social processes: social support and social influence. Both are products of how strongly or weakly individuals are integrated into the society around them. Integration in the form of ties to social networks or to larger social institutions plays a profound role in an individual's health (Holt-Lunstad et al., 2010).

A fundamental assumption driving the theories and models in this section is the reciprocal influence between cognitions, affect, and behaviors of individuals and the environments around them. This chapter introduces these theories and models, describes their defining characteristics, and discusses some future research directions.

Social Cognitive Theory

Social Cognitive Theory (SCT) addresses the classic tension between human agency and the social structure by emphasizing the construct of *reciprocal determinism*, which suggests that human agency and the environment interact with and influence

Health Behavior: Theory, Research, and Practice, Sixth Edition. Edited by Karen Glanz, Barbara K. Rimer, and K. Viswanath.
© 2024 John Wiley & Sons, Inc. Published 2024 by John Wiley & Sons, Inc.
Companion website: www.wiley.com/go/glanz/healthbehavior6e

each other, leading to individual and social change. As Mantey, Hunt, Hoelscher, and Kelder explain in Chapter 9, underlying SCT is the proposition that individuals have the capacity to change or even build the environment. By emphasizing the *dynamism in the interactions* among human behavior, personal cognitive factors, and social-environmental influences, SCT moves away from an exclusive focus on one level or the other and has been one of the most influential theories in health behavior.

The various key SCT constructs and the relationships among them are detailed in the chapter, but it is worth noting that many researchers have tested only selective concepts from the theory rather than the entire theory. A few deserve particular attention: self-efficacy and its counterpart, collective efficacy, and observational learning or modeling. *Self-efficacy* is one of the most widely used constructs by health behavior theorists and practitioners and some have gone so far as to argue that it is the "central mechanism of behavior change" (Cervone, 2000). Self-efficacy has been applied to many domains of health behavior and has been adopted for use in other theories, such as the Health Belief Model (Chapter 5), the Theory of Planned Behavior, Integrative Behavioral Model, and Reasoned Action Approach (Chapter 6). *Collective efficacy*, a community-level concept, has been argued by some as promoting social cohesion and reducing health disparities (Butel & Braun, 2019). A major appeal of the concepts of self-efficacy and collective efficacy is that they are modifiable factors.

The concept of *observational learning* (or *modeling*) proposes that behavior change may occur as a result of observing others. This idea has been a deep vein mined in a variety of disciplines that explain phenomena such as media violence, intervention skills to address substance abuse, and adapting new behaviors and skills.

Models of Social Support and Health

Holt-Lunstad and Proctor (Chapter 10) provide a clear conceptualization of social support and summarize the empirical evidence linking social support to good health. A key point they make is that there is an important distinction between perceived support and received support. *Perceived support*, or the expectation that others will provide support if it is needed, has been consistently associated with better health. *Received support*, or the actual provision of support by another person, has a more complicated association with health. Sometimes received support has a positive association with good health, but other times it has been linked with adverse effects on health. It has been suggested that the effect of received support is dependent on whether the support receiver perceives the support to be responsive to their needs.

In view of strong empirical evidence for the health-promoting power of perceived support, consider how interventions to increase behavior-specific perceived support might look. Rather than engaging in provider-driven support, support providers could be trained in (1) how to help support recipients articulate the form of support that they think will be most helpful and (2) how to support individuals attempting to change health behavior. Involving recipients in planning and developing social support programs will likely increase their acceptability and effectiveness. But, of course, even when people in programs can articulate the support they prefer, it is not assured that their supporters will fulfill their needs.

The relationship of social support to loneliness was examined in a meta-analysis which showed that perceived social support is strongly and negatively associated with loneliness, thus identifying one potential solution to the "loneliness epidemic" raised by the US Surgeon General (Zhang & Dong, 2022).

Holt-Lunstad and Proctor raised an intriguing issue in the randomized trials they described, which is whether support recipients must be aware of the support that they are receiving for it to be health promoting. This may be a fruitful line of research for developing and evaluating effective social support interventions.

Social Networks and Health Behavior

A related but distinct concept is *social networks*, whose importance has grown with burgeoning social media in contemporary life (Chapter 22). Social network theory (SNT) focuses on the structure and system-level properties of the web of social relationships within which individuals live. Social network analysis provides tools for understanding how social contexts influence decision-making processes and actions. In Chapter 11, Valente and Piombo define the important components of SNT and social network analysis and provide examples of how they inform health behavior interventions.

Social network analysis quantifies the extent to which members of one's social network endorse certain attitudes or engage in specific behaviors or in other ways influence cognitions, affect, and behaviors. Research suggests that when people are considering how often an unhealthy or risky behavior (such as smoking) is being performed by their peers, they tend to overestimate prevalence. On the other hand, people tend to underestimate the extent to which healthy behaviors are being performed. Social network analysis provides information necessary for an accurate descriptive norm among network members, thus offering data to influence people's behaviors to be more in line with the accurate—and ideally, healthy—behavioral norm (Berkowitz, 2003). By mapping social networks and analyzing individuals' positions within their networks, those who have many ties to others (are highly central network members), and those who bridge between disparate subgroups within a network can be identified and recruited to be change agents for their communities.

Homophily is a critical concept in SNT. SNT posits that when a high proportion of network members are very similar to each other, it is difficult to effect change among network members (Valente, 2010). One key finding from a recent systematic review suggests that *selection* of friends who are similar to themselves in health behaviors (homophily), good or bad, reinforced member behaviors (Montgomery et al., 2020). Social influence, whereby friends influence each other, is another important social process within a network.

Flow of information is another critical feature of networks. A network may include those who consider themselves "health mavens" interested in sharing knowledge among their network members (Hayashi et al., 2020). Their impact on health behaviors requires more work. The role of social networks attained greater importance during the COVID-19 pandemic with the assumption that networks influence information sharing, whether accurate or not, and that network norms may influence adoption of public health prevention behaviors like vaccination (Rabin & Kohler, 2023).

Stress, Coping Adaptation, and Health Behavior

The experience of stress is pervasive, and its potential adverse effects on health are well-known. In Chapter 12, Woods-Giscombe and Bey describe the challenges in studying stress, since it is "referred to as a stimulus, a response, and an interaction."

The authors propose that stress affects health through two pathways. The first, the behavioral pathway, opens possibilities of how the different strategies people use to cope with stress influence the negative or positive impact that stress has on health. They explicitly mention the importance of culture-specific coping strategies. Second is a physiological pathway that affects the body's physiological conditions or systems including hormones and the well-known allostatic load (McEwen, 2012).

New to this edition is the focus on stressors that stem from racism, discrimination, and inequalities (see Chapter 14). Giscombe-Woods and Bey assert that even though the effects of stress on health and the importance of coping strategies to buffer stress's impact on health are well-established, stress among racial and ethnic minorities is understudied. Some exposures to stressors persist for long periods of time while others are of short duration. The experience of racism is often persistent over time and across contexts, resulting in profound physiological and psychological changes (Krieger, 2014; Kwate and Goodman, 2015). In contrast, daily hassles might include getting caught in traffic or having an argument, and these types of stressors usually manifest less intense, shorter-duration responses.

The authors assert that measures of stress that account for stressors from identifying with a racial or ethnic minority group are more robust than generic stress measures. Stress research, including concepts of "weathering" and "John Henryism" provides a more complete understanding of the impact of stress and stressors on health of minorities and health inequities. *Weathering* posits that the impact of stress on African American women is cumulative, stemming from experiences of exclusion from social, political, and economic opportunities. Thus, they argue that stress experienced by African American women is gendered. On the other hand, *John Henryism* draws attention to the adequacy of resources and hypothesizes and high degree of coping through hard work under high stress and limited resources could lead to unhealthy outcomes. Some studies show that the John Henryism type of coping may also be protective. How stress affects different racial and ethnic minorities and how it is gendered remains an important area of inquiry.

The authors also review frameworks that focus on adoption of different types of coping strategies against stress, including contemplative practices, such as mindfulness, positive emotions, spirituality, and religion (Davidson, 2021). Turning to specific interventions, the authors draw on the *Superwoman Schema* (SWS) to explain stress and coping among African American women. The SWS is characterized by expectations to project strength, suppression of emotions, and determination to succeed despite the odds and obligation to help others. High scores on SWS question items are associated with higher stress, and the authors are developing interventions drawing on mindfulness to cope with it.

Future Directions

If there is one defining theme of the chapters in this section, it is that the web of relationships in which we are embedded influences how we learn about the world, our emotional responses and feelings of belonging, the decisions we make, and how we cope with stress. These chapters convey a rich understanding of the influence of interpersonal interactions on health and their underlying mechanisms of action. Even so, some important areas for further research remain. These include matching the best strategy to a given situation; expanding our understanding of the roles of social class, race, and ethnicity; intersectionality; and examining how new information and communication technologies (ICTs) affect social support, networks, and health behaviors. While many strategies to strengthen social relationships are available, there is little research to aid in deciding which strategy to use in any given situation.

The roles of social class, race, and ethnicity provide other fruitful avenues for inquiry. These three factors all influence interpersonal relationships, the support that we receive (or perceive), and the stress that we experience. The combined effect of class and race could be even more devastating to individual health than class or race alone (Williams et al., 2019). However, we are only now beginning to develop an understanding of how the accumulation of daily experiences due to racism or classism or intersections of race and ethnicity, class, place, and gender may affect health. Important questions to explore on this issue include: What are the effects, including cumulative effects, on interpersonal interactions and health at the intersection of class, race and ethnicity, and gender?

Platforms such as online support groups and social media have created important new opportunities for seeking and offering information and other types of support. However, the role of virtual social interactions and internet-based exchange of social support is only beginning to be rigorously explored and evaluated. To what extent will computer-mediated relationships prove to be health promoting? Will online communication increase the number of social relationships but reduce the quality or depth of those networks? Or is it creating an entirely new type of support that is enabled by the online domain? Can all the mechanisms introduced in this chapter for enhancing the health-promoting aspects of social relationships take place in a virtual environment? How should virtual interventions be developed to be optimally effective? The chapter on social media in a later part of this book (Chapter 22) reviews some of this work, but the answers are elusive. Also, there are benefits of giving support, and this area requires further investigation. The entire area of study of ICTs in health can benefit from theories described in the chapters in this section. For whatever reason, research in ICT and health seldom draws from the work described here.

Models and theories of interpersonal influences on health behavior stand at the critical juncture where the social environment molds and modifies intraindividual factors, such as cognitions, emotions, and health behaviors. A thorough understanding and appreciation for issues at this level will assist in developing more effective interventions and policies to enhance individual and population health.

References

Berkowitz, A. D. (2003). Applications of social norms theory to other health and social justice issues. In H. W. Perkins (Ed.) *The social norms approach to preventing school and college age substance abuse: A handbook for educators, counselors, clinicians* (pp. 259–279). San Francisco, CA: Jossey Bass.

Butel, J., & Braun, K. L. (2019). The role of collective efficacy in reducing health disparities: A systematic review. *Family and Community Health*, 42(1), 8–19. https://doi.org/10.1097/FCH.0000000000000206.

Cervone, D. (2000). Thinking about self-efficacy. *Behavior Modification*, 24(1), 30–56. https://doi.org/10.1177/0145445500241002.

Data Reportal. (2023). *Global social media stats*. Datareportal.com. https://datareportal.com.

Davidson R. J. (2021). Mindfulness and more: Toward a science of human flourishing. *Psychosomatic Medicine*, 83(6), 665–668. https://doi.org/10.1097/PSY.0000000000000960.

Hayashi, H., Tan, A. S. L., Kawachi, I., Ishikawa, Y., Kondo, K., Kondo, N., Tsuboya, T., & Viswanath, K. (2020). Interpersonal diffusion of health information: Health information mavenism among people age 65 and over in Japan. *Health Communication*, *35*(7), 804–814. https://doi.org/10.1080/10410236.2019.1593078.

Holt-Lunstad, J., Smith, T. B., & Layton, J. B. (2010). Social relationships and mortality risk: A meta-analytic review. *PLoS Medicine*, *7*(7), e1000316. https://doi.org/10.1371/journal.pmed.1000316.

Krieger, N. (2014). On the causal interpretation of race. *Epidemiology*, *25*(6), 937–938. https://doi.org/10.1097/EDE.0000000000000185.

Kwate, N. O., & Goodman, M. S. (2015). Cross-sectional and longitudinal effects of racism on mental health among residents of Black neighborhoods in New York City. *American Journal of Public Health*, *105*(4), 711–718. https://doi.org/10.2105/AJPH.2014.302243.

McEwen, B. S. (2012). Brain on stress: How the social environment gets under the skin. *Proceedings of the National Academy of Sciences*, *10*(Suppl. 2), 17180–17185.

Montgomery, S. C., Donnelly, M., Bhatnagar, P., Carlin, A., Kee, F., & Hunter, R. F. (2020). Peer social network processes and adolescent health behaviors: A systematic review. *Preventive Medicine*, *130*, 105900. https://doi.org/10.1016/j.ypmed.2019.105900.

Office of the Surgeon General (OSG). (2023). Our epidemic of loneliness and isolation: The U.S. Surgeon General's Advisory on the Healing Effects of Social Connection and Community. US Department of Health and Human Services. https://www.hhs.gov/sites/default/files/surgeon-general-social-connection-advisory.pdf.

Pew Research Center. (2021). Social media use in 2021. https://www.pewresearch.org/internet/2021/04/07/social-media-use-in-2021/.

Putnam, R. (2000). *Bowling alone: The collapse and revival of American community*. New York: Simon & Schuster.

Rabin, Y., & Kohler, R. E. (2023). COVID-19 vaccination messengers, communication channels, and messages trusted among Black communities in the USA: A review. *Journal of Racial and Ethnic Health Disparities*, 1–14. https://doi.org/10.1007/s40615-023-01858-1.

Valente, T. (2010). *Social networks and health: Models, methods and applications*. New York: Oxford University Press.

Williams, D. R., Lawrence, J. A., & Davis, B. A. (2019). Racism and health: Evidence and needed research. *Annual Review of Public Health*, *40*, 105–125. https://doi.org/10.1146/annurev-publhealth-040218-043750.

Zhang, X., & Dong, S. (2022). The relationships between social support and loneliness: A meta-analysis and review. *Acta Psychologica*, *227*, 103616. https://doi.org/10.1016/j.actpsy.2022.103616.

CHAPTER 9

SOCIAL COGNITIVE THEORY AND HEALTH BEHAVIOR

Dale S. Mantey
Ethan T. Hunt
Deanna M. Hoelscher
Steven H. Kelder

KEY POINTS

This chapter will:

- Define and describe the history and concepts of Social Cognitive Theory (SCT)

- Describe how SCT concepts explain health-promoting/compromising behaviors and can guide intervention design.

- Illustrate the application of key SCT concepts and principles in two case studies: electronic cigarette (e-cigarette) use prevention in a diverse population of adolescents and obesity prevention among pregnant women at Federally Qualified Health Centers (FQHCs)

Vignette

Marcos is in sixth grade and recently joined the science club. He notices that several older kids, and even some in his grade, started using e-cigarettes (vaping). They are using flavors of mint and green apple, and he does not want to stick out for turning it down if one of the older kids offers him their e-cigarette; he's not sure how he'd say "no" in that situation. Marcos also remembers that when his older brother was caught vaping at school, he was grounded for a long time and had to miss a few basketball games.

What forces are at play as Marco decides what to do? Marcos may notice that many of his peers are vaping, and he wants to fit in. That is, he holds positive social norms toward e-cigarette use as a result of seeing his peers vaping and has positive outcome expectations of vaping (enjoying the flavors; fitting in). Further, Marcos may not yet have the confidence and capacity to refuse offers to vape in all situations. SCT refers to these feelings and beliefs as a gap in self-efficacy and skills to resist e-cigarette use.

Marcos may also be concerned that he could lose his spot in the science club as a possible negative consequence of using e-cigarettes—that is, he also has negative outcome expectations. The negative perceptions of vaping held by Marcos are not rooted in his own personal vaping experience but are, instead, a consequence of observational learning from seeing what happened to his brother as a consequence of e-cigarette use. Marcos' dilemma can thus be interpreted through the lens of several important Social Cognitive Theory (SCT) constructs.

Background

SCT originated with simple experiments to understand how individuals learn new behaviors and is now a leading behavioral theory for research and practice. Early versions of social learning theory include Miller and Dollard's work on imitation of behavior among animals and humans (Miller, & Dollard, 1941); Rotter's application

Health Behavior: Theory, Research, and Practice, Sixth Edition. Edited by Karen Glanz, Barbara K. Rimer, and K. Viswanath.
© 2024 John Wiley & Sons, Inc. Published 2024 by John Wiley & Sons, Inc.
Companion website: www.wiley.com/go/glanz/healthbehavior6e

of learning principles to clinical psychology (Rotter, 1954, 1966) that focused on reinforcement; and Mischel's emphasis on cognitive constructs in learning theory (Mischel, 1973).

In 1977, Dr. Albert Bandura published a groundbreaking textbook (Bandura & Walters, 1977) and a seminal article (Bandura, 1977) on self-efficacy, the fundamental construct of SCT. Bandura expanded on theories of learning and cognition, which, at the time, theorized behavior acquisition and behavior enactment largely as conditioned responses to stimuli (Pavlov, 1927) and positive or negative reinforcement (Skinner, 1953). Bandura's articulation of SCT proposed that: (1) individuals, through their cognitions, are engaged actively in the relationship between stimulus (reinforcement) and response (behavior) (Bandura, 2001); and (2) an individual's cognitions (thoughts or perceptions) about the relationship between stimulus and response can be learned through observation of *social role modeling*, even without the direct experience of receiving reinforcement (Bandura, 1977; Bandura & Walters, 1977). This understanding has implications for health behaviors and health.

SCT has been adopted widely as a guiding theory to develop effective public health interventions that inform, enable, guide, and facilitate health-promoting behaviors (Bandura, 2004). Through the core construct of *reciprocal determinism*, SCT provides guidance to identify predictors of behavior and design behavioral change strategies within the context of the social and environmental determinants of health. SCT explains how individuals may observe and subsequently adopt risky or health-compromising behaviors as a result of exposure to mass media and communication influencing norms and behavior (Bandura, 2009), even across cultures (Ferguson et al., 2017; Lorenzo-Blanco et al., 2019). For example, SCT has been used to develop adolescent health interventions targeting adolescents *and* their parents, schools, and other influential *social role models* (Perry et al., 1992; Sly et al., 2005; Thomas et al., 2013, 2015).

SCT-guided interventions have been used to prevent and reduce adolescent tobacco use when delivered in both English and Spanish language versions in the United States (Prokhorov et al., 2008, 2010, 2012) and other countries (Nădăşan et al., 2017; Prokhorov et al., 2012; Tamí-Maury et al., 2019; Vishwakarma et al., 2021).

This chapter describes the concepts, constructs, and hypothesized causal mechanisms of SCT and provides two case studies of interventions found to be feasible and show evidence of effectively influencing health behaviors in different populations (pregnant women; infants; adolescents) and across various settings (low-income healthcare safety net clinics; sociodemographically diverse schools).

Major Constructs

SCT proposes that behavior is the product of a dynamic, multidirectional interaction between (1) personal cognitive influences, (2) social/environmental influences, and (3) supporting behavioral factors. The three domains of behavioral influences have a shared, mediating relationship defined as *reciprocal determinism* (Figure 9.1). *Reciprocal determinism* assumes that each determinant of behavior is changing (or changeable) while also influencing (and being influenced by) the remaining determinants. Reciprocal determinism is a foundational concept of SCT and provides a framework for

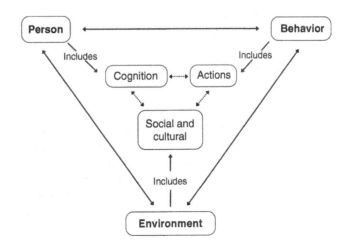

Figure 9.1 Reciprocal Determinism

understanding influences on behavior and behavior change. The concepts of SCT are translated into several major constructs to observe and target determinants of behavior.

Initiation of substance use is a health-compromising behavior that provides an excellent lens through which to understand the application of SCT and reciprocal determinism. For example, if the targeted behavioral outcome is resisting peer pressure to drink alcohol, an SCT-guided intervention would focus on: (1) practicing refusal skills to deflect peer pressure to use alcohol (supporting behavior), (2) increasing self-efficacy to strengthen refusal skills to resist peer pressure toward alcohol use (person), and (3) correcting normative beliefs about the social and physical consequences of use and the acceptability of resisting peer pressure toward alcohol use (environment). This section will describe the major constructs of SCT and their application in understanding and influencing health behavior. The constructs, their definitions, and examples are summarized in Table 9.1.

Table 9.1 Major Constructs from Social Cognitive Theory

Human behavior is explained by SCT in terms of *reciprocal determinism*. An individual's behavior is determined by a triadic, dynamic, and reciprocal relationship with cognitive processes, and the physical or social environment.

Personal Cognitive Influence on Behavior: Mental abilities for processing information, applying knowledge, and changing preferences and behaviors.

Construct	Definition	Illustration
Self-Efficacy	A person's confidence in their ability to perform a behavior that leads to an outcome.	Confidence is enhanced through mastery experiences, social modeling, verbal persuasion, and practicing under stress-free conditions.
Collective-Efficacy	A person's belief about a group of individuals' abilities to perform organized actions striving to achieve an outcome.	Group efficacy is enhanced by shared goals, open communication, teamwork, and prior success.
Knowledge	The knowledge necessary to perform a behavior.	Knowledge is often broken into specific steps; e.g., to cook a healthy meal one needs to know a recipe, where to purchase healthy ingredients, and methods of preparation.
Outcome Expectations	Beliefs about the expected consequence, positive and negative, of one's own behavior.	Expected consequences can be divided into *physical* (condoms protect against STD's) or *social* (if I'm kind and generous I'll have more friends).
Value Expectation	The value, positive or negative, that an individual ascribes to the outcome of a behavior.	Also known as the *functional meaning* of a behavior; e.g., when people see me smoke cigarettes they think I'm cool, or cooking healthy meals for my children means I'm a good parent.

Social and Environmental Influence on Behavior: The physical and social factors in an individual's environment that affect a person's behavior.

Construct	Definition	Illustration
Observational Learning	A type of learning in which a person learns new information and behaviors by observing the behaviors of others.	Accomplished by observing a peer leader or influential role model performing a behavior and achieving a positive or negative outcome. Methods include social media, mass media, behavioral journalism, or dramatic performances such as TV, plays, and movies.
Normative Beliefs	Cultural norms and beliefs about the social acceptability of a behavior.	Interventions often seek to correct normative beliefs such as adolescents' common misperceptions about how many of their peers smoke cigarettes, drink alcohol, or have risky sex.
Social Support	Belief one is cared for, has assistance available from other people, and is part of a supportive social network.	Interventions often seek to provide informational, instrumental, or emotional support to improve the development and adherence to healthy behavior changes.
Opportunities and Barriers	Tools, resources, and attributes of the social or physical environmental that make behaviors harder or easier to perform.	In many situations, it is possible to modify behaviors through *opportunities* (e.g., required daily physical education) and *barriers* (e.g., restricted access to tobacco).

Supporting Behavioral Factors: Individual actions that can be categorized as *health-enhancing* (leading to improved health) or *health-compromising* (leading to poorer health).

Construct	Definition	Illustration
Behavioral Skills	The skills needed to successfully perform a behavior. *Behavioral capacity* is the combination of knowledge and skills.	Many behaviors require the development of a repertoire or specific set of skills to be successfully enacted. Examples include safe driving, planning to avoid high-risk situations, safe sex, playing a sport, or preparing a healthy meal.
Intentions	The intention to add a new behavior or to modify an existing behavior.	By setting a goal, an individual is intending to develop a behavioral skill (or set of skills) to achieve a desired outcome. This is often accomplished by writing or verbalizing goals.
Reinforcement and Punishment	Behavior can be increased or extinguished through the provision or removal of rewards and punishments.	Rewards and punishments can be either *tangible* (e.g., money, goods, trophies) or *social* (e.g., praise, approval, recognition, attention).

Personal Cognitive Influences on Behavior

Personal cognitive influences on behavior include four constructs: (1) self-efficacy, (2) collective efficacy, (3) outcome expectations, and (4) knowledge. These constructs are rooted in the concept that individuals play an active role (they have *agency*) in their environments and behaviors (Bandura, 2001, 2018). Individuals exercise *agency* when they set goals and establish plans to reach their expected outcomes (*forethought*), shift their goals, objectives, and outcome expectations (*self-regulation*), and, most importantly, reflect on their self, capacities, and actions (*self-reflection*) (Bandura, 2005, 2018).

Self-Efficacy

Self-efficacy is a cognitive process defined as one's *confidence* in the ability to exercise agency to achieve an outcome. Self-efficacy is the seminal construct of SCT (Bandura, 1977; Bandura & Walters, 1977) and is related directly to setting a behavioral goal, the level of effort needed to master new skills, and the sustainability of this effort in the face of personal setbacks and environmental barriers. Like all SCT constructs, self-efficacy varies from behavior to behavior and environment to environment. Someone may be experienced and justifiably confident in their ability to prepare a meal (self-efficacy for cooking) but have little experience and confidence in preparing meals that adhere to the dietary restrictions needed to manage chronic health conditions like diabetes or kidney disease. To sustain behavior change, interventions must target *situational* self-efficacy, such as self-efficacy to incorporate dietary restriction into an existing repertoire of meal preparation skills.

Self-efficacy is developed through: (1) previous mastery experiences, (2) vicarious experience, (3) social persuasion, and (4) emotional arousal. Through experience, a person develops behavior-related skills and becomes familiar with the expected outcomes of engaging in the behavior. Active learning strategies can increase self-efficacy by coaching a person through the incremental steps needed to develop behavioral mastery. Active learning strategies include using nutrition labels to create healthy meals, demonstrating proper condom use for safer sex practices, and practicing refusal skills to resist peer pressure for substance use.

Self-efficacy is also impacted by observing the experiences of others, or *vicarious learning experiences*. Individuals watch the behaviors and corresponding outcomes of other people and incorporate these vicarious experiences into their confidence and agency toward engaging in those behaviors. An individual is likely to gain (or lose) confidence in their ability to undertake a behavior upon observing a behavior modeled by someone with a shared degree of agency and behavioral capacity. Similarly, observing people of similar (or aspirational) social status more strongly influences the impact of the modeled behavior. Thus, behavioral modeling efforts must be relevant to the target audience's demographics, culture, economics, and environment.

Social persuasion speaks to the perceived cultural norms and beliefs, social support, and reinforcement of a behavior. Direct encouragement or discouragement is a common form of social persuasion. Influential experts and social role models impact self-efficacy by persuading others to recognize the benefits of a behavior, support the expected and realized outcomes, and reinforce the benefits of behavioral change. School teachers can be influential experts who increase their students' self-efficacy to remain tobacco-free by normalizing the perceptions that most youths do not use tobacco (normative beliefs toward peers), and that using tobacco results in short- and long-term social consequences and physical addiction (reinforcement of use).

The impact of social persuasion on self-efficacy is influenced heavily by the status, influence, and proximity of the source. For example, the same school-based interventions that incorporate teachers as influential experts also rely on credible classroom same-age role models to transmit social information via small-group discussions and role play. Role models can be particularly effective at increasing self-efficacy for certain health behaviors when they demonstrate behavioral change and navigate similar cultural norms and beliefs, social support, barriers/opportunities, and reinforcement as the individual who wants to change behavior (Brown et al., 2016, 2019; Huang & Shen, 2016; Koniak-Griffin et al., 2015; O'Brien et al., 2010).

Self-efficacy is influenced by the emotional arousal of direct and vicarious experiences. Strong emotional arousal in response to specific behavioral cues elicits cognitions of anticipated failure or success, affecting an individual's confidence and agency (self-efficacy) to engage in behavior. Interventions that target emotional arousal must be relevant to their target population with an authentic approach to health education. For example, messages designed to increase emotional arousal toward the negative health consequences of substance use (addiction; incarceration) are unlikely to effectively impact behavior without also addressing the *situational* self-efficacy needed to avoid substance use (for example, self-efficacy to resist peer pressure).

These four sources of self-efficacy, previous mastery experiences, vicarious experience, social persuasion, and emotional arousal help explain behavioral motivation, and can be incorporated into health behavior change strategies designed to improve confidence, agency, and self-efficacy. The impact of these four sources of self-efficacy varies from person to person, environment to environment, and behavior to behavior, although mastery experience is considered the most influential source of self-efficacy: one must know how to engage in a behavior to exhibit that behavior (Bandura et al., 1999).

Collective Efficacy

Collective efficacy, like self-efficacy, is fundamental to understanding cognition and behavior because many goals and objectives are achievable only through group action (Bandura, 2018). Collective efficacy describes how individuals perceive the capacity of a group or organization to act toward achieving a shared agenda (Hipp, 2016), including withstanding opposition and discouraging setbacks (Bandura, 2000). Collective efficacy is developed through the same cognitive processes as self-efficacy—mastery experiences; vicarious experience; social persuasion; and emotional arousal—but at a group collective level. Groups and communities have used collective action to address social determinants of health through improved working conditions, increased economic opportunities, and equitable regulatory policies (Hagedorn et al., 2016; Malinowski et al., 2015). Interventions can improve collective efficacy through activities on the individual level (direct education and training), group level (self-help groups; family-to-family engagement), and community level (media campaigns), often led by community coalitions comprised of local leaders and interested parties (Butel & Braun, 2019).

Knowledge

In SCT, knowledge includes an understanding of the significance (health risk/benefits) and components (scope/sequence) of a behavior. Most important is instrumental knowledge, or the "how-to" information, as distinct from etiologic information. Individuals gain knowledge by learning the significance and step-by-step processes of engaging in a behavior through direct education and vicarious experiences. To change behavior, knowledge is necessary but not sufficient—it is a cognitive prerequisite, but knowledge alone does not explain or change behavior (Bandura, 2004). Instead, knowledge of a behavior's outcome and processes must be combined with the *skills* to engage in that behavior in order to develop the *capacity* to conduct and sustain the behavior (Table 9.1). The development and role of skills and behavioral capacity are discussed later in this chapter.

Outcome Expectations

Outcome expectations are the anticipated consequences of a behavior. They are situational (setting/context) and directional (positive/negative). Youth may hold positive outcome expectations about using e-cigarettes, including the anticipated social benefit of engaging in a behavior perceived as common and acceptable or due to misperceptions about the physical benefits of nicotine (such as weight management or mood regulation). However, youth may also recognize that nicotine is addictive, and that they are socially or legally prohibited from vaping, resulting in negative outcome expectations of e-cigarette use. Interventions sometimes need to balance multidimensional outcome expectations.

Value Expectations

Individuals ascribe outcome expectations to a behavior, then they evaluate those outcomes as positive or negative. Behavior is an evolving process resulting from comparing outcome expectation with internal and external standards (self-evaluative outcome expectations). Behaviors can be reinforced by feelings of satisfaction, pride, joy, and belonging. Conversely, behaviors can be punished through an individual's negative cognitions: emotional feelings of disillusionment, shame, sadness, disgust, or rejection. Interventions targeting outcome expectations that are not relevant to the motivations of a specific behavior such as initiation of nicotine, alcohol, or other substances, are unlikely to change behavior. For example, some prevention programs that do not address perceived positive outcome expectations and instead overemphasize only the adverse health effects and punitive consequences of substance use have been found ineffective for preventing adolescent substance use (e.g., Drug Abuse Resistance Education [DARE]) (West & O'Neal, 2004).

Social and Environmental Influences

Behavioral regulation does not occur solely through personal cognitive factors (Bandura, 2004). SCT also recognizes social and environmental influences: the perceived and physical factors that permit, promote, deter or otherwise impede engagement in a particular behavior. SCT characterizes four social and environmental influences: (1) observational learning, (2) normative beliefs, (3) social support, and (4) opportunities and barriers. It also underscores the interactive relationship between social and environmental influences and personal, cognitive influence through reciprocal determinism.

Observational Learning

SCT is rooted in the concept that individuals can learn behavior vicariously by observing others. Understanding the origins, and underlying mechanisms, through which social and environmental influences determine cognition and capacity is essential to understanding and changing behavior (Bandura, 2009). Individuals do not merely mimic what is observed (Bushman & Whitaker, 2012) but apply cognitive processes to observed behavior and its paired response (Bandura, 2008, 2011). Simply observing someone engaged in a behavior can increase knowledge and self-efficacy of that behavior, but it may not result in adopting a behavior (Bandura, 2008, 2013, 2018). Observing that same behavior paired with a relevant reward or consequence can influence an individual's outcome expectations toward a behavior and make undertaking the behavior more likely (Stacey et al., 2015).

The transition from observation to behavior occurs through four cognitive processes: (1) attention; (2) memory; (3) production; and (4) motivation (Bandura, 2008). When viewing a behavior, a person's level of attention depends on the internal functional value of the observed behavior. People are less likely to attend to consequences they do not value. Cognitive retention can depend on a person's intellectual capacity (such as ability to read or readiness to learn), stage of physical growth and maturity, state of inebriation, or psychological impairment. People are not likely to be influenced by observed events if they do not remember them. An important source of self-efficacy from observational learning also comes from remembering past outcomes from behavior and having the ability to reconstruct past events. Production is the level of knowledge, skills, and self-efficacy already possessed (or the level of willingness to learn them) for performing the modeled behavior. The richer the knowledge and repertoire of needed subskills, the easier it is to integrate them into new forms of behavior. Motivation is determined by the expected costs and benefits of the observed behavior.

Individuals are selective in what they choose to observe, retain, consider, and act upon. Thus, interventions must gain their attention, recall, and forethought in order to increase motivation to engage in and sustain a behavior. The impact of observational learning on motivation is impacted by the cost and benefit of a behavior weighed against the individual's personal standards (self-regulation) and actions (self-evaluation) (Bandura, 2013, 2018).

Normative Beliefs

Normative beliefs are the perceived prevalence and corresponding acceptability of a behavior; this construct is similarly a key element in the Theory of Reasoned Action/Theory of Planned Action (see Chapter 6). In SCT, normative beliefs are developed through direct and observed experiences, and exposure to media. Norms begin with the perceived prevalence of a behavior within a population and/or setting (binge drinking among college students, for example). Individuals consider these norms through *self-evaluation* and *social evaluation*. Per SCT, people adopt standards of behavior and regulate their actions through their idealized self-concept (self-evaluation) while balancing the perceived social pressures toward a behavior and the motivation to comply with those pressures (*social evaluation*) (Bandura, 2004).

SCT-guided interventions can apply normative change strategies focused on correcting misperceptions of the prevalence of a behavior. School-based tobacco prevention programs address student misperceptions about adolescent tobacco use by providing local or national data about tobacco use for the corresponding age and grade-level (Kelder et al., 2021; Thomas et al., 2015). People connect new information related to a behavior to their own social- and self-evaluation of a behavior. A social evaluation may include perceived loss or gain of peer groups due to drinking alcohol. Self-evaluation describes how an individual believes that engaging in a behavior (and the corresponding social evaluations) aligns with their self-image and identity.

Behaviors are reinforced by perceptions of the prevailing, normative beliefs. Behaviors that violate norms can bring social consequences, leading individuals to balance normative influences with their own behavioral standards (self-regulation; self-evaluation). The more one believes that behavior is (dis)encouraged or (dis)approved by significant role models, the more social pressure they feel to adopt community norms. However, individuals also develop a self-concept and identity through considering, establishing, and regulating their behavioral standards, or exercising their agency. Individuals evaluate themselves in relation to those in their social environment, with the most accurate and impactful comparison being those perceived to be most similar to themselves (Schunk & Greene, 2017; Usher & Schunk, 2017). To impact normative beliefs, interventions must target the cognitive processes of social and self-evaluations through health messages delivered by highly regarded social agents. However, no person has mono-cultural normative beliefs, meaning interventions must aim for authenticity in their message content and delivery. Health messages delivered with the requisite social influence to impact how an individual perceives a behavior that aligns with their evaluation of self and social environment should be more successful.

Social Support

Social support is the process by which interpersonal relationships may promote and protect an individual's health and wellness. Creating and sustaining social support is essential for maintaining a behavior. Social support during behavioral acquisition aids in adhering to the desired behavior, allowing individuals to develop self-efficacy, which supports their targeted behavior. Social support is a strong determinant of changes in dietary behavior among adults with diabetes (Ghoreishi et al., 2019; Rad et al., 2013). Social support can be generally categorized into: (1) emotional, including love, caring, and trust; (2) belonging, which includes validation of an individual's beliefs, emotions, and self-concept; (3) informational, which includes advice and counsel; and (4) instrumental, or tangible, support which speaks to the resources (time and money) invested to increase opportunities and reduce barriers for behavioral change. (see Chapter 10 on social support).

Opportunities and Barriers

Behavior is influenced by the opportunities and barriers within a social environment (Bandura, 2008, 2013, 2018). Cognitive barriers to behavior might include low self-efficacy to cook healthy meals or harmful perceived social norms toward preventive health care (COVID-19 masking or immunizations). Barriers are not solely cognitive; the probability (and possibility) of behavioral change is determined in part by attributes of the social and physical environment. Because social and environmental influences are often social and economic in nature (Bandura, 2004), multilevel interventions that address individual and social/environmental determinants of health are optimal (Bandura, 2004). For example, cooking instruction is an effective learning activity to increase self-efficacy and behavior capacity or skills to cook healthy meals. However, cooking requires resources (time and money); thus, to adopt the behavior over time, individuals must be able to purchase the foods and prepare the recipes as directed by the instructions or lessons.

Financial and physical access to medical services and facilities is a strong determinant of health (Bandura, 2004). To effectively change behavior, intervention activities and objectives must be feasible and replicable with the resources available to the target audience (Bandura, 2004, 2005). Some locations lack medical infrastructure and services, resulting in significant impediments to receiving primary and preventive health care and limited emergency medical services

(Frakt, 2019; Gujral & Basu, 2019; Miller et al., 2020). These resource constraints can result in poorer health outcomes, particularly in rural populations. Thus, clinically based health interventions can only effectively address health behaviors if the population has access to these requisite medical infrastructures.

Supporting Behavioral Factors

Supporting behavioral factors include a person's existing repertoire of behavioral capacities (*skills*), goals to acquire or change a behavior (*intentions*), and *reinforcement* for engaging in a behavior. These factors influence and mediate cognitive and social environment influences on behavior.

Behavioral Skills

Behavioral skills are the skills necessary to successfully perform a behavior. SCT proposes that behavioral skills are acquired through five cognitive processes: (1) self-monitoring, described as the systematic observation of one's own behavior; (2) goal setting, identification of desired changes; (3) feedback on performance with methods of improvement; (4) self-reward, which can be tangible or intangible; and (5) self-instruction, described as re-evaluation before and during performance of a behavior.

Behavioral capacity reflects an individual's *skills* combined with their understanding of the significance and components of engaging in a behavior (*knowledge*). Naturally, an individual must possess the requisite knowledge to engage in a behavior if they are to succeed in trialing and adopting the behavior. Individuals gain knowledge and skills (behavioral capacity) through direct and vicarious experiences; the same processes as other SCT constructs. Consequently, improvements in behavioral capacity through increased knowledge and skills can subsequently increase an individual's self-efficacy to engage in a particular behavior.

Goal Setting

Goal setting is central to establish the intentions needed to achieve behavior change (see Chapter 6). Behavioral intentions are an indication of an individual's readiness to perform a given behavior and are assumed to be an antecedent to behavior. Intentions are shaped by forethought (planning the future) and are established through internal standards for behavior (self-evaluation). When developing intentions to engage in a behavior, individuals set behavioral goals to increase their agency, self-efficacy, and behavioral capacity upon achievement or completion of their goals. In SCT, goals and intentions are influenced by a person's motivations to engage in a behavior. Interventions that target the underlying motivations for behavior change are more likely to influence behavioral intentions and encourage goal setting. SCT-guided interventions focus beyond short-term behavioral change and, instead, are designed so that participants gain the motivations, goals, and intentions toward sustained behavioral change after the conclusion of an intervention (i.e., self-management). (Bandura, 2005).

Positive and Negative Reinforcement

Reinforcement is the primary construct from stimulus-response theories of learning (operant conditioning) and involves strengthening a behavior due to its repeated linkage to a stimulus. Reinforcers are the stimuli that strengthen (positive reinforcer) or weaken (negative reinforcer) the association between behaviors and stimuli. Positive reinforcement occurs when a rewarding stimulus is given after the performance of a specific behavior, so that the behavior increases. For example, offering extra recess time as a reward for eating a specific number of fruits and vegetables on a given day can reinforce healthful eating. Conversely, negative reinforcement occurs when an aversive stimulus is removed as a result of a specific behavior, also in an effort to increase the behavior.

Per SCT, individuals develop outcome expectations for a specific behavior not only through pairing reinforcers with behaviors but also through the lens of cognitive and environmental influences on behavior. In other words, individuals have their own cognitions about the pairing of behavior and reinforcer. SCT notes that the degree to which a reinforcer incentivizes behavior will vary by person and situational context. By incorporating cognition into our understanding of the stimulus-response process, SCT provides a more detailed explanation for the origins of outcome expectations as well as a complete roadmap to assist in adding and maintaining new behaviors.

Case Study 1: Healthy Eating Living (HEAL)

Obesity is a significant public health and medical problem in the US, with about 74% of adults aged 20 years and older overweight or obese (Stierman et al., 2021). In 2019, an estimated 29.0% of women were obese prior to pregnancy (Fryar et al., 2018). Excess weight during pregnancy can lead to increased maternal morbidity and mortality (Wang et al., 2021), problems with labor and delivery, and infants who are large-for-gestational age (Averett & Fletcher, 2016; Catalano & Shankar, 2017).

The Healthy Eating Active Living (HEAL) program is a multicomponent program intended to break this cycle by encouraging healthy behaviors during pregnancy. Objectives of HEAL are to achieve healthy weight gain during pregnancy for mothers, improve birth outcomes, and prevent childhood obesity later in life (Sharma et al., 2018). HEAL was developed using an SCT-based approach proposed by Nader and colleagues (Catalano & Shankar, 2017; Nader et al., 2012; Serpas et al., 2013) that focuses on obesity prevention at the earliest stages of development and uses a systems-level approach to intervene.

The HEAL intervention framework draws on concepts from SCT (Bandura, 2001) with three major targeted behaviors: healthy eating, physical activity, and breastfeeding. Major SCT constructs used in the development of HEAL were knowledge, outcome expectations, self-efficacy, goal setting, and social support (Sharma et al., 2018) (Table 9.2).

HEAL program participants were Medicaid-eligible pregnant women. The Medicaid 1115 Transformation Waiver program allowed the state of Texas to implement innovative prevention programs integrated within clinical practices to improve health outcomes and address gaps in service among low-income populations. The program was offered to predominantly African American and Hispanic/Latino women in southeast Texas. Because preliminary developmental work for HEAL was conducted in a Hispanic/Latino population in California (Serpas et al., 2013),

Table 9.2   Operationalization of Individual-Level SCT Constructs in the Healthy Eating Active Living (HEAL) Program

Construct	HEAL-Specific Intervention Application and Strategy	Example of Measurement Item	Response Categories	Scale
Behavioral Capability	*Physical activity knowledge*: participants were taught about the benefits of physical activity	I think the relationship between physical activity and health is important	5-point Likert scale, ranging from strongly disagree to strongly agree	One item
Outcome Expectations	*Outcome expectations*: participants were taught about the benefits and results of consuming fruits and vegetables	I may develop health problems like type 2 diabetes if I do not eat fruits and vegetables	5-point Likert scale, ranging from "strongly disagree" to "strongly agree"	3-item scale
Intentions	*Intention to breast-feed*: participants engaged in one-on-one sessions with dietitians to learn about breastfeeding	How do you plan to feed your baby in the first few weeks?	4-point scale with responses of "breastfeed only, formula feed only, both breast and formula feed, don't know"	N/A; 4 related questions
Self-Efficacy	*Cooking self-efficacy*: participants watched cooking demonstrations of culturally friendly foods and engaged in recipe tasting	How sure are you that you can prepare root vegetables (e.g., beets, sweet potatoes)?	5-point Likert scale ranging from "not at all sure" to "extremely sure"	5-item scale
Self-Efficacy	*Pregnancy exercise self-efficacy*: participants engaged in physical activity with Community Health Worker (CHW) leaders	I am sure that I can find the means and ways to exercise during pregnancy.	5-point Likert scale ranging from "strongly disagree" to "strongly agree"	8-item scale
Goal Setting	*Goals for eating healthful foods*: participants completed a goal-tracking sheet weekly to set HEAL-related behavioral goals, such as cooking at home for a certain number of days per week	N/A	N/A	N/A
Environment	*Social support*: Community Health Workers (CHWs) provided social support for HEAL-related behaviors during sessions, as well as linking participants to community resources, such as local food banks/pantries and federal food assistance programs	N/A	N/A	N/A

the program was adapted for a diverse population including African Americans and Non-Hispanic White individuals. The program included culturally appropriate recipes for cooking demonstrations, hiring and training community health workers (CHWs) with demographics similar to the priority populations, and culturally relevant physical activities.

The HEAL multicomponent program included six sessions over a six-week period, a one-on-one session with a dietitian, and five follow-up group sessions facilitated by a CHW at a community location. The sessions revolved around four themes: (1) communicating effectively during prenatal appointments (patient-provider engagement), (2) physical activity and stress relief during pregnancy, (3) understanding and improving the food environment to make healthy choices, and (4) preparing for breastfeeding. Group sessions were non-didactic, thus enabling experiential adult learning rooted in behavior change, to prepare pregnant women for healthy gestational weight gain (Miller & Rollnick, 2002). A typical group session lasted 90 minutes and began with 30 minutes of CHW-facilitated discussion around the weekly topic areas, followed by a cooking demonstration, recipe tasting, and physical activity. Each week for six weeks, women participating in the program also received approximately 20–25 lbs. (or 50 servings) of donated fresh produce, nutrition education materials, and recipe cards to take home during the education sessions.

Application of SCT Concepts and Constructs

Reciprocal Determinism

A good example of reciprocal determinism can be seen in the interplay between the intervention strategies for HEAL. Fresh vegetables and fruits were made available to the families through collaboration with a local food bank and a local non-profit organization, Brighter Bites. (Sharma et al., 2015). The produce gave the women instrumental support and the opportunity to practice healthy cooking while using skills and knowledge learned through the classes, which further increased their self-efficacy to engage in these behaviors at home as well as reinforcing the outcome expectations that healthy food can taste good and be easy to prepare. Recipes provided through the class were culturally friendly and centered around ingredients in the weekly produce allocation. Program participants shared their successes and received social support and positive reinforcement at their weekly classes as well as through clinic visits.

Knowledge

HEAL sessions involved cooking demonstrations and recipe tastings to provide pregnant women with best practices on how to easily prepare healthy meals on a regular basis. The one-on-one sessions with the dietitian provided an assessment of the woman's current eating patterns, information on a healthy diet, and individualized dietary goals. CHWs led physical activity sessions providing pregnancy-safe ideas for physical activity. Providing recipes and focusing on cooking skills through the cooking demonstrations increased individual knowledge about various aspects of maintaining a healthy body weight. Other sessions focused on shopping and preparing healthy meals, healthy sleeping patterns, breastfeeding techniques, and stress reduction. The importance of consistent family routines was also emphasized since behaviors such as a consistent child bedtime have been associated with better weight outcomes and more healthful diets (Haidar et al., 2021).

Outcome Expectations

Throughout the duration of HEAL, pregnant women were able to develop outcome expectations for healthy eating and physical activity, largely through engaging in these behaviors during the classes and experiencing tasty, healthy food and fun physical activities. Information regarding healthy gestational weight gain through dietary practices (healthy weight gain) and physical activity behaviors (meeting physical activity guidelines) helped pregnant women understand both the positive and negative consequences of behaviors throughout pregnancy. Cooking classes provided foods that were healthy and tasty, and that reinforced the concept that healthy food can taste good. Benefits of breastfeeding such as a healthier baby, cost savings compared to formula, and convenience were incorporated into class discussions.

Self-Efficacy

HEAL sessions included components on building self-efficacy for physical activity, dietary behaviors, and breastfeeding. Pregnant women were provided tools from CHWs during sessions to increase their confidence in their ability to be active, consume fruits and vegetables as snacks, and cook and prepare food from basic healthy ingredients, such as roasting root vegetables. For example, a 10- to 15-minute physical activity consisting of various pregnancy-safe, fun, low-impact aerobics, strength-conditioning, stretching, and yoga-based activities was implemented weekly, encouraging the women to participate in guided practice to achieve mastery and improve their self-efficacy to perform the behaviors.

Goal Setting

Participants were encouraged to complete a goal-tracking sheet every week to set healthy goals centered around HEAL components and to develop behavioral intentions to practice new behaviors. Example goals centered on eating more fruits and vegetables on a daily basis, cooking at home for a certain number of days per week, being physically active during several days of the week, and having an intention to breastfeed after birth.

Social Support

The CHWs provided social support for dietary, breastfeeding, and physical activity through leading discussion-type sessions on how to prepare healthy meals, breastfeeding techniques, and how to fit physical activity in their lives. CHWs are especially effective in this role, as they are recruited from similar populations as the program participants and can often address cultural and other barriers in a relevant manner (Katigbak et al., 2015). Women also enjoyed the peer support offered in these sessions.

The CHWs also provided social support by linking participants to available community resources such as local food banks and pantries. They assisted with enrollment in federal assistance programs such as Women, Infants, Children (WIC), and Supplemental Nutrition Assistance Program (SNAP). Enrollment in federal assistance programs in Texas can be difficult and must be renewed frequently, so having the CHWs serve as patient navigators was crucial.

Program Evaluation and Outcomes

A one-group pre-post evaluation was conducted to examine program outcomes for this demonstration study (Milstein & Wetterhall, 1999). Of the 210 women who completed the pre- and post-program evaluations, over 80% attended four or more of the six sessions. Dose of the intervention (e.g., number of sessions attended) was positively associated with perceived benefits of breastfeeding for the baby ($p < 0.05$) and intention to breastfeed exclusively ($p < 0.001$).

Secondary outcomes of the intervention were positive. The program yielded significant increases in participants' daily consumption of fruits and vegetables ($p < 0.001$). Pre-post differences in physical activity following the completion of the HEAL program were also examined as a secondary outcome. Results demonstrated a 15% increase in the number of women reportedly active for at least 30 minutes per day 3+ days per week, and a 14% increase in the number of women who reported they could walk for at least 10 minutes 5+ days a week, with greater increases pre-to-post intervention among women who attended more HEAL sessions ($p < 0.01$). HEAL also showed a trend toward an increased food security of +8.3% ($p = 0.056$). There were improvements, albeit not significant, in interactions between attendance and increased self-efficacy for cooking from basic ingredients and eating fruits and vegetables every day (Sharma et al., 2018).

Results from this study illustrate the feasibility of incorporating a robust integrated program that targets health behaviors in mothers. Over 80% of participants attended ≥4 sessions and approximately 91% of participants found the sessions helpful. Currently, the HEAL program is still being implemented in University of Texas Physicians clinics, although a larger evaluation has not been conducted. The HEAL study highlights the importance of obesity prevention interventions that begin during pregnancy, with benefits for both the mother and the child when using culturally appropriate strategies and supports. In addition, the results highlight the importance of SCT constructs in program design, implementation, and evaluation for diverse, historically underserved populations.

Case Study 2: Catch My Breath

In 2014, e-cigarettes became the most commonly used tobacco/nicotine product among middle and high school students (~12–17 years of age) in the United States, introducing a host of known and unknown health consequences, and threatening 50 years of public health progress. In response to the rise of e-cigarettes among youth, the CATCH research team began developing an SCT-guided intervention, named *CATCH My Breath* (CMB). The CMB program has been found to significantly reduce the risk of e-cigarette initiation from 6th to 7th grade, under a quasi-experimental pilot testing (Kelder et al., 2021). The CMB program has been tested by others whose findings confirm that SCT constructs are relevant to e-cigarette use during adolescence, such as outcome expectations, normative beliefs, and behavioral intentions (Bteddini et al., 2023; Moosbrugger et al., 2023).

Application of SCT Concepts and Constructs

The CMB program targets cognitive and social/environmental influences of behavior while building behavioral capacity and intentions to prevent the initiation and escalation of e-cigarette use. The content and activities of CMB are designed to impact multiple SCT constructs, simultaneously. In this, the CMB program incorporates *reciprocal determinism*, which states that impacting one construct (knowledge, self-efficacy) will correspond with changes to other constructs (outcome expectations. normative beliefs). An overview of these constructs, and their theorized reciprocal relationship, is provided below.

Knowledge

CMB is comprised of four modules, each pairing educational content with active learning exercises. The modules begin with students forming small groups, followed by teachers introducing age-appropriate information about e-cigarettes to the groups to increase knowledge related to health and social consequences of using e-cigarettes and other tobacco products. The four lessons of CMB aim to correct common misperceptions about e-cigarettes reported by youth, including: (1) that e-cigarettes do not deliver "water vapor" but, instead, an aerosol consisting of several chemical (glycerol, propylene glycol. flavored additives) that are combined with the addictive stimulant nicotine; (2) the vast majority of kids their age (middle school) do *not* use e-cigarettes or any form of tobacco; (3) the social and legal consequences of underage e-cigarette use; and (4) the numerous ways tobacco companies market and promote e-cigarettes to youth. The information delivered by CMB is designed to increase knowledge and health-compromising outcomes of e-cigarette use, which will then influence the cognitive processes that determine SCT constructs such as self-efficacy, outcome expectations, and normative beliefs.

CMB pairs the information delivered by the teacher with small group activities which provide students the opportunity to apply (thus reinforce) their knowledge of e-cigarettes. Each group of students is given a worksheet. A volunteer peer facilitator raises questions related to e-cigarette use, collects the groups' thoughts and answers, and then shares them back to the larger class. The small group framework is designed to elicit culturally relevant and local language-specific group responses. This framework also enables students to connect to the content so that lessons learned will more easily be retrieved after the program is over. In this vein, and to extend CMB program contact hours, an essential activity assignment is for students to interview their parent or caregiver with a list of questions to discuss their own experiences with smoking, negative social and physical consequences of smoking, challenges overcoming addiction, and a statement for the family rules about smoking and vaping.

Goals and Self-Efficacy

Intentions to use e-cigarettes are a strong determinant of subsequent initiation (Bold et al., 2017; Carey et al., 2019). Consequently, CMB modules focus largely on self-efficacy and goal setting, each a fundamental construct of SCT. Knowledge and learning exercises of CMB facilitate cognitive processes (self-evaluation, motivation) that positively influence self-efficacy and behavioral intentions. Students apply their knowledge of e-cigarettes to discuss things like peer pressure (to use e-cigarettes) as well as practice their skills to refuse peer pressure. These active learning exercises impact self-efficacy to resist peer pressure by allowing students to gain mastery experiences of the requisite refusal skills. At the conclusion of the core CMB lessons, youth make a public commitment to abstain from using e-cigarettes, thus clearly stating their own goals while socially reinforcing the goals of their peers, who made the same public commitment. The CMB lessons and activities are designed to provide each student with the information and skills needed to maintain their public commitment to not use e-cigarettes or other tobacco products.

Outcome Expectations

Youth learn the possible health consequences and the social and legal ramifications of e-cigarette use. These include risk for nicotine dependence (Benowitz, 2010, 2014; Benowitz et al., 2009) and combustible tobacco cigarette smoking (Chan et al., 2021; Harrell et al., 2022). This knowledge, in theory, influences the student's perceived negative ramifications of e-cigarette use (i.e., outcome expectations). However, the evidence does not support a unidimensional approach to addressing outcome expectations, and thus CMB modules also address and counter the perceived positive outcomes of e-cigarette use. Students gather in small groups and discuss the possible motivations and reasons people use e-cigarettes (such as curiosity, popularity, nicotine stamina boost, addiction) and then list alternatives to using e-cigarettes.

Normative Beliefs

Exposure to new information can result in changes in knowledge, which can then facilitate cognitive processes such as social- and self-evaluation. Youth typically overestimate the true prevalence of health-compromising behaviors, including nicotine use, among their peers. CMB modules are designed to teach middle school students that the vast majority of kids their age do not use e-cigarettes, citing national prevalence data. Youth may experience a change in their perceptions of e-cigarette use among their peers (normative beliefs). In addition, activities are designed to develop a strong intention not to experiment with or use e-cigarettes.

Behavioral Capacity

To counter the influences of e-cigarette marketing, CMB builds knowledge of e-cigarette marketing and advertisement strategies and practices. Students then join small groups to identify and discuss social and environmental influences toward e-cigarette use, including marketing and promotions. With this combination of knowledge and skills (*behavioral capacity*), students then recognize, analyze, and evaluate the pressures toward e-cigarettes in order to resist the attempts of the normalization of e-cigarette use attempted by marketing campaigns. The students also discuss the ethics of marketing an addictive substance to children and, as a group activity, create counter-vaping messages similar to that found in tobacco prevention media campaigns (Noar et al., 2020).

Parent Involvement

Parent involvement is facilitated by a five-page parent tool kit, each with a brief explanatory video. Each week, parents digitally receive a page of the toolkit and corresponding video, covering: (1) what e-cigarettes look like and their social and physical health consequences (outcome expectations); (2) how youth are at risk for experimentation with e-cigarettes (normative beliefs, vicarious learning, and role modeling); (3) methods for parental monitoring, such as knowing the location of their children, who they are with and their phone numbers, the parents of the kids socializing with their children and their phone numbers; and (4) establishing home rules about vaping and reasonable consequences for their infraction (normative beliefs; outcome expectations).

Physical Education

CMB lessons designed to be taught during physical education combine movement and peer-to-peer interaction to provide the core content. This is thought to be helpful because being active has been identified as a method to improve executive function in youth (Biddle & Asare, 2011; Verburgh et al., 2014). It may improve recall of lessons learned after the program.

Efficacy of Catch My Breath (CMB)

CMB is currently being tested in an NIH-funded efficacy study using a group-randomized controlled trial design in 21 middle schools to determine the prevention effects of the program in youth from 6th to 9th grade. Results will be available in 2024.

In addition, with a strong endorsement from the Substance Abuse and Mental Health Services Administration (SAMHSA), CMB became a popular choice for schools facing the vaping crisis. The CATCH research team responded with the development of elementary school lessons for 4th and 5th graders and high school lessons. The team also used Diffusion of Innovation strategies (see Chapter 16) to accelerate the adoption and implementation of CMB (Kelder et al., 2021). As of summer 2023, the program has been adopted in all 50 states, parts of Canada, the Dominican Republic, and Columbia, reaching an estimated 2 million students annually.

Discussion

SCT provides a framework for understanding the complexities of human behavior. According to SCT, prevention programs that rely too heavily on didactic, knowledge-based strategies and place too little emphasis on developing *behavioral capacity* are unlikely to generate meaningful or sustainable results. It is a straightforward task to deliver health knowledge, but far more difficult to change perceptions of self-efficacy, outcome expectations, social support, and barriers/opportunities toward a target behavior. Further, SCT-guided interventions often focus primarily on individual behavior change, overlooking or not adequately considering the environmental influences of behavior during intervention design. SCT constructs are *situational* and must be considered with careful delineation, tailoring, measurement, and application to the target population, setting, and behavior. Thus, it is essential to consider the multiple levels of the social and physical environment as well as individual-level determinants of behavior described by SCT (Bandura, 2008, 2013, 2018). The breadth of the socioeconomic model provides a framework for exploring SCT constructs within various domains (e.g., family, community, school). Laws and their corresponding administration (i.e., public policy) are significant determinants of behavior. As one example, CDC Best Practices for Comprehensive Tobacco Control recommends several policy changes to reduce tobacco use, particularly among youth, such as increased excise taxes and enhanced enforcement of tobacco sales (Centers for Disease Control and Prevention, 2014).

Technological advances have and will continue to heavily influence the application, evaluation, and evolution of SCT. Digital and online technologies (e.g., wearable technology; digital surveys) and measurement methods (e.g., ecological momentary assessments) expand the contextual information and setting through which we can measure SCT constructs. Such innovative applications of SCT can improve the development of effective, theory-driven health interventions. However, the profound impact of technological advances on SCT extends beyond methods of data collection. SCT is rooted in the concept that human thoughts and behaviors are heavily influenced by observing the actions and consequences of others (vicarious experience). SCT was developed in the 1960s when television was becoming a popular method of communication (Bandura et al., 1961). Originally, television content was largely standardized across homes, with few channels and sporadic programming. Now, users can select from a myriad of content for which to observe—and engage—through a single, handheld device. SCT emerged during the technological revolution of the mid-20th century and must continue to evolve through the 21st century and beyond.

Summary

SCT is an action-oriented approach to understanding the influence and interaction of cognitive, social-environmental, and supporting behavioral factors on behaviors. SCT has broad utility in the pursuit of public health, with an extensive history of effectively addressing health-enhancing and health-compromising behaviors through individual and collective action. SCT has been extensively applied in the development and evaluation of theory-based, behavioral health interventions. When applying SCT, the number of theoretical constructs can seem overwhelming, and the processes of change do not necessarily seem linear or even logical. However, the first step for public health practitioners is to carefully review the SCT-oriented risk factor literature for the selected behavioral outcomes (e.g., goal setting, predicting physical activity) and to examine relevant intervention literature to determine the strongest evidence-based combination of intervention components. A key step is to identify the most relevant and effective SCT constructs associated with the targeted behavior with consideration of the appropriateness and relevance for the intended audience and setting. Another important step usually involves facilitating the use of SCT and the tenets of reciprocal determinism with community partners. In the words of Albert Bandura (2004): "As you venture forth to promote your own health and that of others, may the efficacy force be with you!"

Acknowledgments

Disclosure: CMB is offered to schools in the United States without charge due to a generous gift from CVS Pharmacy and other philanthropy organizations. In addition, the CATCH research team has relinquished their intellectual property rights and does not receive any payments. CMB is distributed by the CATCH Global Foundation, a Texas nonprofit.

References

Averett, S. L., & Fletcher, E. K. (2016). Prepregnancy obesity and birth outcomes. *Maternal and Child Health Journal, 20*(3), 655–664.

Bandura, A. (1977). Self-Efficacy: Toward a unifying theory of behavioral change. *Psychological Review, 84*(2), 191.

Bandura, A. (2000). Exercise of human agency through collective efficacy. *Current Directions in Psychological Science, 9*(3), 75–78.

Bandura, A. (2001). Social cognitive theory: An agentic perspective. *Annual Review of Psychology, 52*(1), 1–26.

Bandura, A. (2004). Health promotion by social cognitive means. *Health Education & Behavior, 31*(2), 143–164.

Bandura, A. (2005). The primacy of self-regulation in health promotion. *Applied Psychology, 54*(2), 245–254.

Bandura, A. (2008). Observational learning. In W. Dornsbach, *The international encyclopedia of communication.* John Wiley & Sons.

Bandura, A. (2009). Social cognitive theory of mass communication. In J. Bryant & M. B. Oliver, *Media Effects* (3rd ed.) (pp. 110–140). Routledge.

Bandura, A. (2011). The social and policy impact of social cognitive theory. In M. Mark, S. Donaldson, & B. Campbell (Eds.), *Social psychology and evaluation*, (pp. 33–70). Guilford Press.

Bandura, A. (2013). The role of self-efficacy in goal-based motivation. In E. A. Locke & G. A. Latham (Eds.), *New developments in goal setting and task performance* (pp. 147–157). Routledge.

Bandura, A. (2018). Toward a psychology of human agency: Pathways and reflections. *Perspectives on Psychological Science, 13*(2), 130–136.

Bandura, A., Freeman, W. H., & Lightsey, R. (1997). *Self-efficacy: The exercise of control.* WH Freeman.

Bandura, A., Ross, D., & Ross, S. A. (1961). Transmission of aggression through imitation of aggressive models. *The Journal of Abnormal and Social Psychology, 63*(3), 575.

Bandura, A., & Walters, R. H. (1977). *Social learning theory* (vol. 1). Prentice Hall.

Benowitz, N. L. (2010). Nicotine addiction. *New England Journal of Medicine, 362*(24), 2295–2303.

Benowitz, N. L. (2014). Emerging nicotine delivery products. Implications for public health. *Annals of the American Thoracic Society, 11*(2), 231–235.

Benowitz, N. L., Hukkanen, J., & Jacob, P. (2009). Nicotine chemistry, metabolism, kinetics and biomarkers. In Jack E. Henningfield, Edythe D. London, Sakire Pogun (Eds.), *Nicotine psychopharmacology* (pp. 29–60): Springer.

Biddle, S. J., & Asare, M. (2011). Physical activity and mental health in children and adolescents: A review of reviews. *British Journal of Sports Medicine, 45*(11), 886–895.

Bold, K. W., Kong, G., Cavallo, D. A., Camenga, D. R., & Krishnan-Sarin, S. (2017). E-cigarette susceptibility as a predictor of youth initiation of e-cigarettes. *Nicotine and Tobacco Research, 20*(1), 140–144.

Brown, H., Atkin, A., Panter, J., Wong, G., Chinapaw, M. J., & Van Sluijs, E. (2016). Family-based interventions to increase physical activity in children: A systematic review, meta-analysis and realist synthesis. *Obesity Reviews, 17*(4), 345–360.

Brown, T., Moore, T. H., Hooper, L., Gao, Y., Zayegh, A., Ijaz, S., O'Malley, C., Waters, E., Summerbell, C. D. (2019). Interventions for preventing obesity in children. *Cochrane Database of Systematic Reviews, 7*, CD001871.

Bteddini, D. S., LeLaurin, J. H., Chi, X., Hall, J. M., Theis, R. P., Gurka, M. J., Polansky, C. J. (2023). Mixed methods evaluation of vaping and tobacco product use prevention interventions among youth in the Florida 4-H program. *Addictive Behaviors, 141*, 107637.

Bushman, B. J., & Whitaker, J. (2012). Media influence on behavior. In V. S. Ramachandra, *Encyclopedia of human behavior* (2nd ed., pp. 571–575): Elsevier Inc.

Butel, J., & Braun, K. L. (2019). The role of collective efficacy in reducing health disparities: A systematic review. *Family & Community Health*, *42*(1), 8–16.

Carey, F. R., Rogers, S. M., Cohn, E. A., Harrell, M. B., Wilkinson, A. V., & Perry, C. L. (2019). Understanding susceptibility to e-cigarettes: A comprehensive model of risk factors that influence the transition from non-susceptible to susceptible among e-cigarette naïve adolescents. *Addictive Behaviors*, *91*, 68–74.

Catalano, P. M., & Shankar, K. (2017). Obesity and pregnancy: Mechanisms of short term and long term adverse consequences for mother and child. *BMJ*; 356 https://doi.org/10.1136/bmj.j1

Centers for Disease Control and Prevention. (2014). *Best practices for comprehensive tobacco control programs.* U.S. Department of Health and Human Services, Centers for Disease Control and Prevention, National Center for Chronic Disease Prevention and Health Promotion, Office on Smoking and Health.

Chan, G. C., Stjepanović, D., Lim, C., Sun, T., Shanmuga Anandan, A., Connor, J. P., Leung, J. (2021). Gateway or common liability? A systematic review and meta-analysis of studies of adolescent e-cigarette use and future smoking initiation. *Addiction*, *116*(4), 743–756.

Ferguson, G. M., Tran, S. P., Mendez, S. N., & Van De Vijver, F. J. (2017). Remote acculturation: Conceptualization, measurement, and implications for health outcomes. In S. J. Schwartz, J. Unger (Eds.), *Oxford handbook of acculturation and health* (pp. 157–173). Oxford University Press.

Frakt, A. B. (2019). The rural hospital problem. *Journal of the American Medical Association*, *321*(23), 2271–2272.

Fryar, C. D., Carroll, M. D., & Ogden, C. L. (2018). *Prevalence of overweight, obesity, and severe obesity among children and adolescents aged 2–19 Years: United States, 1963-1965 through 2015-2016.* National Center for Health Statistics.

Ghoreishi, M.-S., Vahedian-Shahroodi, M., Jafari, A., & Tehranid, H. (2019). Self-care behaviors in patients with Type 2 diabetes: Education intervention base on social cognitive theory. *Diabetes and Metabolic Syndrome: Clinical Research and Reviews*, *13*(3), 2049–2056.

Gujral, K., & Basu, A. (2019). *Impact of rural and urban hospital closures on inpatient mortality (No. w26182).* National Bureau of Economic Research.

Hagedorn, J., Paras, C. A., Greenwich, H., & Hagopian, A. (2016). The role of labor unions in creating working conditions that promote public health. *American Journal of Public Health*, *106*(6), 989–995.

Haidar, A., Sharma, S. V., Durand, C. P., Barlow, S. E., Salahuddin, M., Butte, N. F., & Hoelscher, D. M. (2021). Cross-sectional relationship between regular bedtime and weight status and obesity-related behaviors among preschool and elementary school children: TX CORD study. *Childhood Obesity*, *17*(1), 26–35.

Harrell, M. B., Mantey, D. S., Chen, B., Kelder, S. H., & Barrington-Trimis, J. (2022). Impact of the e-cigarette era on cigarette smoking among youth in the United States: A population-level study. *Preventive Medicine*, *164* (107265), 1–8.

Hipp, J. R. (2016). Collective efficacy: How is it conceptualized, how is it measured, and does it really matter for understanding perceived neighborhood crime and disorder? *Journal of Criminal Justice*, *46*, 32–44.

Huang, Y., & Shen, F. (2016). Effects of cultural tailoring on persuasion in cancer communication: A meta-analysis. *Journal of Communication*, *66*(4), 694–715.

Katigbak, C., Van Devanter, N., Islam, N., & Trinh-Shevrin, C. (2015). Partners in health: A conceptual framework for the role of community health workers in facilitating patients' adoption of healthy behaviors. *American Journal of Public Health*, *105*(5), 872–880.

Kelder, S. H., Mantey, D. S., Van Dusen, D., Vaughn, T., Bianco, M., & Springer, A. E. (2021). Dissemination of CATCH My Breath: A middle school e-cigarette prevention program. *Addictive Behaviors*, *113*, 1–7.

Koniak-Griffin, D., Brecht, M.-L., Takayanagi, S., Villegas, J., Melendrez, M., & Balcázar, H. (2015). A community health worker-led lifestyle behavior intervention for Latina (Hispanic) women: Feasibility and outcomes of a randomized controlled trial. *International Journal of Nursing Studies*, *52*(1), 75–87.

Lorenzo-Blanco, E. I., Arillo-Santillán, E., Unger, J. B., & Thrasher, J. (2019). Remote acculturation and cigarette smoking susceptibility among youth in Mexico. *Journal of Cross-Cultural Psychology*, *50*(1), 63–79.

Malinowski, B., Minkler, M., & Stock, L. (2015). Labor unions: A public health institution. *American Journal of Public Health*, *105*(2), 261–271.

Miller, K. E., James, H. J., Holmes, G. M., & Van Houtven, C. H. (2020). The effect of rural hospital closures on emergency medical service response and transport times. *Health Services Research*, *55*(2), 288–300.

Miller, N. E., & Dollard, J. (1941). *Social learning and imitation*. Yale University Press.

Miller, W. R., & Rollnick, S. (2002). *Motivational interviewing: Preparing people for change* 2nd ed., The Guilford Press.

Milstein, B., & Wetterhall, S. F. (1999). Framework for program evaluation in public health. MMWR. Recommendations and reportse; 48, no. RR-11.

Mischel, W. (1973). Toward a cognitive social learning reconceptualization of personality. *Psychological Review, 80*(4), 252.

Moosbrugger, M., Losee, T. M., González-Toro, C. M., Drewson, S. R., Stapleton, P. J., Ladda, S., & Cucina, I. (2023). Pre-service teachers' perceptions and experiences implementing CATCH My Breath. *American Journal of Health Education, 54*(1), 20–28.

Nădăşan, V., Foley, K. L., Pénzes, M., Paulik, E., Mihăicuţă, Ş., Ábrám, Z., Bálint, J., Csibi, M., & Urbán, R. (2017). The short-term effects of ASPIRA: A web-based, multimedia smoking prevention program for adolescents in Romania: A cluster randomized trial. *Nicotine & Tobacco Research, 19*(8), 908–915.

Nader, P. R., Huang, T. T.-K., Gahagan, S., Kumanyika, S., Hammond, R. A., & Christoffel, K. K. (2012). Next steps in obesity prevention: Altering early life systems to support healthy parents, infants, and toddlers. *Childhood Obesity (Formerly Obesity and Weight Management), 8*(3), 195–204.

Noar, S. M., Rohde, J. A., Prentice-Dunn, H., Kresovich, A., Hall, M. G., & Brewer, N. T. (2020). Evaluating the actual and perceived effectiveness of e-cigarette prevention advertisements among adolescents. *Addictive Behaviors, 109*, 106473–106479

O'Brien, M. J., Halbert, C. H., Bixby, R., Pimentel, S., & Shea, J. A. (2010). Community health worker intervention to decrease cervical cancer disparities in Hispanic 2omen. Journal of General Internal Medicine, 25(11), 1186–1192.

Pavlov, I. (1927). *Conditioning reflexes* (G.V. Anrep, Trans.). Liveright.

Perry, C. L., Kelder, S. H., Murray, D. M., & Klepp, K. I. (1992). Communitywide smoking prevention: Long-term outcomes of the Minnesota heart health program and the class of 1989 study. *American Journal of Public Health, 82*(9), 1210–1216.

Prokhorov, A. V., Kelder, S. H., Shegog, R., Conroy, J. L., Murray, N., Peters, R., Cinciripini, P. M., de Moor, C., Hudmon, K. S., & Ford, K. H. (2010). Project ASPIRE: An interactive, multimedia smoking prevention and cessation curriculum for culturally diverse high school students. *Substance Use & Misuse, 45*(6), 983–1006.

Prokhorov, A. V., Kelder, S. H., Shegog, R., Murray, N., Peters, R., Agurcia-Parker, C., Cinciripini, P. M., de Moor, C., Conroy, J. L., Hudmon, K. D., Ford, K. H., & Marani, S. (2008). Impact of a smoking prevention interactive experience (ASPIRE), an interactive, multimedia smoking prevention and cessation curriculum for culturally diverse high–school students. *Nicotine & Tobacco Research, 10*(9), 1477–1485.

Prokhorov, A. V., Marani, S. K., Calabro, K. S., & Ford, K. H. (2012). Theory- and technology-driven educational curricula addressing tobacco use. *Procedia-Social and Behavioral Sciences, 46*, 4504–4507.

Rad, G. S., Bakht, L. A., Feizi, A., & Mohebi, S. (2013). Importance of social support in diabetes care. *Journal of Education Health Promotion, 2*, 62–68.

Rotter, J. B. (1954). *Social learning and clinical psychology*. Prentice Hall.

Rotter, J. B. (1966). Generalized expectancies for internal versus external control of reinforcement. *Psychological Monographs: General and Applied, 80*(1), 1–28.

Schunk, D. H., & Greene, J. A. (Eds.) (2017). Historical, contemporary, and future perspectives on self-regulated learning and performance. In *Handbook of self-regulation of learning and performance* (pp. 1–15). Routledge.

Serpas, S., Brandstein, K., McKennett, M., Hillidge, S., Zive, M., & Nader, P. R. (2013). San Diego healthy weight collaborative: A systems approach to address childhood obesity. *Journal of Health Care for the Poor and Underserved, 24*(2), 80–96.

Sharma, S., Helfman, L., Albus, K., Pomeroy, M., Chuang, R.-J., & Markham, C. (2015). Feasibility and acceptability of brighter bites: A food co-Op in schools to increase access, continuity and education of fruits and vegetables among low-income populations. *The Journal of Primary Prevention, 36*(4), 281–286.

Sharma, S. V., Chuang, R.-J., Byrd-Williams, C., Danho, M., Upadhyaya, M., Berens, P., & Hoelscher, D. M. (2018). Pilot evaluation of HEAL–A natural experiment to promote obesity prevention behaviors among low-income pregnant women. *Preventive Medicine Reports, 10*, 254–262.

Skinner, B. (1953). *Science and human behaviour*. Simon and Schuster.

Sly, D. F., Arheart, K., Dietz, N., Trapido, E. J., Nelson, D., Rodriguez, R., McKenna, J., & Lee, D. (2005). The outcome consequences of defunding the Minnesota Youth Tobacco-Use prevention program. *Preventive Medicine, 41*(2), 503–510.

Stacey, F. G., James, E. L., Chapman, K., Courneya, K. S., & Lubans, D. R. (2015). A systematic review and meta-analysis of Social Cognitive Theory-based physical activity and/or nutrition behavior change interventions for cancer survivors. *Journal of Cancer Survivorship, 9*(2), 305–338.

Stierman, B., Afful, J., Carroll, M. D., Chen, T. C., Davy, O., Fink, S., Fryar, C. D., Gu, Q., Hales, C. M., Hughes, J. P., & Ostchega, Y. (2021). National health and nutrition examination survey 2017–March 2020 prepandemic data files—development of files and prevalence estimates for selected health outcomes. *National Health Statistics Reports, 158*. https://stacks.cdc.gov/view/cdc/106273

Tamí-Maury, I., Noé-Díaz, V., García, H., Amell, L., Betancur, A., Chen, M., Pérez O., Calabro K. S., Yepes A., Ríos X., Sansores R., & Prokhorov, A. V. (2019). Adapting a computer-based smoking prevention program to Latin American adolescents. *NCT Neumología y Cirugía de Tórax, 78*(4), 342–347.

Thomas, R. E., McLellan, J., & Perera, R. (2013). School-based programmes for preventing smoking. *Evidence-Based Child Health: A Cochrane Review Journal, 8*(5), 1616–2040.

Thomas, R. E., McLellan, J., & Perera, R. (2015). Effectiveness of school-based smoking prevention curricula: Systematic review and meta-analysis. *BMJ Open, 5*(3), e006976.

Usher, E. L., & Schunk, D. H. (2017). Social cognitive theoretical perspective of self-regulation. In D. H. Schunk, & J. A. Greene (Eds.), *Handbook of self-regulation of learning and performance* (pp. 19–35). Routledge.

Verburgh, L., Königs, M., Scherder, E. J., & Oosterlaan, J. (2014). Physical exercise and executive functions in preadolescent children, adolescents and young adults: A meta-analysis. *British Journal of Sports Medicine, 48*(12), 973–979.

Vishwakarma, G., Singh, S., Marani, S. K., Arya, A., Calabro, K., Gupta, G., Mehta, A., & Alexander, V. (2021). Evaluation and impact of ASPIRE: An interactive tobacco prevention curriculum among university students in India. *South Asian Journal of Cancer, 10*(3), 144–150.

Wang, M. C., Freaney, P. M., Perak, A. M., Greenland, P., Lloyd-Jones, D. M., Grobman, W. A., & Khan, S. S. (2021). Trends in prepregnancy obesity and association with adverse pregnancy outcomes in the United States, 2013 to 2018. *Journal of the American Heart Association, 10*(17), e020717.

West, S. L., & O'Neal, K. K. (2004). Project DARE outcome effectiveness revisited. *American Journal of Public Health, 94*(6), 1027–1029.

CHAPTER 10

SOCIAL SUPPORT AND HEALTH

Julianne Holt-Lunstad
Andrew Scot Proctor

KEY POINTS

This chapter will:

- Define social support, including how it is conceptualized and measured, and distinguishing it from related concepts.

- Provide a historical background for the association between social support and health.

- Provide a theoretical framework to understand the association between social support and health.

- Briefly review the empirical evidence for social support's protective and potentially harmful effects.

- Present two examples of social support interventions for promoting health.

Vignette

Don and Nancy had been together for 45 years. They got married in their late thirties and have enjoyed their life filled with travel, meaningful work, and advanced educational opportunities. Don quit smoking in his thirties when Nancy entered the picture. He still smoked a cigar occasionally on vacations, but Nancy could not stand the smell. So, it was a rare occasion. Nancy loved the arts, and Don was an avid baseball fan and loved to go to local games during baseball season. Nancy went to baseball games with Don, and Don went to the museums and plays with Nancy. They walked together daily, no matter the weather. Their relationship enjoyed a lot of harmony because of shared activities. Nancy was also very involved with the community and regularly volunteered at a local soup kitchen for homeless women where she made friends with other volunteers and with some of the homeless women.

Nancy was the oldest of five sisters in her family. Her sisters who lived nearby visited her almost weekly. Don was the only child, and both his parents had passed away 16 years ago. He had a few friends he kept in touch with from work, but since retiring, Don and Nancy had decided to move closer to her family because they did not have children of their own. After the move, Don was hundreds of miles away from his former coworkers.

One night while at a musical performance with Don, Nancy felt faint for no apparent reason. By the end of the performance, Nancy looked pale and was completely drained of energy. She could barely walk to the car without Don's assistance. Don insisted that they go to the emergency room, but Nancy said it was probably just something she ate and that she just needed to rest. They went home and Nancy went straight to bed. The next day she felt even worse, and Don realized that she could not speak correctly. He took her to the hospital where the ER doctor said that she had experienced a severe stroke. Over the next week, Nancy had multiple visitors at the hospital from her sisters and friends at the soup kitchen, including some of the soup kitchen's clients. Despite Nancy's inability to communicate verbally, she had tears of gratitude in her eyes with every visit. Nancy passed away a week after suffering the stroke.

Don was heartbroken, and the grief was the heaviest burden he had ever experienced in his life. After the first few weeks of Nancy being gone, Don awoke to the

Health Behavior: Theory, Research, and Practice, Sixth Edition. Edited by Karen Glanz,
Barbara K. Rimer, and K. Viswanath.
© 2024 John Wiley & Sons, Inc. Published 2024 by John Wiley & Sons, Inc.
Companion website: www.wiley.com/go/glanz/healthbehavior6e

reality of his isolation. He was not interested in starting a new relationship in his late 70s and lived too far from the only friends he still had from work, with whom he rarely interacted since moving. Don stopped going on walks without Nancy and instead stayed home most days all day. His diet changed dramatically, and even his interest in baseball seemed lower without someone to go to the games with him. Without Nancy around, Don returned to smoking. Nancy's sisters stopped by around the holidays but did not regularly come by because of the grief they faced being around Nancy's old home. Don's mobility started to decline, but he was not motivated to visit the doctor regularly. By the time Don was 78, he had developed lung cancer and was showing signs of heart disease. Don died at age 79.

This fictional vignette illustrates three approaches to research on social relationships and health: functional, structural, and quality. After reading more about these in this chapter, we suggest that you return to this vignette later and ask yourself how Don's health was impacted by aspects of each of these three different approaches to social support and health.

Robust evidence links social support to better mental health (Harandi et al., 2017) and reduced risk for morbidity and mortality from certain diseases and conditions (Holt-Lunstad et al., 2010; NASEM, 2020; Olaya et al., 2017; Vila, 2021). Understanding the nature and types of social support and the pathways through which it is associated with health is essential to guide effective interventions. Although many questions remain, theories and evidence suggest that social support is a wide-ranging concept, with multiple pathways through which social support may influence mental and physical health. In this chapter, we first provide a review of different conceptualizations of support, the evidence linking social support to health outcomes, and the major theoretical models relating social support to health. We end by focusing on the implications for intervention and describe two recent applications of social support to modify health outcomes.

Definition and Conceptualizations of Social Support

Social support, social networks, and social integration are often used interchangeably but are distinct concepts. Although the influence of social relationships has been conceptualized and measured in diverse ways, they can be divided into three broad categories: the structure, functions, and quality of social relationships (Berkman et al., 2000; Holt-Lunstad, 2021; NASEM, 2020; Uchino, 2006). Generally, these three approaches distinguish the dimensions of social networks, the support that they provide, and their quality.

Figure 10.1 illustrates the three approaches. Structural aspects of relationships refer to the extent to which individuals are situated within or integrated into social networks. Social networks describe connections between individuals and their relationships or network ties (see Chapter 11). Measures of social networks typically assess the density, size, and/or number of social contacts. Social integration describes the extent of an individual's participation in a broad range of social relationships, including active engagement in various social activities or relationships and a sense of communality and identification with one's social roles. In contrast, functional measures focus on the specific functions served by relationships, and they are measured by the actual or perceived availability of support, aid, or resources from these relationships.

Additionally, quality of support measures the sense of connection to others based on positive or negative qualities such as relationship satisfaction, strain, or degree of perceived ambivalence regarding a relationship. Epidemiological studies that have linked social relationships to mortality can be categorized according to the specific measurement approaches described in Table 10.1.

The breadth of these three approaches—structural, functional, and quality—has been both a strength and weakness of research on social relationships and health. On the one hand, a broad approach more fully describes how aspects of social relationships may influence health and the potential interconnection among these constructs. On the other hand, such an approach makes it difficult to identify which particular aspects are related to health outcomes and through which pathways. It is also challenging to reconcile conflicting evidence when different measures are used to measure social support. This chapter focuses primarily on the perspective that social support is the functional aspect of relationship processes when describing specific mechanisms and outcomes.

Functional social support describes the functions served by social relationships (Table 10.2). Supportive individuals make available or provide what can be termed emotional support (e.g., expressions of caring), informational support (e.g., information that might be used to deal with stress), tangible support (e.g., direct material aid, also referred to as instrumental, practical, or financial support), and belonging support (e.g., having others to engage with in social activities) (Cohen et al., 1985; Cutrona & Russell, 1990; Uchino et al., 2018). Factor analyses have shown that these support

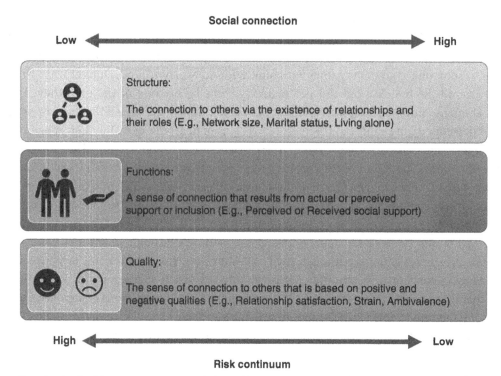

Figure 10.1 Social Connection as a Continuous Multifactorial Risk Factor with Components Related to Structure, Function, and Quality. Note: Low levels of these components are Associated with Risk and High Levels are Associated with Protection (Holt-Lunstad, 2021)

Table 10.1   Measurement Approaches Used to Assess Social Relationships

Type of Measure	Description
Structural	*The existence of and interconnections among differing social ties and roles*
Marital Status	Married versus other (never married, divorced, or widowed)
Social Networks	Network density or size; number of social contacts
Social Integration	Participation in a broad range of social relationships, including active engagement in a variety of social activities or relationships, and a sense of communality and identification with one's social roles
Complex Measures of Social Integration	A single measure that assesses multiple components of social integration, such as marital status, network size, and network participation
Living Alone	Living alone versus living with others
Social Isolation	Pervasive lack of social contact or communication, participation in social activities, or confidants
Functional	*Functions provided by or perceived to be available from social relationships*
Received Support	Self-reported receipt of emotional, informational, tangible, or belonging support
Perceptions of Social Support	Perceptions of availability of emotional, informational, tangible, or belonging support if needed
Perceptions of Loneliness	Feelings of isolation, disconnectedness, and not belonging
Quality	*The Sense of Connection to Others That Is Based on Positive and Negative Qualities*
Relationship Satisfaction	The degree to which one is satisfied with a relationship
Relationship Strain	Strain on a relationship due to difficult circumstances
Ambivalence	A relationship that is both positive and negative
Combined	*Assessment of both structural, functional, and quality measures*
Multifaceted Measurement	Multiple measures obtained that assess more than one of the above conceptualizations

Table 10.2 Definition and Examples of Dimensions of Functional Support

Type of Support	Definition	Example
Perceived Support	The expectation that others will provide support if needed	Perceiving that your friends will be there for you no matter the circumstance
Received Support	The actual provision of support by another	Your friend directly provides you with support to handle an important problem
Emotional	Expressions of comfort and caring	Someone who makes you feel better just because they listen to your problems
Belonging	Shared social activities, sense of social belonging	A friend who you enjoy simply "hanging out" with
Tangible[a]	Provision of material aid	A family member who could give you a personal financial loan
Informational	Provision of advice and guidance	A person who can give you trusted advice and guidance on an issue

[a] This is also referred to as instrumental support.

components are distinct lower-order processes that together make up the higher-order concept of social support (Cutrona & Russell, 1990). These functions also can be differentiated based on whether social support is perceived or received (Dunkel-Schetter & Skokan, 1990; Uchino et al., 2018). Perceived support refers to the perception that others will be available to provide support if needed. Received support is the actual support provided by others. Perceived support is correlated only moderately with received support. Hence, they are distinct constructs (Wills & Shinar, 2000).

A relatively large body of literature links social support to health-relevant outcomes, including health behaviors (e.g., smoking cessation), adherence to medical regimens (e.g., medication), development of and the course of specific chronic conditions (e.g., cardiovascular disease), and all-cause mortality (Barth et al., 2010; DiMatteo, 2004; Hill et al., 2016; Holt-Lunstad et al., 2010; Magrin et al., 2015; Olaya et al., 2017; Vila, 2021). Overall, there is good epidemiological evidence that distinct measures of social support are related to positive health outcomes. More specific findings will be described later, but a meta-analysis by Holt-Lunstad et al. (2010) found that those reporting greater social connection (averaged across different measurement approaches utilized in studies) were associated with 50% increased odds of survival relative to those lacking social connection. Additionally, drawing on data from four nationally representative longitudinal samples of US population, Yang et al. (2016) found that higher levels of social integration (structural support) were associated with lower risk of physiological dysregulation in a dose–response manner in both early and later life.

Among measurements of social connection (e.g., structure, function, quality), the 2010 meta-analysis found that perceived functional support was a significant predictor of lower mortality. Received support did not predict mortality risk significantly. This lack of significance was likely due to large heterogeneity across studies, suggesting that some kinds of support may be more effective than others. These data are consistent with studies finding that perceived support is a more consistent predictor of mental and physical health outcomes than received support (Haber et al., 2007; National Academies of Sciences, Engineering, and Medicine, 2020; Uchino, 2009; Wills & Shinar, 2000). As will be discussed later, this is a significant theoretical issue as interventions aimed at increasing support often try to increase the receipt of social support without considering whether it responds to the individual's needs or is perceived as supportive.

Historical Perspectives

The study of social relationships and physical health has a long research tradition. One early influence was the renowned French sociologist Émile Durkheim. In his classic analysis of suicide rates across social classes, cultures, religious affiliations, and genders, he argued that suicide rates were tied closely to the social environment (Durkheim et al., 1951). For instance, he argued that egoistic suicide—suicide committed by individuals who were social outcasts and saw themselves as being alone or outsiders—resulted from excessive individualism and lack of integration of the individual into society or family life. These individuals were left to face life's challenges on their own. Durkheim's analysis was compelling and led to a subsequent focus on more specific aspects of social relationships related to health outcomes.

In 1976, two influential reviews were published that emphasized the health relevance of the qualitative aspects of social networks. They gave rise to an emphasis in health psychology on the functional support that social networks may provide. Cobb (1976) defined social support as information from others that one is cared for, loved, esteemed, and part of a mutually supportive network. Cobb reviewed evidence suggesting that these social support resources were important in dealing with stressful life events, such as pregnancy, hospitalization, and bereavement. Cassell (1976) focused more on the biological processes linking support to health. He argued that social support might be seen as a protective factor, and he reviewed studies suggesting that such a relationship factor might modify bodily processes (e.g., blood pressure or endocrine activity) in health-relevant ways. These two reviews highlighted the important role that functional social support might play in physical health outcomes.

A few years after these groundbreaking reviews, one of the first population-based longitudinal research studies linking social relationships to mortality was published. Lisa Berkman and Leonard Syme (1979) examined survey responses of nearly 7,000 residents of Alameda County, California. More specifically, they linked answers to questions about the extent of people's social connections to overall mortality and found that people with fewer social ties had higher mortality rates. This classic paper was groundbreaking because it ruled out possible alternative explanations (e.g., results due to poorer initial health status) and provided highly compelling evidence for the link between social relationships and mortality.

While Berkman and Syme (1979) focused on the structure of social relationships, one of the first community-based epidemiological studies linking functional support to health was conducted by Dan Blazer (1982) in a community sample of older adults in Durham County, North Carolina. Even when adjusting for standard control variables, such as physical health status and smoking, his analyses showed that perceptions of greater functional support predicted lower mortality rates. These results also held when accounting for structural measures of social integration, such as those used by Berkman and Syme (1979), thereby showing an association between perceptions of support and physical health regardless of the size of one's network.

Finally, in 1988, James House and his colleagues published a paper titled "Social Relationships and Health" in the journal *Science* (House et al., 1988). After examining evidence from the available, prospective studies, the authors concluded that being socially integrated had an independent protective effect on mortality. These effects were of similar magnitude to those found for blood pressure, smoking, and physical activity. This review's careful analysis of well-designed prospective studies stimulated further research on the links between more specific aspects of support and health outcomes.

Theoretical Models

Since the 1970s, there has been growing interest and subsequent systematic research examining the impact of social support on health. General models emerging from this work suggest that social support can be health-promoting by influencing both psychological and behavioral processes (Hostinar, 2015; Uchino, 2006). For instance, relevant psychological pathways include stress appraisals, and behavioral pathways include health behavior change. These pathways were thought to influence health-relevant biological pathways that ultimately influence either the development or course of physical health problems. An overarching framework that highlights these general pathways but incorporates more specific models (e.g., direct effect, stress-buffering models) is highlighted in Figure 10.2.

As shown in Figure 10.2, functional support can have both a stress-related and a direct effect on health outcomes but via distinct theoretical pathways. The *direct effect pathway* highlights the generally health-enhancing influence of social support. The *stress-buffering pathway*, in comparison, suggests that social support diminishes the adverse health

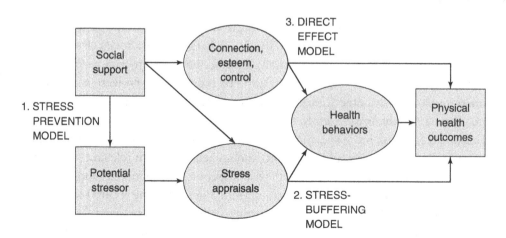

Figure 10.2 Theoretical (Stress Prevention, Direct Effect, and Stress Buffering) Models and Pathways Linking Social Support to Physical Health Outcomes

effects of stress (Cohen & Wills, 1985). A *stress prevention pathway* is also included, as it was highlighted in an early review by Gore (1981), who pointed to the importance of a stress-preventive function of support. As such, the pathways depicted in Figure 10.2 are not necessarily competing perspectives but highlight different contexts and processes by which social support operates (Uchino, 2006). Where they converge is in the "downstream" processes that ultimately link them to health. That is, the final common pathways include health behaviors such as exercise, diet, drug use, and sleep patterns, which in turn can influence health-relevant outcomes. These outcomes range from health-relevant biomarkers (e.g., blood pressure, inflammation) to clinical disease endpoints such as hypertension. The model also suggests that social support can directly impact physical health outcomes.

Social Support as a Buffer for Stress

One of the earliest models of social support in relation to health, the stress prevention model, focuses on the possibility that social support might decrease exposure to adverse life events (Gore, 1981). As shown in Figure 10.2, this model suggests that social support is beneficial because network members may provide resources to avoid or reduce exposure to some types of stressors. Social support may reduce our exposure to stress through several intriguing pathways. First, social support may influence cognitive processes so that people are less likely to appraise or interpret a situation as threatening or challenging (Cohen, 1988) (Also see Chapter 12). Second, social support that encourages proactive coping—including, for example, informational support on planning for a rainy day—can help individuals make informed decisions that minimize subsequent exposure to stress (Aspinwall & Taylor, 1997). Finally, adequate social support in one context may decrease exposure to *secondary stressors* (Pearlin, 1989). For instance, stress at work can lead to conflict at home. However, if spousal support reduces work stress, it may effectively eliminate potential spillover of work stress into marital interactions and reduce exposure to such secondary stressors (Pearlin, 1989).

The best-known stress-related model is the stress-buffering model of support (Cohen & Wills, 1985). As shown in Figure 10.2, this model differs from the stress prevention model in that individuals might still experience stress, but social support is predicted to decrease the strength of the association between stress and physical health outcomes (Cohen & Wills, 1985). This model is based on the hypothesis that stressors have an adverse influence on health behaviors and physical health outcomes but that appropriate support can minimize such links. Consistent with Figure 10.2, Cohen postulated that this stress buffering occurs through a cognitive appraisal process (interpretation of the situation and one's coping resources), which can, in turn, weaken or "buffer" the typically robust association between stress and health-related outcomes (Cohen, 1988).

A major variant of the stress-buffering model is what has been called the *matching hypothesis* (Cutrona & Russell, 1990). This hypothesis predicts that stress buffering is most effective when the type of support matches the needs or challenges of the stressful event. More specifically, it predicts that informational and tangible support should be most effective for controllable events (such as preparing for a job interview), whereas emotional and belonging support should be most effective for uncontrollable events (such as being laid off from a job) (Cutrona & Russell, 1990). This version of the stress-buffering model is one of the few theoretical models of social support that highlights how different functional components of support might be related to outcomes based on the nature of the stressor (such as its controllability).

Overview of the Direct Effect Model

The direct effect model postulates that social support is effective more generally, regardless of stress levels (Cohen & Wills, 1985). Cohen and Wills's (1985) review found that structural support measures were more likely to demonstrate direct effects. The direct effect of structural measures was seen as representing the influence of social support on social identity via direct (e.g., demands from others to behave more healthily) or indirect (e.g., behaving more healthily because relationships add greater life meaning) social control processes (Umberson, 1987). However, there is now evidence that functional support also can directly affect outcomes by promoting a sense of connection, self-esteem, and control over life, due to knowing that one is cared for and supported by others (Lakey & Orehek, 2011; Thoits, 2011).

Lakey and Orehek (2011) extended the direct effect model by proposing the relational regulation theory (RRT) to account for the direct effects of social support on mental health outcomes. According to RRT, everyday interactions (e.g., talking about events of a typical day, gossip) help individuals generalize their relationship representations to stressful contexts (i.e., is this person I am comfortable with likely to be supportive during stress?). These researchers have been able to forecast which relationships might be most beneficial months later, based on analyses of brief (e.g., 10-minute) lab-based general discussions (Veenstra et al., 2011).

Empirical Evidence Supporting the Models

The stress-buffering model has been tested in several well-controlled laboratory studies, many of which examine cardiovascular reactivity (CVR) as the outcome. In these studies, either a friend or a stranger (the experimenter or a confederate) provides the participant with support while the person is undergoing a standardized task designed to induce stress, such as giving a speech in front of a confederate. Most of these studies find that social support is associated with lower CVR (Creaven et al., 2020; Teoh & Hilmert, 2018). Some emerging evidence examining threat arousal via brain activation has shown that perceived social support is associated with lower activation of the hypothalamic-pituitary-adrenal (HPA) region of the brain (Coan et al., 2017), which is partially responsible for stress response regulation (Brown et al., 2017).

There is much less research evaluating links between the other stress-related models and processes in these models. The matching hypothesis has received some support in terms of psychological and relational outcomes (Cutrona & Russell, 1990; Lee et al., 2020), but has been tested less frequently in epidemiological and physical health studies. Some studies examining objective health outcomes also provide some supportive evidence of the matching hypothesis. For example, one study of 41 American Indian/Alaska Native and Native Hawaiian patients with diabetes examined five types of support offered and found that emotional and esteem social support messages from healthcare providers accounted for 32.5% of the variance in diabetic patient glycemic control (Robinson et al., 2017). Though it was unclear why the patients only benefited from emotional and esteem social support, these findings raise the question of whether proactively matching support to patient needs may optimize benefits—the key contention of the matching hypothesis.

The stress prevention model is the least tested of the stress-related models in the health domain despite the fact that longitudinal studies are consistent with its basic premise. One longitudinal study of 301 older adults found that individuals with limited social support experienced more depressive symptoms 12 months later, and that the effect was both direct and indirect (Russell & Cutrona, 1991).

The direct effect model suggests that social support should affect physical health outcomes directly. There is strong evidence that perceived social support is related directly to beneficial influences on biological function (Howard et al., 2017; Uchino et al., 2018; Lutgendorf et al., 2005). Consistent with a health behavior link, there is also consistent evidence linking perceived support to health-promoting behaviors, including more exercise, less smoking or alcohol consumption, and better sleep quality (Ailshire & Burgard, 2012; Kent de Grey, 2018; Laird et al., 2016; Stewart et al., 2011). Finally, a comprehensive meta-analysis shows that social support is also associated with better patient cooperation with treatment regimens in chronic disease populations (DiMatteo, 2004; Magrin et al., 2015).

The overall model in Figure 10.2 posits that only part of the link between social support and health is due to health behaviors, as shown in prior studies. One study, for example, reported that the link between social support and cardiovascular disease was mediated by poor sleep among women but not men (Nordin et al., 2008). Thus, there is both a direct and indirect link (through health behaviors) between social support and physical health, though future studies will have to directly test such association using more robust tests of mediation (Rucker et al., 2011).

Empirical Evidence of the Health Effects of Social Support

Evidence for the Protective Influence of Social Support

Overall, there is strong evidence for the protective effect of social support on health, with stronger evidence for perceived support than received support (see Uchino's 2009 review).

This evidence comes from laboratory, field, and epidemiological studies across morbidity and mortality outcomes. The evidence for the effects of social support on heart disease and the evidence of a protective effect on overall mortality is summarized below. We focus on these two particular outcomes because the evidence is the strongest in terms of both the number and quality of studies.

Coronary Heart Disease

There is substantial evidence linking low levels of social support to coronary heart disease (CHD), the leading cause of death in most industrialized countries. Barth et al.'s (2010) systematic review and meta-analysis examined prospective studies that measured both structural and functional social support and cardiovascular outcomes. These included studies of CHD etiology, development of CHD in previously healthy individuals, and CHD prognosis, including individuals with preexisting CHD (Barth et al., 2010; Lett et al., 2005, 2007). In a 13-year longitudinal study, low functional support and depression were found to be predictive of CHD as well (Liu et al., 2017).

Across multiple studies, there is evidence for the beneficial cardiovascular effects of functional support. Higher levels of functional social support were associated with lower risk of incident hypertension (incident rate ratio 0.64, [95% CI 0.41–0.97]) (Harding et al., 2022). Perceived social support is associated with better psychosocial adjustment in people diagnosed with CHD (Karataş & Bostanoğlu, 2017). By extension, lack of social support is a significant predictor of rehospitalization, and greater support predicts lower mortality in heart failure patients (Luttik et al., 2005), and it can have a direct effect on physical health when looking at quality of life for CHD patients (Lee et al., 2012; Wang et al., 2013). Another meta-analysis also found that social support and social integration were associated with lower levels of inflammation, pointing to one pathway by which social support may contribute to cardiovascular outcomes (Uchino et al., 2018).

Higher levels of social support are also associated with lower loneliness and social isolation ($r = -0.39$), according to a recent meta-analysis (Zhang & Dong, 2022). With that in mind, one cross-sectional study suggested that being lonely, even with high levels of social support, poses the greatest risk for hypertension, a major risk factor for CHD (Yazawa et al., 2022). In a secondary analysis of 11,486 community-dwelling Australians aged 70 and above, individuals who had poor scores on measures of social health—defined as an individual's ability to form satisfying and meaningful relationships, their ability to adapt in social situations, and their interactions and perceived support from other people, institutions and services—were 42% more likely to develop CHD and twice as likely to die from CHD, even when initially free of CHD (Freak-Poli et al., 2021). The same study showed that social isolation and low social support, but not loneliness, were more salient risk factors when it comes to CHD. Valtorta et al. (2016) conducted a meta-analysis that found that poor social relationships were associated with a 29% increase in risk of incident CHD and a 32% increase in risk of stroke.

Although fewer studies have been conducted in developing countries, evidence suggests the protective effects of social support may extend to less industrialized regions. For example, among Vietnamese patients with hypertension, larger network size and the provision of informational, emotional, and instrumental illness-related support were associated with lower odds of uncontrolled hypertension (Thuy et al., 2021).

Mortality

There is now substantial evidence for the protective effect of social connections on risk for all-cause mortality. Some of the first epidemiological evidence was highlighted in the review by House et al. (1988). They summarized data from five prospective studies: the Alameda County (Berkman & Syme, 1979), Evans County, Tecumseh, Eastern Finland, and Gothenburg studies. These studies examined large community samples of initially healthy individuals, assessed their social relationships, and then followed them over several years to determine whether the level of social integration predicted who would still be alive. Indeed, the evidence confirmed that those with lower social integration had significantly higher age-adjusted mortality risk (Steptoe et al., 2013).

Since that time, the number of studies examining the influence of social relationships (both functional and structural) and mortality has grown exponentially. One recent study ($n = 388,973$ from the years 1998–2014) showed that all-cause mortality risk was 45% higher among adults 18–64 years old living alone compared to those who were living with others (Lee & Singh, 2021). Multiple meta-analyses have linked social support and mortality. In a meta-analysis of 148 independent prospective studies with data from 308,849 individuals followed for an average of 7.5 years, results indicated that individuals with greater social connections (averaged across the different measures shown in Table 10.1) have a 50% greater likelihood of survival than those with fewer social connections (Holt-Lunstad et al., 2010). The effect was consistent across gender, age, initial health status, and causes of mortality. This meta-analysis provided evidence of the directional effect of social relationships influencing mortality. Most

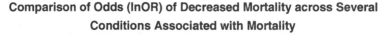

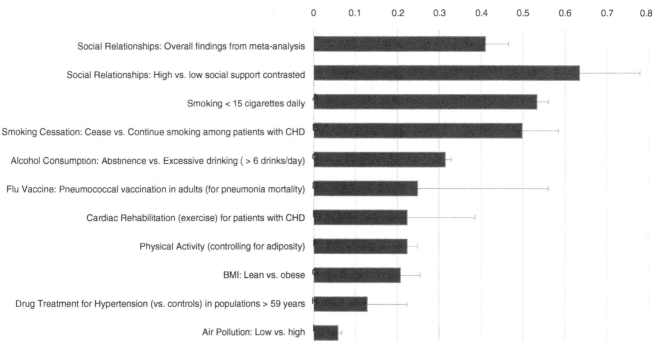

Note. Effect size of zero indicates no effect. The effect sizes were estimated from meta analyses: ; A = Shavelle, Paculdo, Strauss, and Kush, 2008; B = Critchley and Capewell, 2003; C = Holman, English, Milne, and Winter, 1996; D = Fine, Smith Carson, Meffe, Sankey, Weissfeld, Detsky, and kapoor, 1994; E = Taylor, Brown, Ebrahim, Jolliffe, Noorani, Rees et al, 2004; F,G = Katzmarzyk, Janssen, and Ardern, 2003; H = Insua, Sacks, Lau, Lau, Reitman, Pagano, and Chalmers, 1994; I = Schwartz, 1994.

Figure 10.3 Benchmark Data Comparing the Magnitude of Effect of Social Support on Odds of Decreased Mortality Relative to Other Factors
Source: Holt-Lunstad, Smith & Layton, 2010

studies were population-based, and, thus, examined initially healthy participants. However, even among those who were ill, greater social connectedness (that is, having large amounts of both structural and functional support) was associated with greater odds of survival. Thus, regardless of initial health status, those who were more socially connected lived longer. Most notably, the overall magnitude of the effect of social connections on risk for mortality was comparable with and, in many cases, exceeded the effect of many well-established risk factors for mortality. For instance, lacking social connectedness carries a risk equivalent to smoking up to 15 cigarettes per day and is greater than that for alcohol abuse, physical inactivity (sedentary lifestyle), obesity, and air pollution (see Figure 10.3) (Holt-Lunstad et al., 2010).

Across studies, the influence of social relationships was measured in diverse ways, including both functional and structural aspects (Table 10.1). The magnitude of risk reduction differed significantly across types of measurement approaches examined. Although both structural (OR = 1.57, 95% CI [1.46, 1.70]) and functional measures (OR = 1.46, 95% CI [1.28, 1.66]) were associated significantly with greater odds of survival, specific measurement approaches within these broader categorizations varied in their predictive utility. Within functional support measures, perceived support was a significant predictor of longevity (OR = 1.35, 95% CI [1.22, 1.49]), whereas received support was not (OR = 1.21, 95% CI [0.91, 1.63]). When examining structural measures, living alone (OR = 1.19, 95% CI [0.99, 1.44]) was the poorest predictor, and complex measures of social integration were the best predictors (OR = 1.91, 95% CI [1.63, 2.23]), with assessments that considered the multidimensional aspects of social relationships associated with 91% increased odds of survival. Taken together, these data suggest the importance of both social networks and the social support they provide.

A more recent summary of 23 meta-analyses published between 1994 and 2021 that included 1,187 longitudinal and cross-sectional studies (*n* = 1.458 million people in many countries and multiple continents) was highly consistent with the above meta-analysis, pointing to a predicted link between social support and reduced disease and mortality (Vila, 2021).

Across all these studies and meta-analyses, overall effects of social relationships on mortality may be a conservative estimate. Most studies adjusted for initial health and other lifestyle risk factors to establish the independent influence of social connections on risk for mortality. However, social relationships are linked inextricably with multiple pathways, behaviors, and risk factors known to be associated with mortality (Holt-Lunstad, 2021; Liu & Newschaffer, 2011; Pantell et al., 2013). For example, excessive alcohol consumption is associated with poor social support; and individuals with more positive social relationships engage in fewer risky health behaviors (Hsieh et al., 2017; Umberson & Karas Montez, 2010).

This means they are more likely to exhibit behaviors, such as not smoking, using seatbelts, getting adequate sleep, healthy diet, regular exercise, and good dental hygiene (Brummett et al., 2006; Fuemmeler et al., 2006). Therefore, these analyses eliminate one of the pathways through which social relationships may influence risk for mortality. The overall effect may also be a conservative estimate because most studies failed to measure relationship quality. Thus, estimates likely include both high- and poor-quality relationships (potential detrimental influences of poor-quality relationships are discussed in the next section).

Factors That May Moderate the Influence of Social Support

Perceived and Received Support

Although social support generally is related to better health, in some circumstances, received support is unrelated or is even linked to negative health outcomes (Holt-Lunstad et al., 2010; Uchino, 2009; Uchino et al., 2018). Many of the studies reviewed above that found links between social support and physical health are based upon measures of perceived support. In prior work, the concepts of perceived and received support have been used interchangeably, with the assumption that individuals high in perceived support also receive greater support (Dunkel-Schetter & Bennett, 1990; Uchino, 2009). However, measures of perceived and received support are only moderately correlated and, hence, seem to represent distinct constructs (Haber et al., 2007).

Recent research has distinguished more clearly between perceived and received support. Several recent studies have found that perceived support protects against negative outcomes, while received support often is unrelated to outcomes (Hartley & Coffee, 2019; Kaniasty, 2020; Szkody et al., 2020). Consistent with this possibility, a complicated set of findings emerges throughout these studies when examining measures of received support on health outcomes. For instance, several prospective epidemiological studies examining received support (especially tangible support) found it to be associated with higher subsequent mortality rates (Forster & Stoller, 1992; Krause, 1997). This is also consistent with cross-sectional laboratory studies in which receiving support appears to cause stress (Bolger & Amarel, 2007). Although a simple plausible explanation, based on the concept of support mobilization, is that individuals who are more dependent on receiving support are siply more physically impaired to begin with, these studies do not appear to support this explanation because most considered the influence of initial health status prospectively. A balance between the support provided and the support received was associated with a lower risk of all-cause mortality compared to either disproportionately receiving more support from others, or disproportionately providing more support to others than they received (Chen et al., 2021).

It has been argued that the links between received support and health might be more contextual. Hence, stressor factors (e.g., a match between stressor and support type), provider factors (e.g., relationship quality), and recipient factors (e.g., threats to independence) are important considerations (Bolger & Amarel, 2007; Dunkel-Schetter & Skokan, 1990; Uchino, 2009). All these factors can influence whether recipients see received support as responsive, and it has been argued that this is a key factor in the efficacy of received support (Maisel & Gable, 2009). Consistent with this possibility, the Midlife in the United States (MIDUS) study found that only when received support was viewed as unresponsive was it associated with higher mortality rates (Selcuk & Ong, 2013). This is an important finding, and future interventions should consider such issues in designing effective interventions. In fact, responsiveness/unresponsiveness is the component of received tangible support that appears to be most consistently related to higher mortality (Forster & Stoller, 1992; Kaplan et al., 1994).

Relationship Quality

Another important issue is relationship quality. Much of the epidemiological evidence that has established the health relevance of social support did not consider the quality of relationships and assumed that all relationships are positive. However, even though relationships may be caring, considerate, and sources of warmth and love, they can also be sources of conflict and stress. Although the stress-buffering model suggests that relationships can buffer the negative health effects of stress, it is also possible that some relationships may be sources of stress. Among the few epidemiological studies that examined relationship quality, findings indicate that negativity in social relationships predicts a greater risk for mortality (Friedman et al., 1995). For instance, a study that followed 2,264 breast cancer patients for an average of 10.8 years found that, while network support is associated with better prognosis, poor quality and burden in family relations were associated with higher risk of all-cause mortality (Kroenke et al., 2012).

Relationship distress may be particularly salient in the context of marriage, given its importance. Indeed, a growing body of research among couples shows that despite the health advantage of marital status, distressed marriages are associated with greater morbidity and risk for mortality (Robles et al., 2014; Whisman et al., 2018). Relationship distress also has been associated with deleterious health-relevant processes, including immune dysregulation and delayed wound healing (Kiecolt-Glaser, 2005), high ambulatory blood pressure, and metabolic syndrome (Birmingham et al., 2019; Troxel et al., 2005). There is also evidence that unsupportive behavior and partner distress are associated with poorer quality of life among women with breast cancer (Manne et al., 2005).

Likewise, interpersonal stress may be more impactful than other sources of stress. For instance, the Stockholm Female Coronary Risk Study found that after controlling for standard risk factors, marital distress was associated with nearly a threefold increase in risk of recurrent coronary events, whereas work stress was unrelated (Orth-Gomer et al., 2000). (For more on stress and coping, see Chapter 12.)

Technology and Social Support

Within the last decade, advancements in technology have led to dramatic shifts in the way social support is communicated (Antonucci et al., 2017; Canale et al., 2021; Hunter et al., 2022; Zhou & Cheng, 2022). Use of the Internet and smartphones is widespread in most developed nations and is now the primary form of communication. Research is now exploring equivalencies between technology-mediated and face-to-face communication and the potential, unique benefits of each modality for social support. There is some evidence to support both potential advantages and disadvantages of online compared to face-to-face support.

Beyond merely connecting individuals at a distance, technology-mediated social support may have potential advantages. For example, those with stigmatized conditions can seek Internet-mediated support that allows them to remain anonymous (Malik & Coulson, 2008); users of online forums can search previous posts for informational and emotional support, thereby reducing the burden for both provider and recipient (Wright & Bell, 2008); individuals who are able to connect across geographic distances can create support networks around their specific support needs (Rainie & Wellman, 2012); and older adults who experience regular depression as a result of social isolation may mitigate symptoms using social media (Wu & Chiou, 2020). Overall, these data point to the general utility of communicating informational and emotional support online (Dare & Green, 2011). Evidence also has emerged that participation in social support groups contributes to experiencing a sense of belonging (Smit et al., 2021). Likewise, there is some evidence to suggest that individuals participate in online support groups to help others (Rimer et al., 2005), thereby increasing provision of support.

Some forms of technology-communicated social support may be less effective than other forms of support or even have deleterious effects under some circumstances. For instance, there is evidence that text messages, despite having similar effects psychologically to talking with someone about a stressful event, do not have similar physiological effects (Seltzer et al., 2012). Similarly, research examining use of the Internet for support after a traumatic event found that despite perceptions of benefit, there was no evidence of an effect on psychological well-being (Vicary & Fraley, 2010). The same technology that can facilitate support from others across geographic distances can also interfere with face-to-face support. For instance, the presence of a mobile phone in social settings may reduce closeness and quality of interactions, interfering with social support and relationships (Przybylski & Weinstein, 2012). A recent study examining remote contact as a replacement for in-person contact to protect mental health among a nationally representative sample of older adults found that in-person contact cannot be replaced by remote means of contact for maintaining mental health. The participants in the study experienced depression, reductions in happiness, and loneliness despite increases in remote contact (Hawkley et al., 2021). Future research that directly examines the links between perceived and received Internet-mediated support and physical health outcomes will be needed to make this final link, and it may operate differently in various situations.

Taken together, this evidence has important implications for social support interventions. First, we should consider several contextual factors: stress-related factors that may influence efficacy of support, support provider factors and characteristics, and support recipient factors and support desires. Second, the data on relationship quality show that researchers and practitioners must assess both positivity and negativity in the context of social support. Interventions aimed at increasing social support may have unintended detrimental effects if they fail to account for negativity in relationships and the responsivity of the support provided. Likewise, by reducing negativity and increasing responsiveness, interventions may have larger effects than previously estimated. Finally, when designing interventions using online tools, it should not be assumed that online support will be equivalent to face-to-face support.

Social Isolation During the COVID-19 Pandemic

The COVID-19 pandemic has had far-reaching impacts on public health beyond the virus itself, contributing to secondary impacts on physical and mental health. Social distancing and other restrictions made accessing both informal and formal social support difficult. This was particularly true for older adults and those in residential housing where such restrictions were often strictly enforced. Meta-analytic data gathered from 32 longitudinal studies confirmed increases in both the severity and prevalence of loneliness during the pandemic (Ernst et al., 2022). A review of 35 years of studies examining factors influencing susceptibility to upper respiratory infectious illness via viral challenges found that, among other factors, social integration and social support decreased risk of upper respiratory illness after exposure to the viruses (Cohen, 2020).

Nonetheless, many studies examined whether social support buffered pandemic-related stressors. Results from hundreds of surveys have been published to understand who was most resilient and what factors were associated with greater risk during various phases of the global pandemic. Multiple reviews and meta-analyses have found that better social support was associated with better outcomes and poorer social support was associated with worse outcomes among healthcare workers (Muller et al. 2020; Serrano-Ripoll et al., 2020; Spoorthy 2020). While many studies show that poor social support has been associated with worse mental health, well-being, and poorer health-related behaviors, understanding some of the longer-term health effects may require longer follow-up. Future research carefully and systematically documenting social factors, following individuals and populations for decades, will be needed to understand the full scope and ramifications of the COVID-19 pandemic on social support and health.

Health Behavior Applications

Theoretical models linking social support to health highlight the potential role of behavior (e.g., medical cooperation and health behaviors) in linking support to disease outcomes (Uchino, 2006). The next section describes evidence from two research areas to illustrate modifiable consequences of social support on health behaviors. The first application summarizes evidence for the link between social connection and opioid misuse, and the second describes evidence pointing to social support interventions for suicide prevention.

Application 1: Social Connection and Opioid Misuse

Earlier research has brought to light evidence that endogenous opioids play a significant role in social bonding in humans and other primates (Machin & Dunbar, 2011; Inagaki et al., 2016). Christie (2021) has theorized that there is a temporal connection between higher levels of social isolation and greater levels of opioid misuse. Albertín and Íñiguez (2008) found that people who used opioids reported that the drug replaced the need for sexual intimacy, and the human need to socially connect by spending time with friends. When these participants were forced to choose between use of opioids and relationships, they were more likely to choose opioid use.

A systematic review of 29 studies found that social connection was a correlate to opioid misuse; however, the directionality was not consistent, and associations were both negative and positive (Cance et al., 2021). A study of 371 methadone maintenance treatment (MMT) patients aged 18 and older (Polenick et al., 2019) found that the gender of the patient was the moderator in the association between illicit opioid use and loneliness. "Severe loneliness was associated with higher odds of using illicit opioids among women (OR = 3.00, 95% CI [1.19, 7.57], p = 0.020) but lower odds of using illicit opioids among men (OR = 0.35, 95% CI [0.14, 0.87], p = 0.024), accounting for age, marital status, work status, depressive symptoms, and MMT characteristics (treatment episode, treatment duration, and methadone dose)." In a nationally representative sample of 6,017 older adults (aged 65 and above), loneliness was a strong predictor of higher use of pain medications, such as opioids and NSAIDs. In this study, loneliness was related to higher pain medication use and more than two times the frequency of use of antidepressants, sleep medications, and benzodiazepines (Kotwal et al., 2021).

More research is needed to understand the relationship between opioid misuse and levels of social isolation and lack of perceived social support. The psychobiological mechanistic function of endogenous opioids for bonding may provide clarity as to why opioid misuse leads to lower levels of social connection in those who use opioids.

Application 2: Social Support Intervention for Suicide Prevention

The rate of suicide in the United States increased by 30% between 2000 and 2018 but decreased between 2019 and 2020 (CDC, 2022). Though suicide was no longer listed as one of the top ten causes of death in the United States in 2020 during the COVID-19 pandemic, it is still a leading cause with 45,979 deaths by suicide in 2020 (Centers for Disease Control and Prevention, 2020). Suicide and other nonfatal self-harm cost the US economy close to $490 billion in amelioration for medical bills, costs of work loss, quality of life costs, and other estimated costs (Peterson et al., 2021).

Of the nine protective factors against suicide that the Centers for Disease Control and Prevention (CDC) identified (Centers for Disease Control and Prevention, 2022), seven are directly related to social support or broader social determinants of health:

- Effective coping and problem-solving skills

- Reasons for living—for example: family, friends, pets

- Strong sense of cultural identity

- Support from partners, friends, and family

- Feeling connected to others

- Feeling connected to school, community, and other institutions

- Availability of high-quality and consistent physical and mental health care

- Cultural and religious beliefs that discourage suicide

- Reduced access to lethal means

Several social support interventions for preventing suicide have been developed and evaluated. One study focused on a sample from Chennai, India, where over 153,000 deaths by suicide occurred in 2020, more than any other country in the world (National Crime Records Bureau, n.d.). This randomized controlled study found that brief intervention and contact (BIC) was effective in reducing subsequent suicidal behavior among people who attempted suicide (Vijayakumar et al., 2011). Researchers randomly assigned 680 individuals who had attempted suicide and were admitted to Government Royapettah General Hospital in Chennai to either the BIC group (n = 320) or the treatment-as-usual (TAU) group (n = 360). During each visit, the subjects in the BIC group were asked how they were feeling and whether they needed any support. If they indicated needing support, they were referred to an agency that would provide outpatient mental health care.

Completed and attempted suicide was significantly lower in the BIC group after the intervention at an 18-month follow-up compared to the TAU group, with eight attempted and only one completed suicide in the BIC group, 17 attempted and 9 completed suicides in the TAU group, and 65% of the participants in the BIC group considering the visits to be helpful and supportive. These findings showed that a brief intervention session, combined with systematic long-term contact after discharge, can have a positive impact on preventing subsequent suicide and suicide attempts. While there are many possible factors involved, BIC may have acted as an added social support network, enhancing a feeling of connectedness or feeling more cared for by others.

A recent meta-analysis that examined 22 intervention studies (including the above study) found a 52% reduction in suicides in the BIC intervention groups. The analysis concluded that social support interventions may reduce the risk of using lethal means and therefore reduce deaths by suicide, but not suicide attempts (Hou et al., 2021).

People with greater perceived and received social support have a decreased likelihood of lifetime suicide attempts (Kleiman & Liu, 2013). While cognitive reasons for death by suicide are difficult to study, research suggesting that social support is protective against suicidal ideation and attempts is promising. Social support is a behavior that can be modified and can be used globally to bolster suicide prevention programs around the world.

Future Directions for Research and Practice

Several conceptual issues need greater attention in future research and interventions on social support and health. As noted earlier, received support can be associated with negative influences on health if that support is not seen as responsive (Stanton et al., 2019). Interventions that seek to mobilize support from either similar peers or family and friends should be sure that support is responsive to individuals in order to provide either direct or stress-related beneficial links to health behaviors and related outcomes (see Figure 10.2).

Quality of relationships is another factor that can influence the responsiveness of support that has not been considered strongly in prior work. A recent study found that among US adults, high-quality social relationships functioned as a buffer between psychosocial stress and depressive symptoms (Kaveladze et al., 2020). However, while relationships with others may be sources of warmth and love, these social relationships can also be sources of conflict and stress, resulting in relationships that have a mix of both positive and negative qualities (i.e., ambivalent relationships) (Holt-Lunstad & Uchino, 2019). This work suggests that such ambivalent ties are related to less effective support provision and greater biological risk for disease (Holt-Lunstad & Uchino, 2019). Future work should consider the quality of relationships, given that it may affect health-relevant support processes.

Future research also should consider social support in the context of a changing social climate. Despite the increases in technology that would presumably foster social connections, people are reporting greater social isolation and loneliness. When surveyed during the height of the 2020 pandemic, an estimated 36% of American respondents reported experiencing serious loneliness within the past four weeks, making loneliness one of the most widespread mental health conditions in the country (Weissbourd et al., 2021). Hawkley et al. (2021) found that remote social contact does not replace in-person contact to protect mental health of older adults. Future research should explore the nuanced impact of digital technology to enhance perceived and received social support.

Given the increase in the extent to which individuals rely on digital communication (in the form of online social networking, texting, telehealth, etc.), there is a need for greater attention to the health relevance of online social support. Although this is a burgeoning area of research, there are still important gaps in our understanding. For instance, research must distinguish between social support gained from exclusively online relationships (e.g., online support groups and chat groups) and support from friends and look at how in-person and online social support can and should complement each other, especially when looking at older generations versus younger generations (Benvenuti et al., 2020; Cole et al., 2017). Moving forward, it will be important to examine what pathways may be capitalized on, and what pathways may be absent, when individuals seek or provide support using online tools.

Finally, future research should consider the stress-buffering effects of social support in racial/ethnic minority groups where discrimination that has acute and chronic negative health outcomes has been historically present (see also Chapter 12).

Summary

There is robust evidence that social support significantly and positively influences health and longevity and that the effects of social support can occur through multiple types of support and various pathways. On the other hand, a lack of social connectedness carries a risk of similar magnitude as many of the factors prioritized in public health, for example, smoking, alcohol abuse, physical inactivity, obesity, and air pollution. Epidemiological and experimental research also suggests that not all aspects of social support are equally effective and that we need a more nuanced approach to social support. A new generation of research is currently considering the role of technology in interpersonal functioning, the use of social support, and the implications of that role for public health. Careful attention to these issues is needed in developing effective social support interventions.

References

Ailshire, J. A., & Burgard, S. A. (2012). Family relationships and troubled sleep among U.S. adults: Examining the influences of contact frequency and relationship quality. *Journal of Health and Social Behavior, 53*(2), 248–262. https://doi.org/10.1177/0022146512446642

Albertín, P., & Íñiguez, L. (2008). Using drugs: The meaning of opiate substances and their consumption from the consumer perspective. *Addiction Research & Theory, 16*(5), 434–452. https://doi.org/10.1080/16066350802041455

Antonucci, T. C., Ajrouch, K. J., & Manalel, J. A. (2017). Social relations and technology: Continuity, context, and change. *Innovation in Aging, 1*(3), igx029. https://doi.org/10.1093/geroni/igx029

Aspinwall, L. G., & Taylor, S. E. (1997). A stitch in time: Self-regulation and proactive coping. *Psychological Bulletin, 121*(3), 417–436. https://doi.org/10.1037/0033-2909.121.3.417

Barth, J., Schneider, S., & von Känel, R. (2010). Lack of social support in the etiology and the prognosis of coronary heart disease: A systematic review and meta-analysis. *Psychosomatic Medicine, 72*(3), 229–238. https://doi.org/10.1097/psy.0b013e3181d01611

Benvenuti, M., Giovagnoli, S., Mazzoni, E., Cipresso, P., Pedroli, E., & Riva, G. (2020). The relevance of online social relationships among the elderly: How using the web could enhance quality of life? *Frontiers in Psychology, 11*, 551862. https://doi.org/10.3389/fpsyg.2020.551862

Berkman, L. F., & Syme, S. L. (1979). Social networks, host resistance, and mortality: A nine-year follow-up study of Alameda County residents. *American Journal of Epidemiology, 109*(2), 186–204. https://doi.org/10.1093/oxfordjournals.aje.a112674

Berkman, L. F., Glass, T., Brissette, I., & Seeman, T. E. (2000). From social integration to health: Durkheim in the new millennium. *Social Science & Medicine (1982), 51*(6), 843–857. https://doi.org/10.1016/s0277-9536(00)00065-4

Birmingham, W. C., Wadsworth, L. L., Hung, M., Li, W., & Herr, R. M. (2019). Ambivalence in the early years of marriage: Impact on ambulatory blood pressure and relationship processes. *Annals of Behavioral Medicine, 53*(12), 1069–1080. https://doi.org/10.1093/abm/kaz017

Blazer, D. G. (1982). Social support and mortality in an elderly community population. *American Journal of Epidemiology, 115*(5), 684–694. https://doi.org/10.1093/oxfordjournals.aje.a113351

Bolger, N., & Amarel, D. (2007). Effects of social support visibility on adjustment to stress: Experimental evidence. *Journal of Personality and Social Psychology, 92*(3), 458–475. https://doi.org/10.1037/0022-3514.92.3.458

Brown, C. L., Beckes, L., Allen, J. P., & Coan, J. A. (2017). Subjective general health and the social regulation of hypothalamic activity. *Psychosomatic Medicine, 79*(6), 670–673. https://doi.org/10.1097/psy.0000000000000468

Brummett, B. H., Babyak, M. A., Siegler, I. C., Vitaliano, P. P., Ballard, E. L., Gwyther, L. P., & Williams, R. B. (2006). Associations among perceptions of social support, negative affect, and quality of sleep in caregivers and non-caregivers. *Health Psychology, 25*(2), 220–225. https://doi.org/10.1037/0278-6133.25.2.220

Canale, N., Marino, C., Lenzi, M., Vieno, A., Griffiths, M. D., Gaboardi, M., Giraldo, M., Cervone, C., & Massimo, S. (2021). How communication technology fosters individual and social wellbeing during the Covid-19 pandemic: Preliminary support for a digital interaction model. *Journal of Happiness Studies, 23*(2). https://doi.org/10.1007/s10902-021-00421-1

Cance, J. D., Saavedra, L. M., Wondimu, B., Scaglione, N. M., Hairgrove, S., & Graham, P. W. (2021). Examining the relationship between social connection and opioid misuse: A systematic review. *Substance Use & Misuse, 56*(10), 1–15. https://doi.org/10.1080/10826084.2021.1936056

Cassel, J. (1976). The contribution of the social environment to host resistance. *American Journal of Epidemiology, 104*(2), 107–123. https://doi.org/10.1093/oxfordjournals.aje.a112281

Centers for Disease Control and Prevention. (2020). Deaths. Wonder.cdc.gov. https://wonder.cdc.gov/Deaths-by-Underlying-Cause.html

Centers for Disease Control and Prevention. (2022). Risk and protective factors. www.cdc.gov. https://www.cdc.gov/suicide/factors/index.html

Chen, E., Lam, P. H., Finegood, E. D., Turiano, N. A., Mroczek, D. K., & Miller, G. E. (2021). The balance of giving versus receiving social support and all-cause mortality in a US national sample. *Proceedings of the National Academy of Sciences, 118*(24), e2024770118.

Christie, N. C. (2021). The role of social isolation in opioid addiction. *Social Cognitive an Affective Neuroscience*, 16(7): 645–656. https://doi.org/10.1093/scan/nsab029

Coan, J. A., Beckes, L., Gonzalez, M. Z., Maresh, E. L., Brown, C. L., & Hasselmo, K. (2017). Relationship status and perceived support in the social regulation of neural responses to threat. *Social Cognitive and Affective Neuroscience*, 12(10), 1574–1583. https://doi.org/10.1093/scan/nsx091

Cobb, S. (1976). Social support as a moderator of life stress. *Psychosomatic Medicine*, 38(5), 300–314. https://doi.org/10.1097/00006842-197609000-00003

Cohen, S. (2020). Psychosocial vulnerabilities to upper respiratory infectious illness: Implications for susceptibility to coronavirus disease 2019 (COVID-19). *Perspectives on Psychological Science*, 16(1), 174569162094251. https://doi.org/10.1177/1745691620942516

Cohen, S., & Wills, T. A. (1985). Stress, social support, and the buffering hypothesis. *Psychological Bulletin*, 98(2), 310–357. https://doi.org/10.1037/0033-2909.98.2.310

Cohen, S., Mermelstein, R., Kamarck, T., & Hoberman, H. M. (1985). Measuring the functional components of social support. *Social Support: Theory, Research and Applications*, 8(11), 73–94. https://doi.org/10.1007/978-94-009-5115-0_5

Cole, D. A., Nick, E. A., Zelkowitz, R. L., Roeder, K. M., & Spinelli, T. (2017). Online social support for young people: Does it recapitulate in-person social support; can it help? *Computers in Human Behavior*, 68, 456–464. https://doi.org/10.1016/j.chb.2016.11.058

Creaven, A.-M., Higgins, N. M., Ginty, A. T., & Gallagher, S. (2020). Social support, social participation, and cardiovascular reactivity to stress in the midlife in the United States (MIDUS) study. *Biological Psychology*, 155, 107921. https://doi.org/10.1016/j.biopsycho.2020.107921

Cutrona, C. E., & Russell, D. W. (1990). Type of social support and specific stress: Toward a theory of optimal matching. In B. R. Sarason, I. G. Sarason, & G. R. Pierce (Eds.), *Social support: An interactional view* (pp. 316–366). John Wiley & Sons. https://psycnet.apa.org/record/1990-97699-013

Dare, J., & Green, L. (2011). Rethinking social support in women's midlife years: Women's experiences of social support in online environments. *European Journal of Cultural Studies*, 14(5), 473–490. https://doi.org/10.1177/1367549411412203

DiMatteo, M. R. (2004). Social support and patient adherence to medical treatment: A meta-analysis. *Health Psychology*, 23(2), 207–218. https://doi.org/10.1037/0278-6133.23.2.207

Dunkel-Schetter, C., & Bennett, T. L. (1990). Differentiating the cognitive and behavioral aspects of social support. In B. R. Sarason, I. G. Sarason, & G. R. Pierce (Eds.), *Social Support: An Interactional View* (pp. 267–296). John Wiley & Sons. https://psycnet.apa.org/record/1990-97699-011

Dunkel-Schetter, C., & Skokan, L. A. (1990). Determinants of social support provision in personal relationships. *Journal of Social and Personal Relationships*, 7(4), 437–450. https://doi.org/10.1177/0265407590074002

Durkheim, E., Spaulding, J. A., & Simpson, G. (1951). Suicide: A study in sociology. *American Journal of Sociology*, 57(1), 100–101. https://doi.org/10.1086/220884

Ernst, M., Niederer, D., Werner, A. M., Czaja, S. J., Mikton, C., Ong, A. D., Rosen, T., Brahler, E., & Beutel, M. E. (2022). Loneliness before and during the COVID-19 Pandemic: A systematic review with meta-analysis. *American Psychologist*, 77(5), 660. https://doi.org/https://doi.org/10.1037/amp0001005

Fasihi Harandi, T., Mohammad Taghinasab, M., & Dehghan Nayeri, T. (2017). The correlation of social support with mental health: A meta-analysis. *Electronic Physician*, 9(9), 5212–5222. https://doi.org/10.19082/5212

Forster, L. E., & Stoller, E. P. (1992). The impact of social support on mortality: A seven-year follow-up of older men and women. *Journal of Applied Gerontology*, 11(2), 173–186. https://doi.org/10.1177/073346489201100204

Freak-Poli, R., Ryan, J., Neumann, J. T., Tonkin, A., Reid, C. M., Woods, R. L., Nelson, M., Stocks, N., Berk, M., McNeil, J. J., Britt, C., & Owen, A. J. (2021). Social isolation, social support and loneliness as predictors of cardiovascular disease incidence and mortality. *BMC Geriatrics*, 21(1). https://doi.org/10.1186/s12877-021-02602-2

Friedman, H. S., Tucker, J. S., Schwartz, J. E., Tomlinson-Keasey, C., Martin, L. R., Wingard, D. L., & Criqui, M. H. (1995). Psychosocial and behavioral predictors of longevity: The aging and death of the "Termites". *American Psychologist*, 50(2), 69–78. https://doi.org/10.1037/0003-066x.50.2.69

Fuemmeler, B. F., Mâsse, L. C., Yaroch, A. L., Resnicow, K., Campbell, M. K., Carr, C., Wang, T., & Williams, A. (2006). Psychosocial mediation of fruit and vegetable consumption in the body and soul effectiveness trial. *Health Psychology*, 25(4), 474–483. https://doi.org/10.1037/0278-6133.25.4.474

Gore, S. (1981). Stress-buffering functions of social supports: An appraisal and clarification of research models. *Stressful Life Events and Their Context*, 202–222.

Haber, M. G., Cohen, J. L., Lucas, T., & Baltes, B. B. (2007). The relationship between self-reported received and perceived social support: A meta-analytic review. *American Journal of Community Psychology, 39*(1–2), 133–144. https://doi.org/10.1007/s10464-007-9100-9

Harding, B. N., Hawley, C. N., Kalinowski, J., Sims, M., Muntner, P., Young, B. A., Heckbert, S. R., & Floyd, J. S. (2022). Relationship between social support and incident hypertension in the Jackson Heart Study: A cohort study. *BMJ Open, 12*(3), e054812. https://doi.org/10.1136/bmjopen-2021-054812

Hartley, C., & Coffee, P. (2019). Perceived and received dimensional Support: Main and stress-buffering effects on dimensions of burnout. *Frontiers in Psychology, 10*, 1724. https://doi.org/10.3389/fpsyg.2019.01724

Hawkley, L. C., Finch, L. E., Kotwal, A. A., & Waite, L. J. (2021). Can remote social contact replace in-person contact to protect mental health among older adults? *Journal of the American Geriatrics Society, 69*(11), 3063–3065. https://doi.org/10.1111/jgs.17405

Hill, T. D., Uchino, B. N., Eckhardt, J. L., & Angel, J. L. (2016). Perceived social support trajectories and the all-cause mortality risk of older Mexican American women and men. *Research on Aging, 38*(3), 374–398. https://doi.org/10.1177/0164027515620239

Holt-Lunstad, J. (2021). The major health implications of social connection. *Current Directions in Psychological Science, 30*(3), 251–259. https://doi.org/10.1177/0963721421999630

Holt-Lunstad, J., & Uchino, B. N. (2019). Social ambivalence and disease (SAD): A theoretical model aimed at understanding the health implications of ambivalent relationships. *Perspectives on Psychological Science, 14*(6), 941–966. https://doi.org/10.1177/1745691619861392

Holt-Lunstad, J., Smith, T. B., & Layton, J. B. (2010). Social relationships and mortality risk: A meta-analytic review. *PLoS Medicine, 7*(7), e1000316. https://doi.org/10.1371/journal.pmed.1000316

Hostinar, C. E. (2015). Recent developments in the study of social relationships, stress responses, and physical health. *Current Opinion in Psychology, 5*, 90–95. https://doi.org/10.1016/j.copsyc.2015.05.004

Hou, X., Wang, J., Guo, J., Zhang, X., Liu, J., Qi, L., & Zhou, L. (2021). Methods and efficacy of social support interventions in preventing suicide: A systematic review and meta-analysis. *Evidence-Based Mental Health, 25*(1), 29–35. ebmental-2021-300318. https://doi.org/10.1136/ebmental-2021-300318

House, J., Landis, K., & Umberson, D. (1988). Social relationships and health. *Science, 241*(4865), 540–545. https://doi.org/10.1126/science.3399889

Howard, S., Creaven, A.-M., Hughes, B. M., O'Leary, É. D., & James, J. E. (2017). Perceived social support predicts lower cardiovascular reactivity to stress in older adults. *Biological Psychology, 125*, 70–75. https://doi.org/10.1016/j.biopsycho.2017.02.006

Hsieh, H.-F., Heinze, J. E., Lang, I., Mistry, R., Buu, A., & Zimmerman, M. A. (2017). Violence victimization, social support, and Papanicolaou smear outcomes: A longitudinal study from adolescence to young adulthood. *Journal of Women's Health, 26*(12), 1340–1349. https://doi.org/10.1089/jwh.2016.5799

Hunter, J. F., Jones, N. M., Delgadillo, D., & Kaveladze, B. (2022). The influence of technology on the assessment and conceptualization of social support. In Katarzyna Wac, Sharon Wulfovich. *Quantifying Quality of Life: Incorporating Daily Life Into Medicine* (pp. 373–394). Cham: Springer International Publishing. https://doi.org/10.1007/978-3-030-94212-0_15

Inagaki, T. K., Ray, L. A., Irwin, M. R., Way, B. M., & Eisenberger, N. I. (2016). Opioids and social bonding: Naltrexone reduces feelings of social connection. *Social Cognitive and Affective Neuroscience, 11*(5), 728–735. https://doi.org/10.1093/scan/nsw006

Kaniasty, K. (2020). Social support, interpersonal, and community dynamics following disasters caused by natural hazards. *Current Opinion in Psychology, 32*, 105–109. https://doi.org/10.1016/j.copsyc.2019.07.026

Kaplan, G. A., Wilson, T. W., Cohen, R. D., Kauhanen, J., Wu, M., & Salonen, J. T. (1994). Social functioning and overall mortality: Prospective evidence from the Kuopio Ischemic Heart Disease Risk Factor Study. *Epidemiology, 5*(5), 495–500. https://pubmed.ncbi.nlm.nih.gov/7986863/

Karataş, T., & Bostanoğlu, H. (2017). Perceived social support and psychosocial adjustment in patients with coronary heart disease. *International Journal of Nursing Practice, 23*(4), e12558. https://doi.org/10.1111/ijn.12558

Kaveladze, B., Diamond Altman, A., Niederhausen, M., Loftis, J. M., & Teo, A. R. (2020). Social relationship quality, depression and inflammation: A cross-cultural longitudinal study in the United States and Tokyo, Japan. *International Journal of Social Psychiatry, 68*(2), 253–263. https://doi.org/10.1177/0020764020981604

Kiecolt-Glaser, J. K., Loving, T. J., Stowell, J. R., Malarkey, W. B., Lemeshow, S., Dickinson, S. L., & Glaser, R. (2005). Hostile marital interactions, Proinflammatory cytokine production, and wound healing. *Archives of General Psychiatry, 62*(12), 1377. https://doi.org/10.1001/archpsyc.62.12.1377

Kleiman, E. M., & Liu, R. T. (2013). Social support as a protective factor in suicide: Findings from two nationally representative samples. *Journal of Affective Disorders, 150*(2), 540–545. https://doi.org/10.1016/j.jad.2013.01.033

Kotwal, A. A., Steinman, M. A., Cenzer, I., & Smith, A. K. (2021). Use of high-risk medications among lonely older adults. *JAMA Internal Medicine, 181*(11), 1528–1530. https://doi.org/10.1001/jamainternmed.2021.3775

Krause, N. (1997). Received support, anticipated support, social class, and mortality. *Research on Aging, 19*(4), 387–422. https://doi.org/10.1177/0164027597194001

Kroenke, C. H., Quesenberry, C., Kwan, M. L., Sweeney, C., Castillo, A., & Caan, B. J. (2012). Social networks, social support, and burden in relationships, and mortality after breast cancer diagnosis in the Life After Breast Cancer Epidemiology (LACE) Study. *Breast Cancer Research and Treatment, 137*(1), 261–271. https://doi.org/10.1007/s10549-012-2253-8

Laird, Y., Fawkner, S., Kelly, P., McNamee, L., & Niven, A. (2016). The role of social support on physical activity behaviour in adolescent girls: a systematic review and meta-analysis. *International Journal of Behavioral Nutrition and Physical Activity, 13*(1). https://doi.org/10.1186/s12966-016-0405-7

Lakey, B., & Orehek, E. (2011). Relational regulation theory: A new approach to explain the link between perceived social support and mental health. *Psychological Review, 118*(3), 482–495. https://doi.org/10.1037/a0023477

Lee, H., & Singh, G. K. (2021). Social isolation and all-cause and heart disease mortality among working-age adults in the United States: The 1998–2014 NHIS–NDI Record Linkage Study. *Health Equity, 5*(1), 750–761. https://doi.org/10.1089/heq.2021.0003

Lee, D. T. F., Choi, K. C., Chair, S. Y., Yu, D. S. F., & Lau, S. T. (2012). Psychological distress mediates the effects of socio-demographic and clinical characteristics on the physical health component of health-related quality of life in patients with coronary heart disease. *European Journal of Preventive Cardiology, 21*(1), 107–116. https://doi.org/10.1177/2047487312451541

Lee, D. S., Jiang, T., Canevello, A., & Crocker, J. (2020). Motivational underpinnings of successful support giving: Compassionate goals promote matching support provision. *Personal Relationships, 28*(2), 276–296. https://doi.org/10.1111/pere.12363

Lett, H. S., Blumenthal, J. A., Babyak, M. A., Strauman, T. J., Robins, C., & Sherwood, A. (2005). Social support and coronary heart disease: Epidemiologic evidence and implications for treatment. *Psychosomatic Medicine, 67*(6), 869–878. https://doi.org/10.1097/01.psy.0000188393.73571.0a

Lett, H. S., Blumenthal, J. A., Babyak, M. A., Catellier, D. J., Carney, R. M., Berkman, L. F., Burg, M. M., Mitchell, P., Jaffe, A. S., & Schneiderman, N. (2007). Social support and prognosis in patients at increased psychosocial risk recovering from myocardial infarction. *Health Psychology, 26*(4), 418–427. https://doi.org/10.1037/0278-6133.26.4.418

Liu, L., & Newschaffer, C. J. (2011). Impact of social connections on risk of heart disease, cancer, and all-cause mortality among elderly Americans: Findings from the Second Longitudinal Study of Aging (LSOA II). *Archives of Gerontology and Geriatrics, 53*(2), 168–173. https://doi.org/10.1016/j.archger.2010.10.011

Liu, R. T., Hernandez, E. M., Trout, Z. M., Kleiman, E. M., & Bozzay, M. L. (2017). Depression, social support, and long-term risk for coronary heart disease in a 13-year longitudinal epidemiological study. *Psychiatry Research, 251*, 36–40. https://doi.org/10.1016/j.psychres.2017.02.010

Lutgendorf, S. K., Sood, A. K., Anderson, B., McGinn, S., Maiseri, H., Dao, M., Sorosky, J. I., De Geest, K., Ritchie, J., & Lubaroff, D. M. (2005). Social support, psychological distress, and natural killer cell activity in ovarian cancer. *Journal of Clinical Oncology: Official Journal of the American Society of Clinical Oncology, 23*(28), 7105–7113. https://doi.org/10.1200/JCO.2005.10.015

Luttik, M. L., Jaarsma, T., Moser, D., Sanderman, R., & van Veldhuisen, D. J. (2005). The importance and impact of social support on outcomes in patients with heart failure. *The Journal of Cardiovascular Nursing, 20*(3), 162–169. https://doi.org/10.1097/00005082-200505000-00007

Machin, A. J., & Dunbar, R. I. M. (2011). The brain opioid theory of social attachment: A review of the evidence. *Behaviour, 148*(9–10), 985–1025. https://doi.org/10.1163/000579511x596624

Magrin, M. E., D'addario, M., Greco, A., Miglioretti, M., Sarini, M., Scrignaro, M., . . . & Crocetti, E. (2015). Social support and adherence to treatment in hypertensive patients: a meta-analysis. *Annals of Behavioral Medicine, 49*(3), 307–318.

Maisel, N. C., & Gable, S. L. (2009). The paradox of received social support. *Psychological Science, 20*(8), 928–932. https://doi.org/10.1111/j.1467-9280.2009.02388.x

Malik, S. H., & Coulson, N. S. (2008). Computer-mediated infertility support groups: An exploratory study of online experiences. *Patient Education and Counseling, 73*(1), 105–113. https://doi.org/10.1016/j.pec.2008.05.024

Manne, S. L., Ostroff, J., Winkel, G., Grana, G., & Fox, K. (2005). Partner unsupportive responses, avoidant coping, and distress among women with early stage breast cancer: Patient and partner perspectives. *Health Psychology, 24*(6), 635–641. https://doi.org/10.1037/0278-6133.24.6.635

Muller, A. E., Hafstad, E. V., Himmels, J. P. W., Smedslund, G., Flottorp, S., Stensland, S. Ø., Stroobants, S., Van de Velde, S., & Vist, G. E. (2020). The mental health impact of the covid-19 pandemic on healthcare workers, and interventions to help them: A rapid systematic review. *Psychiatry Research*, *293*, 113441. https://doi.org/10.1016/j.psychres.2020.113441

National Academies of Sciences, Engineering, and Medicine. (2020). Social isolation and loneliness in older adults. National Academies Press. https://doi.org/10.17226/25663

National Crime Records Bureau. (n.d.). Accidental deaths and suicides in India. https://ncrb.gov.in/en/accidental-deaths-suicides-in-india

Nordin, M., Knutsson, A., & Sundbom, E. (2008). Is disturbed sleep a mediator in the ssociation between social support and myocardial infarction? *Journal of Health Psychology*, *13*(1), 55–64. https://doi.org/10.1177/1359105307084312

Olaya, B., Domènech-Abella, J., Moneta, M. V., Lara, E., Caballero, F. F., Rico-Uribe, L. A., & Haro, J. M. (2017). All-cause mortality and multimorbidity in older adults: The role of social support and loneliness. *Experimental Gerontology*, *99*, 120–126. https://doi.org/10.1016/j.exger.2017.10.001

Orth-Gomér, K., Wamala, S. P., Horsten, M., Schenck-Gustafsson, K., Schneiderman, N., & Mittleman, M. A. (2000). Marital stress worsens prognosis in women with coronary heart disease. *JAMA*, *284*(23), 3008. https://doi.org/10.1001/jama.284.23.3008

Pantell, M., Rehkopf, D., Jutte, D., Syme, S. L., Balmes, J., & Adler, N. (2013). Social isolation: A predictor of mortality comparable to traditional clinical risk factors. *American Journal of Public Health*, *103*(11), 2056–2062. https://doi.org/10.2105/AJPH.2013.301261

Pearlin, L. I. (1989). The sociological study of stress. *Journal of Health and Social Behavior*, *30*(3), 241. https://doi.org/10.2307/2136956

Peterson, C., Miller, G. F., Barnett, S. B. L., & Florence, C. (2021). Economic cost of injury—United States, 2019. *MMWR. Morbidity and Mortality Weekly Report*, *70*(48), 1655–1659. https://doi.org/10.15585/mmwr.mm7048a1

Polenick, C. A., Cotton, B. P., Bryson, W. C., & Birditt, K. S. (2019). Loneliness and illicit opioid use among methadone maintenance treatment patients. *Substance Use & Misuse*, *54*(13), 2089–2098. https://doi.org/10.1080/10826084.2019.1628276

Przybylski, A. K., & Weinstein, N. (2012). Can you connect with me now? How the presence of mobile communication technology influences face-to-face conversation quality. *Journal of Social and Personal Relationships*, *30*(3), 237–246. https://doi.org/10.1177/0265407512453827

Rainie, H., & Wellman, B. (2012). *Networked: The new social operating system*. Mit Press.

Rimer, B. K., Lyons, E. J., Ribisl, K. M., Bowling, J. M., Golin, C. E., Forlenza, M. J., & Meier, A. (2005). How new subscribers use cancer-related online mailing lists. *Journal of Medical Internet Research*, *7*(3), e32. https://doi.org/10.2196/jmir.7.3.e32

Robinson, J. D., Turner, J. W., Tian, Y., Neustadtl, A., Mun, S. K., & Levine, B. (2017). The relationship between emotional and esteem social support messages and health. *Health Communication*, *34*(2), 220–226. https://doi.org/10.1080/10410236.2017.1405476

Robles, T. F., Slatcher, R. B., Trombello, J. M., & McGinn, M. M. (2014). Marital quality and health: A meta-analytic review. *Psychological Bulletin*, *140*(1), 140–187. https://doi.org/10.1037/a0031859

Rucker, D. D., Preacher, K. J., Tormala, Z. L., & Petty, R. E. (2011). Mediation analysis in social psychology: Current practices and new recommendations. *Social and Personality Psychology Compass*, *5*(6), 359–371. https://doi.org/10.1111/j.1751-9004.2011.00355.x

Russell, D. W., & Cutrona, C. E. (1991). Social support, stress, and depressive symptoms among the elderly: Test of a process model. *Psychology and Aging*, *6*(2), 190–201. https://doi.org/10.1037/0882-7974.6.2.190

Selcuk, E., & Ong, A. D. (2013). Perceived partner responsiveness moderates the association between received emotional support and all-cause mortality. *Health Psychology*, *32*(2), 231–235. https://doi.org/10.1037/a0028276

Seltzer, L. J., Prososki, A. R., Ziegler, T. E., & Pollak, S. D. (2012). Instant messages vs. speech: Hormones and why we still need to hear each other. *Evolution and Human Behavior*, *33*(1), 42–45. https://doi.org/10.1016/j.evolhumbehav.2011.05.004

Serrano-Ripoll, M. J., Meneses-Echavez, J. F., Ricci-Cabello, I., Fraile-Navarro, D., Fiol-deRoque, M. A., Moreno, G. P., Castro, A., Ruiz-Pérez, I., Campos, R. Z., & Gonçalves-Bradley, D. (2020). Impact of viral epidemic outbreaks on mental health of healthcare workers: A rapid systematic review and meta-analysis. *Journal of Affective Disorders*, *277*. https://doi.org/10.1016/j.jad.2020.08.034

Smit, D., Vrijsen, J., Groeneweg, B., Vellinga-Dings, A., Peelen, J., & Spijker, J. (2021). A qualitative evaluation of a newly developed online peer support community for depression (Depression Connect): Qualitative study. *Journal of Medical Internet Research*, *23*(7), e25917. https://doi.org/10.2196/25917

Spoorthy, M. S. (2020). Mental health problems faced by healthcare workers due to the COVID-19 pandemic–A review. *Asian Journal of Psychiatry*, *51*, 102119. https://doi.org/10.1016/j.ajp.2020.102119

Stanton, S. C. E., Selcuk, E., Farrell, A. K., Slatcher, R. B., & Ong, A. D. (2019). Perceived partner responsiveness, Daily negative affect reactivity, and all-cause mortality. *Psychosomatic Medicine*, *81*(1), 7–15. https://doi.org/10.1097/psy.0000000000000618

Steptoe, A., Shankar, A., Demakakos, P., & Wardle, J. (2013). Social isolation, loneliness, and all-cause mortality in older men and women. *Proceedings of the National Academy of Sciences*, *110*(15), 5797–5801. https://doi.org/10.1073/pnas.1219686110

Stewart, D. W., Gabriele, J. M., & Fisher, E. B. (2011). Directive support, nondirective support, and health behaviors in a community sample. *Journal of Behavioral Medicine*, *35*(5), 492–499. https://doi.org/10.1007/s10865-011-9377-x

Szkody, E., Stearns, M., Stanhope, L., & McKinney, C. (2020). Stress-buffering role of social support during COVID-19. *Family Process*, *60*(3), 1002–1015. https://doi.org/10.1111/famp.12618

Teoh, A. N., & Hilmert, C. (2018). Social support as a comfort or an encouragement: A systematic review on the contrasting effects of social support on cardiovascular reactivity. *British Journal of Health Psychology*, *23*(4), 1040–1065. https://doi.org/10.1111/bjhp.12337

Thoits, P. A. (2011). Mechanisms linking social ties and support to physical and mental health. *Journal of Health and Social Behavior*, *52*(2), 145–161. https://doi.org/10.1177/0022146510395592

Thuy, L. Q., Thanh, N. H., Trung, L. H., Tan, P. H., Nam, H. T. P., Diep, P. T., An, T. T. H., Van San, B., Ngoc, T. N., & Van Toan, N. (2021). Blood pressure control and associations with social support among hypertensive outpatients in a developing country. *BioMed Research International*, *2021*, 1–10. https://doi.org/10.1155/2021/7420985

Troxel, W. M., Matthews, K. A., Gallo, L. C., & Kuller, L. H. (2005). Marital quality and occurrence of the metabolic syndrome in women. *Archives of Internal Medicine*, *165*(9), 1022. https://doi.org/10.1001/archinte.165.9.1022

Uchino, B. N. (2006). Social support and health: A review of physiological processes potentially underlying links to disease outcomes. *Journal of Behavioral Medicine*, *29*(4), 377–387. https://doi.org/10.1007/s10865-006-9056-5

Uchino, B. N. (2009). Understanding the links between social support and physical health: A life-span perspective with emphasis on the separability of perceived and received support. *Perspectives on Psychological Science: A Journal of the Association for Psychological Science*, *4*(3), 236–255. https://doi.org/10.1111/j.1745-6924.2009.01122.x

Uchino, B. N., Bowen, K., Kent de Grey, R., Mikel, J., & Fisher, E. B. (2018). Social support and physical health: Models, mechanisms, and opportunities. *Principles and Concepts of Behavioral Medicine: A Global Handbook*, 341–372.

Umberson, D. (1987). Family status and health behaviors: Social control as a dimension of social integration. *Journal of Health and Social Behavior*, *28*(3), 306. https://doi.org/10.2307/2136848

Umberson, D., & Karas Montez, J. (2010). Social relationships and health: A flashpoint for health policy. *Journal of Health and Social Behavior*, *51*(Suppl), S54–S66. https://doi.org/10.1177/0022146510383501

Valtorta, N. K., Kanaan, M., Gilbody, S., Ronzi, S., & Hanratty, B. (2016). Loneliness and social isolation as risk factors for coronary heart disease and stroke: Systematic review and meta-analysis of longitudinal observational studies. *Heart*, *102*(13), 1009–1016. https://doi.org/10.1136/heartjnl-2015-308790

Veenstra, A. L., Lakey, B., Cohen, J. L., Neely, L. C., Orehek, E., Barry, R., & Abeare, C. A. (2011). Forecasting the specific providers that recipients will perceive as unusually supportive. *Personal Relationships*, *18*(4), 677–696. https://doi.org/10.1111/j.1475-6811.2010.01340.x

Vicary, A. M., & Fraley, R. C. (2010). Student reactions to the shootings at Virginia Tech and Northern Illinois University: Does sharing grief and support over the Internet affect recovery? *Personality and Social Psychology Bulletin*, *36*(11), 1555–1563. https://doi.org/10.1177/0146167210384880

Vijayakumar, L., Shujaath Ali, Z., Kesavan, K., Umamaheswari, C., & Devaraj, P. (2011). Intervention for suicide attempters: A randomized controlled study. *Indian Journal of Psychiatry*, *53*(3), 244. https://doi.org/10.4103/0019-5545.86817

Vila, J. (2021). Social support and longevity: Meta-analysis-based evidence and psychobiological mechanisms. *Frontiers in Psychology*, *12*, 717164. https://doi.org/10.3389/fpsyg.2021.717164

Wang, W., Lau, Y., Chow, A., Thompson, D. R., & He, H. G. (2013). Health-related quality of life and social support among Chinese patients with coronary heart disease in mainland China. *European Journal of Cardiovascular Nursing*, *13*(1), 48–54. https://doi.org/10.1177/1474515113476995

Weissbourd, R., Batanova, M., Lovison, V., & Torres, E. (2021). Loneliness in America: How the pandemic has deepened an epidemic of loneliness and what we can do about it. Making Caring Common Project. Harvard Graduate School of Education. https://mcc.gse.harvard.edu/reports/loneliness-in-america

Whisman, M. A., Gilmour, A. L., & Salinger, J. M. (2018). Marital satisfaction and mortality in the United States adult population. *Health Psychology*, *37*(11), 1041–1044. https://doi.org/10.1037/hea0000677

Wills, T. A., & Shinar, O. (2000). Measuring perceived and received social support. In S. Cohen, L. G. Underwood, & B. H. Gottlieb, (Eds.), *Social support measurement and intervention* (pp. 86–135). Oxford University Press. https://doi.org/10.1093/med:psych/9780195126709.001.0001

Wu, H.-Y., & Chiou, A.-F. (2020). Social media usage, social support, intergenerational relationships, and depressive symptoms among older adults. *Geriatric Nursing*, *41*(5), 615–621. https://doi.org/10.1016/j.gerinurse.2020.03.016

Yang, Y. C., Boen, C., Gerken, K., Li, T., Schorpp, K., & Harris, K. M. (2016). Social relationships and physiological determinants of longevity across the human life span. *Proceedings of the National Academy of Sciences*, *113*(3), 578–583. https://doi.org/10.1073/pnas.1511085112

Yazawa, A., Inoue, Y., Yamamoto, T., Watanabe, C., Tu, R., & Kawachi, I. (2022). Can social support buffer the association between loneliness and hypertension? A cross-sectional study in rural China. *PLoS One*, *17*(2), e0264086. https://doi.org/10.1371/journal.pone.0264086

Zhang, X., & Dong, S. (2022). The relationships between social support and loneliness: A meta-analysis and review. *Acta Psychologica*, *227*, 103616. https://doi.org/10.1016/j.actpsy.2022.103616

Zhou, Z., & Cheng, Q. (2022). Relationship between online social support and adolescents' mental health: A systematic review and meta-analysis. *Journal of Adolescence*, *94*(3), 281–292. https://doi.org/10.1002/jad.12031

CHAPTER 11

SOCIAL NETWORKS AND HEALTH BEHAVIOR

Thomas W. Valente
Sarah E. Piombo

Vignette: COVID-19 and Social Networks

Maria was an average high school student. She liked learning but did not care for the hours spent sitting inside classrooms listening to teachers drone on about things she really did not care about. It was early March 2020, and Maria was looking forward to finishing her junior year of high school. There were a lot of new things to look forward to, like junior prom, visiting potential colleges and having the freedom to visit friends after getting her driver's license. When news started circulating about a strange and concerning new disease called COVID that she heard could be fatal to older and other vulnerable people. Maria did not think much of it and assumed it would not be a huge deal. The following week, though, her school sent everyone home, and now, they would be doing school online.

Maria was depressed. Yes, she hated school, but now realized how much she missed seeing her friends every day and hanging out between classes and during lunch. She even missed seeing the people she barely knew and the random conversations that sometimes happened in the classroom. She knew she needed to keep her distance from everyone, because if she contracted COVID, she could give it to more vulnerable family members. Maria's grandmother lived in their home, and Maria certainly did not want to accidentally expose her and get her sick.

She now realized this strange paradox. Being with her friends could put her and her loved ones at risk for a potentially fatal disease. Yet, not seeing these friends was making her feel stress, depression, and overall bored and bummed out. Maria found herself spending all her time online: in classes via Zoom, on Instagram sending memes and random pictures to her friends, scrolling through TikTok, and simultaneously Snapchatting with her friends to stay in contact. These online connections helped relieve her boredom, but they also brought her attention to messages and videos being shared online that said COVID was a hoax and no reason for concern.

Some of Maria's friends were secretly hanging out together and said COVID was no big deal, but they did not have grandparents or older family members in their households. Maria was conflicted. Her friends insisted there was nothing to be worried about, but she wanted to protect her grandmother. When one of her

KEY POINTS

This chapter will:

- Provide a brief review of the history of social network theory (SNT) and social network analysis (SNA) and their importance for health behaviors.

- Describe and articulate the main components of SNT and SNA.

- Present examples of how SNT is applied to two health behaviors: contraceptive use and adolescent e-cigarettes use.

- Briefly describe statistical tools for SNA.

Health Behavior: Theory, Research, and Practice, Sixth Edition. Edited by Karen Glanz, Barbara K. Rimer, and K. Viswanath.
© 2024 John Wiley & Sons, Inc. Published 2024 by John Wiley & Sons, Inc.
Companion website: www.wiley.com/go/glanz/healthbehavior6e

friends got very sick from COVID, Maria realized it was a real threat, and she started sharing accurate information with her friends via her social media and also in group chats. She was worried that if people did not begin to take things seriously, it might be a long time before life went back to "normal."

Introduction

Evidence that people's relationships with friends, family members, colleagues, and others—collectively known as *social networks*—act as important conduits for health information, sources of support, and determinants (both good and ill) of health behaviors has come from many studies and decades of empirical research. Whether these social networks are in-person or online, they are both important influences on, as well as influenced by, many health behaviors.

Whether research about social networks constitutes a theory or a method to measure other theoretical constructs is a subject of debate. The word theory is used when describing the mechanisms by which networks influence behavior, and when describing endogenous network processes, such as the tendency for friends of friends to become friends. Social Network Theory (SNT) stresses the importance of connections or relations for understanding health and/or behaviors of individuals (Valente, 2010). Researchers might thus use SNT to model health outcomes as a function of network processes.

Social Network Analysis (SNA) is used when network methods are incorporated into other health behavior theories, sometimes, as a central component, such as in the diffusion of innovations (Valente, 1995) and, sometimes, peripherally, as in efforts to understand how networks influence normative beliefs. Social network methods have proliferated across the physical and social sciences. This rapidly expanding research paradigm shifts the focus of study from individuals to their relationships with others (Borgatti, et al., 2013; Valente, 2010). Relationships vary widely, including friendships among adolescents in schools, trade among nations, and communications over social media. These relational data are analyzed using models and tools distinct from those traditionally employed by statisticians and epidemiologists, though the approaches may converge (Valente, 2010). Network data, aided by visualization, mathematical algorithms, and computational tools, typically provide an in-depth view of how communities, organizations, settings, and systems are structured and relate to each other. SNA enables researchers to conduct a mathematical ethnography—that is, a quantitative description—of the behavior or system(s) being studied. Consequently, network research is simultaneously deceptively simple and maddeningly complex.

This chapter focuses on how networks influence health behaviors and reviews the research to date that shows a strong and powerful influence of networks on individual, organizational, community, and system-related health behavior and outcomes. It focuses only on social networks and not on social support, a branch of social network research that measures the support resources individuals have in their social networks. These resources typically are classified as the emotional, cognitive, tangible, and physical support that an individual receives from others (see Chapter 10). SNA, in contrast, measures relationships, such as friendships or other task- or work-oriented relationships (which may or may not provide support) and treats these directional ties themselves as objects of study (Valente, 2010; Valente & Pitts, 2017). Throughout this chapter, social networks will be described as relationships (ties) among people, but most statements also apply to networks of organizations, governments, websites, and any other unit or "actors" (nodes) as well.

Table 11.1 at the end of the chapter defines key terms used throughout this chapter.

History

Many social scientists employed network research methods and the use of mathematics and graph theory in their research prior to 1930 (Freeman, 2004). Most scholars, however, trace the beginning of modern social network research to Jacob Moreno (1934) who was one of the first to develop a program of research studying social networks and outcomes, usually among elementary school students (Moreno, 1934). By the 1950s, various research groups had begun to create a field called SNA or Sociometry. The group dynamics center at the University of Michigan Institute for Social Research is credited with training scholars on early uses of graph theory to understand social networks. Several noted social psychologists, such as Heider, Cartwright, Homans, Festinger, and many others, conducted studies on social networks in workplaces and communities.

Table 11.1   Social Network Analysis Terms

Key Term	Definition
Social Networks	The connections or relationships among people, organizations, political entities, or other units.
Social Network Theory	A theoretical perspective for understanding the connections in social networks and their impact on behaviors.
Social Network Analysis	Using network methods and analytic techniques to understand the role of networks in the social and physical sciences. (for example, integrating social networks into health behavior research.)
Node	The actors in a network. Actors are usually people, organizations, agencies, or states but can be anything.
Tie	A link or relationship between two nodes.
Dyad	A pair of nodes with a tie.
Ego	The focal individual in a network study. Typically, egos are the respondents in a network study but also a term used to refer a focal individual.
Alter	A person named by a respondent in response to a network question. A person's direct tie.
Influence	When an individual changes their behavior to be the same as their network partners.
Selection	When an individual changes their network to be compatible with their behavior.
Opinion Leader	Those who influence others in the network, which is measured as those high in centrality. In-degree centrality is the preferred measure.
Semantic Network	A network of relations among words or phrases, often from the text in documents and/or manuscripts.
Individual measures	
Bridge	A person or link that spans different groups or subsections of a network.
Centrality	The degree to which a person occupies a prominent or significant position in a network. There are three main centrality scores.
• Degree	Number of ties a person has. Out-degree is the number of outgoing ties and in-degree the number of incoming ties for each person (or node).
• Betweenness	Extent to which a node lies on the shortest path connecting other nodes in the network.
• Closeness	The inverse of the distance each node is to all other nodes.
Network Exposure	Percentage or count of the people in an individual's personal network who have some behavioral property.
Threshold	The theoretical level of exposure in one's network that an individual would need to have before adopting a behavior.
Network Structural Properties	
Homophily	The tendency for people connected in networks to have similar characteristics. Example: boys are more likely to name other boys as friends.
Heterophily	The tendency for people connected in networks to have different characteristics. Example: a tendency of boys to name girls as friends.
Reciprocity	A link in one direction implies it exists in the other direction.
Density	The number of links in a network expressed as a proportion of the number possible.
Centralization	The degree links in the network are focused around one or a few nodes.
Transitivity	A link from A to B and one from B to C implies one from A to C.
Small World Property	The phenomenon by which distance between any two people in a network is less than what would be expected in a random network of the same size and density. This network property was demonstrated in the classic Milgram study which coined the term "six degrees of separation."

Two SNA research communities emerged by the beginning of the 1960s (Scott, 2017): the Manchester Anthropologists (from Manchester, United Kingdom) and the Harvard structuralists (centered around sociologist Harrison White). By the mid-1970s, two academic meetings were held in Hawaii to bring together the various scholars interested in studying social networks. These meetings culminated in the launch of the International Network for Social Network Analysis (INSNA) and a commitment to hold an annual meeting starting in 1981. The journal *Social Networks* was launched and a bulletin/journal, *Connections*, was created. INSNA provided a venue to develop SNA methods, theories, and applications, and support the growth of network scholarship. At least a few more social network journals have been created since then: *Journal of Social Structure*, *Network Science*, and *Social Network Analysis and Mining*.

By the mid-to-late 1980s, SNA scholars had begun to develop a library of social network algorithms for measuring key constructs and a culture of scientific exchange, collegiality, and cooperation. UCINET, a widely used computer program for SNA, was first released in the mid-1980s. The advent of the AIDS epidemic and an influx of public health researchers eager to use these tools for investigating important public health issues helped bolster the viability of the network science community in the early 1990s. Now, no longer a nascent community, the SNA field began to develop more powerful and user-friendly computer tools and programs. The explosive growth of the worldwide web, Internet, and computer communications made networks and networking both explicit and ubiquitous, bringing even more attention to SNA from many different disciplines. Consequently, there was a dramatic growth in applications of SNA, outpacing theoretical developments.

Recent Developments

Importance of Networks and Disease Transmission

SNA is critical to understanding infectious (communicable) disease transmission. Infectious diseases can be spread by person-to-person contact or through vectors that carry diseases. SNA has been used to study the transmission of many communicable diseases, including HIV/STIs, hepatitis, and H1N1 influenza (Cauchemez et al., 2011). The dynamics of COVID-19 transmission have been studied on multiple levels using SNA, from close personal networks to global networks. Most people are now familiar with the concept that social contact/social networks directly affect the risk of disease transmission or infection, as illustrated in this chapter's opening vignette. Having a larger network or more frequent social contact increases risk of contracting or spreading COVID-19.

Contact tracing is an important public health tool based in SNT for controlling the spread of disease during pandemics, especially in its early phases when spread can be controlled. With contact tracing, individuals who test positive for an infectious disease, such as COVID-19, are asked for information about their contacts within a certain period prior to their positive test result. These individuals are then contacted about their potential exposure, tested, and quarantined if positive. Research suggests that timely and thorough contact tracing has important potential for disease containment (Kretzschmar et al., 2020).

Networks for Disseminating Accurate Information and Misinformation

In addition to the spread of disease, social networks have played a critical role in the spread of information (and misinformation) regarding COVID-19. Information can spread in a way that mimics viral transmission. People often are influenced by the opinions and behaviors of individuals in their personal networks. This has led to the diffusion of behaviors, information, and beliefs surrounding COVID-19 by social networks. A study examining vaccine hesitancy in the United States, for example, found that people were significantly more likely to refuse vaccination if they had not known anyone who was infected by, hospitalized for, or had died of COVID-19 (Khubchandani et al., 2021). Social networks via social media also play an important role in the diffusion of ideas and beliefs. Misinformation regarding disease contagion, vaccines, and even conspiracy theories can spread rapidly through online platforms (Ahmed et al., 2020). The widespread dissemination of misinformation is both problematic and concerning for public health officials. At the same time, however, network interventions can be used to combat the spread of misinformation and connect individuals with trusted information sources (Young et al., 2021).

Agent-based Models and Simulations of Social Networks

Network simulation models can model network dynamics to understand how networks form and grow; and how health behavior interventions may impact, and be impacted by, social networks. Agent-based simulation models have been used during the COVID-19 pandemic, for example, to model the impact of nonpharmaceutical interventions, such as mask-wearing, social distancing, and other policy measures. Such simulation studies have shown that network interventions can be effective in reducing the spread of COVID-19. One simulation study demonstrated that dividing (having different groups of people accessing school or work on different days or times) and balancing (redirecting individuals or setting occupancy limits at stores to reduce physical contact) networks can reduce transmission while still sustaining economic activity (Nishi et al., 2020). This simulation also showed that combining these strategies would effectively reduce the COVID-19 disease spread to a tolerable level.

Another series of models using real COVID-19 data from Los Angeles County showed that the risk of severe illness and death from COVID-19 varies both between and within age groups, based on other comorbidities, such as obesity and smoking status, thus demonstrating significant differences in risk probabilities across subpopulations (Horn et al., 2021). This research examined individual attributes, such as age, ethnicity, and socioeconomic status (SES), to show how health inequities interact with social networks in contributing to COVID-19 risk. These types of models are important both in identifying high-risk groups and in informing policy decisions and population-level interventions during disease outbreaks (Valente et al., 2019).

Social Networks and Technological Developments

In the first decade of the 21ˢᵗ century, SNT and SNA were applied to substantive issues in many disciplines. Today big data (Lazer et al., 2009) and powerful new computing technologies mean that network research is no longer confined to small groups and communities, but rather can be applied to whole populations and large, naturally occurring communities. Researchers now can study social networks through the lens of health inequities as well. The concept of big data and refinement of visualization tools to understand data have made analysis of social networks more feasible and meaningful. Nonetheless, researchers should be conscious of the problem of data absenteeism that occurs when there is inadequate representation from disadvantaged or vulnerable groups (Lee & Viswanath, 2020).

Research methods in network analysis are evolving rapidly alongside other technological advances, such as artificial intelligence (AI), natural language processing (NLP), and machine learning (ML). These evolving methods extract meaning from massive, passive data sources and often rely on SNA techniques to display and analyze the data.

Artificial Intelligence

There is no one definition of AI, but most agree that it consists of a constellation of technologies that enable machines to analyze data and apply algorithms to make sense of data. There are multiple applications of AI for public health and health promotion. For example, AI allows researchers to analyze Google search terms to monitor disease prevalence, monitor search terms used by different people to send them targeted health promotion messages, or detect individual trends such as blood pressure variations using data captured from wearable sensors.

Natural Language Processing

NLP is the act of numerically analyzing text documents (such as books, plays, and narratives) to quantify them both in terms of sentiment and the interrelationship of words/phrases. NLP can be used to analyze social media data sources such as Twitter, Reddit, Facebook, and online health forums and has already been applied to explore communicable diseases, mental health, and the use of substances including tobacco, alcohol, marijuana, and opioids (Conway et al., 2019). Using NLP to examine text-based communication and conduct semantic analysis between members of an online network, for example, can identify community structures in that network. ML algorithms can also be used to classify posts, identify themes, and extract meaningful information in online communications. One such study used ML on Twitter data for its relevance to vaping, commercial nature, and sentiment (pro-vaping or not) (Visweswaran et al., 2020). Implementing ML methods for Twitter surveillance can provide insight into the effects of tobacco control policies. A study of a tobacco-cessation online community, for example, integrated behavior change theory with SNA to understand which user characteristics were associated with certain behavior change techniques when members tried to quit (Manas et al., 2019)—providing information potentially useful in designing technology-based interventions as well as in connecting users with one another to share strategies and social support.

These techniques are not limited to analyzing social media data or communications between individuals. They also can be applied to examine communication patterns between organizations, governments, and other entities. One study used NLP, for example, to examine how countries adopting the WHO Framework Convention on Tobacco Control treaty interacted, and how these interactions influenced each country's ratification of the treaty. Text-based analysis using data from GLOBALink, an international online discussion forum of tobacco control advocates, showed how countries in different adoption stages interacted with one another. Semantic network analysis was used to identify common themes and topics in the online discussions. There was evidence of supportive information-sharing between countries but also unshared ideas that did not spread between countries, potentially slowing treaty diffusion (Chu et al., 2017).

Today, network research is one of the most vibrant and exciting scientific fields, with potential to contribute substantially to scientific knowledge. These developments have enabled SNA researchers to craft specific axioms that have led to an identifiable SNT.

Social Network Theory

SNT has three main components, each of which is discussed below: (1) network environment; (2) a person's position in a network, and (3) network structure. A final component of SNT is that there is a dynamic relationship between the micro and macro levels of network analysis; that is, choices by individual members (or nodes) of a network give rise to larger level network structures. Thus, micro-level interactions between people who become friends with friends of current friends create macro-level network clusters of friends.

Network Environment

A basic tenet of SNT is that people or actors (e.g., organizations, states, collectives) take actions based on their network environment: their set of relationships, or *ties*, with other people or actors, both direct and indirect. SNT predicts that these network environmental *influences* are powerful determinants of behavior. An individual's network environment is that individual's set of direct relationships.

The network in Figure 11.1 depicts relationships of who knew whom in one organization, with the nodes shaped by individual departments. Persons 23 and 32 are the most central, receiving the most incoming ties, named by others frequently, and the most central on other centrality measures such as betweenness and closeness. Person 31 acts as a bridge connecting subgroups 8, 16, 22, 24, 28, and 31. The dyad consisting of 10 and 12 are disconnected from the larger group and only know one another; whereas 18, 27, and 38 are isolates whom no one knew, and who knew no one. The overall network density is 10%, indicating that 10% of all possible ties exist, and the average path length, the number of steps between people was 2.77 (with the assumption that nodes that are unreachable are assumed to be six steps apart, which is one plus the maximum path distance in the connected part of the network).

We can use SNT to make many predictions about how health behaviors would spread in this network. For example, the central nodes should have a large influence on what is considered normative, and what behaviors might spread easily in the network. The bridging node controls the flow of information and influence from the larger group to the subgroup; and the disconnected dyad (nodes 10 and 12), and isolates will be immune to influence from the larger group. There is homophily in department membership, meaning that people in the same department are more likely to know one another than those in different departments and that similarly shaped nodes are more likely to be connected than dissimilar ones.

Such homophily is derived from at least two network processes: influence and selection. *Influence* occurs when an individual changes his/her behavior to be the same as their network partners. *Selection* occurs when an individual changes their network to be compatible with their behavior. In the case of e-cigarette use, influence occurs when a person decides to start vaping because their friends vape; selection occurs when a person decides to vape and then makes new friendships with vapers.

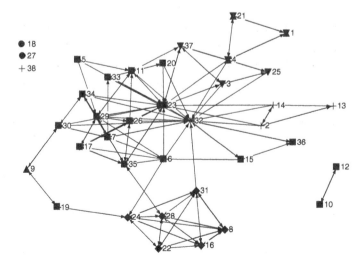

Figure 11.1 Network of Who Knew Whom in One Organization, Shapes Indicate Department Affiliations. Each Symbol and Corresponding Number Refers to a Person and the Arrow Indicates the Direction of the Nomination. For Example, Persons 10 and 12 Nominated Each Other, Whereas Person 7 Named 15 but 15 did not Name 7

Because SNT predicts that individuals are influenced by their immediate social networks both in their behaviors and their network choices, influence and selection effects are considered *environmental effects*. Network theory has developed many extensions of these environmental, or exposure, effects, including weighing them by (1) tie strength, (2) tie distance (including indirect ties), (3) connectivity to the same third parties, (4) degree of equivalence in network position, (5) centrality of ties (see next section), (6) extent of participation in joint activities (such as being on the same sports team), or (7) network attributes that may alter effects (such as gender, age, or education level). SNT also predicts that individuals vary in the extent to which they are influenced by their personal networks. Some individuals, for example, may have low thresholds for taking action and so change behaviors even if few others in their network do so, while other individuals may have high thresholds and wait until the majority have engaged in a behavior before acting (Valente, 2010).

Position in Networks

Another core tenet of SNT is that a person's position in a network influences their behaviors. Several positions have been identified as important: central, bridging, and peripheral. Central individuals occupy prominent positions in the network as indicated by high scores on algorithms that identify nodes that have the potential to influence many other nodes or play other important roles in the network. People can be central if they receive a lot of nominations (degree centrality), for example, but also if they occupy strategic positions in the network such as closeness centrality, which means being on average, fewer "steps" from everyone else in the network or lying on the shortest path connecting other nodes in the network (betweenness centrality) (Freeman, 1979). Being central can also make individuals more sensitive to community norms and values that may either promote or inhibit innovation and/or change, suggesting that the central nodes should have a large influence on what is considered normative, and what behaviors might spread easily in the network. Central individuals learn about new ideas sooner and can have access to information earlier than less central people. The central position can be advantageous if the information received is valuable; however, when it comes to the spread of diseases, being central can be a liability as it exposes that person to viruses and bacteria earlier than noncentral members (Christakis & Fowler, 2010).

Bridging individuals, people who connect otherwise disconnected groups—also can be associated with behavior in a network for several reasons: (1) bridging provides access to different subgroups in the network, (2) bridging individuals may be less beholden to the *status quo* than central individuals, and (3) bridges are less constrained by their immediate personal network. Granovetter's (1973) influential paper on the strength of weak ties argued that people who are weakly connected often exchange valuable information because they are linked to different people and thus have access to different information. Network theory highlights the importance of bridges for linking disparate groups and enabling or hindering collective action.

Being peripheral also can influence behaviors. Peripheral individuals are free from social norms in the community or network; thus, they may be less constrained in their behavior and freer to innovate. They also might have more connectivity to other groups and networks in which case they would be bridges between networks but peripheral in one of them. There also is evidence that being peripheral in a network may be associated directly with health behaviors. Research has shown that social isolation is associated with poor physical health, for example, and that loneliness in particular is associated with poor physical health among adolescents and young adults (Christiansen, et al., 2021) (see Chapter 10).

Structural or Network Properties

SNT also makes predictions at the macro, or whole network, level, using indicators such as the rates of homophily and reciprocity, and the levels of density, transitivity (clustering), and centralization in the network. In Figure 11.1, *homophily* is more apparent as people are more likely to be connected if they are from the same department. There is also homophily in behavior such that vapers are friends with other vapers. SNT predicts this homophily will occur in many networks and that networks with high rates of homophily will be more resistant to change.

Transitivity also occurs at higher rates in many networks such that friends of friends are, or become friends. If Angela names Mary as a friend, and Mary names Beth as a friend, then Angela will likely become friends with Beth.

In Figure 11.1, persons 2, 13, and 14 have a transitive triad as 2 names 14, and both 14 and 2 name 13. *Clustering* is the degree of transitivity in a network and so highly clustered networks have pockets of dense interconnectivity that accelerates behavior change within clusters but slows it between different clusters.

As mentioned earlier, people vary in the number of their ties, making some people central and others peripheral. The overall distribution of these ties is an indication of a network's *centralization*. Centralized networks, characterized by the extent to which ties are focused around one or a few nodes are thought to be more effective because the central hubs can coordinate activities for the network. Evidence also suggests that centralized networks are less sustainable, in part, (1) because centralized networks have hubs that are very important, and their removal can have profound consequences, and (2) people are often less satisfied working in centralized networks in which they have little control or input into decision-making.

A final, well-known structural property of networks is the *"small world" property*. That is, the distance between any two people in the network is less than what would be expected in a random network of the same size and density (the number of links in the network). Milgram (1967) conducted the classic "small world study," which found that any two people in the US chosen at random are separated by six steps or the well-known six degrees of separation.

These five structural properties—homophily, reciprocity, transitivity, centralization, and their small-world character—are properties that enable us to describe and compare different networks; and make predictions about how networks emerge and evolve over time. Once attributes of the nodes—such as sex, race and ethnicity, age, and other characteristics of people—are added, we can make even more profound and powerful predictions about how networks evolve and how they influence behavior.

Individual Network-Level Interactions

Individual- and network-level properties interact to influence behavior. For example, being central in a centralized network affords one more power and control than being central in a decentralized network. A person with a *heterophilous* tie (a tie to someone with different characteristics) in a network with high rates of homophily is unusual and so may feel increased pressure to sever that tie or may have access to information and resources at a greater rate than other individuals. Therefore, to fully understand how networks influence behavior, one must simultaneously consider both the individual (micro) and network (macro) levels of analysis.

Diversity and Equity in Social Networks

The advantages of having a homophilous network, where individuals have ties with others similar to themselves, or a heterophilous network, where individuals have ties with others who are different from themselves, are dependent on the behavior being studied. A heterophilous social network can be advantageous if one is seeking exposure to new information and ideas or looking to grow and diversify connections. On the other hand, a heterophilous network can be disadvantageous when it comes to public health issues like disease containment. For example, having a heterophilous network of sexual partners can increase the transmission of sexually transmitted infections or make it challenging to contain an outbreak within a social network.

Variation in size and composition of social networks is sometimes related to individual attributes, community settings, or socioeconomic factors. Early work examining diversity in social networks was conducted by Peter Marsden using data from the 1985 General Social Survey (Marsden, 1987). He analyzed the variations in core discussion networks of Americans by age, education level, race/ethnicity, sex, and setting. In general, he found that the heterogeneity of social networks increases with age, and having a diverse network results in access to different social groups, which provides advantages, such as access to new information or resources. At the time of the survey (1985), social networks were relatively homophilous with regard to race/ethnicity, with white respondents having more homophilous networks than African Americans and Hispanic/Latinx respondents. Higher education and urban residence were also associated with larger, more heterophilous networks.

More than 25 years after the 1985 General Social Survey, some aspects of social networks have changed while others remain the same. People still tend to associate with others who are like themselves, resulting in homophilous social networks (McPherson et al., 2001). However, homophily limits exposure to new ideas, attitudes, beliefs, and behaviors.

Further, the tendency toward homophily can exacerbate divisions between groups. More recent research has taken a closer look at the impact of SES, diversity, and equity in social networks.

Access to social capital, or the resources accessed in social networks, may vary based on group membership and network position. Since higher-SES individuals generally have larger and more diverse networks, they are more likely to attain higher status and access to more resources, educational advancement, and employment opportunities. Cross-SES ties, where low-SES and high-SES individuals are connected, can bridge homophilous SES groups and benefit lower-SES individuals by increasing their social capital. These friendships can positively influence norms, aspirations, education outcomes, and career opportunities (DiMaggio & Garip, 2012). Increasing heterophily in social networks during childhood and adolescence could thus potentially benefit lower-SES students by providing access to more resources, positioning these students for greater socioeconomic attainment. Unfortunately, existing social structures tend to exacerbate social capital inequalities rather than ameliorate them (Chetty et al., 2022).

Social Media

Communities are increasingly being formed on the Internet, which removes the constraints of geography and time by enabling like-minded people to communicate, share, collaborate, and coordinate on many levels. Technological developments have given rise to a new era of social media and online networks (see Chapter 22). To understand the role of these developments in SNA, we must first distinguish between the concepts of *social networks* and *social networking*. Social networks are the real-life connections or ties between people or entities, while social networking is interacting with others using social media sites, such as Twitter (now called "X"), Facebook, and Instagram. There is significant overlap between the two terms, however, as most people interact on social media with others they know in real life or use social media to build new connections. One advantage of online social networks is that they are not limited by physical distance or proximity. They offer opportunities for people to connect with others, seek information and advice, and receive social support from virtually any location.

SNA tools are useful to study and understand the role of social media in society and its subsequent impact on public health. Several scientists capitalized on the availability of these tools and conducted experiments to determine whether network effects can be replicated online and whether marketers can accelerate diffusion using online networks (Hinz et al., 2011). They found that online networks can stimulate behavior changes and that these effects are stronger when influences on behavior come from close friends (Bond et al., 2012). Although the effect sizes were less than those achieved via face-to-face interactions, the scale that is achievable on social media magnifies those effects substantially.

SNA can play an important role in characterizing and interpreting the online environment surrounding public health issues. Such analysis, for example, can help us understand the marketing strategies that tobacco companies use on social media platforms to advertise e-cigarettes and related products (Chu et al., 2018). SNA also can use online networks to examine the differences between social networks of smokers and those of nonsmokers (Fu et al., 2017), provide insight into public perceptions of vaping products (Allem et al., 2018), and even understand the reasons that people use tobacco or e-cigarettes (Ayers et al., 2017). Without physical limitations, online network-based interventions can be designed to reach a wider audience. Network strategies can be used to design interventions to combat e-cigarette marketing through targeted public health messaging and education campaigns on social media platforms (Chu et al., 2019).

While social media and other online networks offer many advantages, they can also negatively impact public health by spreading misinformation. A recent systematic review found evidence of online misinformation pertaining to smoking products and drugs, vaccines, diets, and diseases. In this study, Twitter (now "X") was identified as the site with the highest prevalence of misinformation (Suarez-Lledo & Alvarez-Galvez, 2021). These network problems require network solutions (Young et al., 2021).

Applications

SNT has been applied to many health areas and other domains. SNA can be applied to any discipline or health issue, including individual behavior, organizational performance, interorganizational relations, policy diffusion, service delivery improvements, community-based participatory research, and so on. SNA also provides useful tools for measuring key constructs in other theories. For example, the Theory of Reasoned Action and the Theory of Planned Behavior include constructs, such as normative beliefs, that influence decisions to engage in behaviors (see Chapter 6). In this chapter, network theory is applied to contraceptive decision-making among women in developing countries and adolescent tobacco/nicotine use, two important public health issues.

Contraception Decision-Making in Developing Countries

Many factors influence whether and how many children a couple will have. These factors can be classified into "supply versus demand" or "economic versus sociocultural." People may know how babies are made, but regulating how many children to have has been an evolving concept, one most effectively aided by use of modern contraceptives. The development, supply, and diffusion of contraceptives are of major public health importance and have generated considerable academic study. Social networks are also a frequently cited source of information and influence on contraceptive choices.

An early, foundational, study applying SNT to understand the adoption and diffusion of contraceptive use was conducted among women in 25 Korean villages. This study showed that individual contraceptive use by individuals was correlated with use by their network partners (Rogers & Kincaid, 1981). In alignment with these findings, subsequent studies have continued to demonstrate that women's social networks influence their decisions to use contraceptive methods in many developing countries (Comfort et al., 2021). These studies show that women are aware of and use the same methods as their friends (Valente et al., 1997), and women who report being encouraged to use methods by their friends are more likely to use them (Gayen & Raeside, 2010; Valente et al., 1997). Since contraception use is not easily or directly observable by researchers, information about how women obtain and use contraception must often be transmitted via informal conversations.

A person's close social network and larger community network also can influence other factors related to family planning, such as when to have children. A study exploring high rates of adolescent pregnancy in Honduras examined network factors associated with adolescent childbirth in 176 villages (Shakya et al., 2019, 2020). Each village was considered its own network, from which the researchers collected complete census data on social network connections, attitudes, and norms regarding adolescent pregnancy. Participants were asked questions about their social relationships and to name individuals in their village. They were then asked normative questions about pregnancy, such as, "At what age is it OK for a girl to have her first baby?" The outcome of interest, adolescent childbirth, included any female participants who had given birth before age twenty.

Several personal and community network factors were associated with increased risk of adolescent childbirth in these villages. First, village norms regarding adolescent childbirth were associated significantly with an adolescent's risk of pregnancy, but there were differences based on network cohesion. Cohesion, or density of a social network, is calculated as the number of social ties out of the total number of possible ties (Valente, 2010). In low-cohesion villages, if 40% of the community supported or approved of adolescent childbirth, then, an adolescent woman's risk was 17%; however, in high-density villages with the same level of approval, an adolescent woman's risk was 35% (Shakya et al. 2019).

Second, a woman's personal social network also was associated with her probability of pregnancy. Even when controlling for village-level norms, if someone in a woman's proximal social network gave birth as an adolescent, this increased her own risk for adolescent childbirth. This association was stronger for closer relationships and social contacts closer in age. However, if a woman still had a father in her social network, this was a protective factor and reduced her probability of adolescent pregnancy (Shakya et al., 2020). These studies illustrate how the attitudes and behaviors of individuals in our personal networks can affect health risks and outcomes. They also suggest the importance of considering the larger social network in which people are embedded, as societal norms can also strongly influence perceptions and behaviors.

Adolescent E-Cigarette Use

Electronic nicotine delivery systems, also known as e-cigarettes, e-cigs, or vapes, have become extremely popular recently and are a global public health concern. According to results from the Global Youth Tobacco Surveys, the overall pooled estimates for adolescent e-cigarette awareness and ever-use were 56.7% and 20.2%. The World Health Organization (WHO) regions with the highest e-cigarette ever-use rates among youth were the European Region (34.5%), the South-East Asian Region (20.5%), and the Region of the Americas (18.7%) (Sreeramareddy et al., 2022).

E-cigarette use has continued to increase rapidly and is the most used tobacco product among adolescents. In the United States, 14.1% of high school students and 3.3% of middle school students reported being current e-cigarette users in 2022 (Cooper et al., 2022).

E-cigarettes are not only detrimental to health but are also correlated with initiation of combustible cigarette use among adolescents and young adults (Barrington-Trimis et al., 2016). E-cigarettes can contain higher levels of nicotine, are more addictive, and are often marketed to young audiences. Adolescents have more positive attitudes toward e-cigarettes and perceive them as less harmful and more socially acceptable than combustible cigarettes. Evidence shows that e-cigarettes are addictive and that e-cigarette dependence strongly predicts continuation of use (Vogel et al., 2020).

SNA can help us understand the social mechanisms driving e-cigarette use among adolescents and yield information that might be valuable in developing network-based interventions. E-cigarette use is likely driven by a combination of psychological, social, environmental, and systemic factors. During adolescence, the importance of friendships, social connections, and the desire to fit in may exacerbate the effects of friends' opinions and behaviors on individual behavior. Prior social network research has shown that having friends who smoke is associated with individuals' cigarette use (Alexander et al., 2001; Mercken et al., 2010). One of the first studies to demonstrate this association by Cheryl Alexander and colleagues showed that the risk of adolescent smoking increases with smoking prevalence in one's social network. The odds of smoking are twice as high if one or two of a person's best friends smoke (Alexander et al., 2001). E-cigarettes are now more prevalent and popular than combustible tobacco among adolescents, which suggests that there are distinct differences in the social dynamics driving e-cigarette use.

Understanding social network dynamics is key to implementing effective interventions and curtailing the use of tobacco products among adolescents (Valente, 2012). Preliminary studies have also begun to show potential for peer-led interventions to reduce e-cigarette use (Chu et al., 2021). A recent study recruited peer leaders in schools to model healthy norms and reduced acceptability or approval of vaping (Wyman et al., 2021). The leaders' messages had relatively good exposure, but some vulnerable students, nonusers who reported being susceptible to e-cigarette use, viewed the peer leaders' message as less impactful. Recent vapers had greater exposure to other high-risk students and to students who viewed vaping as minimally harmful, whereas students who had more peer-leader friends were less likely to report recent vaping (Wyman et al., 2021). Understanding network dynamics is essential to designing effective interventions. In this study, network analysis revealed that clustering of high-risk students might reinforce acceptability toward vaping. It also showed that students who are isolated from adults were at higher risk, and more likely to be recent e-cigarette users. SNA provides insight into the diffusion of vaping attitudes and behaviors in the network and helps inform creation of interventions that strategically engage high-risk groups.

The network plot in Figure 11.2 shows vaping prevalence among high school students at two time points from a network study. At the first time point, prevalence of vaping in the network was 42%, and at follow-up, it had risen to 52%. The plot below shows students' friendship networks and indicates which students have ever vaped (gray nodes) and which never vaped (clear nodes). Over time, vaping behavior has diffused through the network resulting in a 10-percentage-point increase at follow-up.

Figure 11.3 highlights two individuals in the high school, 191 and 133. Student 191 had no vaping friends at baseline yet became a vaper at time 2 and named 5 friends, all of whom vape. Student 133 named four friends at baseline all of whom were vapers. Subsequently, this student became a vaper at time two and named two new friends who were also vapers. These micro-level analyses illustrate the role of network influence and network selection.

Network Statistics

Although these two applications provide ample evidence for network effects on health behaviors, there is still much work to be done. Estimating network influences can be a challenge due to the nonindependent nature of network data. Statistical regression approaches typically expect each unit in the database to be independent, and not connected to any other unit in the data. For network data, this assumption is explicitly violated. The problem is further compounded by the network properties of reciprocity, transitivity, and homophily, each of which provides alternative explanations for network effects. For example, if the data show that a smoker is more likely to have smoking friends, it does not necessarily indicate that the friends' smoking has caused the smoking of the individual. Rather this smoking homophily could be a function of ethnicity if both the individual and network are homophilous with respect to ethnicity and smoking rates vary by ethnicity.

Friendship ties and vaping at T1   Friendship ties and vaping at T2

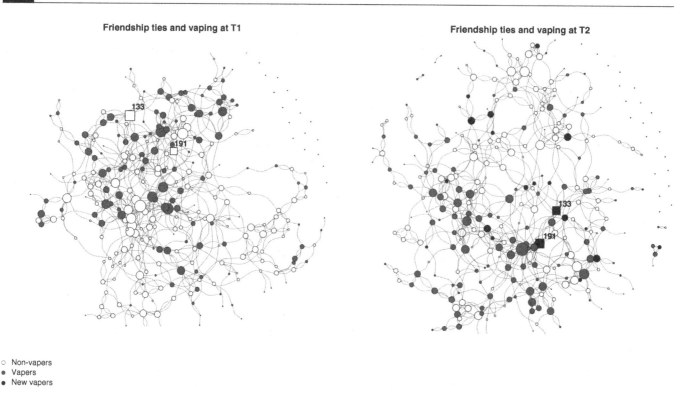

○ Non-vapers
● Vapers
● New vapers

Figure 11.2 Friendships Ties Between Students in One High School with Vaping Behavior Depicted by Shading, Clear, Nonvapers; Gray, Vapers; Black, New Vapers

To address these issues, network statisticians have developed several approaches that account for network structure in the estimation of network effects. The critical insight was to make the network the dependent variable, the outcome, and the behavior the independent variable. The two tools developed using this approach are exponential random graph models (ERGMs) (Robins et al., 2007), and stochastic actor-oriented models (SAOMs) implemented in Rsiena (Simulation Investigation for Empirical Network Analysis) (Snijders et al., 2010). Both models are implemented in the open-source statistical system, R (CRAN).

To estimate an ERGM, the researcher specifies the network and attributes of the nodes in the network, and optionally, attributes of the relationships in the network. For example, the network is a link list of the ID numbers for each relationship and separate fields for the type or strength of the relationship. In a separate file, the researcher stores the attributes of the nodes, characteristics such as age, sex, ethnicity, smoking status, and so on. The researcher then specifies a model of the theoretical relationships thought to be contained in the data such as whether there is reciprocity, transitivity, and homophily on various characteristics. The ERGM software as implemented in STATNET or PNET will indicate the magnitude and statistical significance of the effects specified in the model. SAOMs are estimated similarly, though the model specification process is a bit more complicated due to the longitudinal nature of the data. The science and theory of social networks have expanded greatly with the development of these tools because they have extended our theoretical thinking about how networks influence health behaviors and how network structure and behaviors co-evolve.

Discussion and Conclusion

This brief introduction to SNT and SNA has described the many ways that social networks influence behavior and the challenges inherent in estimating these effects. These effects can be simple, such as being more likely to gain weight when exposed to overweight peers, or complex, such as being resistant to adopting radical innovations when occupying a central position in a centralized network. And, although social network concepts and diagrams can be quite intuitive, often considerable mathematical and computational methods undergird the work. The website for the INSNA can be a helpful starting point (www.insna.org).

The important takeaway from this chapter is that systems (including human ones) are composed of units that interact and are connected by many varying relations. These relations have patterns and structures that are increasingly well

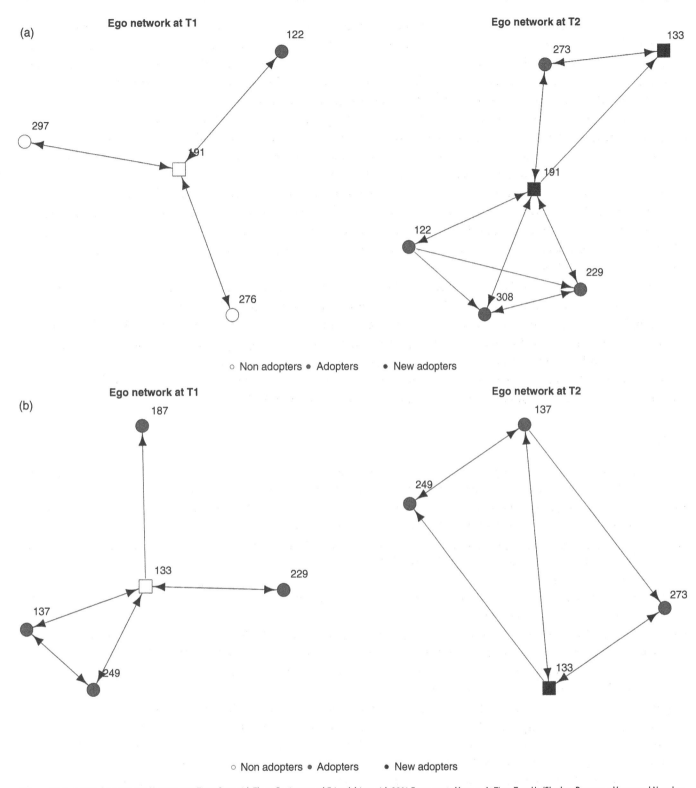

Figure 11.3 (a) Student 191 is a Nonvaper at Time One with Three Reciprocated Friendships with 33% Exposure to Vapers. At Time Two He/She has Become a Vaper and Now has Named Five Friends who all Vape; (b) Student 133 is a Nonvaper at Time One with Four Friendships with 100% Exposure to Vapers. At Time Two He/She has Become a Vaper

understood and shown to have profound and enduring influences on health behaviors. Studies and programs that ignore these relations miss out on the opportunity to advance the science of human behavior and, for interventions, potentially fall short of their true capacity to improve outcomes. SNT specifies the conditions under which people are more likely to be connected and influence one another. It also makes similar claims for organizations, states, inanimate objects, and many other entities. Applying this theory to other theories and to a vast array of health-related domains promises to improve our understanding of how we can make populations healthier and more productive.

Much work remains to be done. The COVID-19 pandemic exposed our limitations in instituting network interventions to slow the spread of the virus, and new pathogens will similarly challenge us in the future. In addition, the widespread use of social and other media to spread misinformation resulted in countless unnecessary infections and subsequent deaths. These experiences suggest that improving public health will require combatting misinformation by making more effective use of social network and social networking interventions.

SNT and SNA can also be used more fully to address equity, diversity, and inclusiveness across private and public sectors and help in understanding barriers and opportunities to create a just and equitable society. As our attitudes and behaviors regarding justice are strongly influenced by our social networks, we must tap into these influences to work toward a level playing field for members of disadvantaged communities.

Meanwhile, we need to continue basic research in network measures, processes, and effects across new and old public health challenges. For example, a cigarette use has emerged as a major public health threat, and emerging evidence indicates that, as with combustible tobacco use, social networks strongly influence its initiation and continued use. Also desperately needed are network interventions to promote healthcare access to reproductive health services and care being jeopardized in recent years.

Finally, we noted that SNT specifies how individual network choices affect macro-level network structures. The converse, however, is also true: macro-level policies and forces also have an impact on micro-level network dynamics. For example, real-estate racial segregation minimizes opportunities for cross-racial social ties and can thus increase racial animosity. Macro-level forces such as segregation policies, climate change, systemic racism, and poverty also have impacts on micro-level network choices and structures, thus impacting individual health.

The road ahead will continue to be challenging, but the new tools of network analysis, combined with ML, AI, NLP, and big data offer opportunities to meet those challenges with tools up to the task.

References

Ahmed, W., Vidal-Alaball, J., Downing, J., & López Seguí, F. (2020). COVID-19 and the 5G conspiracy theory: Social network analysis of twitter data. *Journal of Medical Internet Research*, 22(5), e19458. https://doi.org/10.2196/19458

Alexander, C., Piazza, M., Mekos, D., & Valente, T. W. (2001). Peer networks and adolescent cigarette smoking: An analysis of the national longitudinal study of adolescent health. *Journal of Adolescent Health*, 29(1), 22–30.

Allem, J. P., Dharmapuri, L., Unger, J. B., & Cruz, T. B. (2018). Characterizing JUUL-related posts on Twitter. *Drug and Alcohol Dependence*, 190, 1–5. https://doi.org/10.1016/j.drugalcdep.2018.05.018

Ayers, J. W., Leas, E. C., Allem, J. P., Benton, A., Dredze, M., Althouse, B. M., Cruz, T. B., & Unger, J. B. (2017). Why do people use electronic nicotine delivery systems (electronic cigarettes)? A content analysis of Twitter, 2012-2015. *PLoS One*, 12(3), e0170702. https://doi.org/10.1371/journal.pone.0170702

Barrington-Trimis, J. L., Urman, R., Berhane, K., Unger, J. B., Cruz, T. B., Pentz, M. A., Samet, J. M., Leventhal, A. M., & McConnell, R. (2016). E-cigarettes and future cigarette use. *Pediatrics*, 138(1), e20160379. https://doi.org/10.1542/peds.2016-0379

Bond, R. M., Fariss, C. J., Jones, J. J., Kramer, A. D. I., Marlow, C., Settle, J. E., & Fowler, J. H. (2012). A 61-million-person experiment in social influence and political mobilization. *Nature*, 489(7415), 295–298.

Borgatti, S. P., Everett, M. G. & Johnson, J. C. (2013). *Analyzing social networks.* London: Sage Publications.

Cauchemez, S., Bhattarai, A., Marchbanks, T. L., Fagan, R. P., Ostroff, S., Ferguson, N. M., Swerdlow, D., & Pennsylvania, H. N. w. g. (2011). Role of social networks in shaping disease transmission during a community outbreak of 2009 H1N1 pandemic influenza. *Proceedings of the National Academy of Sciences*, 108(7), 2825–2830. https://doi.org/10.1073/pnas.1008895108

Chetty, R., Jackson, M. O., Kuchler, T., Stroebel, J., Hendren, N., Fluegge, R. B., Gong, S., Gonzalez, F., Grondin, A., Jacob, M., Johnston, D., Koenen, M. Laguna-Muggenburg, E., Mudekereza, F., Rutter, T., Thor, N., Townsend, W., Zhang, R., Bailey, M., & Wernerfelt, N. (2022). Social capital I: Measurement and associations with economic mobility. *Nature*, 608, 108–121. https://doi.org/10.1038/s41586-022-04996-4

Christakis, N., & Fowler, J. (2010). Social network sensors for early detection of contagious outbreaks. *PLoS One*, 5(9), e12948.

Christiansen, J., Qualter, P., Friis, K., Pedersen, S. S., Lund, R., Andersen, C. M., Bekker-Jeppesen, M., & Lasgaard, M. (2021). Associations of loneliness and social isolation with physical and mental health among adolescents and young adults. *Perspectives in Public Health*, 141(4), 226–236.

Chu, K. H., Allem, J. P., Unger, J. B., Cruz, T. B., Akbarpour, M., & Kirkpatrick, M. G. (2019). Strategies to find audience segments on Twitter for e-cigarette education campaigns. *Addictive Behaviors*, 91, 222–226. https://doi.org/10.1016/j.addbeh.2018.11.015

Chu, K. H., Colditz, J. B., Primack, B. A., Shensa, A., Allem, J. P., Miller, E., Unger, J. B., & Cruz, T. B. (2018). JUUL: Spreading online and offline. *Journal of Adolescent Health*, *63*(5), 582–586. https://doi.org/10.1016/j.jadohealth.2018.08.002

Chu, K. H., Pitts, S. R., Wipfli, H., Valente, T. W. (2017). Coding communications across time: Documenting changes in interaction patterns across adopter categories. *Network Science (Camb Univ Press)*, *5*(4), 441–460. https://doi.org/10.1017/nws.2017.28

Chu, K.-H., Sidani, J., Matheny, S., Rothenberger, S. D., Miller, E., Valente, T., & Robertson, L. (2021). Implementation of a cluster randomized controlled trial: Identifying student peer leaders to lead E-cigarette interventions. *Addictive Behaviors*, *114*, 106726–106726. https://doi.org/10.1016/j.addbeh.2020.106726

Comfort, A. B., Harper, C. C., & Tsai, A. C., et al. (2021). Social and provider networks and women's contraceptive use: Evidence from Madagascar. *Contraception*, *104*(2), 147–154. https://doi.org/10.1016/j.contraception.2021.04.013

Conway, M., Hu, M., & Chapman, W. W. (2019). Recent advances in using natural language processing to address public health research questions using social media and consumer generated data. *Yearbook of Medical Informatics*, *28*(1), 208–217. https://doi.org/10.1055/s-0039-1677918

Cooper, M., Park-Lee, E., Ren, C., Cornelius, M., & Jamal, A., Cullen, K. A. (2022). Notes from the field: E-cigarette use among middle and high school students—United States, 2022. *Morbidity and Mortality Weekly Report*, *71*, 1283–1285. http://dx.doi.org/10.15585/mmwr.mm7140a3

DiMaggio, P., & Garip, F. (2012). Network effects and social inequality. *Annual Review of Sociology*, *38*(1), 93–118. https://doi.org/10.1146/annurev.soc.012809.102545

Freeman, L. (1979). Centrality in social networks: Conceptual clarification. *Social Networks*, *1*, 215–239.

Freeman, L. (2004). *The development of social network analysis: A study in the sociology of science.* Vancouver, BC: Empirical Press.

Fu, L., Jacobs, M. A., Brookover, J., Valente, T. W., Cobb, N. K., & Graham, A. L. (2017). An exploration of the Facebook social networks of smokers and non-smokers. *PLoS One*, *12*(11), e0187332. https://doi.org/10.1371/journal.pone.0187332

Gayen, K. & Raeside, R. (2010). Social networks and contraception practice of women in rural Bangladesh. *Social Science & Medicine*, *71*(9), 1584–1592.

Granovetter, M. S. (1973). The strength of weak ties. *American Journal of Sociology*, *78*(6), 1360–1380.

Hinz, O., Skiera, B., Barrot, C., & Becker, J. U. (2011). Seeding strategies for viral marketing: An empirical comparison. *Journal of Marketing*, *75*(6), 55–71. https://doi.org/10.1509/jm.10.0088

Horn, A. L., Jiang, L., Washburn, F., Hvitfeldt, E., de la Haye, K., Nicholas, W., Simon, P., Pentz, M., Cozen, W., Sood, N., & Conti, D. V. (2021). An integrated risk and epidemiological model to estimate risk-stratified COVID-19 outcomes for Los Angeles County: March 1, 2020-March 1, 2021. *PLoS One*, *16*(6), e0253549. https://doi.org/10.1371/journal.pone.0253549

Khubchandani, J., Sharma, S., Price, J. H., Wiblishauser, M. J., & Webb, F. J. (2021). COVID-19 morbidity and mortality in social networks: Does it influence vaccine hesitancy? *International Journal of Environmental Research and Public Health*, *18*(18), 9448. https://www.mdpi.com/1660-4601/18/18/9448

Kretzschmar, M. E., Rozhnova, G., Bootsma, M. C. J., van Boven, M., van de Wijgert, J., & Bonten, M. J. M. (2020). Impact of delays on effectiveness of contact tracing strategies for COVID-19: A modelling study. *The Lancet Public Health*, *5*(8), e452–e459. https://doi.org/10.1016/S2468-2667(20)30157-2

Lazer, D., Pentland, A., Adamic, L., Aral, S., Barabasi, A.-L., Brewer, D, Christakis, N., Contractor, N., Fowler, J., Gutmann, M., Jebara, T. King, G., Macy, M., Roy, D., & Van Alstyne, M., (2009). Computational social science. *Science*, *323*(5915), 721–723.

Lee E. W. J., & Viswanath, K. (2020). Big data in context: Addressing the twin perils of data absenteeism and chauvinism in the context of health disparities research. *Journal of Medical Internet Research*, *22*(1), e16377.

Manas, S., Young, L. E., Fujimoto, K., Franklin, A., & Myneni, S. (2019). Exploring the social structure of a health-related online community for tobacco cessation: A two-mode network approach. *Studies in Health Technology and Informatics*, *264*, 1268–1272. https://doi.org/10.3233/shti190430

Marsden, P. V. (1987). Core discussion networks of Americans. *American Sociological Review*, *52*(1), 122–131.

McPherson, M., Smith-Lovin, L., & Cook, J. M. (2001). Birds of a feather: Homophily in social networks. *Annual Review of Sociology*, *27*(1), 415–444. https://doi.org/10.1146/annurev.soc.27.1.415

Mercken, L., Snijders, T. A. B., Steglich, C., Vertiainen, E., & de Vries, H. (2010). Smoking-based selection and influence in gender-segregated friendship networks: A social network analysis of adolescent smoking. *Addiction*, *105*(7), 1280–1289.

Milgram, S. (1967). The small world problem. *Psychology Today*, *2*, 60–67.

Moreno, J. L. (1934). *Who shall survive? A new approach to the problem of human interrelations.* Washington, DC: Nervous and Mental Disease Publishing.

Nishi, A., Dewey, G., Endo, A., & Young, S. D. (2020). Network interventions for managing the COVID-19 pandemic and sustaining economy. *Proceedings of the National Academy of Sciences, 117*(48), 30285–30294. https://doi.org/10.1073/pnas.2014297117

Robins, G., Pattison, P. Kalish, Y., & Lusher, D. (2007). An introduction to exponential random graph (p*) models for social networks. *Social Networks, 29*(2), 173–191.

Rogers, E. M., & Kincaid, D. L. (1981). *Communication networks: A new paradigm for research.* New York: Free Press.

Scott, J. (2017). *Network analysis: A handbook.* (3rd ed.). Newbury Park, CA: Sage.

Shakya, H. B., Darmstadt, G. L., Barker, K. M., Weeks, J., & Christakis, N. A. (2020). Social normative and social network factors associated with adolescent pregnancy: A cross-sectional study of 176 villages in rural Honduras. *Journal of Global Health, 10*(1), 010706. https://doi.org/10.7189/jogh.10.010706

Shakya, H. B., Weeks, J. R., & Christakis, N. A. (2019). Do village-level normative and network factors help explain spatial variability in adolescent childbearing in rural Honduras? *SSM Population Health, 9*, 100371. https://doi.org/10.1016/j.ssmph.2019.100371

Snijders, T. A. B., van de Bunt, G. G., & Steglich, C. E. G. (2010). Introduction to stochastic actor-based models for network dynamics. *Social Networks, 32*(1), 44–60.

Sreeramareddy, C. T., Acharya, K. & Manoharan, A. (2022). Electronic cigarettes use and 'dual use' among the youth in 75 countries: Estimates from Global Youth Tobacco Surveys (2014–2019). *Scientific Reports 12*, 20967. https://doi.org/10.1038/s41598-022-25594-4

Suarez-Lledo, V., & Alvarez-Galvez, J. (2021). Prevalence of health misinformation on social media: Systematic review. *Journal of Medical Internet Research, 23*(1), e17187. https://doi.org/10.2196/17187

Valente, T. W. (1995). *Network models of the diffusion of innovations.* Cresskill, NJ: Hampton Press.

Valente, T. W. (2010). *Social networks and health: Models, methods, and applications.* New York: Oxford University Press.

Valente, T. (2012). Network interventions. *Science, 337*(6090), 49–53.

Valente, T. W., & Pitts, S. (2017). An appraisal of social network theory and analysis as applied to public health. *Annual Review of Public Health, 38*, 103–118.

Valente, T. W., Pitts, S. R., Wipfli, H., & Yon, G. G. V. (2019). Network influences on policy implementation: Evidence from a global health treaty. *Social Science and Medicine, 222*, 188–197.

Valente, T. W., Watkins, S., Jato, M. N., Van der Straten, A., & Tsitsol, L. M. (1997). Social network associations with contraceptive use among Cameroonian women in voluntary associations. *Social Science & Medicine, 45*(5), 677–687.

Visweswaran, S., Colditz, J. B., O'Halloran, P., Han, N. R., Taneja, S. B., Welling, J., Chu, K. H., Sidani, J. E., & Primack, B. A. (2020). Machine learning classifiers for twitter surveillance of vaping: Comparative machine learning study. *Journal of Medical Internet Research, 22*(8), e17478. https://doi.org/10.2196/17478

Vogel, E. A., Cho, J., Mcconnell, R. S., Barrington-Trimis, J. L., & Leventhal, A. M. (2020). Prevalence of electronic cigarette dependence among youth and its association with future use. *JAMA Network Open, 3*(2), e1921513. https://doi.org/10.1001/jamanetworkopen.2019.21513

Wyman, P. A., Rulison, K., Pisani, A. R., Alvaro, E. M., Crano, W. D., Schmeelk-Cone, K., Keller Elliot, C., Wortzel, J., Pickering, T. A., & Espelage, D. L. (2021). Above the influence of vaping: Peer leader influence and diffusion of a network-informed preventive intervention. *Addictive Behaviors, 113*, 106693. https://doi.org/10.1016/j.addbeh.2020.106693

Young, L. E., Sidnam-Mauch, E., Twyman, M., Wang, L., Xu, J. J., Sargent, M., Valente, T. W., Ferrara, E., Fulk, J., & Monge, P. (2021). Disrupting the COVID-19 misinfodemic with network interventions: Network solutions for network problems. *American Journal of Public Health, 111*(3), 514–519. https://doi.org/10.2105/ajph.2020.306063

CHAPTER 12

STRESS, COPING, ADAPTATION, AND HEALTH BEHAVIOR

Cheryl L. Woods-Giscombe
Ganga Bey

Vignette

Candace is a 42-year-old African American mother of two sons. She was married to her sons' father for 16 years before he unexpectedly died of a heart attack 3 years ago. Candace and her husband were both career-oriented and successful. Her husband was an engineer, and Candace is a television producer. Over the past three years, Candace has been managing her household while raising her very active teenage sons. She spends her evenings taking her sons to and from athletics, music, and leadership-related activities after school. Once her sons go to bed, Candace takes care of last-minute work-related tasks, and she repeats her routine each day. Candace has benefited from the strong support system at church and in her women's clubs, in the context of raising her sons as a widowed mother. Candace and her sons adjusted to the loss of Candace's husband and their father through the support of friends and family. Candace's parents live in her neighborhood, and she benefited from their consistent support. However, over the past 18 months, Candace's life took a challenging turn as both of her aging parents became ill.

Despite needing help from her friends, Candace tried everything she could possibly do to make it work on her own, unassisted by others. She eventually made an appointment with a counselor after one of the pastors at her church encouraged her to reconsider her assumptions about seeking therapy. The counselor was a faith-based therapist who encouraged Candace to enroll in a mindfulness course to learn new skills for responding to chronic stress. After only four weeks of the course, Candace noticed feeling like she had more space to think and exist. She began to view the overall situation as an opportunity for growth and development for her and her sons. Candace was also able to return to regular church services, which provided her with additional resources for coping, such as prayer and music, to promote relaxation and acceptance, in addition to the mindfulness practices that helped her be more mentally and physically healthy.

The accumulation of interpersonal and life stress experienced by Candace can be understood and managed in the context of theories of stress, coping, and health described in this chapter. These theory-based constructs also inform how she responded to stress, and her use of coping resources to manage contextual stressors that were adversely influencing her health.

KEY POINTS

This chapter will:

- Provide an overview of foundational and emerging theories and research related to stress, coping, and health.

- Summarize historical stress, coping, and health frameworks, including the General Adaptation Syndrome and the Transactional Model of Stress and Coping.

- Discuss biobehavioral theoretical extensions of stress, coping/adaptation, and health, including psycho-neuroendocrinology, psychoimmunology, and additional stress-influenced cognitive-emotional-behavioral responses across the life course.

- Describe the contribution of stress, coping, and related contextual factors (such as workplace stress, racism/discrimination experiences, sociodemographic factors, and adverse childhood events) to racial and ethnic disparities in health.

- Describe factors that promote adaptation, resilience, well-being, health, and longevity.

- Illustrate applications of classic and newly emerging models of stress, coping, and health to the design and testing of interventions to improve health and health equity.

This chapter heavily emphasizes examples of stressors related to racial and ethnic disparities and health equity. These themes are very important in contemporary health behavior and public health. However, we do not mean to suggest that they are the only sources of stress, which can also include stressors in relationships from illness and other concerns.

Health Behavior: Theory, Research, and Practice, Sixth Edition. Edited by Karen Glanz, Barbara K. Rimer, and K. Viswanath.
Companion website: www.wiley.com/go/glanz/healthbehavior6e

Historical Overview of Stress and Coping Research

The definition of stress is conceptually complex. The term "*stress*" has been referred to as a stimulus, a response, and an interaction (Brannon & Feist, 2004). As early as 1950, Hans Selye described what he referred to as the "General Adaptation Syndrome" or GAS. Selye later updated this description, referring to it as the "stress response." Selye introduced the terms "distress" and "eustress" to describe negative and positive stress, respectively (Selye, 1950). Considered one of the foundational, modern-day frameworks for stress and coping, GAS developed in three stages: (1) alarm reaction; (2) stage of resistance; and (3) stage of exhaustion. As a physician and a chemist, Selye's pioneering research and description of biological stress focused on the physiologic characteristics of the alarm-reaction stage and the stress-reactive processes of both defense and damage, including actions of the nervous, hormonal, and adrenal systems leading to catabolism of tissue, gastrointestinal disruptions, adrenal cortex secretory discharge, hypoglycemia, and the work the body endured to maintain what French physiologist Claude Bernard described as *milieu interior* (Bernard, 1974; Holmes, 1986). Implications for stress-related health conditions were described, including (but not limited to) vascular damage, inflammatory and immune dysfunction, as well as cardiac, kidney, renal, and lymphatic dysfunction. Selye dedicated his research career to integrating American physiologist Walter Cannon's previously articulated concepts of "homeostasis" and "fight-or-flight" (coined as early as 1915) (Cannon, 1941) to "better understand life and the treatment of disease" (Selye, 1950, p. 1). Selye identified what we now refer to as the hypothalamic-pituitary axis system, and "diseases of adaptation," including rheumatoid arthritis, allergies, dermatitis, diabetes, lupus erythematosus, alcoholism, and hypertension. Selye identified the challenges of chronic stress in limiting adaptability to stress.

The social sciences were not included in Selye's list of necessary multidisciplinary fields needed to understand stress and disease, although they are prominent in present-day understanding of social determinants of health, stress, and coping. Yet, Selye wisely contextualized his initial definition of GAS by proclaiming it would take years, if not generations, to comprehensively understand the concepts of stress and adaptation. He also declared that his preliminary conceptualization was knowingly incomplete and perhaps even incorrect, but it was an attempt to begin the important operationalization of the influence of stress, adaptive processes, and disease states. The term "*stressor*" refers to the environmental demand, event, threat, or stimulus to which an individual is exposed. The term "*distress*" refers to an adverse state evidenced by physical or psychological symptoms, including tension, worry, weakness, or headaches, influenced by exposure to environmental demands in the context of inadequate resources (Dohrenwend & Dohrenwend, 1974).

Another influential stream of stress research in the 1960s and 1970s focused on identifying and quantifying potential stressors or stressful life events. Holmes & Rahe (1967) developed the Social Readjustment Rating Scale (SRRS), a tool to measure stressful life events to understand how they might cause illness. Studies showed that people with high scores on the SRRS had more illness episodes than those with low scores. This scale stimulated a substantial body of research that continues to the present day. Selye and psychiatrists Holmes and Rahe were oriented primarily toward understanding biological mechanisms of stress and adaptation and how stress influences illness.

Pathways Through Which Stress Influences Health

There are two major pathways through which psychological stress can influence health: the *stress-behavioral coping pathway* and the *stress-physiology pathway* (American Psychological Association [APA], 2017; Epel, 2009). Cognitive-emotional responses to stress can affect the impact that stress has on both physiology and behaviors.

Psychological stress and its potential adverse effects in the context of inadequate resources have been documented (APA, 2017). Exposure to stressors can affect psychological well-being and physical health negatively. Physical effects of stress on health may result from changes in lifestyle and health behaviors, such as diet, exercise, nicotine use, and other forms of substance use. If experienced chronically, stress can impair coping-related health behaviors and increase risk for long-term adverse health conditions (APA, 2017).

Transactional Model of Stress and Coping

Psychologists Richard Lazarus and Susan Folkman integrated psychological, emotional, cognitive, and behavioral factors into the conceptualization of stress and adaptation or coping. According to the Transactional Model of Stress and Coping, stress is a subjectively perceived discrepancy between environmental demands or threats and an individual's

Table 12.1 Transactional Model of Stress and Coping, with Extensions: Definitions and Applications

Concept	Definition	Applications
Primary Appraisal	Evaluation of the significance of a stressor or threatening event	Perceptions of an event as threatening can cause distress. If an event is perceived as positive, benign, or irrelevant, little negative threat is felt
Secondary Appraisal	Evaluation of the controllability of the stressor and available coping resources	Perceiving the ability to change the situation, manage emotional reactions, and/or cope effectively can lead to successful coping and adaptation
Coping Efforts	Actual strategies used to mediate primary and secondary appraisals	
Problem Management	Strategies aimed at changing a stressful situation	Strategies include active coping, problem-solving, and seeking information
Emotional Regulation	Strategies aimed at changing the way of thinking or feeling about a stressful situation	Strategies include venting feelings, behavioral avoidance, disengagement, denial, and seeking social support
Meaning-Based Coping	Coping processes that produce positive emotions, which in turn sustain the coping process by allowing re-enactment of problem- or emotion-focused coping	Positive reappraisal of the stressor, revised goals, spiritual and religious beliefs, and focusing on positive events
Outcomes of Coping (adaptation)	Emotional well-being, functional status, health behaviors	Coping strategies may result in short- and long-term positive or negative adaptation
Dispositional Coping Styles	Generalized ways of behaving that can affect emotional or functional reaction to a stressor; relatively stable across time and situations	
Optimism	Tendency to have generalized positive expectancies for outcomes	Optimists can experience fewer symptoms and/or faster recovery from illness
Benefit Finding	Identification of positive life changes that have resulted from major stressors	Benefit finding may be related to the use of positive reappraisal and active coping
Information Seeking	Attentional styles that are vigilant (monitoring) versus those that involve avoidance (blunting)	Monitoring may increase distress and arousal; it may also increase active coping. Blunting may mute excessive worry but may reduce adherence

Source: Wethington, Glanz & Schwartz (2015)/John Wiley & Sons.

biological, psychological, and social resources for coping (Lazarus & Folkman, 1984). According to this model, stress is a process. One of the most important elements is perception, or what individuals may think about the environmental demands or threats and their ability to meet these demands. This is commonly referred to as stress *appraisal* (Lazarus & Folkman, 1984). When an individual is confronted with or exposed to an environmental demand or threat, he or she engages in a cognitive appraisal process to assess the meaning, relevance, and potential danger of this demand (*primary appraisal*) and the presence of resources to manage it (*secondary appraisal*). The degree of stress an individual experiences depends on the dynamic relationship between the individual and their environment. An individual's perceptions, including their worldview and perceived availability of supportive resources, influence the appraisal of events as stressful or not (Folkman et al., 1986) (Lazarus & Folkman, 1984). Table 12.1 summarizes key concepts, definitions, and applications of the Transactional Model of Stress and Coping and the key extensions discussed in this chapter. Figure 12.1 illustrates the interrelationships among these concepts.

Behavioral Pathways: Definition and Concept of Coping

Coping is a transactional process that has been conceptualized as an individual's cognitive, behavioral, and emotional efforts in response to demands, internal or external, or stressors appraised as exceeding existing resources (Folkman & Lazarus, 1988; Folkman et al., 1986). According to this theory, the availability of adequate coping resources minimizes stress.

There are two types of coping (Folkman et al., 1986). *Problem-focused coping* involves the targeted reduction or removal of the underlying cause of a stressor. Problem-focused coping, such as problem-solving, can be most beneficial in situations that are within the individual's control to change the stressor, such as using better time-management skills, changing jobs, or moving to a more comfortable home or safer community. When a situation is beyond control of the individual, such as emotional loss, or if problem-focused coping strategies are not financially or socially accessible, problem-focused coping is less beneficial. Emotion-focused coping can be potentially adaptive (e.g., meditation, prayer,

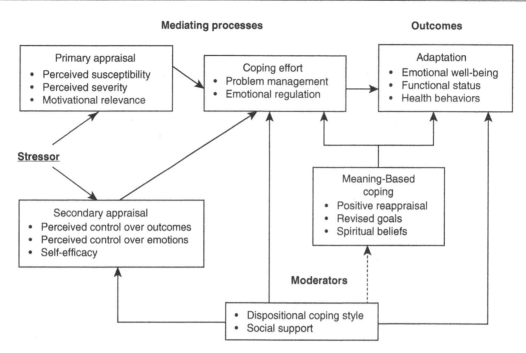

Figure 12.1 Transactional Model of Stress and Coping and Its Major Extensions
Source: Wethington et al. (2015)/John Wiley & Sons

emotional disclosure, writing) or maladaptive (e.g., emotional eating, substance abuse, risk-taking behaviors, or emotional avoidance), depending on the degree to which these strategies are used and their long-term impact on health and well-being. Emotion-focused coping can be helpful when demands or stressors are less amenable to direct control by the individual.

A cumulative body of research suggests that coping strategies mediate the impact of stress on biopsychosocial processes that can lead to adverse health conditions. For example, journaling or written emotional expression (Petrie Booth & Pennebaker, 1998) was identified as a coping strategy that could influence immunoprotective outcomes. Research by Utsey (1999) and Mattis (2002) emphasized the importance of including culture-specific coping strategies, and the limitations of placing coping strategies in exclusive problem- or emotion-focused categories. Collective coping, religious and spirituality-centered coping, and cognitive-emotional debriefing are considered to be both problem- and emotion-focused coping strategies that buffer associations between stressful life experiences and adverse psychological or physical health.

Physiological Stress Pathways: Foundational Research

Stress can alter physiology, the aging process, and health status *directly* (APA, 2017; Epel & Lithgow, 2014). Some major pathways through which stress exerts influence on health include:

Neuroendocrine pathway: Corticotropin-releasing hormone (CRH) plays a pivotal role in the activity of the hypothalamic–pituitary–adrenal axis and in physiological responses to stress (McEwen, 2007). Corticotropin stimulates secretion of cortisol by the adrenal cortex. Emotional or physical stress can interrupt this negative feedback loop, resulting in an overproduction of cortisol. Excessive and unlimited cortisol secretion is associated with depression, hypertension, immunosuppression, insulin resistance, and cerebrovascular disease (Epel, 2009; McEwen, 2007).

Vascular pathway: The association between stress and increased risk for cardiovascular disorders, such as hypertension, has been well documented (Kivimäki & Steptoe, 2018; Steptoe & Kivimäki, 2012). Cardiovascular reactivity to stress may result from functional changes in neuroendocrine and autonomic nervous system mechanisms.

Immune pathway: A third physiological pathway involves immunosuppression and infection (Dhabhar, 2014; Straub & Cutolo, 2018). Alterations in immune functioning resulting from stress adversely affect health, including respiratory functioning, and wound-healing degradation (Kiecolt-Glaser et al., 2002).

Inflammatory pathway: Acute and chronic stress are associated with higher levels of pro-inflammatory cytokines, including Interleukin-6, tumor necrosis factor alpha, and C-reactive protein (Marsland et al., 2017). All are thought to be risk factors for cardiovascular disease, type 2 diabetes, depression, osteoporosis, autoimmune conditions, and other diseases of inflammation.

Allostatic load: Allostatic load describes comprehensive and cumulative risk across multiple physiological regulatory systems resulting from chronic exposure to life challenges or stressors that influence health outcomes across the life span (McEwen, 2007, 2017). Allostasis, the body's ability to maintain homeostasis and adapt to acutely stressful events, is challenged in situations of chronic or frequent stress when there is excessive demand on the body's regulatory systems (McEwen, 2017). Indices of cardiovascular activity, the sympathetic nervous system, metabolism, and neuroendocrine function are used to calculate allostatic load (e.g., Seeman et al., 2002), which predicts increased risk for mortality, physiological dysfunction, the incidence of cardiovascular disease, and cognitive decline (McEwen, 2017).

Workplace Stress and Health

Work-related factors are significant sources of stress among working adults (National Institute for Occupational Safety and Health, 2014). Workplace stress is a major source of demands influencing coping behaviors that increase risk for morbidity, including alcohol use, cigarette smoking, and burnout-related sedentary behavior (The American Institute of Stress, n.d.). About 63% of the American population is employed (United States Department of Labor, Bureau of Labor Statistics, 2018), and these adults spend most of their active daily lives in workplace settings. Furthermore, workplace stress has increased over time; about 83% of workers report work-related stress, and nearly one million are absent from work due to stress-related symptoms (American Institute of Stress, 2023). The CDC suggests that workplace wellness initiatives to address work-related stress may be an optimal population health approach to target stress, coping, and risk-related health behaviors. Workplace wellness strategies can contribute to reductions in work-related adverse physical and mental health conditions across the lifespan (CDC, 2019). For example, promising research suggests that chronic health conditions, such as cardiovascular disease, can be prevented through workplace mindfulness-based stress reduction programs and other related mind-body interventions (Woods-Giscombe & Gaylord, 2022).

Stress and Health Inequities

Despite the strong evidence that supports a relationship between stress and health, the experience of psychological stressors among racial/ethnically diverse populations, the effects of stress on emotional and physical well-being, and related coping strategies have been underexplored in stress and coping research. Influential research on stress and coping in diverse populations identified stress as a potential factor influencing health disparities, defined as "differences in the incidence, prevalence, mortality, and burden of diseases and other adverse health conditions that exist among specific population groups in the United States" (Carter-Pokras et al., 2002, p. 430). Blacks/African Americans, Hispanics/Latinos, Native Americans, Alaskan Natives, Asian Americans, Native Hawaiians, Pacific Islanders, and other medically underserved groups are considered health disparity populations (NIH, 2015). Clark et al. (1999) were among the first research teams to identify racial discrimination as a stressor. Previous conceptualizations of stress were generic and did not include sources of stress related to race, culture, or gender nor the possibility that different groups may respond to the same stressors in different ways. Research by Woods-Giscombe and Lobel (2008) later provided evidence that operationalizations of stress that include race and gender were more comprehensive and predictive of psychological and physiological symptoms of distress compared to operationalizations of stress that included more generic experiences of stress alone.

Grounded in the bioecological framework (Bronfenbrenner & Ceci, 1994), expanded conceptualizations of stress included contextual, historical, developmental, structural, and social determinants that influence individual experiences and responses to stress (APA, 2017). In alignment with this *bioecological approach* (Bronfenbrenner & Ceci, 1994), concepts such as Weathering (Geronimus et al., 2019) and John Henryism (James, 1994), described below, provide a more comprehensive understanding of how stress and stress-coping responses influence health and health inequities.

The accumulating evidence on the mechanisms of Weathering and John Henryism emphasizes the importance of including culturally relevant concepts in research on stress and coping.

Weathering

The weathering framework (see Geronimus et al., 2019) suggests that African American women experience health decrements because of "the cumulative impact of repeated experience with social, economic, or political exclusion" throughout their lifetimes (Geronimus, 2001, p. 133). Like allostatic load, the concept of "*weathering*" (Geronimus et al., 2019) provides an explanation for potentially greater susceptibility to stress. Research on weathering has been focused on African American women to identify mechanisms through which stress influences the disproportionately high rates of stress-related chronic illness they experience compared with European American women. Support for the concept of weathering includes evidence that health disparities between African American and European American women become amplified after age 25 and are most evident from ages 35 to 64 (Geronimus, 2001; Simons et al., 2021). African American women's unique experiences of racism and discrimination, which include both racism and gendered stress, contribute to weathering and greater potential for chronic disease.

John Henryism Active Coping

The *John Henryism Hypothesis* (James 1994) proposed that African American men who exhibited high effort coping under high demands with insufficient resources have a higher risk for cardiovascular disease. Psychosocial and historically influenced high-effort coping in response to stressors can result in poor health—particularly among those with inadequate resources to manage stress (James 1994). John Henryism characteristics include hard work, self-sufficiency, and determination despite challenging circumstances. Recent research has examined John Henryism and its mechanisms in both men and women from various racial/ethnic backgrounds. In some, mixed results were found; John Henryism Active Coping strategies have been identified as resilience factors that are protective against the chronic health risks associated with stress (Robinson & Thomas Tobin, 2021).

Frameworks that Inform Strategies to Foster Adaptive Coping, Resilience, and Well-Being

Existing and emerging frameworks detail factors that foster adaptive coping, resilience, and well-being including spirituality, social connectivity, and self-care practices, such as healthy eating, physical activity, self-regulation, and positive reappraisal (Felix et al., 2022). In this section, we discuss three models that use stress theory to focus on promoting improved stress-management strategies: the *Relaxation Response*, the *Broaden-and-Build Theory of Positive Emotions*, and the *Identity Vitality-Pathology Framework*.

Relaxation Response

The relaxation response, described by Benson and Klipper (2000), is a strategy for coping that can be induced to interrupt or counteract potential adverse effects of psychological stress. Through activating physiological mechanisms of parasympathetic activity, including reduced blood pressure, slowed respiratory rate, slowed digestion, increased blood flow, and muscle relaxation, the body can be protected from adverse impacts of stress. Repeating words, sounds, prayers, or yoga can help induce the relaxation response, which can be beneficial for immune, inflammatory, cardiovascular, respiratory, and cognitive functioning (Jacobs, 2001; Wallace et al., 1971). These techniques do not change the underlying causes of stress, but they can reduce the deleterious effects when they are used.

A solid body of evidence demonstrates broad effectiveness of meditation and mindfulness-based practices in reducing stress through enhanced self-regulation, positive reappraisal of stressful experiences, and self-compassion, as well as compassion for others (Zhang et al., 2021).

The Broaden-and-Build Theory of Positive Emotions

The Broaden-and-Build Theory posits that happiness and other positive emotions facilitate the development of awareness, novel thoughts, and novel actions, which help foster skills-building and enhance the availability of psychological resources (Frederickson, 1998) in response to stress. According to the framework, positive appraisal of situations can be cyclical and can increase well-being, positive emotions, creativity, resilience, flourishing, and deeper life satisfaction (Fredrickson, 2003). Practices that can enhance positive emotions include meditation, writing about positive experiences, and religious or spiritual practices (Fredrickson, 2003, 2004; Van Cappellen et al., 2016).

Identity Vitality-Pathology Model

The Identity Vitality-Pathology (IVP) Model (Bey, 2022) is an emerging theoretical framework that links self-concept to health through identity-related beliefs about worth and social status which are hypothesized to influence how individuals appraise and respond to stress, both physiologically and behaviorally. The model describes this set of modifiable identity beliefs that may be influential in stress appraisal and coping as an *identity state*, which is characterized by the ways individuals primarily conceptualize: (1) an internalized, stable identity, (2) the value of living beings, and (3) whether concepts of self-worth are attached to external evaluations. The IVP framework builds on existing theory and evidence on the roles of inclusive identities (Cross Jr. & Vandiver, 2001; Myers et al., 1991), loving compassion (Kahana et al., 2021; Myers et al., 1991), and inherent self-worth in well-being (Crocker & Knight, 2005), positing that modulation of stress by the three factors comprising one's identity state has direct implications for the physiological processes underlying both mental and physical health.

The IVP framework is distinct from other stress and coping frameworks relevant to health inequities in that it hypothesizes an additional source of disease risk and resilience—pathological or vitalized identity states—as a modifiable target for bringing people closer to ideal states of health Identity states, as defined by the IVP model, exist on a spectrum from "vitalized" to "pathological" which can be captured using a scale, the recently developed IVP Scale. Individuals in "vitalized" identity states are hypothesized to have a reduced likelihood of appraising a high level of stress associated with identity-based stressors such as race or gender discrimination (Figure 12.2).

On the other end of the identity state spectrum is identity pathology (distinct from the psychopathologies previously described as identity pathology by Kaufman & Crowell, 2018). Identity pathology is a pathogenic state characterized by

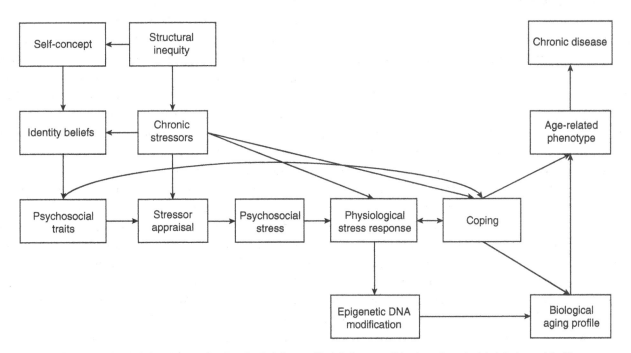

Figure 12.2 Applied Identity Vitality-Pathology Framework to Describe the Influence of Socially Constructed Identity on Stress Appraisal, Coping, and Health
Source: Bey (2022) (adapted)

an identity grounded in physical traits, and the belief that a person's worth depends on their social position. In this pathologized identity state, individuals are more likely to appraise identity-based stress within the social environment (such as is associated with perceived discriminatory treatment or displacement from rightfully filled positions) that triggers harmful conditioned stress responses and exacts a physiological toll.

Rather than conceptualizing identity states as inherent and independent of context, IVP theory names the specific social structures, including structurally embedded systems of hegemony, that shape the cultural, political, and social norms foundational to the construction and adoption of identity. Ultimately, the IVP model extends the fundamental assertions of the Transactional Model of Stress and Coping (TMSC) to propose novel methods for improving well-being on a population level.

Stress, Coping, Adaptation, and Health Behavior: Applications to Current and Emerging Research

The application of frameworks that consider how environmental factors, discrimination, or adverse childhood experiences (APA, 2017) influence stress and coping mechanisms may provide critically important information to inform the development of individual- and system-level interventions to prevent or reduce stress and promote adaptive coping responses.

Emerging research on moderators and mediators of the relationships of stress, coping, and well-being can offer promise for developing effective interventions across the lifespan. In this section, we discuss examples of how research on stress, coping, and health has been applied empirically toward this goal. We describe the value of mindfulness-based approaches to address stress responses and stress-related biobehavioral risk factors for adverse health conditions (Woods-Giscombe & Gaylord, 2014; Woods-Giscombe et al., 2019b).

Superwoman Schema Conceptual Framework

The Superwoman Schema (SWS) Conceptual Framework and the subsequently developed SWS Questionnaire were informed by Woods-Giscombe's series of quantitative and qualitative investigations of stress, coping, and health (Giscombe & Lobel, 2005; Woods-Giscombe, 2010). The framework grew out of research on contextually relevant operationalizations of stress and coping (Woods-Giscombe & Gaylord, 2014; Woods-Giscombe & Lobel, 2005, 2008), and has led to the development of culturally tailored, mind-body interventions to reduce risk for chronic illness. Early observational research with 189 African American women from diverse socioeconomic backgrounds demonstrated how stress related to racism and gender-related stress contribute to outcomes that include psychological and physical symptoms (Woods-Giscombe & Lobel, 2008). This research suggested that interventions to reduce stress-related disparities may be more effective if they specifically target race-related and gender-related stressors. Gender-related stress was defined not just as sexism, but as a culturally nuanced interaction between exposure to stressors and historical and socially sanctioned reactions to stress that influence coping responses such as perceived obligations to project an image of strength and the suppression of emotions—collectively described as the SWS.

According to the SWS framework, historical and sociocultural events in the United States related to gender and race have resulted in the development of five characteristics among African American women that manifest as a superwoman role, including (1) a perceived obligation to manifest an image of strength; (2) a perceived obligation to suppress emotions; (3) resistance to being vulnerable or dependent; (4) determination to succeed, even in the face of limited resources; and (5) a perceived obligation to help others. More specifically, this framework posits that factors such as a historical legacy of racial or gender stereotyping or oppression, lessons from foremothers about how to manage these experiences, a history of disappointment or abuse influenced by chronic socioeconomic deprivation, and spiritual values all contribute to the development of the SWS and role manifestation. The SWS characteristics help women with the preservation of self, family, and community. Otherwise stated, SWS is a survival tactic.

SWS characteristics are associated with objectively measured physiological and behavioral risk factors for chronic health conditions, such as cardiovascular, metabolic, and autoimmune conditions (Allen et al., 2019; Woods-Giscombe et al., 2019a). Endorsement of SWS characteristics has been associated with adverse outcomes such as postponement of self-care, stress-related eating, interpersonal conflict, disturbance in sleep quality or quantity, psychological distress, anxiety, and depression (Sheffield-Abdullah & Woods-Giscombe, 2021; Woods-Giscombé, 2010).

Culturally Relevant Mind-Body Interventions for Stress-Related Adverse Health Outcomes

The emergence of mind-body practices such as Mindfulness-Based Stress Reduction, Relaxation Response (described above) (Benson & Klipper 2000; Kabat-Zinn, 2005) and the promotion of positive emotions as a method of fostering healthy coping and well-being (Frederickson, 1998) can be used as a foundation for health-promoting interventions. These concepts have been translated into community-based programs and population-level interventions, with the aim of reducing stress-related risk factors and health inequities among racial minorities and other marginalized groups (Woods-Giscombe et al., 2019a).

The "We Can Prevent Diabetes" study (Woods-Giscombe et al., 2019b) was a randomized controlled, feasibility study that integrated mindfulness meditation into a conventional behavioral lifestyle intervention. This study examined whether addressing psychological stressors with a mindfulness-based intervention would improve individuals' ability to engage in and sustain healthy eating and physical activity. Sixty-eight African American adults were randomized into one of two groups that each participated in a 4-hour retreat, eight weekly intervention sessions, and six weekly booster sessions (a total of 33 hours). The control group focused on information and behavior change skills, while the mindfulness program included an adapted mindfulness-based stress reduction training component in addition to conventional diabetes risk-reduction education.

Findings showed that both groups had reduced hemoglobin A1C, indicating successful risk reduction. However, respondents who also received the mindfulness-stress management component reported trends toward enhanced peacefulness; lower stress; and lower fat, carbohydrate, and calorie intake; and lower body mass index (Woods-Giscombe et al., 2019b). The SWS Conceptual Framework and the subsequently developed SWS Questionnaire were informed by Woods-Giscombe's series of quantitative and qualitative investigations of stress, coping, and health (Giscombe & Lobel, 2005; Woods-Giscombe, 2010; Woods-Giscombe & Lobel, 2008).

Findings from this study were used to develop a more nuanced, culturally tailored behavioral lifestyle program called "Harmony" to reduce biobehavioral factors associated with cardiometabolic risk factors in African American women. The "Harmony" intervention program is being tested in a randomized trial with 200 women to assess its efficacy for self-care and behavioral change to reduce stress-related risk factors for chronic illness in African American women over 10 months of intervention (Woods-Giscombe & Gaylord, 2022). We hypothesize that the evidence-based, culturally tailored "Harmony" intervention will support women's goals to be healthier by enhancing their abilities to practice mindfulness, self-compassion, and self-care in the context of social stressors known to increase risk for cardio-metabolic conditions.

Critiques and Knowledge Gaps in Stress and Coping Research

Trends in Conceptualization of Stress and Coping

Building on early models of stress including General Adaptation Syndrome (Selye, 1956) and stress as a stimulus (Holmes & Rahe, 1967), Lazarus and Folkman's TMSC (Lazarus & Folkman, 1987) addressed many of the theoretical shortcomings of early stress research. They incorporated the role of individual psychological characteristics, previous life experiences, and the environment in the experience of stress (Lazarus & Folkman, 1984, 1987). To date, many of the fundamental assumptions and assertions of TMSC have been empirically demonstrated in diverse populations (Giurgescu et al., 2015; Sanguanklin et al., 2014). Stress research largely has moved away from the development of new theory toward clarifying the complex relationship between the individual and their environment outlined by TMSC.

This shift has allowed for a much more expansive and impactful conceptualization of the role of stress in health outcomes. Chronic stressors such as economic deprivation, caregiver burden, and increasingly, experiences of racism, prejudice, and discrimination have been identified as key contributors to a wide array of mental and physical health outcomes (Berjot & Gillet, 2011). Attention to the individual characteristics (e.g., gender, race, personality, trauma history) influencing stressor appraisal and coping response has further highlighted mechanistic pathways from stress exposure to health disparities (Bey et al., 2019; Lee et al., 2020).

Knowledge Gaps

The body of health research grounded in stress theory could be further strengthened by addressing several persistent gaps. One of the most prominent of these growth areas is the need for a more nuanced understanding of common *sources* of stress (such as discrimination and other social determinants of stress) and methods of coping across racially diverse and other marginalized populations. For example, prominent stress frameworks do not specifically identify the role of structural inequity in shaping the stress process for populations across different social positions, even as they may acknowledge prejudice and discrimination as stressors (Clark et al., 1999). As a rule, moreover, prevailing stress frameworks do not consider the mechanisms by which structural racism and other social determinants act to influence the experience of stress and coping behavior across differently racialized groups, highlighting the need to integrate minority-stress hypotheses into the core tenets of stress theory.

Few efforts have been directed toward elucidating how the disproportionate and unjust accumulation of social and material resources, including wealth and political capital, may impose psychological pressures to which individuals do not have adequate resources to adapt (Bey et al., 2019). Addressing this deficit, emerging theories (Bey, 2022) and growing evidence support the assertion that hierarchical social dynamics facilitating maladaptive behaviors in response to these psychological pressures may partially explain racialized and gendered patterns in antisocial tendencies such as the perpetuation of mass shootings, trophy hunting, domestic violence, and child sexual abuse (Alegria et al., 2013; Batavia et al., 2019), which may be triggered by acute and/or chronic exposure to stressors as noted in the diathesis-stress model (Broerman, 2017; Levi, 1974). Failure to identify these predilections as correlates of dominant social status may be attributable to the tendency within the health disciplines to normalize the pathologies of members of dominant status groups (Bey, 2022).

Opportunities

The field of stress research could also contribute more to resolving growing tensions regarding best practices for reducing and eliminating health inequities (see Chapter 14). The core tenets of what is often referred to as positive psychology within the psychological disciplines (Frederickson, 2004; Seligman & Csikszentmihalyi, 2000) provide a foundation for a growing interest in identifying sources of both community- and individual-level resilience rather than focusing solely on risk within the health research literature (Boehm & Kubzansky, 2012; Taylor & Carr, 2021). Modifiable psychosocial factors, such as optimism, and culturally rooted practices such as spirituality, modulate the effects of stress exposure on health behaviors and outcomes (Boehm & Kubzansky, 2012; Laubmeier et al., 2004). However, an increased interest in resilience has met with resistance from some health-equity researchers questioning the utility of such approaches for long-term improvements in health at the population level. Approaches focused on promoting adaptive coping and resilience as a viable intervention strategy for population-level, stress-driven health outcomes often are positioned as, at worst, counter to and, at best, tangential to those focused primarily on eradicating structural inequity as a stressor through policy and other structural interventions (Bailey et al., 2017; Brown et al., 2019).

In this vein, additional implementation science research is needed to understand the longitudinal effects of interventions. This approach could help to promote adaptive coping, resilience, well-being, and health. While promising evidence from cross-sectional and other observational studies suggests that many interventions on stress-responsive cognition and behavior are accessible, sustainable, amenable to culturally tailored adaptations, and effective across the life course at mitigating the health consequences of prolonged stress exposure (Borgi et al., 2020; Miller-Graff & Campion, 2016; Woods-Giscombe et al., 2019b), these findings largely have not been replicated in the context of rigorous prospective experimental investigation. Well-designed longitudinal randomized controlled trials (RCTs) examining Mind-Body, identity-based, or positive emotion interventions are a necessary next step for the field.

Summary

This chapter provides an overview of historical and emerging theories relating stress and coping to health. Summaries of the growing empirical evidence supporting biobehavioral extensions of traditional stress theory, emphasizing the multisystem pathways emerging as critical to the effects of stress, coping, and adaptation on health outcomes illustrate the complex associations of stress, stress response, coping, and health. Contextual factors, including adverse childhood events and exposure to racism, shape unique experiences of stress, highlighting the need for attention to the cumulative physiological burden resulting from such experiences. Descriptions of established and emerging stress and coping frameworks illustrate the confluence of social, cultural, and historical factors shaping experiences of stress across differentially racialized groups. Stress research can be strengthened, including prioritizing the RCTs and multilevel strategy approaches needed to establish interventions on stress and coping as effective strategies for improving population health and addressing health inequity in ways that produce sustainable health benefits at individual, familial, community, societal, and structural levels.

References

Alegria, A. A., Blanco, C., Petry, N. M., Skodol, A. E., Liu, S. M., Grant, B., & Hasin, D. (2013). Sex differences in antisocial personality disorder: Results from the national epidemiological survey on alcohol and related conditions. *Personality Disorders*, *4*(3), 214–222. https://doi.org/10.1037/a0031681

Allen, A. M., Wang, Y., Chae, D. H., Price, M. M., Powell, W., Steed, T. C., Rose Black, A., Dhabhar, F. S., Marquez-Magaña, L., & Woods-Giscombe, C. L. (2019). Racial discrimination, the superwoman schema, and allostatic load: Exploring an integrative stress-coping model among African American women. *Annals of the New York Academy of Sciences*, *1457*(1), 104–127. https://doi.org/10.1111/nyas.14188

American Institute of Stress. (2023). https://www.stress.org/workplace-stress

American Psychological Association, APA Working Group on Stress and Health Disparities (2017). Stress and health disparities: Contexts, mechanisms, and interventions among racial/ethnic minority and low-socioeconomic status populations. http://www.apa.org/pi/health-disparities/resources/stress-report.aspx

Bailey, Z. D., Krieger, N., Agénor, M., Graves, J., Linos, N., & Bassett, M. T. (2017). Structural racism and health inequities in the USA: Evidence and interventions. *The Lancet*, *389*(10077), 1453–1463.

Batavia, C, Nelson, M. P., Darimont, C. T., Paquet, P. C., Ripple, W. J., Wallach, A. D. (2019). The elephant (head) in the room: A crucial look at trophy hunting. *Conservation Letters*, *12*(1), e12565.

Benson, H., & Klipper, M. Z. (2000). *The relaxation response*. New York: Harper Collins.

Berjot, S. & Gillet, N. (2011). Stress and coping with discrimination and stigmatization. *Frontiers in Psychology*, *2*, 33. https://doi.org/10.3389/fpsyg.2011.00033

Bernard, C. (1974). *Lectures on the phenomena common to animals and plants* (Hoff, H. E., Guillemin, R,, & Guillemin, L., Trans.) Springfield (IL): Charles C Thomas.

Bey, G., Ulbricht, C. M., & Person, S. D. (2019). Theories for race and gender differences in management of social identity-related stressors: A systematic review. *Journal of Racial and Ethnic Health Disparities*, *6*(1), 117–132. https://doi.org/10.1007/s40615-018-0507-9

Bey, G. (2022). The Identity Vitality-Pathology model: A novel theoretical framework proposing "identity state" as a modulator of the pathways from structural to health inequity. *Social Science & Medicine*, *314*, 115495. https://doi.org/10.1016/j.socscimed.2022.115495

Boehm, J. K., & Kubzansky, L. D. (2012). The heart's content: The association between positive psychological well-being and cardiovascular health. *Psychological Bulletin*, *138*(4), 655.

Borgi, M., Collacchi, B., Ortona, E., & Cirulli, F. (2020). Stress and coping in women with breast cancer: Unravelling the mechanisms to improve resilience. *Neuroscience & Biobehavioral Reviews*, *119*, 406–421.

Brannon, L. & Feist, J. (2004). *Health psychology: An introduction to behavior and health* (5th ed.). San Francisco, CA: Thomas/Wadsworth.

Broerman, R. (2017). Diathesis-stress model. In V. Zeigler-Hill & T. K. Shackelford (Eds.), *Encyclopedia of personality and individual differences* (pp. 1–3). Springer International Publishing. https://doi.org/10.1007/978-3-319-28099-8_891-1

Bronfenbrenner, U., & Ceci, S. J. (1994). Nature-nurture reconceptualized in developmental perspective: A bioecological model. *Psychological Review*, *101*(4), 568–586. https://doi.org/10.1037/0033-295X.101.4.568

Brown, A. F., Ma, G. X., Miranda, J., Eng, E., Castille, D., Brockie, T., Jones, P., Airhihenbuwa, C. O., Farhat, T., Zhu, L., & Trinh-Shevrin, C. (2019). Structural interventions to reduce and eliminate health disparities. *American Journal of Public Health*, *109*(S1), S72–S78. https://doi.org/10.2105/AJPH.2018.304844

Cannon, W. B (1941). The body physiologic and the body politic. *Science*, *93*(2401), 1–10.

Carter-Pokras, O., & Baquet, C., & Carter-Pokras, O. (2002). What is a "health disparity?". *Public Health Reports*, *17*(5), 426–434. https://doi.org/10.1093/phr/117.5.426

Centers for Disease Control and Prevention. (2019). Mental health in the workplace. https://www.cdc.gov/workplacehealthpromotion/tools-resources/workplace-health/mental-health/index.html

Clark, R., Anderson, N. B., Clark, V. R., & Williams, D. R. (1999). Racism as a stressor for African Americans. A biopsychosocial model. *The American Psychologist*, *54*(10), 805–816. https://doi.org/10.1037//0003-066x.54.10.805

Crocker, J., & Knight, K. M. (2005). Contingencies of self-worth. *Current Directions in Psychological Science*, *14*(4), 200–203. https://doi.org/10.1111/j.0963-7214.2005.00364.x

Cross Jr., W. E., & Vandiver, B. J. (2001). Nigrescence theory and measurement: Introducing the Cross Racial Identity Scale (CRIS). In J. M. Casas, L. A. Suzuki, C. M. Alexander, & M. A. Jackson (Eds.), *Handbook of multicultural counseling* (2nd ed., pp. 371–393). Sage Publications.

Dhabhar F. S. (2014). Effects of stress on immune function: The good, the bad, and the beautiful. *Immunologic Research*, *58*(2–3), 193–210. https://doi.org/10.1007/s12026-014-8517-0

Dohrenwend, B. S., & Dohrenwend, B. P. (1974). *Stressful life events: Their nature and effects*. Oxford, England: Wiley.

Epel, E. S. (2009). Psychological and metabolic stress: A recipe for accelerated cellular aging?*Hormones (Athens, Greece)*, *8*(1), 7–22. https://doi.org/10.14310/horm.2002.1217

Epel, E. S., & Lithgow, G. J. (2014). Stress biology and aging mechanisms: toward understanding the deep connection between adaptation to stress and longevity. *The journals of gerontology. Series A, Biological sciences and medical sciences*, *69 Suppl 1* (Suppl 1), S10–S16. https://doi.org/10.1093/gerona/glu055

Felix, A. S., Nolan, T. S., Glover, L. M., Sims, M., Addison, D., Smith, S. A., Anderson, C. M., Warren, B. J., Woods-Giscombe, C., Hood, D. B., & Williams, K. P. (2022). The modifying role of resilience on allostatic load and cardiovascular disease risk in the Jackson Heart Study. *Journal of Racial and Ethnic Health Disparities.* https://doi.org/10.1007/s40615-022-01392-6. Advance online publication. https://doi.org/10.1007/s40615-022-01392-6

Folkman, S., & Lazarus, R. S. (1988). *The ways of coping questionnaire*. Palo Alto, California: Consulting Psychologists Press.

DeLongis, A. (1986). Appraisal, coping, health status, and psychological symptoms. *Journal of Personality and Social Psychology*, *50*(3), 571–579. https://doi-org.libproxy.lib.unc.edu/10.1037/0022-3514.50.3.571

Fredrickson, B. L. (1998). What good are positive emotions? *Review of General Psychology*, *2*, 300–319.

Fredrickson, B. L. (2003). The value of positive emotions. *American Scientist*, *91*(4), 330–335. https://doi.org/10.1511/2003.26.865

Fredrickson, B. L. (2004). The broaden-and-build theory of positive emotions. *Philosophical Transactions of the Royal Society, B: Biological Sciences*, *359*(1449), 1367–1378. https://doi.org/10.1098/rstb.2004.1512

Geronimus, A. T. (2001). Understanding and eliminating racial inequalities in women's health in the United States: The role of the weathering conceptual framework. *Journal of the American Medical Women's Association*, *56*(4), 133–150.

Geronimus, A. T., Bound, J., Waidmann, T. A., Rodriguez, J. M., & Timpe, B. (2019). Weathering, drugs, and whack-a-mole: Fundamental and proximate causes of widening educational inequity in U.S. life expectancy by sex and race, 1990-2015. *Journal of Health and Social Behavior*, *60*(2), 222–239. https://doi.org/10.1177/0022146519849932

Giscombé, C. L., & Lobel, M. (2005). Explaining disproportionately high rates of adverse birth outcomes among African Americans: The impact of stress, racism, and related factors in pregnancy. *Psychological Bulletin*, *131*(5), 662–683. https://doi.org/10.1037/0033-2909.131.5.662

Giurgescu, C., Zenk, S. N., Templin, T. N., Engeland, C. G., Dancy, B. L., Park, C. G., Kavanaugh, K., Dieber, W., & Misra, D. P. (2015). The impact of neighborhood environment, social support, and avoidance coping on depressive symptoms of pregnant African-American women. *Women's Health Issues*, *25*(3), 294–302. https://doi.org/10.1016/j.whi.2015.02.001

Holmes, F. L. (1986). Claude Bernard, the milieu intérieur, and regulatory physiology. *History and Philosophy of the Life Sciences*, *8*(1), 3–25.

Holmes, T. H., & Rahe, R. H. (1967). The social readjustment rating scale. *Journal of Psychosomatic Research*, *11*, 213–218.

Jacobs, G. D. (2001). The physiology of mind-body interactions: The stress response and the relaxation response. *Journal of Alternative and Complementary Medicine*, *7*(Suppl. 1), S83–S92. https://doi.org/10.1089/107555301753393841 [Published correction appears in *Journal of Alternative and Complementary Medicine 8*(2), 219.]

James, S. A. (1994). John Henryism and the health of African-Americans. *Culture, Medicine and Psychiatry*, *18*, 163–182.

Kabat-Zinn, J. (2005). *Full catastrophe living: Using the wisdom of your body and mind to face stress, pain, and illness*. New York: Random House.

Kahana, E., Bhatta, T. R., Kahana, B., & Lekhak, N. (2021). Loving others: The impact of compassionate love on later-life psychological well-being. *The Journals of Gerontology: Series B*, *76*(2), 391–402.

Kaufman, E. A., & Crowell, S. E. (2018). Biological and behavioral mechanisms of identity pathology development: An integrative review. *Review of General Psychology*, 22(3), 245–263.

Kiecolt-Glaser, J. K., McGuire, L., Robles, T. F., & Glaser, R. (2002). Psychoneuroimmunology: Psychological influences on immune function and health. *Journal of Consulting and Clinical Psychology*, 70(3), 537–547. https://doi.org/10.1037//0022-006x.70.3.537

Kivimäki, M., & Steptoe, A. (2018). Effects of stress on the development and progression of cardiovascular disease. *Nature Reviews Cardiology*, 15(4), 215–229. https://doi.org/10.1038/nrcardio.2017.189

Laubmeier, K. K., Zakowski, S. G., & Bair, J. P. (2004). The role of spirituality in the psychological adjustment to cancer: A test of the transactional model of stress and coping. *International Journal of Behavioral Medicine*, 11, 48–55. https://doi.org/10.1207/s15327558ijbm1101_6

Lazarus, R. S., & Folkman, S. (1984). *Stress, appraisal, and coping*. New York, NY: Springer.

Lazarus, R. S., & Folkman, S. (1987). Transactional theory and research on emotions and coping. *European Journal of Personality*, 1, 141–169.

Lee, S. Y., Park, C. L., & Pescatello, L. S. (2020). How trauma influences cardiovascular responses to stress: Contributions of post-traumatic stress and cognitive appraisals. *Journal of Behavioral Medicine*, 43(1), 131–142.

Levi, L. (1974). Psychosocial stress and disease. A conceptual model. In E. K. E. Gunderson & R. H. Rahe (Eds.), *Life stress and illness* (pp. 8–33). Springfield, IL: Thomas.

Marsland, A. L., Walsh, C., Lockwood, K., & John-Henderson, N. A. (2017). The effects of acute psychological stress on circulating and stimulated inflammatory markers: A systematic review and meta-analysis. *Brain, Behavior, and Immunity*, 64, 208–219. https://doi.org/10.1016/j.bbi.2017.01.011

Mattis, J. S. (2002). Religion and spirituality in the meaning making and coping experiences of African American women: A qualitative analysis. *Psychology of Women Quarterly*, 26, 308–320. https://doi.org/10.1111/1471-6402.t01-2-00070

McEwen, B. S. (2007). Physiology and neurobiology of stress and adaptation: Central role of the brain. *Physiological Reviews*, 87(3), 873–904. https://doi.org/10.1152/physrev.00041.2006

McEwen, B. S. (2017). Neurobiological and systemic effects of chronic stress. *Chronic Stress*, 1, 2470547017692328. https://doi.org/10.1177/2470547017692328

Miller-Graff, L. E., & Campion, K. (2016). Interventions for posttraumatic stress with children exposed to violence: Factors associated with treatment success. *Journal of Clinical Psychology*, 72(3), 226–248.

Myers, L. J., Speight, S. L., Highlen, P. S., Cox, C. I., Reynolds, A. L., Adams, E. M., & Hanley, C. P. (1991). Identity development and worldview: Toward an optimal conceptualization. *Journal of Counseling & Development*, 70(1), 54–63. https://doi.org/10.1002/j.1556-6676.1991.tb01561.x

National Institutes of Health. (2015). Racial and ethnic categories and definitions for NIH diversity programs and for other reporting purposes. https://grants.nih.gov/grants/guide/notice-files/NOT-OD-15-089.html

National Institute of Occupational Safety and Health. (2014). Stress management in work settings. https://www.cdc.gov/niosh/docs/87-111/87-111.pdf?id=10.26616/NIOSHPUB87111

Petrie, K. J., Booth, R. J., & Pennebaker, J. W. (1998). The immunological effects of thought suppression. *Journal of Personality and Social Psychology*, 75, 1264–1272.

Robinson, M. N., & Thomas Tobin, C. S. (2021). Is John Henryism a health risk or resource?: Exploring the role of culturally relevant coping for physical and mental health among Black Americans. *Journal of Health and Social Behavior*, 62(2), 136–151. https://doi.org/10.1177/00221465211009142

Sanguanklin, N., McFarlin, B. L., Finnegan, L., Park, C. G., Giurgescu, C., White-Traut, R., & Engstrom, J. L. (2014). Job strain and psychological distress among employed pregnant Thai women: Role of social support and coping strategies. *Archives of Women's Mental Health*, 17(4), 317–326. https://doi.org/10.1007/s00737-013-0410-7

Seeman, T. E., Singer, B. H., Ryff, C. D., Love, G. D., & Levy-Storms, L. (2002). Social relationships, gender, and allostatic load across two age cohorts. *Psychosomatic Medicine*, 64, 395–406.

Seligman, M. E., & Csikszentmihalyi, M. (2000). Positive psychology. An introduction. *American Psychology*, 55(1), 5–14. https://doi.org/10.1037//0003-066x.55.1.5

Selye, H. (1950). Stress and the general adaptation syndrome. *British Medical Journal*, 1(4667), 1383–1392. https://doi.org/10.1136/bmj.1.4667.1383

Selye, H. (1956). *The stress of life*. New York: McGraw-Hill.

Sheffield-Abdullah, K. A., & Woods-Giscombe, C. L. (2021). Perceptions of the superwoman role and distress among African American women with pre-diabetes). *Archives of Psychiatric Nursing* – Social Determinants of Health Special Issue, *35*(1), 88–93. doi:10.1016/j.apnu.2020.09.011

Simons, R. L., Lei, M. K., Klopack, E., Zhang, Y., Gibbons, F. X., & Beach, S. (2021). Racial discrimination, inflammation, and chronic illness among African American women at midlife: Support for the weathering perspective. *Journal of Racial and Ethnic Health Disparities, 8*(2), 339–349. https://doi.org/10.1007/s40615-020-00786-8

Steptoe, A., & Kivimäki, M. (2012). Stress and cardiovascular disease. *Nature Reviews Cardiology, 9*(6), 360–370. https://doi.org/10.1038/nrcardio.2012.45

Straub, R. H., & Cutolo, M. (2018). Psychoneuroimmunology-developments in stress research. *Wien Med Wochenschr, 168*, 76–84. doi: 10.1007/s10354-017-0574-2

Taylor, M. G., & Carr, D. (2021). Psychological resilience and health among older adults: A comparison of personal resources. *The Journals of Gerontology: Series B, 76*(6), 1241–1250.

The American Institute of Stress. (n.d.). Workplace stress. https://www.stress.org/workplace-stress

United States Department of Labor, Bureau of Labor Statistics (2018). Databases, tables & calculators by subject website. Labor force statistics from the current population Survey. https://data.bls.gov/timeseries/LNS11300000external icon

Utsey, S. O. (1999). Development and validation of a short form of the index of race-related stress (IRRS): Brief version. *Measuring and Evaluation in Counseling and Development, 32*, 149–167.

Van Cappellen, P., Toth-Gauthier, M., Saroglou, V., & Fredrickson, B. L. (2016). Religion and well-being: The mediating role of positive emotions. *Journal of Happiness Studies, 17*, 485–505. https://doi.org/10.1007/s10902-014-9605-5

Wallace, R. K., Benson, H., & Wilson, A. F. (1971). A wakeful hypometabolic physiologic state. *American Journal of Physiology, 221*(3), 795–799.

Wethington, E., Glanz, K., & Schwartz, M. D. (2015). Stress, coping, and health behavior. In K. Glanz, B. K. Rimer, & K. V. Viswanath (Eds.), *Health behavior: Theory, research, and practice* (5th ed., pp. 223–242). Jossey-Bass/Wiley.

Woods-Giscombé, C. L. (2010). Superwoman schema: African American women's views on stress, strength, and health. *Qualitative Health Research, 20*(5), 668–683. https://doi.org/10.1177/1049732310361892

Woods-Giscombé, C. L., Allen, A. M., Black, A. R., Steed, T. C., Li, Y., & Lackey, C. (2019a). The Giscombe Superwoman Schema Questionnaire: Psychometric properties and associations with mental health and health behaviors in African American women. *Issues in Mental Health Nursing, 40*(8), 672–681. https://doi.org/10.1080/01612840.2019.1584654

Woods-Giscombé, C. L., & Gaylord, S. A. (2014). The cultural relevance of mindfulness meditation as a health intervention for African Americans: Implications for reducing stress-related health disparities. *Journal of Holistic Nursing, 32*(3), 147–160. https://doi.org/10.1177/0898010113519010

Woods-Giscombe, C. L., & Gaylord, S.A. (2022). The HARMONY Study: A culturally-relevant, randomized-controlled, stress management intervention to reduce cardiometabolic risk in African American women. ClinicalTrials.gov identifier: NCT04705779. Updated April 1, 2021. https://clinicaltrials.gov/ct2/show/NCT04705779

Woods-Giscombe, C. L., Gaylord, S. A., Li, Y., Brintz, C. E., Bangdiwala, S. I., Buse, J. B., Mann, J. D., Lynch, C., Phillips, P., Smith, S., Leniek, K., Young, L., Al-Barwani, S., Yoo, J., & Faurot, K. (2019b). A mixed-methods, randomized clinical trial to examine feasibility of a mindfulness-based stress management and diabetes risk reduction intervention for African Americans with prediabetes. *Evidence-based Complementary and Alternative Medicine: Ecam, 2019*, 3962623. https://doi.org/10.1155/2019/3962623

Woods-Giscombe, C.L., & Lobel, M. (2005). Explaining disproportionately high rates of adverse birth outcomes among African Americans: the impact of stress, racism, and related factors in pregnancy. *Psychol Bulletin, 131*, 662–683. doi: 10.1037/0033-2909.131.5.662

Woods-Giscombé, C. L., & Lobel, M. (2008). Race and gender matter: A multidimensional approach to conceptualizing and measuring stress in African American women. *Cultural Diversity & Ethnic Minority Psychology, 14*(3), 173–182. https://doi.org/10.1037/1099-9809.14.3.173

Zhang, D., Lee, E., Mak, E., Ho, C. Y., & Wong, S. (2021). Mindfulness-based interventions: An overall review. *British Medical Bulletin, 138*(1), 41–57. https://doi.org/10.1093/bmb/ldab005

PART FOUR

COMMUNITY AND GROUP MODELS OF HEALTH BEHAVIOR CHANGE

CHAPTER 13

INTRODUCTION TO COMMUNITY AND GROUP MODELS OF HEALTH BEHAVIOR CHANGE

Karen Glanz
Tamara J. Cadet

An understanding of the functioning of groups, organizations, large social institutions, and communities and how they interact with each other is vital to health enhancement. Designing health behavior and policy, systems and environmental (PSE) change initiatives to benefit communities and populations is at the heart of a public health orientation (Bunnell et al., 2012; Glanz & Bishop, 2010; US Department of Health and Human Services, 2016). The collective well-being of communities can be fostered by creating, modifying, or dismantling structures and policies that support or deter healthy lifestyles. These strategies require an understanding of how social systems operate, how change occurs within and among communities and organizations, and how ideas and information spread, including through the Internet and social media.

The chapters in Part Four present theoretically informed approaches to create and support health behavior change through groups, organizations, communities, and social systems. The aims of these chapters are: (1) to demonstrate the utility and promise of a variety of theories and frameworks in health behavior and health behavior change, and (2) to identify important ways to understand and address populations using theoretically grounded models.

In Chapter 14, Bailey builds the case for improving the effectiveness of health behavior theories by proactively integrating concepts of social justice, racism, and health equity. She proposes that integrating racism-related theories and constructs with health behavior models may contribute to more antiracist public health interventions.

In Chapter 15, Keawe Kaholokula and colleagues provide an up-to-date overview of principles and methods of community engagement for health improvement, including community organization and community building, coalitions and partnerships, and community-based participatory research (CBPR). They discuss the concept of community, and the main theoretical and conceptual bases of community engagement, processes, and models for community organization and building for health. They also discuss measurement and evaluation issues and describe a case study that illustrates how community engagement was applied in the Pasifika Prediabetes Youth Empowerment Program (PPYEP) in New Zealand.

In Chapter 16, Ramanadan and Shelton address implementation, dissemination, and diffusion of public health interventions as an approach to enhancing longer-term impact of community and group interventions. They focus on the importance of, the conceptualization of, and strategies for, implementation and dissemination of evidence-based interventions (EBIs) to improve health. Using two widely used models as exemplars, the Diffusion of Innovations and the Consolidated Framework for Implementation Research (CFIR), the chapter provides key terminology in a rapidly evolving area of inquiry and practice—in detail. The chapter includes applications of these models and illustrates components that cut across individual, organizational, and societal levels of context, analysis, and intervention.

In Chapter 17, Gollust and Nagler focus on communication and health behavior in a rapidly changing media environment. In addition to describing longstanding theories, their chapter characterizes emerging issues related to how people receive and use public information and its implications for health communication and health behavior. They illustrate these concepts and issues with two applications: Partisan views regarding COVID-19 vaccines, including the news media's potential to widen health disparities, and the use of tobacco imagery in popular entertainment in India to illustrate the competition that exists for audience attention while considering planned and unplanned approaches to communication for health.

Perspectives on Community, Group, and Organizational Interventions

The central theme of Part Four is that we must understand, predict, and know how to influence the social systems and structures that provide the context for health behaviors. We need models that help those who facilitate or lead change efforts and/or study them to be more effective in their efforts to create healthier institutions and communities. A focus on integrating communities and the importance of their voice, values, and views is central to understanding the interplay between behavior and health. Change within and among systems, organizational processes, and communication channels are apparent across each of the chapters, as are changes in political and information environments. We emphasize implementation of EBIs, scaling up and dissemination to maximize impact while preventing/reducing health disparities and increasing health equity.

Each chapter in this section of the book addresses a broad perspective, approach, or type of strategy—rather than a single theory. The chapters then describe, synthesize, and apply key theories, frameworks, and models that have been found useful for addressing the core issues of the chapter. It is notable that the theories and models focus attention on interpersonal, community/organizational, and policy/environment levels of action, as well as the individual level, as applicable.

Chapters in this section bring together longstanding approaches with new concepts and strategies to understand health behaviors and facilitate positive changes. In Chapter 14, Bailey discusses the differences and impact of race and racism providing a historical context noting that race is a social construct and a symbol or marker of processes of racism, an organized social system where a dominant racial group uses its power to devalue, disempower and differentially allocate societal resources and opportunities to groups they identify as inferior. The difference is important to consider as Bailey suggests that a focus on individual or interpersonal experiences of racism invalidates the broader impact of structural racism that may be captured in existing health behavior models.

In Chapter 15, Keawe'aimoku Kaholokula and co-authors refocus the ideas of models of community organization and community building under the umbrella of *community engagement*. These newer models emphasize community engagement as a health equity strategy that includes both community-based and community-driven principles and actions. The focus is on longer-term community assets and capacity building rather than being solely problem-driven. While this is not a new concept (Minkler, 2000), it is updated in a broader context in this chapter.

Keawe'aimoku Kaholokula and co-authors define community capacity, empowerment and critical consciousness, participation and relevance, and health equity under the umbrella of discussing what is a community, and describe how consideration of each of these principles alone or in combination are strategies to address multiple health-related concerns. Chapter 15 also provides a detailed discussion of CBPR and the need to consider research and measurement issues to test CBPR. Chapter 16 by Ramanadhan and Shelton analyzes major concepts within implementation, dissemination and diffusion of public health innovations, and the critical importance of bridging the gap between health promotion research, policy, and practice. The chapter describes how to understand what an EBI is and the importance of blending individual, organizational, and system change. The authors examine the main types of dissemination and implementation frameworks to understand how innovations can be spread and to simultaneously promote dissemination and implementation of EBIs.

In Chapter 17, Gollust and Nagler discuss both planned and unplanned approaches to communication as we conceptualize audiences and media effects. They consider both the individual-level communication effects along with societal-level communication effects to explore how the public information environment (framing, narratives, agenda setting, and priming) shapes the public's attitudes, beliefs, and consequently their health-related behaviors. These features cut across a range of considerations about mass media: its application in social action and advocacy; and communication regarding health risks, especially those risks with broad public health implications.

Because each chapter in this section draws on multiple theoretical traditions that contribute to important areas of health behavior and health education, rather than presenting single or unified theories, there is much for readers to digest in each chapter. This synthesis focuses on similarities among the models, draws common themes, and critiques their usefulness for research and practice in health behavior and public health.

Multiple Levels of Influence and Action

A central premise of this book is that improvements in health require both understanding the multilevel determinants of health behavior and a range of change strategies at the individual, interpersonal, and macro levels. The view that societal-level changes and supportive environments are necessary to address major health problems successfully *and* to maintain individual-level behavior change is now widely endorsed (Glanz & Bishop, 2010; Paskett et al., 2016). The chapters in this section clearly exemplify a multilevel perspective, which builds on intrapersonal and interpersonal theories to explain and/or affect community change.

The applications described in the four chapters in this section each illustrate how multiple levels of influence interact and require attention to improve conditions and health. In Chapter 14, Bailey explains the challenging concepts of structural systems of inequity, most notably racism, and introduces readers to Ecosocial Theory, Critical Race Theory, and Public Health Critical Race Praxis. She illustrates how applications of these ideas are compatible with the Social Ecological Model and Integrative Behavioral Model, and can be blended to address social justice issues. The example of the PPYEP in Chapter 15 begins with academic partners engaging a Pasifika community member who helped to recruit 41 Pasifika youth to participate in the program to develop the health knowledge and skillsets of the youth to reduce prediabetes risk in the Pasifika adult community. This empowerment program was co-designed with the youth who subsequently implemented an eight-week community-based intervention.

In Chapter 16, the example of the Pool Cool skin cancer prevention dissemination trial illustrates how enhanced strategies for implementation/dissemination can simultaneously target individuals, organizations, and environments (Glanz et al., 2015) and the example of the VA Diabetes Prevention Program illustrates the need for context using CFIR along with implementation strategies can support EBI implementation. In Chapter 17, authors illustrate how the role of information processing theories can shape responses to COVID-19 vaccination messaging and how the role of modeling (positive portrayals of tobacco use) and normative influences (frequent tobacco portrayals) can shape responses to tobacco use among youth in India.

An important message at the heart of these chapters is that the broader, community-, or organization-level models and concepts are not intended to stand alone at the expense of neglecting the individuals who comprise groups, organizations, and communities (Kegler & Glanz, 2008). Important concepts and issues related to health equity are integrated into Chapter 15 in relation to the concepts and principles of community engagement and in Chapter 16 with respect to innovations being "designed for dissemination," which can accelerate successful uptake and promote health equity (Kwan et al., 2022). While macro-level theories are invaluable for understanding the complex environments in which behavior takes place, creating change in these environments still often requires identifying and targeting individual change agents, such as local stakeholders that include target audiences including youth, news gatekeepers, or politicians. In other words, understanding individual behavior will remain integral, especially because proximal behavior targeted is health and requires multiple levels of influence to impact health. While it is collectives of *individuals* who create organizational structures, provide leadership in communities, and choose to engage—or not engage—in community efforts to make decisions about local, state, and federal priorities, it is premature to assume that policy development, social action, and environmental change are sufficient for behavior change across various health topics and populations. The history of tobacco control policies illustrates how important policies and laws can be while underscoring that clinical and individual-level strategies operated synergistically with policies to achieve major reductions in combustible tobacco use (Warner, 2014).

Adoption of Models from Outside the Health Field

In each of these four chapters, the history of various frameworks and models did not emerge within the field of health, medicine, or public health. Concepts and principles of race and social justice have strong roots in sociology. Community engagement and community organization concepts and principles started with social work (Chapter 15). Implementation, dissemination, and diffusion of innovations grew from efforts to spread the use of hybrid seed corn in Iowa—work originally done by rural sociologists working in the field of agriculture. (Chapter 16). The core concepts described in the communications and media come from psychology, social psychology, and sociology (Chapter 17).

The adaptation of these models to address health behavior has brought challenges in measurement and research design. Kaholokula and colleagues point to important issues in the development of measures of process and outcomes for community engagement and CBPR, acknowledging the need for conceptual clarity to measure the goals most valued by a community and/or partner. The CFIR, a framework meant to unify key constructs from many implementation science frameworks, is relatively new in terms of developing measures to assess its core constructs and domains though the literature using CFIR is growing rapidly (Chapter 16).

Research designs to test active strategies for promoting social justice, community engagement, implementation and dissemination, and media communications present shared challenges. First, the foundations for such intervention strategies are usually complex, and when they embrace multiple levels (individual, interpersonal, and group/organization/community), they present challenges for conducting rigorous research and evaluation. However, as illustrated in Chapter 16, there have been cluster-randomized controlled trials of efficacious intervention strategies conducted at churches, medical centers, and swimming pools. Trials of mass media communication have randomized media markets. But, it is not always feasible (e.g., due to the cost of such research) to undertake such ambitious research—leaving practitioners and researchers challenged with optimizing the assessment of process indicators and intermediate outcomes. No doubt, there will continue to be debates about whether it is necessary to assess individual behavior or health outcomes in large, multiorganization and/or multicommunity interventions; or whether endpoints of adoption and implementation of EBIs are sufficient to conclude that positive impacts have occurred.

Future Directions

While all four chapters in this section describe trends and the emergence of new research and public health concerns, none makes these points in a more emphatic and dramatic manner than the chapter on Communication and Media Effects on Health Behavior (Chapter 16). The multiplication of communication platforms, increased grassroots participation, the pace of change, and the persistence of communication inequalities are daunting for public health experts and health behavior researchers. Since the last edition of this book was written, the impact of COVID-19 has highlighted issues relevant to each of these chapters: social justice; community engagement, dissemination, and implementation; and the role of communication and the media underscores each of the other chapters. The influence of health disparities and inequities along with politics have influenced community engagement, EBIs, and dissemination and implementation efforts regarding the risk of COVID-19. This example of the complexity of communication about health foreshadows challenges that health behavior experts will confront.

An understanding of theory, research, and practice in communities, systems, and organizations will be increasingly critical to wide improvement of health in the future. This part of *Health Behavior: Theory, Research, and Practice* provides a diverse set of frameworks and applications for consideration of both researchers and practitioners. Readers should invest time and energy in digesting the complexity of these issues, models, and frameworks.

References

Bunnell, R., O'Neil, D., Soler, R., Payne, R., Giles, W. H., Collins, J., Bauer, U., & Communities Putting Prevention to Work Program Group. (2012). Fifty communities putting prevention to work: Accelerating chronic disease prevention through policy, systems and environmental change. *Journal of Community Health*, *37*, 1081–1090.

Glanz, K., & Bishop, D. (2010). The role of behavioral science theory in development and implementation of public health interventions. *Annual Review of Public Health*, *31*, 399–418.

Glanz, K., Escoffery, C., Elliott, T., & Nehl, E. (2015). Randomized trial of two dissemination strategies for a skin cancer prevention program in aquatic settings. *American Journal of Public Health*, *105*, 1415–1423.

Kegler, M., & Glanz, K. (2008). Perspectives on group, organization and community interventions. In K. Glanz, B. K. Rimer, and K. Viswanath (Eds.), *Health behavior and health education: Theory, research and practice* (4th ed. pp. 389–403). San Francisco, C.A.: Jossey-Bass.

Kwan, B. M., Brownson, R. C., Glasgow, R. E., Morrato, E. H., & Luke, D. A. (2022). Designing for dissemination and sustainability to promote equitable impacts on health. *Annual Review of Public Health*, *43*, 331–353. https://doi.org/10.1146/annurev-publhealth-052220-112457

Minkler, M. (2000). Using participatory action research to build healthy communities. *Public Health Reports*, *115*, 191–197.

Paskett, E., Thompson, B., Ammerman, A. S., Ortega, A. N., Marsteller, J., & Richardson, D. (2016). Multilevel interventions to address health disparities show promise in improving population health. *Health Affairs*, *35*(8), 1429–1434.

US Department of Health and Human Services. (2016). *Public Health 3.0: a call to action to create a 21st century public health infrastructure*. Washington, DC: US Department of Health and Human Services.

Warner, K. E. (2014). Tobacco control policies and their impacts: past, present, and future. *Annals of the American Thoracic Society*, *11*(2), 227–230.

CHAPTER 14

RACE, HEALTH, AND EQUITY
Integrating Concepts of Social Justice Into Health Behavior Models

Zinzi Bailey

KEY POINTS

- The most often used models of health behavior change seldom explicate or integrate theories about structural systems of injustice, especially racism.

- In interventions focused on health equity, individual and interpersonal health behavior change models can and should be considered in combination with multilevel and structural theories.

- Integrating racism-related theories and constructs with health behavior models may contribute to more antiracist public health interventions. More work is needed to build evidence of how and whether these improve intervention effectiveness.

Vignette: The COVID-19 Pandemic as a Wake-Up Call to Racial/Ethnic Health Inequities

Edna is a 72-year-old Black woman with mobility issues who shares a home with her daughter—an essential worker with a history of severe asthma, kidney disease, and hypertension—and her school-aged granddaughter. On March 11, 2020, the World Health Organization declared COVID-19 a global pandemic, and Edna and her family needed to take action. She tried to keep up with often changing public health advice. When vaccines became available in her city, Edna struggled to find a way to get vaccinated. Because she lived in a racially segregated neighborhood, vaccines were not readily available, and she did not have fast enough Internet service to secure one of the elusive appointments only available online. Her friends and neighbors were in a similar boat. Because Edna was not eligible for vaccination for another few months, she is at high risk herself and confers that risk to her intergenerational household—contracting COVID-19 before she could get vaccinated. Meanwhile, a week into the vaccination rollout, an exclusive, predominantly white, affluent neighborhood nearby had already reached a 40% vaccination rate. Edna's relative disadvantage due to her age, connectivity challenges, and health concerns is exacerbated by racial inequities. By not using a racial equity lens, the initial public health COVID-19 vaccine rollout defaulted to pre-existing inequities, with an impact on people like Edna and her family. In the process, inequities have increased.

In the United States, the COVID-19 pandemic not only shined a light on the glaring inadequacies of our public health and healthcare systems but also laid bare the pre-existing structural inequities that create very different living conditions and constraints across groups of different racial and ethnic, socioeconomic and geographic circumstances. Throughout the pandemic, American Indian and Alaska Native, Black, and Hispanic/Latinx people experienced disproportionately high incidence and mortality from COVID-19 (Ndugga & Artiga, 2021). The uneven spread of COVID-19, delayed and fragmented public health response, and broader social unrest triggered by the murder of George Floyd called attention to the role of

Health Behavior: Theory, Research, and Practice, Sixth Edition. Edited by Karen Glanz, Barbara K. Rimer, and K. Viswanath.
© 2024 John Wiley & Sons, Inc. Published 2024 by John Wiley & Sons, Inc.
Companion website: www.wiley.com/go/glanz/healthbehavior6e

upstream historical and contemporary racism on downstream effects, such as inequities in COVID-19's impact and chronic disease inequities. Not only does racism contribute to Black, Indigenous, and other people of color (often referred to as BIPOC) living in racially and economically segregated communities with substandard or crowded housing conditions, unsafe or limited water, and unhealthy air, but it also affects patterns of access to routine and urgent healthcare, health insurance, and chronic and infectious disease development and progression.

Prominent individual and interpersonal health behavior models are helpful for designing interventions that target the structural vulnerability of historically marginalized communities of color. However, to achieve health equity, interventions to improve the health-related behaviors and outcomes that contribute to structural vulnerability in marginalized communities of color should also incorporate constructs from theories that explicitly address race, racism, and structural inequity.

Rather than highlighting structural vulnerabilities faced by marginalized communities of color, many public health professionals—especially at the beginning of the COVID-19 pandemic—focused on reducing disproportionate risks conferred by individual-level health conditions or behaviors. For instance, obesity was hypothesized as a driver of racial/ethnic disparities, and some experts emphasized programs promoting healthy eating and physical activity (Coleman et al., 2022), without acknowledging the role of eating and activity behaviors constrained by social disadvantage (Dover & Lambert, 2016; Venn & Strazdins, 2017). Consequently, as with other health behaviors and outcomes, behavior change is often prioritized for historically marginalized racial and ethnic groups as populations identified for interventions, without analyzing social determinants of their behaviors. Without carefully considering the larger social, economic, and political policies, systems and environments, interventions can be ineffective or even widen the gaps in chronic and infectious disease rates.

Social Ecological models (SEMs) are increasingly being used to account for social, economic, and political environments (Chapter 3), but with insufficient attention to the theoretical foundations underpinning how one analyzes racial/ethnic inequities, and how interventions can operate on macro levels, including policies, regulations, and systemic transformation. It can be helpful to be more explicit in tapping into the multiple systemic levels of the SEM when trying to target factors that generate and sustain health disparities in disease management and outcomes. One example of a framework that approaches the widespread issue of obesity this way is Shiriki Kumanyika's Framework for Increasing Equity Impact in Obesity Prevention. This framework, which draws on the SEM (Chapter 3) and community participatory frameworks (Chapter 15) directs attention to policy, systems, and environmental changes for developing obesity-prevention interventions, including addressing structural racism (Kumanyika, 2019). Kumanyika specifically notes that observed disparities in obesity are rooted in adverse social circumstances, part of a deeper problem of systemic and structural dynamics. Several health behavior models refer to the social environment, but their applications in intervention design do not necessarily address structural discrimination constraints in the application of those behavior models for health equity. Kumanyika's framework has a strong focus on working with communities to build capacity and empower and partner with communities (Kumanyika, 2019).

This chapter will (1) discuss theoretical foundations that focus on race and racism, and (2) propose ways of integrating racism-focused theory into two key behavior change theories: the SEM and the Integrative Behavior Model.

Race and Racism in Health Behavior: Definitions and Theoretical Foundations

Race and Racism

In public health, health behavior, and health promotion, it is often assumed that there is a common understanding of what race is and is not. For example, health professionals often reference racial and ethnic disparities in health—"preventable differences [by race and ethnicity] in the burden of disease, injury, violence, or opportunities to achieve optimal health that are experienced by socially disadvantaged populations" (Division of Population Health, National Center for Chronic Disease Prevention and Health Promotion, 2017). Across many measures of health status, Black, Hispanic/Latinx, American Indian or Alaska Native, and Native Hawaiian and Other Pacific Islander people fare worse than their white counterparts (Mahajan et al., 2021; Zimmerman & Anderson, 2019). In 2019, Black people in the United States had a life expectancy of four years less than non-Hispanic/Latinx white people, with the lowest life expectancy among Black men. By 2021, during the second year of the COVID-19 pandemic, these disparities had widened;

Black people's life expectancy was 5.6 fewer years than non-Hispanic/Latinx white people (Arias et al., 2022). Similarly, non-Hispanic/Latinx American Indian and Alaska Native people were expected to live seven fewer years than their white counterparts in 2019 and 11.2 fewer years than their white counterparts in 2021 (Arias et al., 2022). However, these numbers do not explain structural factors driving these disparities.

Rooted in sociological theory, concepts of race and racism are inextricably linked (Bonilla-Silva, 1997; Feagin, 2006; Omi & Winant, 1994; Smedley & Smedley, 2005). Fundamentally, race is a social construct whose meaning stems from complex historical and contemporary social ideology, whereby people are categorized by physical appearance, skin color, and (real or perceived) ancestry based on society-specific and time-specific contexts. The conceptualization of race as a social construct developed over time. In the United States, for instance, the concept of race has evolved from the settler-colonial origins of the nation—"othering" by way of genocide and slavery. However, historians contend that the inferior social status that came to be associated with African ancestry was not a given, but "a deliberate choice the English elites came to over time" (Kauanui, 2017; Morgan, 1975; Wolfe, 2016). For instance, in early 17th-century colonial Virginia, many Africans were sold into forced indentured servitude alongside poor European immigrants, bound by specific contracts rather than legalized slavery (Kauanui, 2017; Morgan, 1975; Takaki, 2008). Between 1619 (when the first Africans were forced onto American land) and 1661, Africans lived in Virginia without laws legalizing chattel slavery, and there is historical record of free Africans who owned property (Kauanui, 2017; Takaki, 2008). However, the construction and evolution of racial meaning—racialization—quickly began to be legally and administratively codified to reflect historical social dynamics, including labor organizing and threats of insurrection (e.g., social dynamics leading to Bacon's Rebellion). The 1660s ushered in a period of codification of race-based chattel slavery in Virginia, with a law defining enslaved African people as property (Kauanui, 2017; Takaki, 2008).

Through racialization over time—"the extension of racial meaning to … previously racially unclassified relationship[s], social practice[s], or group[s]," cultural, historical, ideological, geographic, and legal influences—primarily racist influences—have driven the importance ascribed to phenotypic and genetic characteristics (Omi & Winant, 1994). Race derives its meaning through the differentiation of groups rather than any intrinsic, precise measure of characteristics associated with any one group (Gonzalez-Sobrino & Goss, 2019; Omi & Winant, 1994; Smedley & Smedley, 2005). In fact, there are more genetic differences within races (or geographic ancestral groups) than across races (or geographic ancestral groups) (Duello et al., 2021; Sirugo et al., 2021). In short, race is a symbol or marker of processes of racialization and racism. In the words of Ta-Nehisi Coates, "race is the child of racism, not the father" (Coates, 2015). Race and racism have essential implications for the distribution of biological mechanisms, psychosocial mechanisms, health behaviors, and health outcomes. In fact, when racial/ethnic disparities in health are considered, discussions of race must be grounded in society- and time-specific experiences of racism on multiple levels.

Theoretical Foundations of Race and Racism

Much of the theory surrounding race and racism stems from a sociological tradition, including Michael Omi and Howard Winant's racial formation theory (Omi & Winant, 1994), Joe Feagin's systemic racism (Feagin, 2006), and Bonilla-Silva's racialized social systems (Bonilla-Silva, 1997). Racism is not a collection of isolated acts. On the contrary, it is "an organized social system in which the dominant racial group, based on an ideology of inferiority, categorizes and ranks people into social groups called 'races' and uses its power to devalue, disempower, and differentially allocate valued societal resources and opportunities to groups defined as inferior" (Williams et al., 2019).

Eduardo Bonilla-Silva's theory of the racialized social system emphasizes a structural approach to racism that has a historical progression with key starting points and evolutions over time and over different geographies (Bonilla-Silva, 1997; National Academy, 2022). Racism is not static over time and does not operate in the same ways in different places. Most obviously, racism across different racialized societies may operate through different institutions and different material implications across different groups. For example. the so-called "one-drop rule"—the classification of anyone with even one Black ancestor as "Black"—operating in the United States through much of its history can be contrasted with colorism and (unfounded) ideologies of racial democracy that often influence racial hierarchies in Latin American societies, like Brazil and Cuba, where racial identities and conflict have been downplayed in favor of a broader national identity (Burdick, 1992; de la Fuente, 1999; Hickman, 1997; Hollinger, 2005; Peña et al., 2004; Winant, 1999).

However, racism—particularly, the structural components of racism—can occur differently in distinct local contexts. For example, Black-white racism has been experienced strongly across the United States, with Southeastern states legally enforcing the structural racism of Jim Crow (Fredrickson, 2015; Packard, 2003), more operationally similar to South African apartheid (Maylam, 2017), while other states imposed racism in other ways (e.g., restrictive covenants, residential markets) (Jones-Correa, 2000; Rothstein, 2017).

Structural racism can be defined as "the totality of ways in which societies foster racial and ethnic discrimination, via mutually reinforcing inequitable systems [...] that in turn reinforce discriminatory beliefs, values, and distribution of resources," also described as "über discrimination" by Barbara Reskin and as "systemic racism" by Joe Feagin (Bailey et al., 2017; Feagin, 2006; Reskin, 2012). Structural racism reinforces discriminatory beliefs, including—perhaps most destructively on an organizational or systemic level—the normalization and legitimization of adverse outcomes for people of color, resulting in the color-blind enforcement of a racialized social system, even by seemingly "innocent" or "colorblind" actors (Bailey et al., 2017; Bonilla-Silva, 1997). Focusing more narrowly on individual or interpersonal experiences of racism negates the broader impact of structural racism, which constrains and facilitates health behavior.

Ecosocial theory is a health-equity-focused population-level approach that comprehensively assesses the relationship between discrimination and health. First proposed by Nancy Krieger in 1994, the theory describes and explains causal relationships in disease distribution, namely development of health inequities (Krieger, 2012). One of its key concepts is that material and social conditions are embodied biologically to produce inequities in health. This embodiment occurs through key pathways, including economic and social deprivation, exposure to environmental toxins, inadequate healthcare, targeted marketing of harmful substances and practices, and forced migration. Harmful exposures are cumulative, synergistic, and continually interact with individual susceptibility and resistance across the life course and generations. Furthermore, this approach emphasizes the role of accountability and agency, that is, the concept that we can and should act to disrupt inequitable systems (Table 14.1). While potential policy and system changes might be based on these analyses, it is important to note that Ecosocial Theory is not intended as a foundation for intervention development.

Critical Race Theory (CRT) and the associated Public Health Critical Race Praxis (PHCRP) provide foundational theoretical bases for considering race and racism in the study of racial/ethnic inequities. CRT, originally developed in the legal field, primarily by scholars of color, drew attention to the practices and cultures that embed racism in institutions, laws and structures (Bell, 1995; Crenshaw & Gotanda, 1995; Delgado & Stefancic, 2005; Lawrence III, 1995; Matsuda, 2018; Taylor, 1998; Williams, 1991). The PHCRP, drawn from CRT, is focused on answering two main questions: (1) How is racialization relevant to the problem? and (2) How is racialization relevant to the production of knowledge about the problem? (Ford, 2016; Ford and Airhihenbuwa, 2010a).

The PHCRP is based on four focus areas (Table 14.2): contemporary patterns of racial relations, knowledge production, conceptualization and measurement, and action. It also espouses 10 major principles: race consciousness; primacy of racialization; race as a social construct; ordinariness of racism; structural determinism; social construction of knowledge; critical approaches; intersectionality; disciplinary self-critique; and voice (Ford & Airhihenbuwa, 2010a, b) (see Table 14.2). Given the comprehensive nature of the framework, the applications of PHCRP in empirical work vary widely but are most often used to design, analyze, and interpret observational research, and not to design interventions. Two such applications are discussed at the end of the chapter.

Table 14.1 Ecosocial Theory

Main Components of ecosocial theory	Embodiment: how material and social world is incorporated in one's biology.
	Pathways of embodiment: ways in which we incorporate the material and social world influenced by societal arrangements of power and property.
	Cumulative interplay between exposure, susceptibility, and resistance: the multilevel and multidomain nature of each factor in pathways of embodiment.
	Accountability and agency: the recognition of decision-making and choice in the construction of social inequities in health as well as a reflexive practice of scientists to utilize appropriate theoretical foundations of their research.

Table 14.2   Principles of Public Health Critical Race Praxis (PHCRP)

Key Principles	Explanation
Race Consciousness	Awareness of one's racial position and how racial stratification occurs
Primacy of Racialization	Understand that racial stratification is an essential contributor to societal problems
Race as a Social Construct	Racial categories are derived from historical and contemporary social, economic, and political forces
Ordinariness of Racism	Racism is embedded in society's social fabric
Structural Determinism	Tendency for dominant group members and institutions to safeguard existing social stratification, systems, and policies
Social Construction of Knowledge	Idea that the research enterprise is not immune to racism
Critical Approaches	Actively identify and oppose racism to promote racial equity
Intersectionality	Overlap and reinforcement of the systems of stratification and how they experienced by individuals in their multiple, co-occurring identities
Disciplinary Self-Critique	Understanding biases in knowledge production process, including how such knowledge privileges existing power structures
Voice	Prioritize the voices and perspectives of socially marginalized groups

Integrating Racism-Focused Constructs into Health Behavior Models

Health equity-focused theoretical foundations can be incorporated into applications of individual, interpersonal, or community health behavior change models, though this can be challenging. At the extreme, health behavior change models can overemphasize individual level factors, such as self-efficacy, self-control, and intention, while population-level theories can undervalue individual and collective agency. The lack of inclusion of structural constraints perpetuates an inequitable status quo, while a sole focus on structures limits the role of agency. Therefore, the work of achieving health equity should be to integrate theories of structural injustice, namely race, racialization, and racism into traditional health behavior change models. To explore approaches to doing this, this section discusses two widely used health behavior models exploring (1) how social environments can be better integrated into theories and (2) how each model's constructs may be contextualized within racialized social systems.

Social Ecological Model

The SEM (Chapter 3) is one of the most widely used health behavior change models for designing and/or adapting interventions, especially for incorporating social and policy contexts. This model emphasizes a multilevel and interconnected ecological system that affects human development and behavior (Bronfenbrenner, 1979; Bronfenbrenner & Morris, 2007). At the intrapersonal level, each person has unique biological and psychological characteristics that influence behavior. Behavior and behavior change are influenced and constrained by interpersonal, familial, community-level, and societal-level factors.

Considering childhood obesity prevention as an example, numerous obesity researchers have identified factors at the biological, household, social, environmental, and policy levels that interact to explain patterns of childhood overweight/obesity and eating behaviors (Quick et al., 2017; Story et al., 2008). In a review of studies published between 1984 and 2018 on determinants of childhood obesity by SEM level, Pereira and colleagues found that most studies using SEM models to guide research on determinants of childhood obesity focused predominantly on individual and family-level factors. They concluded that "… more evidence is needed about the role of the community, environmental, and policy level determinants," which were included in only between 20% and 40% of studies included in their review (Pereira et al., 2019). The review did not examine interventions.

Thus, a substantial minority of studies on childhood obesity in the review focused on factors at levels higher than the individual level. Furthermore, the SEM does not explicitly incorporate inequitable power dynamics—namely, systems of oppression—into how these levels influence behavior. Systems of oppression are "discriminatory institutions, structures, norms, to name a few, that are embedded in the fabric of our society," including racism, classism, sexism, heterosexism, and ablism (Simon Fraser Public Interest Research Group, 2023). These systems of oppression often constrain behavior and act as barriers to the implementation of behavior change interventions at the individual and population levels. It is likely that the researchers who conducted many of the studies in Pereira's review did not have access to, and thus did not consider, incorporating measures of racism and related power dynamics.

Kumanyika's Framework for Increasing Equity Impact in Obesity Prevention seeks to prioritize equity when pursuing policy, systems, and environmental change (Kumanyika, 2019, 2022). The premise is that disparities related to obesity and other health problems cannot be remedied without attention to underlying inequities. Approaches to address underlying inequities include increasing healthy options, such as health-promoting built environments and retail food stores, reducing deterrents like discrimination and higher costs, improving social and economic resources through legal services and nutrition assistance programs, and building on community capacity through strategic partnerships and behavior change, knowledge, and skills. For instance, in addition to its more individually focused obesity prevention and disease management programs, building on almost a decade of efforts to work with food retailers, in 2012 the New York City Health Department launched the Shop Healthy program to increase access to healthy food in neighborhoods with high levels of obesity and poorer nutritional options, namely disinvested communities of color (Adjoian et al., 2017; Arevalo, 2017; Dannefer et al., 2016; Del Signore Dresser et al., 2023). Over time, there were directed efforts to counteract racialized practices, like targeted corporate marketing of unhealthy food and beverages and distributors' assumptions of unhealthy food consumption in disinvested neighborhoods of color. The Shop Healthy program's approach moves beyond individual behavior to consider systemic constraints that contribute to health disparities. Results were modest (e.g., in terms of purchases of healthier food choices and reductions in unhealthy advertisements), however, and there remains a pressing need to study long-term impacts of novel, anti-racism interventions. If they work, they should be implemented widely; and if not, evaluators should study the obstacles to success and develop more promising approaches.

Integrative Behavioral Model

The Integrative Behavioral Model, first published in 2000 (Fishbein, 2000), builds on constructs from several previously developed health behavior models, including the Theory of Reasoned Action and Theory of Planned Behavior (Chapter 6). Key constructs are hypothesized to contribute to an individual's intention or decision to perform a behavior, with a range of "other factors" modifying the key constructs and behavior itself beyond intention. Considerations for incorporating race and racism theory can be applied to the IM constructs.

An individual's emotional response to getting a colonoscopy after a positive stool-based screening test result and the beliefs about the outcomes associated with getting a colonoscopy are structurally patterned, with perceived norms based on real social norms that may have structural bases. For instance, perceived norms around colonoscopies may be rooted in stigma related to the invasiveness of the procedure, historical experiences of late-stage diagnosis of health conditions with poor prognoses, or out-of-pocket costs disproportionately experienced by Black and Latinx patients. Personal agency is based on evaluation of real structural, racialized barriers, including insurance coverage, work constraints, and childcare constraints. The salience of the desired behavior is rooted in a complex context of competing desired behaviors and structural barriers. This can be broadly characterized, especially through social and material deprivation, forced migration, resource scarcity, and other pathways between racism and health. These issues should be considered when scheduling colonoscopy screenings when they are completed, and when results are given to patients. New, patient-centered communication and education approaches that take these factors into account should be developed and evaluated.

In essence, the argument is that health behavior theories that focus on individual and interpersonal factors can accommodate issues stemming from structural racism, thus making them more robust in their explanation and allowing for the development of interventions that can be applied to address health disparities.

Applications of PHCRP and CRT to Public Health

This section discusses two applications that use PHCRP and CRT to address health disparities.

At a 793-bed academic medical center in Boston, MA, PHCRP was used to design a quality improvement (QI) intervention aimed at eliminating disparities in quality of care for patients with congestive heart failure (Osuagwu et al., 2023). Black and Latinx patients with congestive heart failure were less likely to be admitted for diagnosis-indicated specialty care (cardiology service vs. general medicine service) compared to white patients, resulting in comparatively poor rates of cardiology follow-up and higher 30-day readmission rates. The initiative explicitly drew upon PHCRP to engage QI teams and other key stakeholders in design of the QI intervention. The intervention included but was not limited to enhanced nurse education, social work consultation for patients, electronic referrals for cardiology follow-up, and templates for progress notes including criteria for cardiology consultation, guideline-directed therapy, and guideline-concordant discharge documentation in the electronic health record. While the sample size was smaller than anticipated and therefore not disaggregated, there was a significant improvement in 30-day readmission rates (post: 19.0% versus pre: 24.8%, $p = 0.024$) and scheduling 14- and 30-day post-discharge cardiology appointments among chronic heart failure patients admitted to general medicine service (Osuagwu et al., 2023). The authors argued that the inclusion of "racism-conscious framework" in typical QI approaches is feasible.

Another application of PHCRP focused on identifying the root causes of excessive use of force by police among Black men, offering an alternative framework by which to interpret the research focused on their criminalization, justifications for over-surveillance of segregated Black communities, the reification of stereotypes of violence-prone Black neighborhoods, and the continued disinvestment in Black communities (Gilbert & Ray, 2016). This application not only identifies different lines of empirical inquiry and intervention but also suggests a direction for community mobilization and intervention. The PHCRP is one empirical model/approach for systematically investigating the macro-level structural determinants that are often loosely discussed or ignored in commonly used health behavior models. As PHCRP continues to be utilized, there may be further empirical support for this conceptual and methodological orientation.

Discussion and Conclusions

To achieve health equity, it is important to consider behavior change not in isolation, divorced from pre-existing systems of oppression, like racism, and to examine not just outcomes but also the processes. Interventions to address health inequities can be conceptualized as occurring upstream, downstream, or somewhere in between. Downstream determinants occur at individual levels, including individual biology and specific risk factors and behaviors. Intervening on that level will help individuals, perhaps in a clinical context, but does not address upstream factors that drive patterns—that is, inequities—in health behaviors, outcomes, and biology. Further upstream are living conditions—which include physical residential conditions, social environments, work environments, and services—and the inequities that emerge from them.

The question of why some living conditions are more prevalent in certain communities relates to racial and socioeconomic disadvantage. Often, institutional inequities in the public and private sectors, and in public policy, drive the distribution of social determinants of health. Resource allocation for the structures and space and the absence of universal access to a living wage might drive the living conditions within public housing or a correctional facility; however one has to go farther upstream to social determinants of health inequities—systems of social inequities like racism, sexism, classism, heterosexism, and ablism—to see how access to resources and healthy living conditions are inequitably allocated and distributed, especially institutionally, across pre-existing hierarchies of power. To effect sustainable change, and, specifically, sustainably drive toward health equity, it is critical to consider ways to improve communities farther upstream. Furthermore, interventions that do not get at the root of health inequities may be perceived as metaphorical Band-Aids and/or victim-blaming. To have a real impact on health equity, public health as a field must be committed to dismantling systems of oppression, while health professionals mitigate its impacts on individuals.

Moving beyond cultural competency, *structural competency* "seeks to promote skills … for recognizing how 'culture' and 'structure' are mutually co-implicated in producing stigma and inequality" (Metzl & Hansen, 2014). This requires developing the capacity to recognize influences of structures on individual health, in clinical/programmatic encounters, in clinics and community health organizations, and beyond the clinical or interventional spaces (Neff et al., 2017). While exploring and applying the theoretical foundations underlying structural racism, similar consideration can be given to other systems of oppression, which requires further exploration and investigation. Structural competency enables health professionals to better apply health behavior change models in real-world programs seeking to reduce health inequities. Further, structural competency requires structural humility—"not the hubris of mastery, but the humility to recognize the complexity of the structural constraints that patients, [community residents, health professionals,] and doctors operate within" and continue to learn (Metzl & Hansen, 2014).

Public health experts should think beyond simple health disparities and social determinants of health to social determinants of health inequities, including concrete ways by which racism, sexism, classism, heterosexism, ableism, and other differences constrain and facilitate certain behaviors and actions. Furthermore, it is increasingly important to consider how research, interventions and communications may reinforce inequitable systems, and evaluate which community voices are not being heard and incorporated into the design and implementation of health promotion interventions. Those most impacted by health inequities can offer many of the most promising ideas about systemic improvements.

With that in mind, for theory-based health-behavior interventions to be the most effective in communities with disproportionate needs, it is important to understand the structural constraints from the standpoint of structural humility and design interventions that seek to address multiple levels, or at the very least understanding the level of behavior change within a larger structural ecology. While some interventions may be limited in scope, this focus does not negate capacity-building for facilitating collective action and organizing for social change—within a multilevel intervention by design or in partnership with other community partners.

References

Adjoian, T., Dannefer, R., Willingham, C., Brathwaite, C., & Franklin, S. (2017). Healthy checkout lines: A study in urban supermarkets. *Journal of Nutrition Education and Behavior*, *49*(8), 615–622. https://doi.org/10.1016/j.jneb.2017.02.004

Arevalo, S. (2017). It takes a village to control diabetes. *AADE in Practice*, *5*(3), 28–32.

Arias, E., Tejada-Vera, B., Kochanek, K. D., & Ahmad, F. B. (2022). Provisional life expectancy estimates for 2021. *Vital Statistics Rapid Release, no. 23*. Hyattsville, MD: National Center for Health Statistics.

Bailey, Z. D., Krieger, N., Agénor, M., Graves, J., Linos, N., & Bassett, M. T. (2017). Structural racism and health inequities in the USA: Evidence and interventions. *The Lancet*, *389*(10077), 1453–1463.

Bell, D. A. (1995). Who's afraid of critical race theory. *University of Illinois Law Review*, *4*, 893–910.

Bonilla-Silva, E. (1997). Rethinking racism: Toward a structural interpretation. *American Sociological Review*, *6*(3), 465–480.

Bronfenbrenner, U. (1979). *The ecology of human development: Experiments by nature and design*. Cambridge, Massachusetts: Harvard University Press.

Bronfenbrenner, U., & Morris, P. A. (2007). The bioecological model of human development. In R. M. Lerner, & W. Damon (Eds.), *Handbook of Child Psychology, 1*. Wiley.

Burdick, J. (1992). The myth of racial democracy. *Report on the Americas*, *25*(4), 40–49.

Coates, T.-N. (2015). *Between the world and me*. New York, NY: Spiegel & Grau.

Coleman, P., Barber, T. M., van Rens, T., Hanson, P., Coffey, A., & Oyebode, O. (2022). COVID-19 outcomes in minority ethnic groups: Do obesity and metabolic risk play a role? *Current Obesity Reports*, *11*(3), 107–115. https://doi.org/10.1007/s13679-021-00459-5

Crenshaw, K., & Gotanda, N. (1995). *Critical race theory: The key writings that formed the movement*: The New Press.

Dannefer, R., Adjoian, T., Brathwaite, C., & Walsh, R. (2016). Food shopping behaviors of residents in two Bronx neighborhoods. *AIMS Public Health*, *3*(1), 1.

Delgado, R., & Stefancic, J. (Eds.). (2005). *The derrick bell reader*. New York University Press.

Division of Population Health National Center for Chronic Disease Prevention and Health Promotion. (2017). Health disparities. https://www.cdc.gov/aging/disparities/index.htm

Dover, R. V. H., & Lambert, E. V. (2016). "Choice Set" for health behavior in choice-constrained settings to frame research and inform policy: Examples of food consumption, obesity and food security. *International Journal for Equity in Health*, *15*(1), 48. https://doi.org/10.1186/s12939-016-0336-6

Dresser, I. D. S., Crossa, A., Dannefer, R., Brathwaite, C., Cespedes, A., & Bedell, J. (2023). Marketing sustainability analysis of stores participating in a healthier retail food program. *Journal of Nutrition Education and Behavior*, *55*, 205–214.

Duello, T. M., Rivedal, S., Wickland, C., & Weller, A. (2021). Race and genetics versus 'race' in genetics: A systematic review of the use of African ancestry in genetic studies. *Evolution, Medicine, and Public Health*, *9*(1), 232–245. https://doi.org/10.1093/emph/eoab018

Feagin, J. (2006). *Systemic racism: A theory of oppression*. New York: Routledge.

Fishbein, M. (2000). The role of theory in HIV prevention. *AIDS Care*, *12*(3), 273–278.

Ford, C. L. (2016). Public health critical race praxis: An introduction, an intervention, and three points for consideration. *Wisconsin Law Review*, *2016*(3), 477–491.

Ford, C. L., & Airhihenbuwa, C. O. (2010a). Critical race theory, race equity, and public health: Toward antiracism praxis. *American Journal of Public Health, 100*(S1), S30–S35.

Ford, C. L., & Airhihenbuwa, C. O. (2010b). The public health critical race methodology: Praxis for antiracism research. *Social Science & Medicine, 71*(8), 1390–1398.

Fredrickson, G. M. (2015). *Racism: A short history.* Princeton University Press.

de la Fuente, A. (1999). Myths of racial democracy: Cuba, 1900-1912. *Latin American Research Review, 34*(3), 39–73. https://doi.org/10.1017/S0023879100039364

Gilbert, K. L., & Ray, R. (2016). Why police kill black males with impunity: Applying public health critical race praxis (PHCRP) to address the determinants of policing behaviors and "justifiable" homicides in the USA. *Journal of Urban Health, 93*(1), 122–140. https://doi.org/10.1007/s11524-015-0005-x

Gonzalez-Sobrino, B., & Goss, D. R. (2019). Exploring the mechanisms of racialization beyond the black–white binary. *Ethnic and Racial Studies, 42*(4), 505–510.

Hickman, C. B. (1997). The devil and the one drop rule: Racial categories, African Americans, and the U.S. Census. *Michigan Law Review, 95*(5), 1161–1265. https://doi.org/10.2307/1290008

Hollinger, D. A. (2005). The one drop rule & the one hate rule. *Daedalus, 134*(1), 18–28. http://www.jstor.org/stable/20027957

Jones-Correa, M. (2000). The origins and diffusion of racial restrictive covenants. *Political Science Quarterly, 115*(4), 541–568. https://doi.org/10.2307/2657609

Kauanui, J. K. (2017). Tracing historical specificity: Race and the colonial politics of (in) capacity. *American Quarterly, 69*(2), 257–265.

Krieger, N. (2012). Methods for the scientific study of discrimination and health: An ecosocial approach. *American Journal of Public Health, 102*(5), 936–944. https://doi.org/10.2105/ajph.2011.300544

Kumanyika, S. K. (2019). A framework for increasing equity impact in obesity prevention. *American Journal of Public Health, 109*(10), 1350–1357.

Kumanyika, S. K. (2022). Advancing health equity efforts to reduce obesity: Changing the course. *Annual Review of Nutrition, 42*(1), 453–480. https://doi.org/10.1146/annurev-nutr-092021-050805

Lawrence III, C. R. (1995). Foreword: Race, multiculturalism, and the jurisprudence of transformation. *Stanford Law Review, 47*, 819–847.

Mahajan, S., Caraballo, C., Lu, Y., Valero-Elizondo, J., Massey, D., Annapureddy, A. R., & Krumholz, H. M. (2021). Trends in differences in health status and health care access and affordability by race and ethnicity in the United States, 1999-2018. *JAMA, 326*(7), 637–648. https://doi.org/10.1001/jama.2021.9907

Matsuda, M. J. (2018). *Words that wound: Critical race theory, assaultive speech, and the first amendment.* Routledge.

Maylam, P. (2017). *South Africa's racial past: The history and historiography of racism, segregation, and apartheid.* Routledge.

Metzl, J. M., & Hansen, H. (2014). Structural competency: Theorizing a new medical engagement with stigma and inequality. *Social Science & Medicine, 103*, 126–133. https://doi.org/10.1016/j.socscimed.2013.06.032

Morgan, E. S. (1975). *American slavery, American freedom: The ordeal of colonial Virginia* (1st ed.). New York: Norton.

National Academy of Sciences, Engineering, and Medicine. (2022). *Structural racism and rigorous models of social inequity: Proceedings of a workshop.* Washington, DC.

Ndugga, N., & Artiga, S. (2021). Disparities in health and health care: 5 key questions and answers. https://www.kff.org/racial-equity-and-health-policy/issue-brief/disparities-in-health-and-health-care-5-key-question-and-answers/

Neff, J., Knight, K. R., Satterwhite, S., Nelson, N., Matthews, J., & Holmes, S. M. (2017). Teaching structure: A qualitative evaluation of a structural competency training for resident physicians. *Journal of General Internal Medicine, 32*(4), 430–433. https://doi.org/10.1007/s11606-016-3924-7

Omi, M., & Winant, H. (1994). *Racial formation in the United States: From the 1960s to the 1990s* (2nd ed.). New York, NY: Routledge.

Osuagwu, C., Khinkar, R. M., Zheng, A., Wien, M., Decopain, J., Desai, S., & Schnipper, J. L. (2023). A public health critical race praxis informed congestive heart failure quality improvement initiative on inpatient general medicine. *Journal of General Internal Medicine, 38*, 2236–2244.

Packard, J. M. (2003). *American nightmare: The history of Jim Crow:* Macmillan.

Peña, Y., Sidanius, J., & Sawyer, M. (2004). Racial democracy in the Americas: A Latin and US comparison. *Journal of Cross-Cultural Psychology, 35*(6), 749–762.

Pereira, M. M. C. E., Padez, C. M. P., & Nogueira, H. G. D. S. M. (2019). Describing studies on childhood obesity determinants by Socio-Ecological Model level: A scoping review to identify gaps and provide guidance for future research. *International Journal of Obesity, 43*(10), 1883–1890. https://doi.org/10.1038/s41366-019-0411-3

Quick, V., Martin-Biggers, J., Povis, G. A., Hongu, N., Worobey, J., & Byrd-Bredbenner, C. (2017). A socio-ecological examination of weight-related characteristics of the home environment and lifestyles of households with young children. *Nutrients*, *9*(6), 604. https://www.mdpi.com/2072-6643/9/6/604

Reskin, B. (2012). The race discrimination system. *Annual Review of Sociology*, *38*(1), 17–35. https://doi.org/10.1146/annurev-soc-071811-145508

Rothstein, R. (2017). *The color of law: A forgotten history of how our government segregated America*. Liveright Publishing.

Simon Fraser Public Interest Research Group. (2023). *Systems of oppression. SFPIRG*. https://sfpirg.ca/infohub/systems-of-oppression/

Sirugo, G., Tishkoff, S. A., & Williams, S. M. (2021). The quagmire of race, genetic ancestry, and health disparities. *The Journal of Clinical Investigation*, *131*(11). https://doi.org/10.1172/JCI150255

Smedley, A., & Smedley, B. D. (2005). Race as biology is fiction, racism as a social problem is real: Anthropological and historical perspectives on the social construction of race. *American Psychologist*, *60*(1), 16.

Story, M., Kaphingst, K. M., Robinson-O'Brien, R., & Glanz, K. (2008). Creating healthy food and eating environments: Policy and environmental approaches. *Annual Review of Public Health*, *29*(1), 253–272. https://doi.org/10.1146/annurev.publhealth.29.020907.090926

Takaki, R. (2008). *A different mirror: A history of multicultural America* (Rev. ed.). Boston, MA: Back Bay Books.

Taylor, E. (1998). A primer on critical race theory: Who are the critical race theorists and what are they saying? *The Journal of Blacks in Higher Education 19*, 122.

Venn, D., & Strazdins, L. (2017). Your money or your time? How both types of scarcity matter to physical activity and healthy eating. *Social Science & Medicine*, *172*, 98–106. https://doi.org/10.1016/j.socscimed.2016.10.023

Williams, P. J. (1991). *The alchemy of race and rights*. Harvard University Press.

Williams, D. R., Lawrence, J. A., & Davis, B. A. (2019). Racism and health: Evidence and needed research. *Annual Review of Public Health*, *40*, 105–125.

Winant, H. (1999). Racial democracy and racial identity In M. Hanchard (Eds.), *Racial politics in Contemporary Brazil* (pp. 98–115). Duke University Press.

Wolfe, P. (2016). *Traces of history: Elementary structures of race*. Verso Books.

Zimmerman, F. J., & Anderson, N. W. (2019). Trends in health equity in the United States by race/ethnicity, sex, and income, 1993–2017. *JAMA Network Open*, *2*(6), e196386–e196386. https://doi.org/10.1001/jamanetworkopen.2019.6386

CHAPTER 15

IMPROVING HEALTH THROUGH COMMUNITY ENGAGEMENT: RESEARCH AND PRACTICE

Joseph Keawe'aimoku Kaholokula
John G. Oetzel
Ka'imi A. Sinclair
Ridvan Tupai-Firestone

KEY POINTS

This chapter will:

- Examine the conceptual definition of community that informs community engagement.

- Explore historical and contemporary developments in community engagement and community-engaged research.

- Examine key concepts, principles, applications, and the practice of community engagement.

- Present key theories and models that inform the concepts and practice of community engagement.

- Explain community-based participatory research as a respected community engagement approach for health behavior and health promotion research.

- Examine measurement, evaluation, and research design issues related to community engagement.

- Present a case study application of community engagement that integrates the key principles and approaches of community-engaged research.

Vignette: Taking It to the Pews

African Americans make up nearly half of all new human immunodeficiency virus (HIV) cases in the United States (Centers for Disease Control and Prevention [CDC], 2021). Many go too long living with HIV before being diagnosed and treated because of stigma, discrimination, and homophobia. Not getting HIV treatment when needed increases their chances of developing acquired immunodeficiency syndrome (AIDS) and lowers their chances of survival. Yet, HIV can be prevented with behavior change (e.g., condom use) and effectively treated with antiretroviral therapy.

To improve HIV awareness and screening among African Americans, *Taking It to the Pews* (TIPS) was launched in 2007 (Berkley-Patton et al., 2013) as a community-based participatory research (CBPR) project by researchers from the University of Missouri and leaders of the Black Church—churches predominantly comprised of an African American congregation and leadership—in the greater Kansas City metropolitan area. Church leaders helped set the research agenda, define the partnership, and evaluate and strengthen the church's capacity to address HIV/AIDS. The result was a targeted HIV awareness and screening intervention for delivery by church leaders at multiple levels (e.g., individual, church, and community) to both church and community members.

The TIPS partnership tested its effectiveness by comparing the results between churches that were assigned randomly to either receive the tailored HIV intervention or not (Berkley-Patton et al., 2019). They found that church leaders were effective in delivering the intervention, and that it led to significantly more HIV screenings among the people they served. Because of its success as a community-engaged initiative, the TIPS intervention is being implemented by churches that are part of the Calvary Community Outreach Network to reach the larger African American community in Kansas City. This chapter draws on TIPS throughout to illustrate community engagement in action.

Health Behavior: Theory, Research, and Practice, Sixth Edition. Edited by Karen Glanz, Barbara K. Rimer, and K. Viswanath.
© 2024 John Wiley & Sons, Inc. Published 2024 by John Wiley & Sons, Inc.
Companion website: www.wiley.com/go/glanz/healthbehavior6e

Overview

The US Centers for Disease Control and Prevention (CDC) defines community engagement as ". . . the process of working collaboratively with and through groups of people affiliated by geographic proximity, special interest, or similar situations to address issues affecting the well-being of those people" (CDC, 1997, p. 9). Although over 25 years old, this CDC definition remains the most commonly used definition. This chapter first examines the concept of community, as well as historical and recent developments in community engagement. It then explores key concepts, principles, methods, theories, and models of community engagement and measurement, evaluation, and research-design issues, followed by an example of community engagement in action from the Pasifika Prediabetes Youth Empowerment Program (PPYEP).

Concept of Community

Communities can be characterized by *geographical proximity* (e.g., a neighborhood), *sociocultural proximity* (e.g., race/ethnicity), or *similar situations/experiences* (e.g., exposure to environmental contaminants). Transcending geographical proximity, Fellin (2001) identified three dimensions of communities: (1) *functional spatial units* seeking to meet basic needs (e.g., residents of low-income housing projects mobilized to address food insecurity); (2) *units of patterned social interactions* (e.g., patients and physicians brought together to improve primary care); and (3) *symbolic units of collective identity* (e.g., migrant workers engaged to improve their sexual health). Another dimension is that of social units seeking change on a political level (Minkler et al., 2008).

TIPS' notion of community focused on several community characteristics; African Americans (sociocultural proximity) affected by HIV/AIDS (similar situation) living in the greater Kansas City Metropolitan area (geographical proximity). TIPS also exemplifies Fellin's (2001) symbolic units of collective identity: a community defined by its shared religious affiliation and ethnocultural history. These characteristics and dimensions of a community, and how communities are defined more broadly, are informed by several broad perspectives.

The *ecological systems perspective* (see Chapter 3) focuses on distinct community components, each with its purpose, activities, levels of influence, and boundaries to meet the diverse needs of communities. The *social systems perspective* focuses on the social and political networks (see Chapter 11 on social networks) at multiple levels (e.g., family, community, and geopolitical) that connect individuals, community organizations, and leaders to each other. TIPS exemplifies these perspectives. The organizers designed a multilevel HIV/AIDS intervention built upon the church's natural components—outreach ministry, church services, and group ministry—to reach different segments of their community in different ways (e.g., testimonials and testing events during services), but all with the same goal. In doing so, they leveraged the social connections among African American church members and church leaders and the church's influence in the community.

The *virtual perspective* focuses on computer-mediated forms of communication and networking. Many people connect with others, access information, and seek solutions to their concerns through social media (e.g., Facebook and Twitter) and networking services (e.g., text messaging and e-chat rooms) (see Chapter 22). This has led to virtual communities, or organized groups of people with shared interests, who interact over the Internet or on social media platforms, offering unique ways to engage communities in health promotion and research (Patten et al., 2021).

The *individual perspective* recognizes that people can have multiple and intersecting identities, interests, or conditions that do not fall neatly along geographical, socioeconomic, racial/ethnic lines, or any other single characteristic (McCloskey et al., 2011). No single definition or perspective of a community can capture all the possible ways and reasons people choose to identify, connect, interact, or organize themselves. This is why it is important to understand how communities define themselves.

Historical and Recent Developments

Community engagement has its roots in social justice and social change movements, such as the indigenous land rights, women's rights, civil rights, and environmental justice movements (Minkler et al., 2008). The researchers who developed TIPS engaged leaders of African American churches, in part, because of the Black Church's historical and current role in social justice movements. In this section, we explore the progress of community engagement as an approach to health behavior change and health equity through its endorsement by public health agencies, healthcare organizations, researchers, policymakers, funders, and community leaders. (see Chapter 14 on Race, Health, and Health Equity.)

Since 1948, the World Health Organization (WHO) has promoted the view that "informed opinion and active cooperation on the part of the public are of the utmost importance in the improvement of the health of the people" (World Health Organization, 2022). In 1978, the Declaration of Alma-Ata called for communities to take part in the "... planning, organization, operation, and control of primary health care..." (Kalra et al., 2018). In 1986, the Ottawa Charter for Health Promotion called for community involvement in priority setting, decision-making, and strategic planning and implementation for health promotion (World Health Organization, 1986). WHO's Commission on Social Determinants of Health (2008) called for community engagement to achieve health equity.

In the United States, major federal agencies have encouraged community engagement in public health practice and in research, thus setting the stage for communities and researchers to adopt community-engaged approaches. The CDC has long recognized the importance of community engagement. In 1983, their Planned Approach to Community Health (PATCH) provided a model for state and local public health agencies and local community partners to plan, conduct, and evaluate health promotion and disease prevention programs. Other past CDC programs include the Community Transformation Grants (2011–2014) and the Partnerships to Improve Community Health (2014–2016). For over 20 years, their Racial and Ethnic Approaches to Community Health (REACH) program supported community partnerships to address racial and ethnic disparities in chronic disease burden.

Also in the United States, the National Institutes of Health (NIH) and its institutes have advanced community engagement in research. The National Institute for Environmental Health Sciences was the first at NIH to establish a CBPR grant initiative in 1995. In 2005, the National Center on Minority Health and Health Disparities launched an 11-year CBPR Initiative to support community-academic partnerships to plan, implement, and disseminate interventions to reduce health disparities. The National Cancer Institute funded a Community Networks Program (2005–2014) that involved partnerships with community-based groups to help reduce cancer-related disparities. Today, many of NIH's research infrastructure programs require a community engagement core. These cores are among several fundamental components of research infrastructure grants, with a distinct objective of engaging community-based organizations and practitioners in research and the dissemination of research discoveries.

Due to the SARS-CoV-2 pandemic and inequities in the disease caused by it, COVID-19, public health agencies quickly turned to community engagement as a health equity strategy during the pandemic. CDC called for the engagement of at-risk communities and effective communication with them, data sharing, and partnering for program implementation, dissemination, and evaluation (Michener et al., 2020). NIH took advantage of existing programs with community partnerships to expedite COVID-19 research. For example, NIH formed the Community Engagement Alliance (CEAL). Against COVID-19 Disparities, a network of researchers, policymakers, and community-based organizations to help communities hardest hit by COVID-19 across 21 states (Hunter et al., 2021).

Outside the United States, other countries have endorsed community engagement for health promotion and health equity. For example, the New Zealand Government initiated 11 National Science Challenges in 2014 as a mission-led form of research funding for environmental and social/human health (Prussing & Newbury, 2016). These challenges had the expectation of community engagement to address health equity issues, particularly for Māori (the indigenous people of New Zealand) and Pasifika (a group of people from South Pacific Island nations that include Samoa, Tonga, and Cook Island) communities. The challenges initially were critiqued as centering scientific knowledge production in the context of neoliberalism with Māori researchers reasserting the importance of Māori processes of knowledge production (Prussing & Newbury, 2016). This "pushback" improved the expectations and practice of community engagement in the later stages of these efforts.

Other indigenous populations have expressed similar concerns regarding the recognition of indigenous knowledge and knowledge production (Nicholson et al., 2021) and data sovereignty (McCartney et al., 2022). Guiding principles, recommendations, and processes for engaging indigenous communities in research and data ownership have been developed and implemented, centering on indigenous knowledge and autonomy (Laird et al., 2021). In the United States, many American Indian and Alaska Native tribes, as sovereign nations, have developed protocols for participating in research, which places a greater emphasis on community and cultural benefits, respect for participants, and human-subject protection.

Concepts and Principles

The core concepts and principles of community engagement offer practical guidance and strategies, a foundation for scientific inquiry, and core values that can guide health professionals, researchers, health care providers, community leaders, and organizations in their efforts. They place the notions of respect, trust, equal participation, and integrity at the forefront of working with communities. Understanding how power is negotiated between academic and community partners in community engagement activities is critical to developing respectful, trusting, and equal partnerships (Wallerstein et al., 2019).

In this section, we define four overarching concepts of community engagement with their embedded principles: (1) *community capacity*, with principles of the community as the unit of identity that builds on community strengths; (2) *empowerment and critical consciousness*, with principles that promote co-learning and integrates knowledge and action; (3) *participation and relevance*, with principles to facilitate equitable involvement of all partners in practice and research; and (4) *health inequities* as the focus of change. These concepts and principles are summarized in Table 15.1.

Community Capacity

Community capacity is the development of knowledge, skills, commitment, structures, systems, and leadership to enable effective health promotion (Israel et al., 2013). It is integral to challenging power imbalances and effectively addressing problems. Capacity building involves actions to improve health at three levels: (1) the advancement of knowledge and skills among practitioners; (2) the expansion of support and infrastructure for health promotion in organizations; (3) the development of cohesiveness and partnerships for health in communities (Smith et al., 2006).

Community capacity recognizes the community as a *unit of identity*. Communities' identities often are linked to a sense of emotional connection and relationship to others, shared norms and values, common language and customs, similar goals and interests, and a desire to meet shared needs. There also may be situations in which communities of identity may benefit from involving individuals and groups from outside the community who bring additional needed skills and resources to address communities' concerns.

Community capacity building includes the ability of community members to take action to address their needs and the social and political support that is required for the successful implementation of programs (Israel et al., 1998). As community members actively participate in identifying and solving community issues, they become better able to address future issues collaboratively. While communities may benefit from academic or health professional skills and resources external to the community, recognition of and building on community strengths is critical for effective capacity building,

Table 15.1 Key Concepts/Principles in Community Engagement

Key Concepts	Key Definition	Principles	Application
Community Capacity	The development of knowledge, skills, commitment, structures, systems, and leadership to enable effective health promotion.	Community as a unit of identity. Builds on community strengths and assets.	Community members actively participate in identifying and solving community issues and become better able to address future issues collaboratively.
Empowerment	Social action process for people to gain mastery over their lives and the lives of their communities.	Promotes co-learning. Integrates knowledge and action.	Community members expand their power or challenge power structures to create desired changes.
Critical Consciousness	A consciousness based on praxis: the cycle of reflection and action toward social change.	Involve cyclical and iterative processes. Collaborative mentorship that honors diversity and cultural humility.	Engage people in listening/dialogue/and action that links root causes and community actions.
Participation and Relevance	Community organizing should "start where the people are" and engage community members as equals in their priorities.	Facilitate equitable involvement of all partners in all stages of practice and research. Long-term commitment. Cultural relevance.	Community members create their agenda based on felt needs, shared power, and awareness of resources.
Health Equity	The opportunity for all to obtain their full health potential regardless of social position or socially determined circumstances.	Address inequitable conditions that create health disparities.	Allocate resources to the community, policy, and systems-level changes that challenge inequitable conditions that cause inequities in health and well-being.

and relationships are a precursor to building capacity to achieve mutual goals (Smith et al., 2006). Rather than viewing communities in terms of deficits, communities should be viewed in terms of their assets and resourcefulness.

Empowerment and Critical Consciousness

Empowerment and critical consciousness are embedded deeply within community engagement. Empowerment is "a group-based, participatory, developmental process through which marginalized or oppressed individuals and groups gain greater control over their lives and environment, acquire valued resources and basic rights, and achieve important life goals and reduced societal marginalization" (Maton, 2008, pp. 4–5). Although often used as a catch-all phrase, empowerment remains a central tenet of community organization, community building, and community engagement.

Researchers use empowerment approaches to explore relationships between individuals within specific social, organizational, educational, and political environments (Freire, 2018; Zimmerman, 2000). As a methodology, community empowerment involves both processes and outcomes and focuses on transforming power relations for individuals, the organizations to which they belong, and the community social structure itself. For individuals, psychological empowerment includes perceived control, critical consciousness, political efficacy, and participation in change (Peterson et al., 2006). Organizational empowerment incorporates advocacy processes as well as organizational effectiveness and collective efficacy in policy change (Laverack, 2007).

Community empowerment outcomes include an increased sense of community, or sense of belonging to and iden-tification with a group or geographic area; community capacity; actual changes in policies, transformed conditions, and/or increased resources—all of which can contribute to reducing health inequities (Wallerstein et al., 2020). There is evidence that empowerment is a viable public health strategy, and that empowering initiatives can lead to improve-ment in health outcomes (Wallerstein, 2006). The most effective empowerment strategies are those that build on and reinforce authentic participation and ensure autonomy in decision-making, a sense of community and local bonding, and psychological empowerment of community members (Wallerstein, 2006).

Freire's (2018) notion of *critical consciousness* is a philosophical, theoretical, and practice-based idea. A major tenet of the concept of critical consciousness is empowerment and action to promote equity and social justice. The process of critical consciousness promotes critical reflection on how social determinants of health can impact individual and community health outcomes (Windsor et al., 2022). In essence, reflection and action on social determinants of health can promote health equity by increasing willingness and ability to effectively combat health inequities and may affect individual and community health outcomes (Wallerstein, 2006).

Participation and Relevance

The concepts of participation and relevance represent the core value of working with communities in ways that acknowl-edge the strengths and skills of community partners. The principle of involving communities means equitable involve-ment of all partners in all stages of practice and research, from identifying the problem to implementing and evaluating plans and strategies (Wallerstein et al., 2018). Within this principle is the recognition that fundamental change requires a long-term commitment to tackling complex and multilayered social and health problems.

One of the most important steps in community engagement involves effective differentiation between problems that are troubling and issues that the community feels strongly about (Staples, 2004). Various methods may be used to help a community group obtain data needed to document issues while ensuring their relevance. Face-to-face data collection processes, including focus groups, surveys, and interviews, can be useful in assessing perceived needs and, at the same time, increasing a sense of participation (Duran et al., 2012).

Health Equity

Braveman et al. (2017) define health equity as everyone having a fair and just opportunity to be as healthy as possible. This requires removing obstacles to health, such as poverty, discrimination, and their consequences, including powerlessness and lack of access to good jobs with fair pay, quality education and housing, safe environments, and healthcare. Health equity is the value underlying a commitment to reduce and ultimately eliminate health inequities. Thus, health equity, more broadly, means reducing and ultimately eliminating disparities in health and its determinants that adversely affect excluded or marginalized groups. While efforts to achieve health equity do not originate in community-engaged practice and research and are not important solely in the context of community engagement, health equity has an important role in community-based health behavior efforts. (see Chapter 14 on Race, Health, and Health Equity for more in-depth coverage.)

Health equity also means social justice and reflects ethical and human rights concerns. Equity requires a concerted effort to achieve more rapid improvements among those who were worse off to start, within an overall strategy to improve everyone's health, and not by worsening advantaged groups' health (Braveman et al., 2017). Increasingly, the term "health inequity"—the opposite of health equity—is being used instead of "health disparity" to capture the moral dimension and to emphasize health differences thought to reflect injustice as distinct from health differences in general.

Ideally, partnerships promote co-learning and capacity building among all partners; foster empowerment and power-sharing processes that reduce social and health inequities; and ensure local relevance and participation. It is important for partnerships invested in equity to critically evaluate the extent to which they provide opportunities for meaningful participation and engagement of community members. As Robert K. Ross, President and Chief Executive Officer for The California Endowment, stated, "The path to health equity and healing *begins* with participation in the process," which, indeed, is "the engine that drives" the entire effort (Ross, 2016, p. 1).

Community Engagement in Practice

In addition to the core concepts and principles described thus far, TIPS exemplifies the evolving and dynamic role of community leaders, members, and organizations, and their engagement in all aspects of a public-health research project. The researchers started by seeking input from African American church leaders before the start of the project to collaboratively involve them in needs assessment, capacity building, intervention development, implementation, testing and dissemination efforts. In this section, we show how the practice of community engagement falls on a continuum representing various levels of involvement. We also describe some of the models and frameworks that inform these different levels of engagement.

Community Engagement Continua

Russel et al. (2008) developed the Active Community Engagement (ACE) Continuum to characterize community engagement along a continuum based on how deeply involved the community and experts are in working together on reproductive health and family planning programs. ACE classifies three levels of engagement: (1) *consultative*, (2) *cooperative*, and (3) *collaborative*. Across each level, engagement occurs for five characteristics: (1) community involvement in assessment, (2) access to information, (3) inclusion in decision-making, (4) local capacity to advocate institutions and governing structures, and (5) accountability of institutions to the public. ACE is proposed to characterize engagement such that a given community-engaged relationship or project can be understood as an evolving process.

A similar approach to the continuum of community engagement was published in 2020 by WHO's Health Promotion Department (2020). This continuum articulated four levels of community engagement for universal coverage: Level 1 is *community-oriented*: informing and mobilizing the community to address immediate short-term problems with strong external support. Level 2 is *community-based*: consulting with the community and engaging them to improve access to health services and/or programs by placing interventions inside the community with some external support. Level 3 is *community-managed*: collaborating with community leaders to set priorities and make decisions. Level 4 is *community-owned*: leveraging community assets and empowerment to develop systems for self-governance, establish and set priorities, implement interventions, and develop sustainable mechanisms for health promotion with partners and external support groups as part of a network. This is similar to the ACE Continuum described above and reflects the growing acknowledgment that community engagement occurs with different degrees of co-creation by experts and communities.

Theories and Models that Inform Community Engagement

Concepts of community engagement and its principles and practices are informed by various theoretical perspectives and models, some of which have foundations in individual-level theories and others which are focused on groups and communities. Two theories that have been influential in the area of community engagement have been critical consciousness and self-determination. As described earlier, Freire's (2018) *critical consciousness theory* emphasizes the notion of empowerment to help disenfranchised and oppressed groups gain control over their own lives and environment and effect change. Although not a community engagement theory per se, *self-determination theory* is used to understand an individual's motivation for community engagement. It posits that people are influenced by three basic needs—competency, autonomy, and relatedness—that influence their psychological wellness and engagement with the world by affecting their motivation and aspirations (Ryan & Deci, 2017).

Rothman (2001) developed a widely used typology of a community organization that consists of three models. The process-oriented *locality development model* focuses on community building by engaging a wide range of stakeholders to create an infrastructure and build capacity for activism and action. *Social planning/policy* is task-oriented and focuses on problem-solving through rational and deliberate planning. This model involves fact-finding and analyzing information to make logical decisions about the best ways to address a community problem. The third model, *social action,* assumes there is a disadvantaged or mistreated segment of the community that should organize itself and/or be organized to make demands on the larger community for fair treatment. This model centers around social justice and the redistribution of power, resources, and decision-making to achieve equity.

Rothman's typology of community organization and community building, first conceived over 35 years ago (Rothman, 2001; Rothman & Tropman, 1987), has been widely used and is a foundation for other more recent models (Minkler et al., 2008). The utility of each of the three models depends on the community situation or context and they are not mutually exclusive. They can be used sequentially to move a community from capacity-building to data-driven planning to action-taking. They provide a systematic and pragmatic approach to community organization, building, and engagement.

Measurement, Evaluation, and Research Designs

Robust measurement and evaluation of community engagement concepts and their application are important to determine their value for improving behaviors and health. From the scientific perspective, valid and precise measurement is needed to test theory-informed strategies and theoretical models. From a practice perspective, measurement enables partnerships to reflect on their community engagement and identify strengths and areas for improvement. Measurement for science and practice is most useful when guided by a clearly defined framework that drives the choice of measures and measurement strategies. Research designs circumscribe what can be learned from an empirical evaluation of a program. This section explores major measurement, evaluation, and research design issues associated with community engagement in research and practice, with an emphasis on CBPR strategies.

CBPR Strategies and Models

As originally conceived, CBPR was defined as a research approach on the highly collaborative end of the "engagement" continuum (Israel et al., 1998). TIPS exemplifies this original approach as a CBPR project that engaged church leaders at every stage of research—problem identification and program conception, development, testing, and dissemination—to address HIV/AIDS inequity among African Americans. Various models and frameworks of CBPR have emerged to fit other unique communities. For example, the tribal participatory research model (Richmond et al., 2008) and the *He Pikinga Waiora* (Enhancing Wellbeing) Implementation Framework (Oetzel et al., 2017) translated the principles of CBPR centered on self-determination for American Indian and Alaska Native and Māori and Pacific Islander communities, respectively.

CBPR has evolved from a general research approach to a multidimensional research strategy. Research by leading CBPR scholars has identified and examined the dimensions and concepts of CBPR to describe a CPBR conceptual model (Wallerstein et al., 2018). They developed a visual framework to illustrate important concepts for measurement and practice. It has been applied in a variety of CBPR projects and has a robust evidence base for measurement. Recent research has also advanced the understanding of theoretical mechanisms in the model (Oetzel et al., 2022).

The CBPR conceptual model depicted in Figure 15.1 illustrates relationships among the key constructs of CBPR within four domains: context, partnership dynamics, research/intervention, and outcomes. Context involves community capacity and structural governance factors that shape the CBPR partnership and partnership dynamics. These factors include commitment to collective empowerment (e.g., collective reflection and shared influence) and relational dynamics

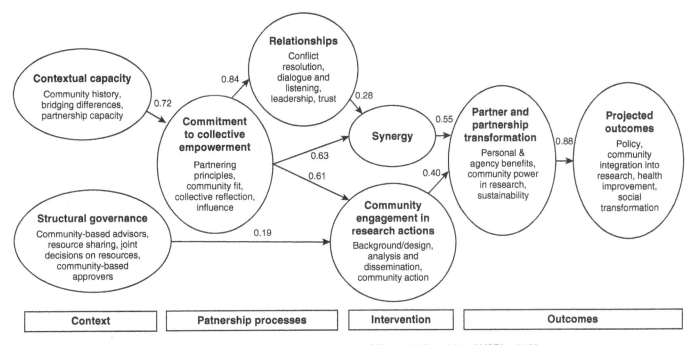

Note: All coefficients are significant at *p* <0.001; Model fit indices: CFI = 0.933, TLI = 0.924, RMSEA = 0.065

Figure 15.1 The Community-Based Participatory Research (CBPR) Conceptual Model (Oetzel et al., 2022, p. 7)
Source: Adapted from Oetzel et al. (2022)

(e.g., participatory decision-making). Partnership dynamics influence the actions of research projects, including the integration of community knowledge into the research design, research processes that empower partners, and community engagement in research actions. These processes produce research outputs that are culturally centered and synergistic of community and academic/scientific expectations. The research processes and outputs then produce intermediate (e.g., power-sharing and capacity building) and distal outcomes (e.g., community transformation and health improvement) for the CBPR partners, partnership, and the targeted community.

This CBPR conceptual model has been developed and revised based on over a decade of research. A two-phased, NIH-funded research project examined how different elements of the CBPR conceptual model were applied in nearly 400 CBPR or community-engaged partnerships in the US and found support for many dimensions of the model (Wallerstein et al., 2018, 2020). A recent study surveyed 453 community and academic partners from 163 CBPR projects regarding their perceptions of context, collective reflection, relational dynamics, research processes (e.g., synergy and community engagement), intermediate outcomes, and projected long-term outcomes). The survey data were analyzed using structural equation modeling with fuzzy-set qualitative comparative analysis, an approach that identifies whether a set of attributes—individually or in some configuration—explain a condition of interest (Lee, 2014). The structural equation model this analysis produced provided support for the relationships identified in the conceptual model. Specifically, it unpacked the structural model by examining which combination of four concepts—context, structural governance, relationships, and collective empowerment—were associated with synergy and community engagement in research actions since these are key mediators of the context/process to health outcomes. The results indicated that *structural governance* was the key mechanism for community engagement in research actions and *collective empowerment* was the key mechanism for synergy; thus, the key reported mechanisms by which CPBR context and processes produced health- and health-related outcomes (Oetzel et al., 2022).

As shown in Figure 15.1, community capacity influences collective empowerment, which in turn, influences both relationships (i.e., relational dynamics) and community engagement in research actions. Structural governance also influences community engagement in research actions. Relationships affect partnerships and partner transformation (i.e., intermediate outcomes) and projected outcomes (distal outcomes) through partnership synergy. Community engagement in research actions directly impacts these outcomes.

Structural governance is how decisions are made and resources are shared for the benefit of the community (Sanchez-Youngman et al., 2021). Collective empowerment is the commitment to CBPR principles and participatory processes to leverage community resilience in health programs and health research. Beyond the fit of the model and identifying these key mechanisms, Oetzel et al.'s (2022) study also illustrates a robust set of measurement tools for researchers and practitioners to consider for evaluation and continual improvement.

Measurement and Evaluation Issues

Despite the robust measurement tools and advances in applying novel analytic methods to CBPR discussed above, reviews of measures of community engagement practices and concepts have identified several important issues in measurement and evaluation that need to be considered (Sandoval et al., 2012; Tigges et al., 2019). One issue is the considerable variation in how particular constructs are conceptualized and measured in research on different community-engaged projects (Luger et al., 2020). There is a need for conceptual clarity about what is being measured, particularly in terms of measuring the goals of a community-engaged project and the goals that are most valued by a community and/or partner (Wallerstein et al., in press). One way to achieve this, as with research based on any model, is by systematically using the chosen model to guide conceptualization and measurement, and ensuring that the measures fit with the needs and values of the community. Key questions to ask are whether they are pragmatic, low-burden, and actionable.

There is debate about the need for standardized measures with psychometric evidence versus a need to have locally derived measures that fit the needs and context of the community (Luger et al., 2020; Tigges et al., 2019). Systematic reviews have revealed limited data about psychometric reliability and validity in community engagement measures (Sandoval et al., 2012; Tigges et al., 2019). For example, Luger et al. (2020) identified 69 measures of context, process, or outcomes in community-engaged research projects, and yet fewer than half had been tested for reliability or validity. Having scientifically validated approaches is important for credibility in the evaluation and to build a robust body of evidence. However, meeting local needs continues to be vital in community-engaged research and practice.

The need to bridge scientific rigor with community needs can be challenging but should also be feasible. Luger et al. (2020) suggest a hybrid approach of using both validated and locally derived measures. This may involve the adaptation of validated measures to fit the local context. It is important to integrate qualitative approaches to measure what communities value and do so in ways that are culturally appropriate and valued (Wallerstein et al., in press). Specific measures and qualitative tools of the CBPR conceptual model can be found in several sources (Boursaw et al., 2021; Wallerstein et al., 2018), which can be adapted to fit local needs and have good psychometric evidence.

Research Design Issues

There is no one definitive way to test CBPR or other forms of community-engaged research. CBPR processes can be studied through nonintervention or descriptive research (e.g., Oetzel et al., 2022). Interventions developed through CBPR, and community-engaged research processes can be studied through pre-experimental (pre-post), quasi-experimental, or experimental designs. With quasi-experimental and experimental designs, the comparative interventions might be done without community engagement or other types of treatment and controls. This section examines some of the key issues around experimental designs of interventions created with CBPR.

Although randomized controlled trial (RCT) designs are the scientific gold standards to establish the efficacy of an intervention, some researchers argue that RCT designs are counter to the values and goals of CBPR because of the degree of control over real-world conditions needed for rigorous testing of interventions (Trickett, 2011). Proponents of CBPR argue that community engagement can improve external or ecological validity because it better reflects real-world applications or conditions (Collins et al., 2018), but it may make replication more challenging.

CBPR and RCT designs can be blended, depending on the goals of the project and the needs of the community. There are many published examples of this. The TIPS partnership successfully conducted an RCT using a CBPR approach (Berkley-Patton et al., 2019). They randomized four comparable churches: two churches to the intervention condition ($n = 235$ participants/respondents) and two to a control condition ($n = 308$ participants). They found that participants at churches in the intervention condition were significantly more likely to get an HIV test in the next 6 months and 12 months than those in the control condition (47% versus 28% and 59% versus 42%, respectively). Other examples of community-academic partnerships that used an RCT to test the efficacy of an intervention in the context of CBPR include a cultural dance program (Kaholokula et al., 2021) and a community-health-worker initiative (Rosenthal et al., 2014).

Goodkind et al. (2017) provide recommendations to address some of the perceived tension between the methods of RCTs and the values and goals of CBPR. They suggest using mixed-method designs to explore the processes, contexts, and power dynamics of intervention implementation to address external validity issues; the consideration of the different forms of evidence valued by researchers and community partners; mutual decision-making to implement an RCT; and conducting group orientations to explain study design before enrollment and public randomization process.

Application: Pasifika Prediabetes Youth Empowerment Program

We illustrate community engagement in action through the PPYEP, a partnership between two Pasifika communities and researchers from Massey University in New Zealand. Pasifika people are individuals from various Pacific Island nations who are residing in New Zealand. Pasifika adults and youth have a much higher prevalence of prediabetes (higher than normal blood sugar levels but not high enough for a diabetes diagnosis) than their non-Pasifika counterparts (Coppell et al., 2013). Thus, PPYEP was started to develop the health knowledge and skillsets of Pasifika youth through an empowerment program to mobilize the community into collective action to reduce prediabetes risk in working-aged NZ Pasifika (Firestone et al., 2021b).

PPYEP is an empowerment program based on Freire's (2018) theory about empowering individual and societal transformation. It uses five strategies to systematize the process of collective engagement between the community and research partners as part of the empowerment process. Table 15.2. summarizes these strategies and illustrates the concepts and principles of community engagement in action. Informed by these strategies, PPYEP includes six empowerment modules and five co-design modules, which are summarized in Table 15.3. The empowerment modules focus on building the youths' capacity and capabilities as agents of social change. The co-design modules help develop the youth's capacity to lead the ideation, planning, implementation, and evaluation of an intervention they help develop.

PPYEP was implemented in a rural and an urban community in New Zealand. At each location, the academic partners engaged a Pasifika community member who helped to recruit 41 Pasifika youth between 15 and 24 years old to participate in the program. Delivered weekly over five months, PPYEP activities provided the youth a knowledge base to view themselves as societal agents of social change, and to recognize that their capacity and capabilities (if channelled under propitious conditions) can affect positive change in their communities. They also helped youth think of health in terms of holistic well-being encompassing physical, mental, emotional, social, and spiritual wellness, strengths in

Table 15.2   Strategies Used to Inform the Development of the Pasifika Prediabetes Youth Empowerment Program

Strategy 1: Empowering Communities
- Engaging communities at all stages of the research.
- Identifying pathways of collaborations (planning stage).
- Exploring and planning for future collaborations (planning and evaluation stages).

Strategy 2: Activating Communities
- Identifying and organizing resources (planning stage).
- Engaging end-user involvement in all program processes (all stages).
- Enabling programs to be culturally focused, community-centered, or community-based.

Strategy 3: Targeted Prevention Programs
- Targeting programs based on current evidence (planning stage).
- Identifying national or regional level health and education policies that highlight the needs and priority of health issues and population groups (planning stage).

Strategy 4: Partnership
- Identifying and using the most appropriate approach to work collaboratively with community partners. The PPYEP used co-design with youth to enable innovation in the planning, implementation, and evaluation of the program (planning stage).

Strategy 5: Culturally Tailoring Interventions for Pasifika Populations
- Facilitating the exploration of ways to develop culturally relevant approaches that matched the lived realities of the participants (planning stage).

Table 15.3   Modular Components of the Pasifika Prediabetes Youth Empowerment Program

Module		Objectives
Empowerment modules		
1	Community contract	To outline the goals and challenges of the program. To outline group values and vision.
2	Historical perspectives of healthy lifestyles for Pasifika peoples	To develop a knowledge base of Pasifika healthy lifestyles from social, cultural, generational, and historical contexts.
3	Leadership compass	To identify personal leadership styles and ways to build effective teams.
4	Heart health	To develop capabilities of measuring and interpreting blood pressure and how heart health connects to noncommunicable diseases.
5	Navigating a supermarket	To explore and compare the costs of food for different socioeconomic realities of Pasifika families and learn how to eat healthily on a budget.
6	Community cooking	To cook and prepare a meal using healthy ingredients on a budget of $20.
7	Mental health and wellness	To introduce a Pasifika model of health and co-develop individualized mental health strategies.
Co-design modules		
8	Root-cause analysis	To brainstorm the systematic causes, supporting problems, and visible impacts of prediabetes specific to Pasifika people.
9	Gift + Issue = Change	To brainstorm community intervention ideas and personal skillsets to contribute to social change.
10	S.M.A.R.T. goals	To refine the ideas using the S.M.A.R.T. Goals framework (specific, measurable, attainable, relevant, time-bound).
11	Seven-steps	To develop community intervention implementation roadmaps ideas using the following seven steps: roles, responsibilities, allies, resources, challenges, possible solutions, timeline.

capacity and capability development, and a collaborative approach to health promotion. They learned about health equity in the context of social justice to affect the social, environmental, and cultural determinants of health. As empowerment focuses on building knowledge and skillsets, it also develops the youth researcher's capability to engage with all antagonists of the community.

Of the 41 Pasifika youth who started PPYEP, 29 (71% retention) completed the program. A formative evaluation of these 29 youths' experiences found that the program offered a safe space to develop their knowledge about health and healthy lifestyles and confidence in their leadership ability to make a social change (Prapaveissis et al., 2022). They also believed they had acquired the skills necessary to develop a culturally centered, prediabetes intervention to benefit their communities.

The Pasifika youth of PPYEP later implemented and evaluated the eight-week, community-based prediabetes interventions they co-designed with the research team for a group of adults. They delivered the interventions to 32 Pasifika adults, ages 25–39, who had excess body weight. The program included lessons on healthy eating and physical activity and a group-based four-kilometer walk. At the end of eight weeks, 26 of the 32 participants (81%) completed the entire intervention. This high retention rate was attributed to the close connection between the youth and their community members. A pre- and post-intervention evaluation of the eight-week program showed significant reductions in percent body weight (an average of 2.43% decrease) and waist circumference (an average of 1.6% decrease), and an increase in the total number of steps taken (an average of 47,252 more steps) over eight weeks (Firestone et al., 2021a). Despite the small size of this program, it demonstrates how community engagement and co-design approaches, together, enable a feasible, culturally acceptable method with short-term effectiveness for improving health while building community capacity to address other health concerns.

Benefits and Challenges of Community Engagement

TIPS and PPYEP illustrate the benefits of community engagement by showing how stakeholder input and active involvement strengthen research efficacy. Their use of CBPR also demonstrates how community engagement can support recruitment and implementation. Clinical trials that used CBPR have been shown to achieve good levels of participation of racial and ethnic minority groups (McFarlane et al., 2022). However, this conclusion is preliminary because CBPR has yet to be compared to approaches without community engagement. A recent meta-analysis found some evidence that programs and studies conducted with substantial community engagement can improve health-related behaviors and outcomes in disadvantaged populations with small to medium effect sizes (O'Mara-Eves et al., 2015).

The TIPS study exemplifies how community engagement can expedite the translation of research findings into public health programs and policies. TIPS now is reaching the larger African American community through its implementation in churches as part of the Calvary Community Outreach Network. Engagement of community stakeholders in the development, implementation, and interpretation of research can ensure they are practical, relevant, and sustainable for successful dissemination and implementation (Estabrooks et al., 2018). (see Chapter 16 on Implementation Science.)

Despite the benefits of community engagement, there are challenges. They include considerable time demands on all partners to develop and foster trusting relationships, reconcile cultural and other differences, resolve ethical concerns, establish expectations for partners and funding agencies, and familiarize or train community partners on research protocols (De las Nueces et al., 2012). All these activities, including compensating community partners for their time, require financial resources and time frames beyond what traditional funding sources usually offer (Cole et al., 2013). The time investment needed to develop and foster trusting and equitable relationships may not immediately satisfy traditional benchmarks of success for academic partners or community partners' desire for swift action (Lowry & Ford-Paz, 2013). There is a need to balance scientific rigor and standards with the needs, expectations, and capacity of the community.

Discussion and Conclusion

Community engagement is a highly valued and widely practiced approach to developing effective and sustainable health behavior and health equity programs and to conducting health-related research with real-world impact. It is a paradigm shift away from the traditional hierarchical approach that privileges the academic and scientific perspective to a collaborative approach that values and recognizes diverse perspectives and the community's autonomy in health promotion and research. It is a strength-based approach to empower and engage communities in building their capacity to address their most pressing health problems and ensure fair and equitable treatment. For these reasons, it is strongly promoted by public health agencies and funders and widely applied by practitioners and researchers from disciplines with a shared goal to improve human health, such as public health, medicine, nursing, psychology, and social work.

At the very core of community engagement is social justice and addressing social determinants of health. It is especially meaningful when it involves marginalized communities, and addresses overarching social issues such as dismantling structural racism, ensuring access to quality health care, promoting neighborhood safety, and obtaining livable wages. It is most effective when the historical and cultural context of the community is respected and integrated; the social determinants of health are targeted for improvement; community partners are engaged before starting a research or health promotion project; a trusting relationship among all partners is built and nurtured over time; and community capacity is assessed and built upon to leverage community assets and resources.

CBPR applies the concepts, principles, and practices of community engagement in the research context. It is a highly collaborative research approach that involves community organizations, leaders, and members in all phases of research—from conceptualization to dissemination—as co-producers of research. Various research designs can be embedded in the CBPR context. CBPR is used to co-design a research agenda and tailor interventions for different populations, settings, and contexts. Although rigorous comparative effectiveness studies of CBPR have yet to be done, CBPR does appear to improve the recruitment and retention of historically underrepresented populations in programs and research (McFarlane et al., 2022), the efficiency and ecological validity of the research (Collins et al., 2018), and targeted psychosocial and health outcomes (O'Mara-Eves et al., 2015).

Despite the prominence of community engagement, there are many practice-related and methodological challenges to community-engaged programs and research. There are also ethical questions to resolve (Glanz et al., 2010). For example, institutional review boards are designed to evaluate the risks and benefits of research to individual participants, but what about the risk and benefits to an entire community? Should entire communities or their governing bodies consent to research? Who should own or have a say in how data from community members should be collected, stored, analyzed, and shared?

Although community engagement involves important challenges, the potential benefits are fundamental to improving health and health equity. Community stakeholders need to be part of the solution—lending their voices, experiences, and skills—to solve their most pressing health concerns in ways that make sense for their community context. In doing so, the solutions developed are more likely to be practicable, acceptable, and sustainable. A popular slogan used by activists for social change—initially attributed to the disability rights movement—sums up the intent of community engagement: "Nothing about us without us."

References

Berkley-Patton, J., Thompson, C. B., Martinez, D. A., Hawes, S. M., Moore, E., Williams, E., & Wainright, C. (2013). Examining church capacity to develop and disseminate a religiously appropriate HIV tool kit with African American churches. *Journal of Urban Health*, *90*(3), 482–499. https://doi.org/10.1007/s11524-012-9740-4

Berkley-Patton, J. Y., Thompson, C. B., Moore, E., Hawes, S., Berman, M., Allsworth, J., Williams, E., Wainright, C., Bradley-Ewing, A., Bauer, A. G., Catley, D. & Goggin, K. (2019). Feasibility and outcomes of an HIV testing intervention in African American churches. *AIDS and Behavior*, *23*(1), 76–90. https://doi.org/10.1007/s10461-018-2240-0

Boursaw, B., Oetzel, J. G., Dickson, E., Thein, T. S., Sanchez-Youngman, S., Peña, J., Parker, M., Magarati, M., Littledeer, L., Duran, B., & Wallerstein, N. (2021). Scales of practices and outcomes for community-engaged research. *American Journal of Community Psychology*, *67*, 256–270. https://doi.org/10.1002/ajcp.12503

Braveman, P., Arkin, E., Orleans, T., Proctor, D., & Plough, A. (2017). *What is health equity? And what difference does a definition make?* Robert Wood Johnson Foundation.

Centers for Disease Control and Prevention (1997). *Principles of community engagement* (1st ed.). CDC/ATSDR Committee on Community Engagement.

Center for Disease Control and Prevention (2021). Estimated HIV incidence and prevalence in the United States, 2015–2019. http://www.cdc.gov/hiv/library/reports/hiv-surveillance.html

Cole, C. A., Edelman, E. J., Boshnack, N., Jenkins, H., Richardson, W., & Rosenthal, M. S. (2013). Time, dual roles, and departments of public health: Lessons learned in CBPR by an AIDS service organization. *Progress in Community Health Partnerships*, *7*(3), 323–330. https://doi.org/10.1353/cpr.2013.0034

Collins, S. E., Clifasefi, S. L., Stanton, J., The Leap Advisory Board, Straits, K. J. E., Gil-Kashiwabara, E., Rodriguez Espinosa, P., Nicasio, A. V., Andrasik, M. P., Hawes, S. M., Miller, K. A., Nelson, L. A., & Wallerstein, N. (2018). Community-based participatory research (CBPR): Towards equitable involvement of community in psychology research. *American Psychologist*, *73*(7), 884–898. https://doi.org/10.1037/amp0000167

Coppell, K. J., Mann, J. I., Williams, S. M., Jo, E., Drury, P. L., Miller, J. C., & Parnell, W. R. (2013). Prevalence of diagnosed and undiagnosed diabetes and prediabetes in New Zealand: Findings from the 2008/09 Adult Nutrition Survey. *New Zealand Medical Journal*, *126*(1370), 23–42. http://journal.nzma.org.nz/journal/126-1370/5555/

De las Nueces, D., Hacker, K., DiGirolamo, A., & Hicks, L. S. (2012). A systematic review of community-based participatory research to enhance clinical trials in racial and ethnic minority groups. *Health Services Research*, *47*(3 Pt 2), 1363–1386. https://doi.org/10.1111/j.1475-6773.2012.01386.x

Duran, B., Wallerstein, N., Minkler, M., Foley, K., Avila, M., & Belone, L. (2012). Initiating and maintaining partnerships. In B. Israel, E. Eng, A. Schulz, & E. Parker (Eds.), *Methods in community based participatory research* (2nd ed., pp. 43–68). Jossey-Bass.

Estabrooks, P. A., Brownson, R. C., & Pronk, N. P. (2018). Dissemination and implementation science for public health professionals: An overview and call to action. *Preventing Chronic Disease*, *15*, E162. https://doi.org/10.5888/pcd15.180525

Fellin, P. (2001). *The Community and the Social Worker* (3rd ed.). F. E. Peacock.

Freire, P. (2018). *Pedagogy of the oppressed* (4th ed.). Bloomsbury Academic.

Firestone, R., Faeamani, G., Okiama, E., Funaki, T., Henry, A., Prapavessis, D., Filikitonga, J., Firestone, J., Tiatia-Seath, J., Matheson, A., Brown, B., Ellison-Loschmann L. (2021a). Pasifika Prediabetes Youth Empowerment Programme: Evaluating the intervention from a participants' perspective. *Kōtuitui: New Zealand Journal of Social Sciences Online*, *16*(1), 210–224. https://doi.org/10.1080/1177083X.2021.1876743

Firestone, R., Matherson, A., Firestone, J., Schleser, M., Yee, M., Tuisano, H., Kaholokula, K. A., & Ellison-Loschmann, L. (2021b). Developing principles of social change as a result of a Pasifika Youth Empowerment Programme: A qualitative study. *Health Promotion Journal of Australia*, *32*(S2),197–205. https://doi.org/10.1002/hpja.395

Glanz, K., Kegler, M. C., & Rimer, B. K. (2010). Ethical issues in the design and conduct of community-based intervention studies. In S. Coughlin, T. Beauchamp, D. Weed (Eds.), *Ethics in epidemiology* (pp. 103–127) (2nd ed.). Oxford University Press.

Goodkind, J. R., Amer, S., Christian, C., Hess, J. M., Bybee, D., Isakson, B. L., Baca, B., Ndayisenga, M., Greene, R. N., & Shantzek, C. (2017). Challenges and innovations in a community-based participatory randomized controlled trial. *Health Education & Behavior*, *44*(1), 123–130. https://doi.org/10.1177/1090198116639243

Hunter, C. M., Chou, W. Y. S., & Webb Hooper, M. (2021). Behavioral and social science in support of SARS-CoV-2 vaccination: National Institutes of Health initiatives. *Translational Behavioral Medicine*, *11*(7), 1354–1358. https://doi.org/10.1093/tbm/ibab067

Israel, B. A., Eng, E., Schulz, A. J., & Parker, E. A. (Eds.). (2013). *Methods for community-based participatory research for health* (2nd ed.). Jossey-Bass.

Israel, B. A., Schulz, A. J., Parker, E. A., & Becker, A. B. (1998). Review of community-based research: Assessing partnership approaches to improve public health. *Annual Review of Public Health*, *19*, 173–202. https://doi.org/10.1146/annurev.publhealth.19.1.173

Kaholokula, J. K., Look, M., Mabellos, T., Ahn, H. J., Choi, S. Y., Sinclair, K. A., Wills, T. A., Seto, T. B., de Silva, M. (2021). A cultural dance program improves hypertension control and cardiovascular disease risk in Native Hawaiians: A randomized controlled trial. *Annals of Behavioral Medicine*, *55*(10), 1006–1018. https//doi.org/10.1093/abm/kaaa127

Kalra, S., Akanov, Z. A., & Pleshkova, A. Y. (2018). Thoughts, words, action: The Alma-Ata Declaration to Diabetes Care Transformation. *Diabetes Therapy*, *9*(3), 873–876. https://doi.org/10.1007/s13300-018-0440-2

Laird, P., Chang, A. B., Jacky, J., Lane, M., Schultz, A., & Walker, R. (2021). Conducting decolonizing research and practice with Australian First Nations to close the health gap. *Health Research Policy and Systems*, *19*(1), 127. https://doi.org/10.1186/s12961-021-00773-3

Laverack, G. (2007) *Health promotion practice: Building empowered communities*. Open University Press.

Lee, S. S. (2014). Using fuzzy-set qualitative comparative analysis. *Epidemiology and Health*, *36*, e2014038. https://doi.org/10.4178/epih/e2014038

Lowry, K. W., & Ford-Paz, R. (2013). Early career academic researchers and community-based participatory research: Wrestling match or dancing partners? *Clinical and Translational Science*, *6*(6), 490–492. https://doi.org/10.1111/cts.12045

Luger, T. M., Hamilton, A. B., & True, G. (2020). Measuring community-engaged research contexts, processes, and outcomes: A mapping review. *The Milbank Quarterly*, *98*, 493–553. https://doi.org/10.1111/1468-0009.12458

Maton, K. (2008). Empowering community settings: Agents of individual development, community betterment, and positive social change. *American Journal of Community Psychology*, *41*(1), 4–21. https://doi.org/10.1007/s10464-007-9148-6

McCartney, A. M., Anderson, J., Liggins, L., Hudson, M. L., Anderson, M. Z., TeAika, B., Geary, J., Cook-Deegan, R., Patel, H. R., & Phillippy, A. M. (2022). Balancing openness with indigenous data sovereignty: An opportunity to leave no one behind in the journey to sequence all of life. *Proceedings of the National Academy of Sciences of the United States*, *119*(4), 3–41. https://doi.org/10.1073/pnas.2115860119

McCloskey, D. J., McDonald, M. A., Cook, J., Heurtin-Roberts, S., Updegrove, S., Sampson, D., Gutter, S. & Eder, M. (2011). Principles of community engagement: Definitions and organizing concepts from the literature. In Clinical and Translational Science Awards Consortium Community Engagement Key Function Committee, Task Force on the Principles of Community Engagement (Ed.), *Principles of community engagement* (2nd ed.). National Institutes of Health.

McFarlane, S. J., Occa, A., Peng, W., Awonuga, O., & Morgan, S. E. (2022). Community-based participatory research (CBPR) to enhance participation of racial/ethnic minorities in clinical trials: A 10-year systematic review. *Health Communication*, *37*, 1075–1092. https://doi.org/10.1080/10410236.2021.1943978

Michener, L., Aguilar-Gaxiola, S., Alberti, P. M., Castaneda, M. J., Castrucci, B. C., Harrison, L., Hughes, L. S., Richmond, A., & Wallerstein, N. (2020). Engaging with communities—Lessons (Re)learned from COVID-19. *Preventing Chronic Disease*, *17*, E65. https://doi.org/10.5888/pcd17.200250

Minkler, M., Wallerstein, N., & Wilson, N. (2008). Improving health through community organization and community building. In K. Glanz, B. K. Rimer, & F. M. Lewis (Eds.), *Health behavior and health education: Theory, research, and practice* (4th ed., pp. 287–312). John Wiley & Sons.

Nicholson, V., Bratu, A., McClean, A. R., Jawanda, S., Aran, N., Hillstrom, K., Hennie, E., Cardinal, C., Benson, E., Beaver, K., Benoit, A. C., Jaworsky, D. (2021). Indigenizing our research: Indigenous community leadership in HIV epidemiology research. *International Journal of Population Data Science*, *6*(1), 1386. https://doi.org/10.23889/ijpds.v6i1.1386

Oetzel, J. G., Boursaw, B., Magarati, M., Dickson, E., Sanchez-Youngman, S., Morales, L., Kastelic, S., Eder, M. M., Wallerstein, N. (2022). Exploring theoretical mechanisms of community-engaged research: A multilevel cross-sectional national study of structural and relational practices in community-academic partnerships. *International Journal for Equity in Health*, *21*, 59. https://doi.org/10.1186/s12939-022-01663-y

Oetzel, J., Scott, N., Hudson, M., Masters, B., Rarere, M., Foote, J., Beaton, A., & Ehau, T. (2017). He Pikinga Waiora Implementation Framework: A tool for chronic disease intervention effectiveness in Māori and other indigenous communities. *International Journal of Integrated Care*, *18*. https://doi.org/10.5334/ijic.s1068

O'Mara-Eves, A., Brunton, G., Oliver, S., Kavanagh, J., Jamal, F., & Thomas, J. (2015). The effectiveness of community engagement in public health interventions for disadvantaged groups: A meta-analysis. *BMC Public Health*, *15*(1), 1352. https://doi.org/10.1186/s12889-015-1352-y

Patten, C. A., Balls-Berry, J. J. E., Cohen, E. L., Brockman, T. A., Valdez Soto, M., West, I. W., Cha, J., Rocha, M. G., & Eder, M. M. (2021). Feasibility of a virtual Facebook community platform for engagement on health research. *Journal of Clinical and Translational Science*, *5*(1), e85. https://doi.org/10.1017/cts.2021.12

Peterson, N. A., Speer, P. W., & Hughey, J. (2006). Measuring sense of community: A methodological interpretation of the factor structure debate. *Journal of Community Psychology*, *34*(4), 453–469. https://doi.org/10.1002/jcop.20109

Prapaveissis, D., Henry, A., Okiama, E., Funaki, T., Faeamani, G., Masaga, J., Brown, B., Kaholokula, K., Ing, C., Matheson, A., Tupai-Firestone, R. (2022). Assessing youth empowerment and co-design to advance Pasifika health: A qualitative research study in New Zealand. *Australian and New Zealand Journal of Public Health*, *46*(1), 56–61. https://doi.org/10.1111/1753-6405.13187

Prussing, E. & Newbury, E. (2016). Neoliberalism and indigenous knowledge: Māori health research and the cultural politics of New Zealand's "National Science Challenges". *Social Science & Medicine*, *150*(C), 57–66. https://doi.org/10.1016/j.socscimed.2015.12.012

Richmond, L. S., Peterson, D. J., & Betts, S. C. (2008). The evolution of an evaluation: A case study using the tribal participatory research model. *Health Promotion Practice*, *9*(4), 368–377. https://doi.org/10.1177/1524839906289069

Rosenthal, E. L., Balcazar, H. G., De Heer, H. D., Wise, S., Flores, L., & Aguirre, M. (2014). Critical reflections on the role of CBPR within an RCT community health worker prevention intervention. *The Journal of Ambulatory Care Management*, *37*(3), 241–249. https://doi.org/10.1097/JAC.0000000000000010

Ross, R. (2016). Preface. In A. Bracho, G. Lee, G. P. Giraldo, R. M. De Prado (Eds.), *Recruiting the heart, training the brain* (pp. ix–xii). Hesperian Health Guides.

Rothman, J. (2001). Approaches to community intervention. In J. Rothman, J. L. Erlich, & J. E. Tropman (Eds.), *Strategies of community intervention* (6th ed., pp. 27–64). Peacock.

Rothman, J., & Tropman, J. E. (1987). Models of community organizing and macro practice perspectives: Their mixing and phasing. In F. M. Cox, J. L. Erlich, J. Rothman, & J. E. Tropman (Eds.), *Strategies of community organization: Macro practice* (pp. 3–25). Peacock.

Russell, N., Igras, S., Kuoh, H., Pavin, M., & Wickerstrom, J. (2008). The active community engagement continuum. *ACQUIRE Project Working Paper*. https://edadm821.files.wordpress.com/2010/11/ace-working-paper-final.pdf

Ryan, R. M., & Deci, E. L. (2017). *Self-determination theory: Basic psychological needs in motivation, development, and wellness.* Guilford Press.

Sanchez-Youngman, S., Boursaw, B., Oetzel, J. G., Kastelic, S., Scarpetta, M., Devia, C., Scarpetta, M., Belone, L. & Wallerstein, N. (2021). Structural community governance: Importance for community-academic research partnerships. *American Journal of Community Psychology*, *67*, 271–283. https://doi.org/10.1002/ajcp.12505

Sandoval, J. A., Lucero, J., Oetzel, J., Avila, M., Belone, L., Mau, M., Pearson, C., Tafoya, G., Duran, B., Iglesias Rios, L., & Wallerstein, N. (2012). Process and outcome constructs for evaluating community-based participatory research projects: A matrix of existing measures. *Health Education Research*, *27*(4), 680–690. https://doi.org/10.1093/her/cyr087

Smith, B. J., Tang, K. C., & Nutbeam, D. (2006). WHO health promotion glossary: New terms. *Health Promotion International*, *21*(4), 340–345. https://doi.org/10.1093/heapro/dal033

Staples, L. (2004). *Roots to power: A manual for grassroots organizing.* Praeger.

Tigges, B., Miller, D., Dudding, K., Balls-Berry, J., Borawski, E., Dave, G., Hafer, N. S., Kimminau, K. S., Kost, R. G., Littlefield, K., Shannon, J., & The Measures of Collaboration Workgroup of the Collaboration and Engagement Domain Task Force, National Center for Advancing Translational Sciences, National Institutes of Health (2019). Measuring quality and outcomes of research collaborations: An integrative review. *Journal of Clinical and Translational Science*, *11*, 261–289. https://doi.org/10.1017/cts.2019.402

Trickett, E. J. (2011). Community-based participatory research as worldview or instrumental strategy: Is it lost in translation(al) research? *American Journal of Public Health*, *101*(8), 1353–1355. https://doi.org/10.2105/AJPH.2011.300124

Wallerstein, N. (2006). What is the evidence on effectiveness of empowerment to improve health? *Health Evidence Network Report.* http://www.euro.who.int/Document/E88086.pdf

Wallerstein, N., Boursaw, B., Eder, M., Kastelic, S., Ward, M., & Oetzel, J. G. (2024) (in press). Community engagement measures and assessments of promising practices. In *Principles of community engagement*, (3rd ed.) National Institutes of Health.

Wallerstein, N., Duran, B., Oetzel, J., & Minkler, M. (Eds.). (2018). *Community-based participatory research for health: Advancing Social and Health Equity* (3rd ed.). Jossey-Bass.

Wallerstein, N., Muhammad, M., Sanchez-Youngman, S., Rodriguez Espinosa, P., Avila, M., Baker, E. A., Barnett, S., Belone, L., Golub, M., Lucero, J., Mahdi, I., Duran, B. (2019). Power dynamics in community-based participatory research: A multiple-case study analysis of partnering contexts, histories, and practices. *Health Education & Behavior*, *46*, 19s–32s. https://doi.org/10.1177/1090198119852998

Wallerstein, N., Oetzel, J. G., Sanchez-Youngman, S., Boursaw, B., Dickson, E., Kastelic, S., Koegel, P., Lucero, J. E., Magarati, M., Ortiz, K., Parker, M., Duran, B. (2020). Engage for equity: A long-term study of community-based participatory research and community-engaged research practices and outcomes. *Health Education & Behavior*, *47*, 380–390. https://doi.org/10.1177/1090198119897075

Windsor, L. C., Jemal, A., Goffnett, J., Smith, D. C., & Sarol, J., Jr. (2022). Linking critical consciousness and health: The utility of the critical reflection about social determinants of health scale (CR_SDH). *SSM Population Health*, *17*, 101034. https://doi.org/10.1016/j.ssmph.2022.101034

World Health Organization (1986). Ottawa charter for health promotion. https://www.who.int/publications/i/item/ottawa-charter-for-health-promotion

World Health Organization (2020). Community engagement: A health promotion guide for universal health coverage in the hands of the people. Licence: CC BY-NC-SA 3.0 IGO.

World Health Organization (2022). Constitution: WHO remains firmly committed to the principles set out in the preamble to the Constitution. https://www.who.int/about/governance/constitution

World Health Organization's Commission on Social Determinants of Health (2008). Closing the gap in a generation: Health equity through action on the social determinants of health. *Final Report of the Commission on Social Determinants of Health*. https://www.who.int/publications/i/item/WHO-IER-CSDH-08.1

Zimmerman, M. (2000). Empowerment theory. In J. Rappaport & E. Seidman (Eds.), *Handbook of community psychology* (pp. 43–63). Springer.

CHAPTER 16

IMPLEMENTATION, DISSEMINATION, AND DIFFUSION OF PUBLIC HEALTH INNOVATIONS

Shoba Ramanadhan
Rachel C. Shelton

KEY POINTS

This chapter will:

- Introduce dissemination and implementation science and practice, including historical foundations and core terminology.

- Present an overview of key theories, models, and frameworks that inform and advance dissemination and implementation science and practice.

- Provide detailed descriptions of two commonly used dissemination and implementation science theories and frameworks: Diffusion of Innovations and the Consolidated Framework for Implementation Research (CFIR).

- Use applications for theories and frameworks in dissemination and implementation research to illustrate key concepts and features.

- Describe study designs and methods common to dissemination and implementation science and practice.

- Identify challenges and opportunities to enhance the impact of dissemination and implementation science and practice.

Vignette

A research team developed an intervention for pediatric medical practices to improve nutrition among elementary-school-age children at risk for diabetes. The program focuses on improving provider communication with families, presenting nutritional guidelines in culturally appropriate ways, and facilitating access to low-cost, healthy foods. It is effective in improving nutrition among children at well-resourced pediatric practices in New York City. However, the team is concerned that the current resource-intensive program will only reach children who regularly see pediatricians in higher-income neighborhood and clinic settings. The team wants to partner with local afterschool programs to broaden the program's reach and impact. They created a manual and provided educational materials and training resources to several afterschool programs.

When the researchers checked in with these sites a few months later, they discovered a range of challenges to using the program. Some program staff said the materials were not culturally appropriate and did not reflect the needs of the children they serve. Others said they did not have the time to run the entire program. So, they just picked a few relevant pieces. A few afterschool site leaders said that they were running the program according to the program manual but were not seeing improvements among participating children. The research team remains committed to making the program work in a broader range of settings but is unsure of how best to address these barriers to program delivery.

This vignette highlights some common barriers and issues that researchers, practitioners, and other program developers encounter when trying to expand the reach, sustainability, and impact of an evidence-based intervention (EBI) or public health innovation. The team must consider how best to disseminate the program (that is, actively support its initial uptake and adoption) for afterschool sites in the community. Additionally, they must consider common barriers to and facilitators of EBI implementation (that is, the integration of the program into the practice site). First, in collaboration with partners, the research team should examine whether program materials and program components should be adapted or refined to better

Health Behavior: Theory, Research, and Practice, Sixth Edition. Edited by Karen Glanz, Barbara K. Rimer, and K. Viswanath.
© 2024 John Wiley & Sons, Inc. Published 2024 by John Wiley & Sons, Inc.
Companion website: www.wiley.com/go/glanz/healthbehavior6e

align with the populations served. Second, researchers should work with site leadership to determine how to support implementation and address barriers to delivery in this setting. The team might also take a closer look at tracking implementation outcomes of interest, such as how many sites or staff have adopted and fully delivered the program. By understanding and addressing these considerations, the team can increase the likelihood of successful implementation and associated improvements in health. Theories and frameworks from dissemination and implementation science can inform understanding, tracking, and planning for the successful adoption, integration, and sustainability of EBIs across a range of topics and diverse community, public health, and healthcare settings.

Introduction to Dissemination and Implementation Science

Despite investments by governments, funders, and others, many health-related EBIs are not widely used across diverse settings. This has major implications for population health. For example, estimates suggest that 44% of global cancer deaths in 2019 could be attributed to a core set of risk factors (e.g., tobacco and alcohol use), highlighting the importance of implementing preventive strategies broadly and equitably (Tran et al., 2022). Dissemination and implementation science seeks to understand how to actively increase the adoption, implementation, and continued use of health-enhancing EBIs and innovations. The designation of EBI can apply to a wide range of entities, such as programs (e.g., behavioral interventions to manage diabetes), practices (e.g., routine screening for social needs in primary care), policies (e.g., smoke-free indoor spaces), and treatments (e.g., the meningitis vaccine).

At the outset, it is essential to distinguish between efforts to establish the effectiveness of interventions from efforts to promote their dissemination and implementation. Often, dissemination and implementation activities begin after an innovation has demonstrated effectiveness for changing health behaviors or health outcomes of interest, highlighted in the example of the nutrition program described in the vignette above. Ideally, innovations in health should be "designed for dissemination," which can accelerate successful uptake and promote health equity (Kwan et al., 2022).

Dissemination involves planned efforts to reach audiences and stakeholders with information about EBIs and strategies to facilitate their adoption or uptake (Baumann et al., 2022). By contrast, *implementation* refers to active and planned efforts to support adoption and integration of EBIs into routine practice in community, clinical, and public health settings. Effectiveness research is a first step in which innovations are tested and, when successful, considered to be EBIs. Implementation research addresses different core questions: How does context influence EBI implementation? What strategies can help implementers use EBIs? And how can we know if implementation efforts are successful? (Curran, 2020; Smith et al., 2020).

With roots in sociology, psychology, organizational behavior, agriculture, and development, dissemination, and implementation science emphasizes the application of evidence-based solutions to public health problems to increase the likelihood of their impact (Brownson et al., 2011). Historically, the work of Georg Simmel and Gabriel Tarde catalyzed conversation in the early 1900s about system-level forces within and across networks and social systems that influence the spread of new ideas and practices (Dearing, 2008). Action research by Lewin (1946), Diffusion of Innovations by Rogers (2003), and practice-based evidence by Green (2008) are important influences on dissemination and implementation science. This work underscores the importance of developing evidence with dissemination and implementation in mind, engaging communities and partners to identify solutions, and examining multilevel influences on the spread of evidence-based solutions.

Dissemination and implementation efforts vary in terms of the time it takes for an EBI to become routinely used, the extent to which services are distributed equitably, and the scale of impact. For example, the development of therapeutics and vaccines during the COVID-19 pandemic showed how innovations can be developed rapidly and disseminated widely; although the underlying science had already been underway for decades, the new vaccines were deployed quickly. The pandemic also highlighted many persistent challenges in facilitating adoption and implementation equitably and at scale (Chambers, 2020). In contrast to this example of rapid translation, commonly cited estimates of the time lag between establishing effectiveness of clinical preventive services and medical treatments to widespread translation in practice are 15–17 years (Balas & Boren, 2000; Khan et al., 2021). Many factors contribute to the time it takes for EBI use to become widely accepted, recommended in guidelines, and part of routine practice. Time to translation (i.e., dissemination and implementation) varies based on the types of EBIs, their costs, and differences in the targets of behavior change and implementation contexts (Morris et al., 2011). Even with such variation in time to adoption, planning for dissemination and implementation can increase the speed of knowledge translation and the likelihood of equitable delivery. There is no available systematic analysis of the time from development to dissemination of behavioral and community-based health interventions, which could parallel clinical services or be faster in the age of the Internet and viral social media.

What is Accepted Evidence for an EBI?

With the goal of spreading EBIs at scale and equitably, researchers and practitioners should reflect on the nature of the evidence base (Brownson et al., 2022). A critical perspective prompts attention to what "counts" as an EBI and the extent to which context, equity, and stakeholder perspectives influence the existing evidence base. Regarding what counts as evidence, often large-scale randomized trials, systematic reviews, and meta-analyses are the basis for determining whether an EBI is effective and ready for widespread dissemination. *The Methods Manual for Community Guide Systematic Reviews* describes a methodology that considers the strength of evidence and execution of efficacy studies as a basis for public health intervention recommendations (Guide to Community Preventive Services, 2023). There are also resources to identify EBIs; databases in the United States include the Evidence-based Cancer Control Programs from the National Cancer Institute (2020) and the Evidence-based Practices Resource Center from the Substance Abuse and Mental Health Services Administration (2022).

Controlled trials provide strong tests of internal validity ("does it work in a controlled study?") but are less helpful in understanding its efficacy when implemented in less-controlled settings. This can limit understanding of where and among whom the EBI is effective and can potentially exclude a range of health issues, populations, and settings. Additionally, most EBIs were not developed and tested in a broad range of settings with variable resources, among diverse populations, and with stakeholder engagement informing the process, which limits the evidence about their potential for broad impact. To attend to these gaps, researchers and program developers can engage early and often with communities so that interventions and implementation strategies are developed and evaluated with an eye toward equity from the outset (Ramanadhan & Viswanath, 2018; Shelton et al., 2024). Funders also should assure that researchers are conducting research with socially disadvantaged and low-resource communities.

As with many growing areas of scholarship, varying terminology is used to refer to dissemination and implementation science. Other terms include knowledge translation, translational research, and knowledge transfer. Table 16.1 provides key terms and definitions. A glossary by Rabin et al. (2008) offers additional detail. Readers may wish to look at additional resources that provide greater detail about the fundamentals of dissemination and implementation research (Brownson et al., 2018).

Conceptualizing Dissemination and Implementation

Dissemination and implementation activities can be thought of as a series of steps, much like the program planning and evaluation process (see Chapter 19 on Planning Models). As seen in Figure 16.1, and described below, dissemination efforts seek to spread EBIs, and implementers engage with EBIs through a series of steps to facilitate their delivery within specific settings.

Dissemination Activities

Since most effective innovations do not spread without planning, persuasion, and action, a "designing for dissemination" lens prompts intervention developers to address the needs and resources of future adopters and implementers (Kwan et al., 2022). In the past, too often, researchers thought about dissemination after demonstrating effectiveness of an intervention. This often is too late because the intervention elements may be valid but not feasible for organizations to adopt. Working with organizations from the beginning can help assure that intervention elements will be adopted, if effective. Such an approach keeps stakeholders at the center of the development and tailoring of strategies to facilitate dissemination. Co-creation of interventions can help assure that community needs are addressed. It is also respectful of communities and other partners. Such a perspective addresses the development of both dissemination products

Table 16.1   Core Terms and Definitions in Dissemination and Implementation Science, in Alphabetical Order

Term	Definition
Diffusion	The passive, untargeted, unplanned, and uncontrolled spread of new interventions. Diffusion is part of the diffusion-dissemination-implementation continuum and it is the least focused and intense approach (Lomas, 1993; MacLean, 1996).
De-implementation	Decreasing or stopping the use of an intervention, e.g., when it is determined to be ineffective, harmful, or low value. This may happen when additional information about the information becomes available or when better alternatives emerge (Norton et al., 2017).
Dissemination	The active approach of spreading EBIs to target audiences using planned strategies (Brownson et al., 2013).
Evidence-Based Interventions (EBIs)	Interventions with proven efficacy and effectiveness; they serve as the focus and foundation of dissemination and implementation activities. EBIs may include programs/interventions, practices, processes, policies, treatments, and guidelines (Rabin et al., 2008).
Fidelity	The extent to which the intervention was delivered as planned. Recently, more attention has focused on (1) preserving the function, rather than the form, of an EBI and (2) examining the fidelity as it relates to the delivery of implementation strategies (Hawe et al., 2004; Shelton et al., 2023).
Implementation	The use of strategies to promote the adoption and integration of EBIs into routine practice in clinical, community, and public health settings (National Institutes of Health, 2019).
Implementation Determinants	Factors at multiple levels that are expected to influence implementation outcomes, e.g., implementers' attitudes towards the EBI influence (Nilsen, 2015).
Implementation Outcomes	The impacts of intentional actions to support EBI implementation. They serve as indicators of implementation success (versus intervention success), support examination of implementation processes, and serve as intermediate outcomes for service and health outcomes (Proctor et al., 2011). Common outcomes include acceptability, fidelity, cost, and sustainability.
Innovation	An idea, practice, or object that is perceived as new by an individual or other unit of adoption (Rogers, 2003)
Implementation Strategies	Approaches to increase the adoption, implementation, and sustainment of EBIs (Powell et al., 2015). They can be individual or bundled strategies that seek to target change among important players in implementation systems, e.g., changing incentives among providers to promote EBI use (Powell et al., 2019).
Sustainability	A state in which after a defined period of time, an EBI and/or implementation strategies continue to be delivered. This supports continued individual behavior change is maintained and the program and behavior change may evolve or adapt while continuing to produce benefits for individuals/systems (Moore et al., 2017).
Knowledge Translation	Knowledge translation occurs within a complex social system of interactions between researchers and knowledge users and with the purpose of improving population health, providing more effective health services and products, and strengthening the health care system. It is a dynamic and iterative process that includes synthesis, dissemination, exchange and application of knowledge (McLean and Tucker, 2013).

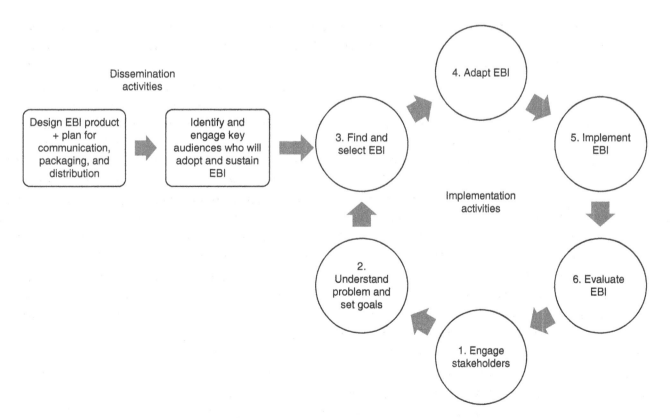

Figure 16.1   Simplified, Illustrative Process for Identifying and Implementing an EBI in Practice Settings, Adapted from the Cancer Prevention and Control Research Network (2017) and the Designing for Dissemination and Sustainability Schema (Kwan et al., 2022). EBI: Evidence-Based Intervention

(e.g., manuals and toolkits with EBI content, tailored to potential adopters in that context) and dissemination activities (e.g., using tailored communication and guidance to support a network of institutions to adopt an EBI). Connecting back to the initial vignette, a designing for dissemination approach might include: (1) establishing the effectiveness of the program for ultimate use in accessible community settings instead of only well-resourced pediatrician's offices, (2) manualizing the program and creating plans to distribute the program, (3) engaging afterschool program leaders and staff who will adopt and sustain the program, and (4) tracking adoption, implementation, and sustainment of the program, particularly with attention to which settings and populations are not reached or able to adopt the program.

Many focused dissemination strategies are used in public health, ranging from databases of EBIs and active outreach by program developers to policy guidelines or targeted communication to policymakers. Additionally, research teams that have developed EBIs may seek dissemination and implementation partners and organizations for more widespread adoption and delivery and may facilitate active dissemination efforts in those settings. Ideally, such partnerships were built into the original program design.

Implementation Activities

Once implementation processes are underway, they should be seen as part of a cyclical and iterative process (see Figure 16.1), with each round of action and learning informing the next to improve evidence-based offerings continually. The following six steps, adapted from the work of the Cancer Prevention and Control Research Network (2017), offer an overview of key implementation activities. The steps may not always be used in a linear manner, but they cover activities that are useful for implementation:

1. *Engage stakeholders:* Researchers or practitioners should start by partnering with relevant stakeholders in the intended implementation settings. Stakeholders may include patients, community members, providers and practitioners, purchasers, organizational leaders, administrators, policymakers, program developers, and researchers (Concannon et al., 2012).

2. *Identify needs and set goals:* Researchers and/or practitioners work with other stakeholders in the setting to identify priority health need(s), goals, and realistic targets for improvement.

3. *Find and select EBI(s):* The implementing organization works with the identified stakeholders to find an EBI that addresses their health concerns. Organizations may select EBIs based on the strength of the underlying evidence, costs, fit with implementation context, appropriateness for the population, and other organizational or contextual factors.

4. *Adapt EBI:* The implementing organization plans and executes adjustments to the EBI to support its delivery and integration. The goal is to balance staying true to the original EBI (or maintaining fidelity to the core components deemed necessary to improve health outcomes) while making strategic adaptations to increase relevance, appropriateness, and acceptability for the new setting or population. It is useful at this stage to understand barriers and facilitators to implementation and identify possible supports that will help implementers and organizations use the EBI within the intended setting (e.g., schools, worksites, clinics). These supports are called implementation strategies and may include identifying champions, providing training or technical assistance, engaging leadership, or changing incentives for practitioners (Powell et al., 2015). Strategies are customized for the implementation setting and specific barriers to delivery for that particular EBI. Thus, training may be critical to support delivery of one EBI, whereas changing incentive structures might be critical for another EBI implemented at the same site.

5. *Implement EBI:* Implementers deliver the EBI according to the implementation plan and monitor this process to make needed refinements to facilitate success. Additional strategies, such as changing staff incentives or aligning with a changing policy environment, may be required if implementation is not going according to plan. It is crucial to track and evaluate the success of implementation strategies, including their impact on key implementation outcomes (e.g., acceptability, adoption, fidelity of delivery, and costs) (Proctor et al., 2011).

6. *Sustain EBI:* The organization where the EBI is implemented can plan for and monitor the ability to institutionalize or maintain the delivery and impact of the program over time. Frameworks and models like the Reach, Effectiveness, Adoption, Implementation, and Maintenance (RE-AIM) extension (Shelton et al., 2020) and the Program Sustainability Assessment Tool (Luke et al., 2014) can be used to inform and track sustainability over time.

Introduction to Key Dissemination and Implementation Frameworks

A variety of theories, models, and frameworks have been developed to understand how innovations spread and to promote dissemination and implementation of EBIs (Explore D&I TMFs, 2023; Tabak et al., 2012). While there are differences between theories, models, and frameworks, these descriptors usually are not strictly defined (see Chapter 2), so "frameworks" is used here as an umbrella term. There are at least three main types of dissemination and implementation frameworks:

Determinant frameworks can help researchers and practitioners understand and intervene in factors influencing the uptake and implementation of innovations and EBIs. These frameworks address characteristics of EBIs, implementers, organizational contexts, and policy environments. The widely used classic theory, Diffusion of Innovations, offers insight from diverse fields to explore the "hows and whys" of dissemination and implementation efforts by characterizing the properties of innovations, adopters, social systems, change agents, and communication (Dearing & Cox, 2018; Rogers, 2003). This theory later evolved into a foundation for promoting and studying active dissemination, as described later in this chapter. The Consolidated Framework for Implementation Research (CFIR) is an example of a commonly used determinant framework (Damschroder et al., 2009; Damschroder et al., 2022b).

Evaluation frameworks support assessment of the impact of implementation efforts, to allow researchers to understand and track interventions such as the adoption of an EBI or innovation among providers across a network of organizations. The RE-AIM planning and evaluation framework is a widely used example (Glasgow et al., 1999, 2019).

Process frameworks can inform steps needed or taken during the implementation process, informing questions such as how to engage stakeholders or adapt the intervention. An example is the Knowledge to Action framework, which outlines processes for stakeholders to use EBIs and integrate them with practice-based evidence to increase impact (Wilson et al., 2011). Some frameworks are *hybrid*, incorporating both determinants and evaluation elements (Nilsen, 2015).

Diffusion of Innovations Theory

Background and Historical Development

Diffusion of Innovations theory focuses on the social processes by which an innovation is communicated through specific channels and among members of a social system over time. An innovation can be an idea, practice, product, or program that actors in a system perceive as new (Rogers, 2002). Diffusion of Innovations is one of the most widely used theories to describe, understand, and accelerate the spread of innovations through a system and has been applied and studied internationally for more than 50 years.

Everett Rogers, trained as a rural sociologist, developed the theory while studying the adoption of a new type of seed in a network of farmers. Many early studies applying this theory assessed the role of change agents and characteristics of innovations and social networks that accelerated adoption. Diffusion concepts that first originated in agriculture have spread to other fields, including health, business, communications, and education. It has had a major impact on health research and has evolved from a theory focused on learning about naturalistic diffusion to a foundation for the practice and study of dissemination (Dearing, 2009).

Key Components of the Theory

At its core, the theory was developed to examine how innovation is communicated through a specific social system, over time, and via distinct channels (Dearing, 2008; Dearing & Cox, 2018; Estabrooks et al., 2018; Rogers, 2003). There are three main stages in the diffusion process: (1) adoption (deciding to take up the innovation), (2) implementation (putting the innovation to use), and (3) institutionalization (long-term integration of the innovation in practice). A key premise of Diffusion of Innovations is that some innovations spread quickly and widely, following an S-shaped curve, with slow initial adoption that increases rapidly and then hits a ceiling.

Also, innovations are adopted at different rates by different individuals, groups, and organizations. Potential adopters are categorized based on the speed with which they adopt *the specific innovation*. First, are the "innovators," individuals who are willing to adopt the innovation even if it has not become common in their social system. The second group includes "early adopters," some of whom serve as influential opinion leaders in their social systems. They have weighed the advantages and disadvantages of the innovation and decided to adopt. The third and fourth groups are the "early majority" and "late majority," respectively, who feel social pressure to adopt the innovation, and may be influenced by early adopters. The final group is labeled "laggards"; they take the longest to adopt and are not compelled by social pressures or norms to take action. This category has sometimes been criticized for not considering that social structural conditions, and not the person or group, may explain the slowness in adopting an innovation. Also, the "laggard" label does not describe people who may appear to be slow to adopt an innovation but are in fact actively opposed to taking action, such as the example of "vaccine deniers."

Diffusion of Innovations Theory focuses on five domains to understand influences on the spread of an innovation (Dearing, 2008; Dearing & Cox, 2018; Estabrooks et al., 2018; Rogers, 2002, 2003):

1. *Innovation characteristics*, including *compatibility* (fit between the innovation and routine processes and values); *complexity* (the extent to which the innovation is perceived to be difficult to understand or use); *observability* (whether or not others can see outcomes or impact); *relative advantage* (the degree to which potential adopters see the innovation as an improvement upon existing ideas or practices); and *trialability* (ability to test the innovation before committing). Increased compatibility, observability, relative advantage, decreased complexity, and greater trialability increase the rate of innovation adoption.

2. *Adopter characteristics*, attributes of adopters influencing the rate of uptake of innovation, including learning style and tolerance for ambiguity.

3. The *social system* in which the innovation will be used, with consideration of the system's social networks, roles and hierarchy, power and resources, pressure to use the innovation, and the influence of organizational settings, norms, and values.

4. The *adoption process*, which takes place in stages, including learning about the innovation, forming an attitude about the innovation, making a decision to adopt or reject, implementing the innovation, and ultimately confirming or rejecting the adoption decision.

5. The *broader diffusion system*, including external change agents who may engage with the adopting system.

Empirical Evidence

Diffusion of Innovations has been cited more than 50,000 times over the past 50-plus years (Tabak et al., 2012) and has one of the most extensive histories of both conceptual and historical study among social science theories (Dearing, 2009). Several recent reviews (Green et al., 2009; Greenhalgh et al., 2004, 2005; Haider & Kreps, 2004) and syntheses (Dearing & Cox, 2018) have quantified the evidence in support of the theory and tracked the evolution of its applications over time.

Perhaps the most comprehensive review of concepts from Diffusion of Innovations theory is found in a "meta-narrative review" of 495 sources (a mix of empirical and nonempirical studies) conducted by Greenhalgh and colleagues (Greenhalgh et al., 2004, 2005). Synthesis of the evidence on this theory across four major disciplines (rural sociology, medical sociology, communications, marketing) largely reinforces the effectiveness and important roles of the attributes in Table 16.2. The Greenhalgh review focuses on the uses and usefulness of Diffusion of Innovations to the organizational and management literature (Greenhalgh et al., 2004) and provides some important insights. First, organizational innovativeness is primarily influenced by structural determinants (e.g., internal division of labor, specialization of the organization). Second, the spread of innovations within and across organizations is strongly influenced by intra- and interorganizational norms. Third, organizations that strongly support on-the-job learning are often more effective in spreading innovations due to their values and goals of supporting the creation and sharing of new knowledge. Fourth, innovative organizations are often those in which new stories can be told that capture and support the idea of "communities of practice" (groups that share a common purpose and interact regularly to improve their practice). And fifth, organizations are complex, and effective diffusion addresses this complexity while maintaining an ability to adapt to change.

Several limitations of Diffusion of Innovations have been identified (Greenhalgh et al., 2004; Oldenburg & Glanz, 2008). These include a major focus on the individual innovation and adopters (perhaps downplaying systems effects), an inherent pro-innovation bias, and the lack of transferability of diffusion research principles from one setting or context to others. Dissemination and implementation science frameworks generally focus on transfer of EBIs, whereas Diffusion of Innovations Theory may examine innovations that are or are not evidence-based. In fact, in some settings,

Table 16.2 Diffusion of Innovations: Concepts, Definitions, and Applications to Public Health and Health Care Delivery

Key Innovation Concepts	Definition	Application
Cost	Perceived cost of adopting and implementing innovation	How much time and effort are required to learn to use the innovation and routinize its use? How long does recouping of costs take?
Relative Advantage (Effectiveness)	The extent to which the innovation works better than that which it will displace	Does a gain in performance outweigh the downsides of cost? Do different stakeholders agree on the superiority of the innovation?
Simplicity	How simple the innovation is to understand	How easy is an evidence-based program for adopters/implementers to understand and/or does it involve a steep learning curve and/or much training before actual implementation?
Compatibility	The fit of the innovation with the intended audience to accomplish goal(s)	How much/little would an evidence-based program disrupt the existing routine and/or workflow of the adopting/implementing organization?
Observability	The extent to which outcomes can be seen and measured	How much and/or how quickly will the results of an evidence-based program become visible to an implementing organization, its clients, funders, and peer organizations?
Trialability	The extent to which the innovation can be tried before the adopter commits to full adoption	Can an evidence-based program be implemented as a pilot project without much investment and be abandoned without incurring much sunk cost?

Source: Adapted from: Oldenburg and Glanz (2008) and Rogers (2003).

the rapid spread of unproven, even harmful, medical treatments and preventive strategies is of great concern, as occurred with some COVID-19 treatments. Even so, understanding how unproven innovations spread can make important contributions to public health science (see Chapter 17 for more on communication of misinformation).

Applications of Diffusion of Innovations

Applications of Diffusion of Innovations in recent health behavior and public health research are noteworthy in their focus on *active* dissemination. In the physical activity field, the SPARK (Sports, Play, and Active Recreation for Kids) and CATCH (Coordinated Approach to Child Health) programs for school-based physical education have been disseminated widely, using some of the core constructs of Diffusion of Innovations to describe dissemination and implementation efforts (Owen et al., 2006).

Body and Soul, a nutrition intervention to increase fruit and vegetable intake and conducted through African-American churches, was disseminated broadly through a partnership with the American Cancer Society, the Centers for Disease Control and Prevention (CDC), and the National Cancer Institute, and was rigorously evaluated (Campbell et al., 2007). It was particularly important that major organizations with responsibility for cancer control collaborated in creating and deploying the dissemination version of the effective nutrition program in the first-generation dissemination. A later study evaluated the results of disseminating Body and Soul without researcher or agency involvement, and found the intervention to be no more effective than a control group (Allicock et al., 2012). The latter findings were somewhat disappointing but underscored the need for both strong partnerships and ongoing evaluation of widely disseminated interventions.

In the cancer control field, the Pool Cool sun-safety program for aquatic settings is an example of a health-behavior-change program that progressed from an efficacy trial to a dissemination-implementation trial conducted in more than 400 pools in 33 metropolitan areas in the United States and Okinawa (Brownson et al., 2015; Glanz et al., 2005, 2015). The Pool Cool Diffusion Trial evaluated the effects of two strategies on implementation, maintenance, and sustainability, and improvements in organizational and environmental supports for sun protection. The enhanced dissemination strategy, which provided additional resources along with goals and rewards for documenting greater implementation, resulted in greater maintenance of the program and significantly greater sun-safety policies over time (Glanz et al., 2015). The Pool Cool program was sustained long-term beyond the end of the dissemination-implementation trial with support from state health departments, cancer agencies, and the CDC. One of the largest and longest-lasting examples of sustainable implementation of Pool Cool is in Kansas, where the Masonic Cancer Alliance has partnered with aquatic councils and swimming pools—training over 4,400 aquatic staff members from 70 different swimming pool sites between 2014 and 2022 (National Cancer Institute, 2023). This illustrates how an effective, easily used intervention blended with a train-the-trainer model and many examples of successful partnerships aligns with Diffusion of Innovation concepts to achieve broad adoption and long-term sustainability.

The Consolidated Framework for Implementation Research

Background and Historical Development

The CFIR was developed by Laura Damschroder and colleagues affiliated with the Department of Veterans Affairs (VA) health system (Damschroder et al., 2009). It grew out of a system-level effort to improve the quality of healthcare for veterans through implementation efforts. A synthesis of the dissemination and implementation science literature informed the selection of domains and constructs in the CFIR framework, including constructs from Diffusion of Innovations theory (Rogers, 2003) and a review of the spread and maintenance of innovations in health service delivery and organizations (Greenhalgh et al., 2004). As the name suggests, this "consolidated" framework was developed by combining well-studied and relevant constructs.

Key Components of the Framework

CFIR is composed of five major domains, each with related constructs. These include *intervention characteristics* (eight constructs including intervention source, relative advantage), *outer setting* (four constructs, including external policies and incentives), *inner setting* (12 constructs, including structural characteristics and culture), *characteristics of individuals involved* (5 constructs), and *implementation process* (8 constructs, including monitoring). Figure 16.2 and Table 16.3 describe the constructs within each CFIR domain and their definitions and applications.

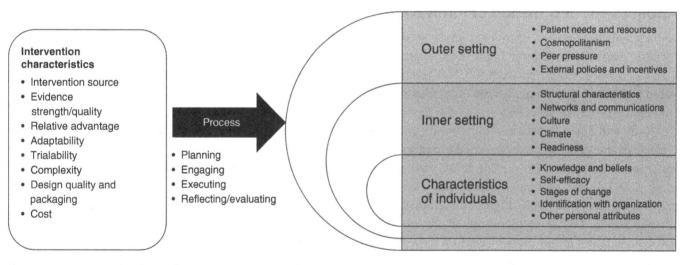

Figure 16.2 Key Constructs from the Consolidated Framework for Implementation Research (Damschroder & Lowery, 2013; Damschroder et al., 2009)

Table 16.3   Consolidated Framework for Implementation Research Domains, Their Definitions, and Their Application to Implementation Research

Domain	Definition	Application
Intervention Characteristics	Key attributes of interventions, which influence the success of implementation	Can the intervention be adapted to our local setting? Will this intervention be better than an alternative?
Outer Setting	Economic, political, and social context within which an organization resides	To what extent is the implementing organization networked with external organizations? Is implementation of the intervention mandated by an external authority?
Inner Setting	Features of structural, political, and cultural contexts	Is the setting in which the intervention is being implemented receptive to change?
Characteristics of Individuals	Characteristics of the individuals involved with the intervention and/or implementation process.	What are the attitudes of individuals responsible for the intervention process toward the intervention?
Implementation Process	Steps to an active change process aimed to achieve individual and organizational level use of the intervention as designed	Who should be involved in implementation, and how can they become engaged in the process?

The CFIR can support development and evaluation of implementation efforts for research and practice. For example, CFIR domains and constructs can inform contextual assessments and formative planning for implementation, which involves assessing multilevel ecological barriers and facilitators to EBI implementation among stakeholders. CFIR constructs also can be used to map the development of implementation strategies that address identified barriers and facilitate EBI delivery. For example, low levels of practitioner knowledge about the EBI may indicate the need for education/training as an implementation strategy (Waltz et al., 2019).

Operational and Analytical Considerations

Given the large number of constructs, it is common for studies guided by CFIR to examine a subset of constructs or domains aligned with the focus of the study (Damschroder et al., 2011). It can be useful to examine differences in CFIR constructs across sites with varying levels of implementation success to determine which constructs or factors have a larger impact on implementation. For example, Damschroder and Lowery (2013) used CFIR to guide qualitative data collection and analysis to evaluate the MOVE! weight management program in VA Medical Centers and compared ratings of CFIR constructs that distinguished between facilities with low versus high program implementation effectiveness. Of the 31 constructs assessed, 10 were significant predictors of implementation. These were mainly inner-setting constructs, reflecting networks and communication or leadership engagement. The study offers empirical support for the impact of organizational context on implementation and illustrates how CFIR may be applied to enhance understanding of which of the core domains and constructs are strongly associated with successful implementation.

Empirical Evidence and Extensions of CFIR

A rapidly growing literature has applied CFIR to various aspects of implementation science studies across various settings and units of analysis, as detailed by a recent review of 26 articles published by January 2015 that meaningfully applied CFIR as a central part of their study design, data collection, and/or analysis (Kirk et al., 2016). They found that as of 2015, much of the research conducted with CFIR was qualitative or mixed-methods work, often focused on organizing study results according to relevant framework domains but without assessment across multiple implementation phases or examination of outcomes.

The evidence base is still developing in terms of which constructs within each of the five domains are most important, though some studies have identified factors from the inner setting as critical (e.g., leadership engagement in the implementing organization) (Damschroder & Lowery, 2013). The clearer linkage of CFIR constructs with each other and with implementation outcomes is a priority for future work (Damschroder et al., 2022a). Given that CFIR is a largely descriptive framework, it can be useful to apply CFIR in combination with other evaluation frameworks to understand the mechanisms linking determinants with implementation or effectiveness outcomes.

A comprehensive set of validated quantitative measures representing all CFIR constructs is not currently available, but measure development is still underway in several areas. Several refinements have been proposed to address existing limitations to CFIR, including applications to promote practice-focused applications or to focus more on health equity. For example, Safaeinili et al. (2020) described a stakeholder-informed pragmatic adaptation of CFIR to evaluate a patient-centered care transformation in a learning health system. Means et al. (2020) evaluated CFIR for use in low- and middle-income countries (LMIC) and proposed a "characteristics of systems" domain and novel constructs to increase compatibility with LMICs (e.g., strategic policy alignment, resource continuity, external funding agent priorities, perceived scalability, community characteristics). Allen et al. (2021) have proposed a racism-conscious adaptation of CFIR that considers how race and racism operate throughout the domains and constructs.

An updated version of the framework (CFIR 2.0) was recently published, informed by empirical evaluation among researchers who have used the original CFIR in their work. The updated version still includes the five core domains and clarifies or expands on constructs that were not well-defined or were missing. For example, "critical incidents" was added in the outer setting to help account for salient, large-scale, often unanticipated events (e.g. floods, pandemic, company buyouts) (Damschroder et al., 2022b).

Application of the Consolidated Framework for Implementation Research

The Diabetes Prevention Program (DPP) is an effective intervention to reduce the incidence of Type 2 Diabetes. Initial research showing that the program was effective was first published in 2002 (Diabetes Prevention Program Research Group, 2002). In the short term, participants showed a 58% reduction in the rate of developing diabetes. Over 15 years, diabetes incidence in the original DPP trial participants was 27% lower among those who had participated in the lifestyle intervention and 18% lower among those taking medication, compared to the placebo group (Diabetes Prevention Program Research Group, 2015). Though the sustained effects were not as large as the original findings, the DPP showed substantial long-term durability.

Since completion of the original trial, the DPP has been implemented widely in YMCAs, churches, and other settings (Ackermann et al., 2008; Aziz et al., 2015). The DPP is a year-long program delivered in person, using web-based tools, or in a hybrid format. The core program includes 16 sessions over the first six months and 6 sessions in the next six months. Trained lifestyle coaches deliver a standardized curriculum. The program goals are to support weight loss through healthier eating and regular physical activity, thereby reducing the risk of developing diabetes. Although it was not originally designed for scale-up in nonclinical settings, the broad translation has increased the reach of the program to diverse populations.

The VA created an in-house version, called the VA-DPP, a 12-month program that, like the original DPP, includes 22 sessions delivered by a CDC-certified coach (Damschroder et al., 2017). For the VA-DPP, a clinical champion gained leadership commitment, the Diabetes Prevention Support Center trained coaches and team members, and sites adapted an implementation protocol. A coordinating center offered support for a uniform approach across five sites. Researchers conducted an implementation assessment and used CFIR to examine implementation barriers and facilitators, the fidelity of delivery, satisfaction among participants, and implementation costs. They also used the RE-AIM planning and evaluation framework (Glasgow et al., 2019) to guide evaluation of the implementation outcomes.

The team conducted semi-structured interviews with VA-DPP team members and other staff members at the sites during early implementation ($n = 15$) and post-enrollment ($n = 23$). The study drew on all five domains of the CFIR (intervention characteristics, outer setting, inner setting, individual characteristics, and implementation process) and the five domains of RE-AIM. The data sources for analysis included participant questionnaires and transcripts, site visit notes, meeting minutes, and communications. VA-DPP staff used a checklist to measure fidelity or the extent to which the program was delivered as intended. Participant satisfaction was measured and implementation costs were also examined, focusing on recruitment/implementation of VA-DPP and conducting sessions. The study identified several contextual barriers and facilitators to implementing the program.

Fidelity for VA-DPP at the site level was high, as was participant satisfaction. The costs of various phases of program delivery were: assessing eligibility ($68 per person), scheduling and supporting continued participation ($328 per person), and delivering the program ($101 per group session or $ 2,220 for the planned 22 sessions). The cost for completed sessions averaged $46 per participant. Overall, the study highlighted a need for multipronged strategies to support successful implementation of VA-DPP and the substantial investment required to engage participants and implement the DPP on a large scale. The study also illustrates how context, assessed in terms of CFIR constructs, links with implementation strategies such as training and using champions to support EBI implementation.

Study Designs and Methodological Approaches in Dissemination and Implementation Science: Some Considerations

Dissemination and implementation research focuses primarily on understanding and supporting the spread and utilization of innovations and EBIs, as distinct from efficacy and effectiveness research, which focuses mainly on studying the impact of intervention strategies on health behaviors, health status, and other outcomes of interest. Dissemination and implementation studies seek to understand the roles of contextual factors, implementation strategies, and implementation outcomes at multiple levels (Mazzucca et al., 2018). Thus, it is useful to understand the types of study designs and methods used in dissemination and implementation science. While a full discussion of research methods for dissemination and implementation is beyond the scope of this chapter, we highlight some key considerations for readers.

As one example, implementation strategies evaluated might address barriers to implementation at multiple levels (e.g., training to address teachers' low knowledge and self-efficacy to deliver the intervention, and organizational resources to facilitate school readiness to implement an EBI) and implementation success might be evaluated at multiple levels (e.g., among students, teachers, and principals). Increasingly, effectiveness and implementation are studied simultaneously using hybrid effectiveness-implementation trials to make it possible to learn about implementation and to what extent the EBIs/innovations achieve the intended results in different contexts and/or when adapted for different populations (Curran et al., 2012).

Dissemination and implementation researchers use a variety of study designs to ensure that their evaluations reflect real-world settings and stakeholders, often with the "cluster" or organizational setting as the main focus (Brown et al., 2017; Mazzucca et al., 2018). Thus, for example, randomized controlled trials (RCTs) of individuals may not be feasible or optimal for dissemination and implementation research. Instead, other designs may be helpful, such as stepped wedge trials. With this design, every site or organization receives the implementation strategy and EBI, but the timing at which they receive it is randomized and staggered. This design, like that of a delayed control group, preserves the focus on assessing outcomes at the site level but also helps avoid ethical concerns due to withholding a beneficial treatment or program (e.g., an EBI that has been found to be effective). Additionally, staggering timing of delivery of implementation strategies and EBIs can address some of the logistical challenges of implementation across a large number of sites or "clusters" (e.g., conducting an implementation trial nationally across 60 primary care practices). A review of recent dissemination and implementation science studies offers a helpful overview of relevant study designs (Mazzucca et al., 2018).

Mixed-method designs that combine and integrate qualitative and quantitative data are becoming increasingly common in dissemination and implementation science. With these designs, qualitative methods support the exploration of phenomena of interest (e.g., implementation context), and quantitative methods allow for testing hypotheses (e.g., which implementation strategies are effective?) (Curran et al., 2012). Reviews and guides of mixed-methods dissemination and implementation research offer additional insight and guidance in applying these approaches rigorously (Palinkas et al., 2011; QualRIS Group, 2019).

Challenges and Future Directions

There are several important challenges for dissemination and implementation science moving forward. First, there is a need for a richer pool of measures that are psychometrically validated, pragmatic, theory-driven, and adaptable to different situations and populations (Mettert et al., 2020). When possible, consistent use of comparable measures across studies will accelerate the growth of the evidence base. Also, new and existing frameworks should be adaptable to different settings, populations, and cultures; there are some examples available, but more are needed to enhance their generalizability and applicability. Diffusion of Innovations has a long history of use in global settings (Rogers, 2003). The CFIR framework has been adapted to address equity, pragmatic applications, and use in LMIC (Allen et al., 2021; Means et al., 2020), and continued adaptation for these contexts is needed.

Additional attention is needed to shorten the often-prolonged timelines and low rates of uptake associated with innovations and EBIs. This will require more academics to actively work and partner in a range of community settings. Participatory and community-engaged research approaches in which community partners engage iteratively with researchers can leverage diverse expertise, co-create solutions, address power imbalances, build capacity, and support the integration of research evidence into communities (Ramanadhan et al., 2023; Shelton et al., 2024). For additional details, see Chapter 15.

Two growing areas of research in dissemination and implementation science warrant more attention. One is de-implementation research, which focuses on discontinuing or reducing EBI delivery when inappropriate, costly, or harmful (Nilsen et al., 2020). Another emerging focus is policy implementation, given the potential for policy change to create change at scale and impact health equity (Emmons & Chambers, 2021).

Last, it is becoming ever more essential that dissemination and implementation frameworks and research focus explicit attention on health equity. Several equity-focused frameworks and refinements of existing frameworks have been developed in recent years, offering a path forward (Baumann & Cabassa, 2020; Shelton et al., 2021; Snell-Rood et al., 2021; Woodward et al., 2019).

Summary

Building on rich traditions of inquiry spanning over 100 years, dissemination and implementation science is an area of growing attention in public health and health behavior. With the focus on understanding how innovations and EBIs can be successfully deployed, the multilevel determinants of implementation, the implementation strategies needed for them to be widely used in practice, and the impacts of these efforts, there are important opportunities to improve the pace, scale, and equity of the spread and use of innovations. Many frameworks are available, addressing context, process, outcomes, or combinations of these components. These frameworks offer the opportunity to build the literature on integrating evidence-based solutions into widespread and routine practice. As the examples of Diffusion of Innovations and CFIR highlighted, a systems perspective prompts engagement of core stakeholders to identify multilevel implementation gaps and potential solutions. Dissemination and implementation science offers a significant opportunity to put evidence-based practice and practice-based evidence to full use and improve health and health equity.

Acknowledgments

We want to thank Savannah Alexander for her support throughout the chapter development process.

References

Ackermann, R. T., Finch, E. A., Brizendine, E., Zhou, H., & Marrero, D. G. (2008). Translating the diabetes prevention program into the community: The DEPLOY pilot study. *American Journal of Preventive Medicine*, *35*(4), 357–363. https://doi.org/10.1016/j.amepre.2008.06.035

Allen, M., Wilhelm, A., Ortega, L. E., Pergament, S., Bates, N., & Cunningham, B. (2021). Applying a race(ism)-conscious adaptation of the CFIR framework to understand implementation of a school-based equity-oriented intervention. *Ethnicity & Disease*, *31*(Suppl. 1), 375–388. https://doi.org/10.18865/ed.31.S1.375

Allicock, M., Campbell, M. K., Valle, C. G., Carr, C., Resnicow, K., & Gizlice, Z. (2012). Evaluating the dissemination of Body & Soul, an evidence-based fruit and vegetable intake intervention: Challenges for dissemination and implementation research. *Journal of Nutrition Education and Behavior*, *44*(6), 530–538. https://doi.org/10.1016/j.jneb.2011.09.002

Aziz, Z., Absetz, P., Oldroyd, J., Pronk, N. P., & Oldenburg, B. (2015). A systematic review of real-world diabetes prevention programs: Learnings from the last 15 years. *Implementation Science*, *10*(1), 172. https://doi.org/10.1186/s13012-015-0354-6

Balas, E. A., & Boren, S. A. (2000). Managing clinical knowledge for health care improvement. In J. Bemmel & A. McCray (Eds.), *Yearbook of medical informaticcs 2000: Patient- centered systems* (pp. 65–70). Schattauer.

Baumann, A. A., & Cabassa, L. J. (2020). Reframing implementation science to address inequities in healthcare delivery. *BMC Health Services Research*, *20*, 190. https://doi.org/10.1186/s12913-020-4975-3

Baumann, A. A., Hooley, C., Kryzer, E., Morshed, A. B., Gutner, C. A., Malone, S., Walsh-Bailey, C., Pilar, M., Sandler, B., Tabak, R. G., & Mazzucca, S. (2022). A scoping review of frameworks in empirical studies and a review of dissemination frameworks. *Implementation Science*, *17*, 53. https://doi.org/10.1186/s13012-022-01225-4

Brown, C. H., Curran, G., Palinkas, L. A., Aarons, G. A., Wells, K. B., Jones, L., Collins, L. M., Duan, N., Mittman, B. S., & Wallace, A. (2017). An overview of research and evaluation designs for dissemination and implementation. *Annual Review of Public Health*, *38*, 1–22. https://doi.org/10.1146/annurev-publhealth-031816-044215

Brownson, R. C., Baker, E. A., Leet, T. L., Gillespie, K. N., & True, W. R. (2011). *Evidence-based public health*. Oxford University Press.

Brownson, R. C., Jacobs, J. A., Tabak, R. G., Hoehner, C. M., & Stamatakis, K. A. (2013). Designing for dissemination among public health researchers: Findings from a national survey in the United States. *American Journal of Public Health*, *103*(9), 1693–1699. https://doi.org/10.2105/AJPH.2012.301165

Brownson, R. C., Tabak, R., Stamatakis, K., & Glanz, K. (2015). Implementation, dissemination, and diffusion of public health interventions. In: K. Glanz, B. Rimer, & K. Viswanath (Eds.), *Health behavior: Theory, research and practice* (pp. 301–325). Wiley.

Brownson, R. C., Colditz, G. A., & Proctor, E. K. (Eds.). (2018). *Dissemination and implementation research in health: Translating science to practice* (2nd ed.). Oxford University Press.

Brownson, R. C., Shelton, R. C., Geng, E. H., & Glasgow, R. E. (2022). Revisiting concepts of evidence in implementation science. *Implementation Science*, *17*, 26. https://doi.org/10.1186/s13012-022-01201-y

Campbell, M. K., Resnicow, K., Carr, C., Wang, T., & Williams, A. (2007). Process evaluation of an effective church-based diet intervention: Body & soul. *Health Education & Behavior, 34*(6), 864–880. https://doi.org/10.1177/1090198106292020

Cancer Prevention and Control Research Network. (2017). Putting public health evidence in action training curriculum. https://cpcrn.org/training

Chambers, D. A. (2020). Considering the intersection between implementation science and COVID-19. *Implementation Research and Practice, 1*(Jan-Dec 2020), 1–4. https://doi.org/10.1177/0020764020925994

Concannon, T. W., Meissner, P., Grunbaum, J. A., McElwee, N., Guise, J. M., Santa, J., Conway, P. H., Daudelin, D., Morrato, E. H., & Leslie, L. K. (2012). A new taxonomy for stakeholder engagement in patient-centered outcomes research. *Journal of General Internal Medicine, 27*(8), 985–991. https://doi.org/10.1007/s11606-012-2037-1

Curran, G. M. (2020). Implementation science made too simple: A teaching tool. *Implementation Science Communications, 1,* 27. https://doi.org/10.1186/s43058-020-00001-z

Curran, G. M., Bauer, M., Mittman, B., Pyne, J. M., & Stetler, C. (2012). Effectiveness-implementation hybrid designs: Combining elements of clinical effectiveness and implementation research to enhance public health impact. *Medical Care, 50*(3), 217–226. https://doi.org/10.1097/MLR.0b013e3182408812

Damschroder, L. J., & Lowery, J. C. (2013). Evaluation of a large-scale weight management program using the Consolidated Framework for Implementation Research (CFIR). *Implementation Science, 8,* 51. https://doi.org/10.1186/1748-5908-8-51

Damschroder, L. J., Aron, D. C., Keith, R. E., Kirsh, S. R., Alexander, J. A., & Lowery, J. C. (2009). Fostering implementation of health services research findings into practice: A consolidated framework for advancing implementation science. *Implementation Science, 4,* 50. https://doi.org/10.1186/1748-5908-4-50

Damschroder, L. J., Goodrich, D. E., Robinson, C. H., Fletcher, C. E., & Lowery, J. C. (2011). A systematic exploration of differences in contextual factors related to implementing the MOVE! weight management program in VA: A mixed methods study. *BMC Health Services Research, 11,* 248. https://doi.org/10.1186/1472-6963-11-248

Damschroder, L. J., Reardon, C. M., AuYoung, M., Moin, T., Datta, S. K., Sparks, J. B., Maciejewski, M. L., Steinle, N. I., Weinreb, J. E., Hughes, M., Pinault, L. F., Xiang, X. M., Billington, C., & Richardson, C. R. (2017). Implementation findings from a hybrid III implementation-effectiveness trial of the Diabetes Prevention Program (DPP) in the Veterans Health Administration (VHA). *Implementation Science, 12,* 94. https://doi.org/10.1186/s13012-017-0619-3

Damschroder, L. J., Reardon, C. M., Opra Widerquist, M. A., & Lowery, J. (2022a). Conceptualizing outcomes for use with the Consolidated Framework for Implementation Research (CFIR): The CFIR Outcomes Addendum. *Implementation Science, 17,* 7. https://doi.org/10.1186/s13012-021-01181-5

Damschroder, L. J., Reardon, C. M., Widerquist, M. A. O., & Lowery, J. (2022b). The updated consolidated framework for implementation research based on user feedback. *Implementation Science, 17*(1), 75. https://doi.org/10.1186/s13012-022-01245-0

Dearing, J. W. (2008). Evolution of diffusion and dissemination theory. *Journal of Public Health Management and Practice, 14*(2), 99–108. https://doi.org/10.1097/01.PHH.0000311886.98627.b7

Dearing, J. W. (2009). Applying diffusion of innovation theory to intervention development. *Research on Social Work Practice, 19*(5), 503–518. https://doi.org/10.1177/1049731509335569

Dearing, J. W., & Cox, J. G. (2018). Diffusion of innovations theory, principles, and practice. *Health Affairs (Project Hope), 37*(2), 183–190. https://doi.org/10.1377/hlthaff.2017.1104

Diabetes Prevention Program Research Group. (2002). Reduction in the Incidence of Type 2 Diabetes with Lifestyle Intervention or Metformin. *New England Journal of Medicine, 346*(6), 393–403. https://doi.org/10.1056/NEJMoa012512

Diabetes Prevention Program Research Group. (2015). Long-term effects of lifestyle intervention or metformin on diabetes development and microvascular complications over 15-year follow-up: The Diabetes Prevention Program Outcomes Study. *The Lancet Diabetes & Endocrinology, 3*(11), 866–875. https://doi.org/10.1016/S2213-8587(15)00291-0

Emmons, K. M., & Chambers, D. A. (2021). Policy implementation science—An unexplored strategy to address social determinants of health. *Ethnicity & Disease, 31*(1), 133–138. https://doi.org/10.18865/ed.31.1.133

Estabrooks, P. A., Brownson, R. C., & Pronk, N. P. (2018). Dissemination and implementation science for public health professionals: An overview and call to action. *Preventing Chronic Disease, 15,* E162. https://doi.org/10.5888/pcd15.180525

Explore D&I TMP. 2023. Dissemination & implementation tools in health. University of Colorado Denver. https://dissemination-implementation.org/tool/explore-di-models/

Glanz, K., Steffen, A., Elliott, T., & O'Riordan, D. (2005). Diffusion of an effective skin cancer prevention program: Design, theoretical foundations, and first-year implementation. *Health Psychology, 24*(5), 477–487. https://doi.org/10.1037/0278-6133.24.5.477

Glanz, K., Escoffery, C., Elliott, T., & Nehl, E. J. (2015). Randomized trial of two dissemination strategies for a skin cancer prevention program in aquatic settings. *American Journal of Public Health, 105*(7), 1415–1423. https://doi.org/10.2105/AJPH.2014.302224

Glasgow, R. E., Vogt, T. M., & Boles, S. M. (1999). Evaluating the public health impact of health promotion interventions: The RE-AIM framework. *American Journal of Public Health, 89*(9), 1322–1327. https://doi.org/10.2105/ajph.89.9.1322

Glasgow, R. E., Harden, S. M., Gaglio, B., Rabin, B., Smith, M. L., Porter, G. C., Ory, M. G., & Estabrooks, P. A. (2019). RE-AIM planning and evaluation framework: Adapting to new science and practice with a 20-year review. *Frontiers in Public Health, 7*, 64. https://doi.org/10.3389/fpubh.2019.00064

Green, L. W. (2008). Making research relevant: If it is an evidence-based practice, where's the practice-based evidence? *Family Practice, 25*(Suppl. 1), i20–i24. https://doi.org/10.1093/fampra/cmn055

Green, L. W., Ottoson, J. M., Garcia, C., & Hiatt, R. A. (2009). Diffusion theory, and knowledge dissemination, utilization, and integration in public health. *Annual Review of Public Health.* https://doi.org/10.1146/annurev.publhealth.031308.100049

Greenhalgh, T., Robert, G., Macfarlane, F., Bate, P., & Kyriakidou, O. (2004). Diffusion of innovations in service organizations: Systematic review and recommendations. *The Milbank Quarterly, 82*(4), 581–629.

Greenhalgh, T., Robert, G., Macfarlane, F., Bate, P., Kyriakidou, O., & Peacock, R. (2005). Storylines of research in diffusion of innovation: a meta-narrative approach to systematic review. *Social Science & Medicine, 61*(2), 417–430.

Guide to Community Preventive Services. (2023). Methods manual for community guide systematic reviews. https://www.thecommunityguide.org/pages/methods-manual.html

Haider, M., & Kreps, G. L. (2004). Forty years of diffusion of innovations: utility and value in public health. *Journal of Health Communication, 9*(S1), 3–11.

Hawe, P., Shiell, A., & Riley, T. (2004). Complex interventions: How "out of control" can a randomised controlled trial be? *BMJ: British Medical Journal, 328*(7455), 1561.

Khan, S., Chambers, D., & Neta, G. (2021). Revisiting time to translation: Implementation of evidence-based practices (EBPs) in cancer control. *Cancer Causes & Control, 32*(3), 221–230. https://doi.org/10.1007/s10552-020-01376-z

Kirk, M. A., Kelley, C., Yankey, N., Birken, S. A., Abadie, B., & Damschroder, L. (2016). A systematic review of the use of the consolidated framework for implementation research. *Implementation Science, 11*, 72. https://doi.org/10.1186/s13012-016-0437-z

Kwan, B. M., Brownson, R. C., Glasgow, R. E., Morrato, E. H., & Luke, D. A. (2022). Designing for dissemination and sustainability to promote equitable impacts on health. *Annual Review of Public Health, 43*, 331–353. https://doi.org/10.1146/annurev-publhealth-052220-112457

Lewin, K. (1946). Action research and minority problems. *Journal of Social Issues, 2*(4), 34–46.

Lomas, J. (1993). Diffusion, dissemination, and implementation: who should do what? *Annals of the New York Academy of Sciences, 703*, 226–235. http://www.ncbi.nlm.nih.gov/entrez/query.fcgi?cmd=Retrieve&db=PubMed&dopt=Citation&list_uids=8192299

Luke, D. A., Calhoun, A., Robichaux, C. B., Elliott, M. B., & Moreland-Russell, S. (2014). The Program Sustainability Assessment Tool: A new instrument for public health programs. *Preventing Chronic Disease, 11*, 130184. https://doi.org/10.5888/pcd11.130184

MacLean, D. R. (1996). Positioning dissemination in public health policy. *Canadian Journal of Public Health, 87*(S2), S40–43. http://www.ncbi.nlm.nih.gov/entrez/query.fcgi?cmd=Retrieve&db=PubMed&dopt=Citation&list_uids=9002342

Mazzucca, S., Tabak, R. G., Pilar, M., Ramsey, A. T., Baumann, A. A., Kryzer, E., Lewis, E. M., Padek, M., Powell, B. J., & Brownson, R. C. (2018). Variation in research designs used to test the effectiveness of dissemination and implementation strategies: A review. *Frontiers in Public Health, 6*, 32. https://doi.org/10.3389/fpubh.2018.00032

McLean R, Tucker J. (2013). *Evaluation of CIHR's knowledge translation funding program.* Ottawa, ON: Canadian Institutes of Health Research.

Means, A. R., Kemp, C. G., Gwayi-Chore, M.-C., Gimbel, S., Soi, C., Sherr, K., Wagenaar, B. H., Wasserheit, J. N., & Weiner, B. J. (2020). Evaluating and optimizing the Consolidated Framework for Implementation Research (CFIR) for use in low-and middle-income countries: A systematic review. *Implementation Science, 15*, 17. https://doi.org/10.1186/s13012-020-0977-0

Mettert, K., Lewis, C., Dorsey, C., Halko, H., & Weiner, B. (2020). Measuring implementation outcomes: An updated systematic review of measures' psychometric properties. *Implementation Research and Practice, 1*(Jan-Dec 2020), 1–29. https://doi.org/10.1177/2633489520936644

Moore, J. E., Mascarenhas, A., Bain, J., & Straus, S. E. (2017). Developing a comprehensive definition of sustainability. *Implementation Science, 12*, 110. https://doi.org/10.1186/s13012-017-0637-1

Morris, Z. S., Wooding, S., & Grant, J. (2011). The answer is 17 years, what is the question: Understanding time lags in translational research. *Journal of the Royal Society of Medicine, 104*(12), 510–520. https://doi.org/10.1258/jrsm.2011.110180

National Cancer Institute. (2020). Evidence-Based Cancer Control Programs (EBCCP): Transforming research into community and clinical practice. https://ebccp.cancercontrol.cancer.gov/index.do

National Cancer Institute. (2023). *Insights from the cancer control field: Pool cool in Kansas*. National Cancer Institute. https://ebccp. cancercontrol.cancer.gov/insights/pool-cool-kansas

National Institutes of Health. (2019). PAR-19-275: Dissemination and implementation research in health (R21 clinical trial optional). https://grants.nih.gov/grants/guide/pa-files/par-19-275.html

Nilsen, P. (2015). Making sense of implementation theories, models and frameworks. *Implementation Science, 10*, 53. https://doi. org/10.1186/s13012-015-0242-0

Nilsen, P., Ingvarsson, S., Hasson, H., von Thiele Schwarz, U., & Augustsson, H. (2020). Theories, models, and frameworks for de-implementation of low-value care: A scoping review of the literature. *Implementation Research and Practice, 1*(Jan-Dec 2020), 1–15. https://doi.org/10.1177/2633489520953762

Norton, W. E., Kennedy, A. E., & Chambers, D. A. (2017). Studying de-implementation in health: An analysis of funded research grants. *Implementation Science, 12*, 144. https://doi.org/10.1186/s13012-017-0655-z

Oldenburg, B., & Glanz, K. (2008). Diffusion of innovations. In K. Glanz, B. Rimer, & K. Vishwanath (Eds.), *Health behavior and health education: Theory, research and practice* (4th ed., pp. 313–334). Jossey-Bass.

Owen, N., Glanz, K., Sallis, J. F., & Kelder, S. H. (2006). Evidence-based approaches to dissemination and diffusion of physical activity interventions. *American Journal of Preventive Medicine, 31*(S4), S35–S44. http://www.ncbi.nlm.nih.gov/entrez/query.fcgi?cmd= Retrieve&db=PubMed&dopt=Citation&list_uids=16979468

Palinkas, L. A., Aarons, G. A., Horwitz, S., Chamberlain, P., Hurlburt, M. S., & Landsverk, J. (2011). Mixed method designs in implementation research. *Administration and Policy in Mental Health, 38*(1), 44–53. https://doi.org/10.1007/s10488-010-0314-z

Powell, B. J., Waltz, T. J., Chinman, M. J., Damschroder, L. J., Smith, J. L., Matthieu, M. M., Proctor, E. K., & Kirchner, J. E. (2015). A refined compilation of implementation strategies: Results from the Expert Recommendations for Implementing Change (ERIC) project. *Implementation Science, 10*, 21. https://doi.org/10.1186/s13012-015-0209-1

Powell, B. J., Fernandez, M. E., Williams, N. J., Aarons, G. A., Beidas, R. S., Lewis, C. C., McHugh, S. M., & Weiner, B. J. (2019). Enhancing the impact of implementation strategies in healthcare: A research agenda. *Frontiers in Public Health, 7*, 3. https://doi. org/10.3389/fpubh.2019.00003

Proctor, E. K., Silmere, H., Raghavan, R., Hovmand, P., Aarons, G., Bunger, A., Griffey, R., & Hensley, M. (2011). Outcomes for implementation research: Conceptual distinctions, measurement challenges, and research agenda. *Administration and Policy in Mental Health and Mental Health Services Research, 38*(2), 65–76. https://doi.org/10.1007/s10488-010-0319-7

QualRIS Group. (2019). Division of Cancer Control and Population Sciences, National Cancer Institute. *Qualitative methods in implementation science*. https://cancercontrol.cancer.gov/IS/docs/NCI-DCCPS-ImplementationScience-WhitePaper.pdf

Rabin, B. A., Brownson, R. C., Haire-Joshu, D., Kreuter, M. W., & Weaver, N. L. (2008). A glossary for dissemination and implementation research in health. *Journal of Public Health Management and Practice, 14*(2), 117–123. https://doi.org/10.1097/01. PHH.0000311888.06252.bb

Ramanadhan, S., & Viswanath, K. (2018). Engaging communities to improve health: Models, evidence, and the participatory knowledge translation (PaKT) framework. In E. B. Fisher, L. Cameron, A. J. Christensen, U. Ehlert, Y. Guo, B. F. Oldenburg, & F. Snoek (Eds.), *Principles and concepts of behavioral medicine: A global handbook* (pp. 679–712). Springer Science & Business Media.

Ramanadhan, S., Davis, M., Donaldson, S., Miller, E., & Minkler, M. (2023). Participatory approaches in dissemination and implementation research. In R. Brownson, G. Colditz, & E. Proctor (Eds). *Dissemination and implementation research in health* (3rd ed., pp. 175–190). Oxford University Press.

Rogers, E. M. (2002). Diffusion of preventive innovations. *Addictive Behaviors, 27*(6), 989–993. https://doi.org/10.1016/ S0306-4603(02)00300-3

Rogers, E. M. (2003). *Diffusion of innovations* (5th ed.). The Free Press.

Safaeinili, N., Brown-Johnson, C., Shaw, J. G., Mahoney, M., & Winget, M. (2020). CFIR simplified: Pragmatic application of and adaptations to the Consolidated Framework for Implementation Research (CFIR) for evaluation of a patient-centered care transformation within a learning health system. *Learning Health Systems, 4*(1), e10201. https://doi.org/10.1002/lrh2.10201

Shelton, R. C., Chambers, D. A., & Glasgow, R. E. (2020). An extension of RE-AIM to enhance sustainability: Addressing dynamic context and promoting health equity over time. *Frontiers in Public Health, 8*, 134. https://doi.org/10.3389/fpubh.2020.00134

Shelton, R. C., Adsul, P., Oh, A., Moise, N., & Griffith, D. M. (2021). Application of an antiracism lens in the field of implementation science (IS): Recommendations for reframing implementation research with a focus on justice and racial equity. *Implementation Research and Practice, 2*(Jan-Dec 2021), 1–19. https://doi.org/10.1177/26334895211049482

Shelton, R. C., Adsul, P., Emmons, K. M., Linnan, L., & Allen, J. D. (2023). Fidelity and its relationship to implementation, effectiveness, and adaptation. In R. C. Brownson, G. A. Colditz, & E. K. Proctor (Eds.), *Dissemination and implementation research in health: Translating science to practice* (3rd ed.). Oxford University Press.

Shelton, R. C., Adsul, P., Baumann, A., & Ramanadhan, S. (2024). Community engagement to promote health equity through implementation science. In *Principles of community engagement*. National Institutes of Health and the Centers for Disease Control and Prevention, in press.

Smith, J. D., Li, D. H., & Rafferty, M. R. (2020). The Implementation Research Logic Model: A method for planning, executing, reporting, and synthesizing implementation projects. *Implementation Science, 15*, 84. https://doi.org/10.1186/s13012-020-01041-8

Snell-Rood, C., Jaramillo, E. T., Hamilton, A. B., Raskin, S. E., Nicosia, F. M., & Willging, C. (2021). Advancing health equity through a theoretically critical implementation science. *Translational Behavioral Medicine, 11*(8), 1617–1625. https://doi.org/10.1093/tbm/ibab008

Substance Abuse and Mental Health Services Administration. (2022). Evidence-based practices resource center. https://www.samhsa.gov/resource-search/ebp

Tabak, R. G., Khoong, E. C., Chambers, D. A., & Brownson, R. C. (2012). Bridging research and practice: Models for dissemination and implementation research. *American Journal of Preventive Medicine, 43*(3), 337–350. https://doi.org/10.1016/j.amepre.2012.05.024

Tran, K. B., Lang, J. J., Compton, K., Xu, R., Acheson, A. R., Henrikson, H. J., Kocarnik, J. M., Penberthy, L., Aali, A., Abbas, Q., Abbasi, B., Abbasi-Kangevari, M., Abbasi-Kangevari, Z., Abbastabar, H., Abdelmasseh, M., Abd-Elsalam, S., Abdelwahab, A. A., Abdoli, G., Abdulkadir, H. A., & Murray, C. J. L. (2022). The global burden of cancer attributable to risk factors, 2010–19: A systematic analysis for the Global Burden of Disease Study 2019. *The Lancet, 400*(10352), 563–591. https://doi.org/10.1016/S0140-6736(22)01438-6

Waltz, T. J., Powell, B. J., Fernández, M. E., Abadie, B., & Damschroder, L. J. (2019). Choosing implementation strategies to address contextual barriers: Diversity in recommendations and future directions. *Implementation Science, 14*, 42. https://doi.org/10.1186/s13012-019-0892-4

Wilson, K. M., Brady, T. J., Lesesne, C., & NCCDPHP Work Group on Translation. (2011). An organizing framework for translation in public health: The Knowledge to Action Framework. *Preventing Chronic Disease, 8*(2), A46.

Woodward, E. N., Matthieu, M. M., Uchendu, U. S., Rogal, S., & Kirchner, J. E. (2019). The Health Equity Implementation Framework: Proposal and preliminary study of hepatitis C virus treatment. *Implementation Science, 14*, 26. https://doi.org/10.1186/s13012-019-0861-y

CHAPTER 17

COMMUNICATION AND MEDIA EFFECTS ON HEALTH BEHAVIOR

Sarah E. Gollust
Rebekah H. Nagler

Vignette: News Media and COVID

The date was February 28, 2020. Only a few dozen COVID-19 ("coronavirus") cases had been identified in the United States, most of which could be linked to international travel. Although the vast majority of US states had yet to document a single case, a handful of new cases recently identified on the West Coast with no known exposure pathway suggested evidence of community spread. Major sports games and concerts had been cancelled, and the US State Department began issuing recommendations against international travel. Anxiety levels among many in the public and health officials were high. In full swing of the election primary season, President Trump held a rally where he devoted much attention to the coronavirus situation. What happened at that rally, and how it would be covered in the news media, was a pivotal moment for the course of health communication over the next months (and years) of the pandemic.

The *New York Times* headline describing the rally was "Trump Accuses Media and Democrats of Exaggerating Coronavirus Threat" (Baker & Karni, 2020). This news article—and the hundreds of others published that week by political journalists charged with reporting on the primary race—recounted that Mr. Trump declared that the coronavirus pandemic was overblown, even going so far as to describe it as a "hoax." Trump explicitly stated that the Democrats were exaggerating the threat as an election-year issue, or "politicizing the coronavirus" (Baker & Karni, 2020). As this chapter aims to make clear, this coverage, and the dynamics of public opinion that followed, exemplify how information in the mass media—traditional broadcast and print news media, as well as social media—has great power to shape the public's attitudes, beliefs, and behaviors about health issues.

Introduction

Health communication theories—and related behavioral theories—can help us make sense of, and even predict, what might result from the news coverage like that *New York Times* article from February 2020, described in the vignette above. This exemplar of downplaying the coronavirus by the most powerful political actor in the country demonstrated how information sources were divided about the

KEY POINTS

This chapter will:

- Describe key features of the current public information environment that are relevant to health and behavior change, using news coverage of the COVID-19 pandemic as an exemplar.

- Introduce a framework for considering media effects in both planned and unplanned applications of health communication.

- Identify the major communication and media effects theories at the individual and societal levels.

- Illuminate the application of these theories with empirical evidence from two cases: COVID-19 vaccination in the United States and use of tobacco imagery in popular entertainment media in India.

severity of the threat (Gollust et al., 2020). Perceived susceptibility to and severity of health risk is a critical component of behavioral change theories, so this claim could signify that Republican listeners would follow Trump and view the threat as less serious, with consequences for their likelihood of taking action (see Chapter 5). It also highlights, explicitly, the way in which information about COVID-19 had become politicized—that is, discourse about the virus had become entangled with political cues. The election year context magnified the potential for information about COVID-19 to become attached to partisan identities. The effects of this discourse rife with partisan cues rather than paying attention to scientific experts increased the likelihood that audiences would incorporate their own political predispositions into their understanding of the virus. This led to dramatic differences by party affiliation in the public's attitudes, beliefs, and behaviors regarding risk mitigation (Gadarian et al., 2022).

This early media portrayal of COVID-19 also illuminates other features of the public information environment that shape the public's response to health information. First, in 2020, there were a multitude of opportunities to learn about COVID-19. No longer did audiences attune mainly to network nightly news or print news for information. By 2020, Americans could get their news from national news outlets, cable news, social media, radio, and a proliferation of other news sites and apps, often, those catering to audiences with particular worldviews (Gottfried & Liedke, 2021). Many local newspapers had closed by 2020, and resources for reporters dedicated to health had shrunk. As a result, the public increasingly relied on health news coverage not by science or medical writers but by reporters from other "beats," such as politics. With traditional, trusted news media no longer a gatekeeper, people also got their COVID-19 information from interpersonal sources (e.g., friends, family) and advertisements (such as public service announcements—PSAs—and political ads in the 2020 election), contributing to competing information about the viral threat and what to do about it.

As scientists learned more about the novel coronavirus, information changed from week to week—and, accordingly, health recommendations evolved, often quite rapidly. Audiences noticed this apparent inconsistency, among politicians and medical experts, with, for instance, differing recommendations emanating from spokespeople at the White House (i.e., Anthony Fauci), the CDC, and state health departments (Nagler et al., 2020). This communication happened within a context of dynamic changes in trust in science and in media (Kennedy et al., 2022).

Also, evidence of racial and socioeconomic disparities in COVID-19 incidence and mortality—as a result of differential exposure to the virus and vulnerability to its consequences because of structural factors—emerged relatively early in the pandemic (Viswanath et al., 2020). This information, combined with renewed attention to racial justice in the summer of 2020 after the killing of George Floyd in Minneapolis, brought more attention to health inequities in the information environment (Xu et al., 2022), although public understanding of these inequities was far from uniform (Gollust et al., 2022).

Finally, this combination of fragmented information outlets, a politically charged environment, and dynamic changes in trust in science and media created a communication environment where misinformation and disinformation could spread quickly (van der Linden, 2022; Vraga & Jacobsen, 2020). One cross-sectional study of a nationally representative sample in 2020 found that endorsement of COVID-19 misinformation was quite common (with 47% of the sample scoring high on misinformation) and that those who relied on conservative sources of news had a higher likelihood of reporting misinformation (Dhawan et al., 2021). The same study showed that those scoring high on misinformation were also less likely to report confidence, or self-efficacy in their ability to perform COVID-19 prevention strategies like social distancing, using face masks, and handwashing (Dhawan et al., 2021).

Each of these dimensions of the information environment at the emergence of COVID-19 in 2020 speaks to the objective of this chapter: to describe communication theories that explain how the public information environment shapes the public's attitudes, beliefs, and, ultimately, their health-related behaviors. Communication theories, combined with an understanding of the trends in media environments outlined above, can offer important predictions for researchers, professional communicators, and public health practitioners on how communication can shape health behaviors, as well as how best to intervene.

Communication and Media Effects Theories

Planned and Unplanned Approaches to Communication for Health: A Framework for Understanding Media Effects in Public Health

There are two primary approaches to studying the role of communication in public health (Figure 17.1). First, communication can be used purposively or intentionally to achieve public health goals, whether these are shifts in health

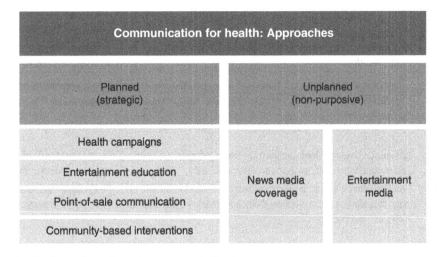

Figure 17.1 Typology of Planned and Unplanned Approaches to Communication for Health

Note. Social media are relevant to both planned (strategic) and unplanned (nonpurposive) approaches to communication. For example, multimedia health campaigns are increasingly disseminated via social media, and social media are also a source of incidental exposure to health information—including mis/disinformation.

beliefs, attitudes, support for public policies, or health behaviors. Historically, one of the most salient of these *planned or strategic uses* of communication for health has been large-scale media campaigns, where the objective is, typically, increasing public awareness and/or promoting behavior change. Other examples of planned communication include: entertainment-education initiatives designed to encourage behavior change through engaging storylines rather than more expository informational approaches; point-of-sale communication of information, such as nutrition labels on foods and beverages or warning labels on tobacco packaging; and community-based interventions that leverage communication technology to improve outcomes, including health literacy and information efficacy.

Communications also are used for health in *unplanned or nonpurposive ways* through the public's routine interactions with the media and broader information environment. These unplanned communications can shape health behavior and its antecedents as much as (if not more than) planned communication efforts, often in unintentional ways. This second approach to communication in public health has become increasingly important in recent years, with widespread availability of health information in both news and entertainment media (e.g., news stories that discuss e-cigarette use among youth, movies that portray tobacco use), alongside greater ability to share such information within both offline and online social networks. Such information diffusion via social ties occurs in both unplanned and planned communication contexts, although inequalities in information sharing across population groups have been identified (Southwell, 2013).

Consider again the case of the COVID-19 pandemic. Between 2020 and 2022, there were countless strategic communication messages to promote mitigation behaviors, such as masking, social distancing, and vaccine uptake—efforts that were spearheaded by a wide range of stakeholders, including local and state health departments, federal agencies like the US Centers for Disease Control and Prevention (CDC), community-based organizations, schools, and universities, and hospitals and health systems. This messaging took the form of full-scale national media campaigns (such as the US Department of Health and Human Services' "We Can Do This" campaign and the Ad Council's "It's Up to You" campaign), as well as more localized efforts in communities, clinical settings, and schools. However, these planned applications of communication to promote COVID-19 prevention measures had to compete with other messages about COVID-19 circulating in the broader information environment, such as news media coverage of debates over vaccine mandates and social media discourse surrounding unproven COVID-19 treatments. As described above, this information ecosystem has been characterized by competing recommendations from health experts and politicians, and rampant mis- and disinformation. Ultimately, then, both planned and unplanned approaches to communication for health are interrelated forces that vie for audience attention and engagement—and although each can be consequential for health behavior, there is increasing concern that competing, inaccurate, and often politicized media content to which the public is routinely and rapidly exposed can undermine public health campaigns and messaging.

Table 17.1   Selected Communication Theories and Approaches at the Individual Level and Societal Level

Theory/Approach	Implication of Theory/Approach for Communication Effects on Public Health	Primary Contexts of the Use of the Theory/ Approach in Research and Practice
Individual and Interpersonal Behavioral Theories Reasoned Action Approach Health Belief Model	Communication can be targeted to the key beliefs and perceptions that underlie a given behavior to change people's behavioral intentions and, in turn, their behavior	Designing persuasive health messages; evaluating health campaigns and other message-based interventions
Social Cognitive Theory	Communication can provide information to enhance people's self-efficacy and/or model other people engaging in the target behavior	Designing and evaluating entertainment-education programs; understanding the effects of media violence
Information Processing Theories Elaboration Likelihood Model Heuristic-Systematic Processing Model Reactance Motivated Reasoning	People will process information in communication messages in different ways, depending on their motivation, ability, and predispositions, including their values and ideology	Designing and understanding how audiences respond to persuasive health messages or news media content
Message Effects Theories Framing (Issue, Gain/Loss) Narrative Persuasion	The ways in which communication messages are packaged—including how issues are framed, and to what extent focal individuals or stories are included—can influence people's beliefs, attitudes, and behavioral intentions	Designing persuasive health messages
Agenda Setting, Priming, and Framing	The communication environment can influence what issues people think are important and how they think about those issues	Understanding how the media cover health and social issues and the effects of such coverage
Cultivation	The communication environment (and television content in particular) can shape people's perceptions of social reality	Understanding how the media cover health and social issues and the effects of such coverage
Communication and Health Equity Knowledge Gap Hypothesis Communication Inequalities	Social groups differ in their ability to access, process, retain, act on, and benefit from information. Organizations also differ in their ability to generate, manipulate, and distribute information	Understanding how audiences differentially respond to persuasive health messages, news media content, or other health information; understanding differences in communication capacity across organizations/institutions

Theories of Communication for Health

Theories provide guidance in efforts to consider how the information environment—including both planned and unplanned communication—influences the public. Theories can help researchers and communication planners understand and make predictions about which key variables might be manipulated and/or affect important outcomes. Communication processes can operate directly, where media exposure influences behavior, and, more often, indirectly, where media exposure influences beliefs, attitudes, norms, and, in turn, behavior. However, no single theory explains and predicts all communication outcomes, and theories can operate on different levels.

For ease of presentation, below, we describe individual-level (micro) and societal-level (macro) communication theories, while acknowledging that there can be interactions across the levels of analysis. While this is not an exhaustive summary of all theoretical constructs that explain communication effects (because these theories come from a broad range of disciplines, including communication, sociology, psychology, and political science), Table 17.1 summarizes the key theories and approaches that are most commonly used to explain health communication effects. The table also points out some of the most common applications of these theories in health communication research and practice, to guide students, researchers, and practitioners.

Individual-Level Explanations of Communication Effects on Health

Much health communication research at the individual level examines the effects of media exposure on a person's beliefs, motivations, cognitions, opinions, attitudes, and behaviors, drawing from a variety of expectancy-value theories, information processing theories, and message effect theories.

Individual and Interpersonal Behavioral Theories

Several theories that are often used in health behavior and health education offer explanations for media effects at the individual level. For example, the *Health Belief Model* (Chapter 5) and *Reasoned Action Approach* (Chapter 6)

propose pathways of behavior change through a finite set of determinants. Specifically, these theories emphasize that people's behaviors (and, in the case of reasoned action, people's behavioral intentions, in particular) are driven by the beliefs they hold about the behavior—including their evaluations of or attitudes toward the behavior, their perceptions of whether the behavior is normative, and their judgments about their capacity to perform the behavior. Communication messages, including those in media, may be targeted to change these beliefs (Fishbein & Yzer, 2003). For example, one study applied the Reasoned Action Approach by randomizing American Indian youth to view a culturally resonant message about tobacco use and then measuring their attitudes (instrumental and experimental), norms (injunctive and descriptive), and perceptions of autonomy and capacity (self-efficacy perceptions)—all theoretical factors known to shape behavioral intentions (Yzer et al., 2021). A campaign related to the Health Belief Model's construct of perceived susceptibility might similarly be used to increase youth's perceptions of the harms of e-cigarettes.

Social Cognitive Theory (SCT) (see Chapter 9)—often considered an "interpersonal" model—suggests that people can learn why and how to perform a behavior by observing others. As part of this process, people rely on their perceptions of outcome expectations (judgments about the consequences of performing a behavior) and self-efficacy (perceived capability or confidence in performing a behavior); cognitive capabilities, such as the ability to derive meaning from symbols, also support learning through observation (Bandura, 1986). Perhaps the most important implications of SCT for understanding the effects of health communication are the concepts of self-efficacy and modeling. For example, as described later in this chapter, actors who smoke on-screen are modeling a risk behavior for young audiences, typically in the absence of negative health consequences.

Information Processing Theories

Information processing theories focus on the cognitive pathways through which media messages may lead to changes in attitudes or reinforce existing attitudes; they also can explain the process through which people select into receiving messages in the first place. There are several relevant theories. The most commonly used are dual process models, such as the *Elaboration Likelihood Model (ELM)* (Petty & Cacioppo, 1986), and the *Heuristic-Systematic Processing Model (HSM)* (Chaiken et al., 1989). Both models suggest that persuasive messages, such as antismoking messages, are processed in either of two ways. A central or a systematic processing route involves the deliberate, thoughtful weighing of message arguments (e.g., the health reasons for quitting smoking), and the attitude changes accompanying such processing are likely to be more enduring (e.g., positive attitudes toward quitting, which can prompt quit attempts). In contrast, peripheral or heuristic processing occurs under conditions of low motivation and ability, where the recipient relies on peripheral cues (e.g., the celebrity status of a spokesperson for a youth antivaping campaign), and any resultant attitude change tends to be shortlived.

Certain individual characteristics, such as personality traits, values, emotional arousal, and ideology or worldviews, can affect how information in communication is processed. Understanding such audience characteristics allows message designers to target messages more effectively. For instance, researchers have examined the match between message content and the values orientation of audiences, generally finding that messages that resonate with particular social or political values are more persuasive (Shen & Edwards, 2005). Research on the concept of *reactance* (Brehm, 1966) suggests that any persuasive message (particularly one that threatens individuals' perceptions of freedom) may arouse a motivation, called reactance, to reject the advocacy (Dillard & Shen, 2005). For example, there is some evidence that smokers' reactance to graphic health warnings on tobacco packaging can weaken the impact of these warnings on intentions to quit smoking (Hall et al., 2018). Psychological reactance has also been found to be related to reduced mask-wearing during the COVID-19 pandemic (Young et al., 2022).

The theory of biased processing (also known as *motivated reasoning*) offers a complementary explanation to reactance, explaining that people are motivated to evaluate the strength and credibility of messages differently depending on their predisposing attitudes and beliefs (Taber & Lodge, 2006). For instance, people respond in different or opposing ways to messages about a sugar-sweetened beverage tax, based on predisposing ideological beliefs about taxation (Gollust et al., 2017). Evidence also suggests that people evaluate messages about breast cancer screening overdiagnosis differently based on their past routines of screening (Nagler et al., 2017). Research also demonstrates biased selection into messages in the media: people seek out media sources that they expect will be more concordant with their worldviews (Stroud, 2011). As we describe below in the COVID-19 application, motivated reasoning also may help explain the emergence of polarized responses to information about COVID-19.

Message Effects Theories

Research on message effects examines how the format and content of messages interact with audience characteristics to influence information processing and impact. Several theoretical approaches—including framing and narrative persuasion—speak to commonly investigated elements of messaging that have major public health implications and applications.

Framing has multiple definitions that originate from multiple disciplines, but communication scholars generally refer to two. First, framing can refer to presenting logically equivalent information in different ways ("*equivalency frames*"), as Tversky and Kahneman did in framing disease risk information in terms of "lives lost" or "lives gained" (Tversky & Kahneman, 1981). This work launched a productive research agenda on gain/loss framing (see, e.g., Rothman et al., 2006) that examines the effects of health messages framed positively or negatively and that continues to this day. Another type of equivalency frame can be seen in a study that showed differences in risk perception by racial group when researchers examined the effects of a health-disparity statistic presented on its own (e.g., risk of sexually transmitted infections (STIs) for Black teen girls) versus presenting that same statistic as a comparison (e.g., risk of STIs for Black versus White teen girls) (Bigman, 2014).

A second common definition of issue framing (also known as "*emphasis framing*") refers to messages that emphasize specific problem definitions, often invoking the cause of, groups affected by, solutions to, and moral valence of a particular issue in society (Entman, 1993). For instance, obesity might be framed as a problem of individuals behaving poorly (failing to diet, failing to exercise) or as a problem of an obesogenic environment characterized by social inequities that constrain individual opportunities to make healthy choices (Barry et al., 2013). Such frames can activate underlying attitudes about who is responsible for addressing the health issue. Another feature of messaging related to emphasis framing is the inclusion of brief anecdotes, which are often included in media depictions of health issues and that can raise similar concerns of contributing to an individualized, versus structural, understanding of social issues.

In contrast to message framing, *narratives* are powerful message structures for packaging more comprehensive health information (Hinyard & Kreuter, 2007). When health information is conveyed in a story (including characters, plot, conflict, and resolution), audiences may be more likely to engage in a target behavior or change their attitudes than when information is communicated through more traditional didactic messages and formats (i.e., statistics or evidence; exhortations or arguments) (Braddock & Dillard, 2016). The persuasive potential of narrative interventions is supported by social cognitive theory (as described briefly above and in Chapter 9): by observing a modeled behavior (even if conveyed as fictional), individuals are more likely to attempt it. Narrative persuasion may be particularly effective for health behaviors that individuals are likely to resist, such as getting vaccines or cancer screenings (Hinyard & Kreuter, 2007). The process of "*transportation*" (Green & Brock, 2000) explains why narratives are likely to be effective: When individuals become immersed in a narrative's plot and/or characters, they are less likely to resist a message because they may not necessarily identify its persuasive intent; also, they become so absorbed by the emotional aspects of the story that they have reduced motivation and ability to counterargue.

Recent research has explored how narratives can communicate about the social determinants of health and health equity while avoiding the trap described earlier of leading readers to overly focus on individual considerations and personal responsibility (Niederdeppe et al., 2008). This body of research suggests that stories have promise in influencing how audiences think about the determinants of health and shape their opinions about policies that target those factors, although these stories must be constructed carefully. For example, these stories should acknowledge individual choices within the context of the social and environmental barriers that shape those choices, explain how the story applies to other people and groups, and articulate policy solutions to the health problems that the narrative's character faces (Niederdeppe et al., 2015, 2021).

There also are other message formats and appeals that have important implications for influencing health behavior. These include, but are not limited to, *normative appeals* (that describe the frequency with which groups engage in a behavior), *emotional appeals* (that use fear, humor, or other emotions in messaging), and *sensation value-enhancing messages* (that feature, for example, music and/or sound effects, intense images, and special visual effects) (Dillard & Shen, 2013).

Societal-Level Explanations of Communication Effects on Health

Media effects also occur at the societal level, where they are not seen as effects on a given individual's cognitions or behavior, but rather, as effects on how society, or people at large, view the world. For example, media exposure can inform what issues people think are important, and how they think about those issues; it can even shape their perceptions of social reality. There are also theoretical perspectives that underscore how communication and media exposure can have differential effects across social groups, directly connecting communication research with health equity priorities. Several of these theories and perspectives are reviewed below and summarized in Table 17.1.

Agenda Setting, Priming, and Framing

While media influence (like framing effects, described above) happens at the individual level, these effects, in aggregate, can also have societal-level implications so they can be considered cross-level phenomena. Communication researchers have long focused on the influence of media on mass public opinion, especially in politics and policymaking. Early media scholars, such as Walter Lippman described the news media's behavior as a "restless searchlight," panning from one issue to the next while seldom lingering on any single issue (Lippman, 1922). Later researchers such as Bernard Berelson noted that while the media influence public opinion, the reverse is also true: public opinion drives what the media report (Berelson, 1948). Paul Lazarsfeld and colleagues noted that media attention confers status upon issues and raises their importance (Lazarsfeld et al., 1968). These insights coalesced in the 1970s, with a focus on the media's powerful role in setting the public agenda of important issues and problems (McCombs & Shaw, 1972). Gerald Kosicki later identified three types of *agenda-setting* research: (1) public agenda setting, which examines the link between media portrayal of issues and issue priorities assigned by the public; (2) policy agenda setting, which examines the connection between media coverage and the legislative agenda of policymakers; and (3) media agenda setting, which focuses on factors that influence whether and how the media cover certain issues (Kosicki, 1993). Subsequent research further refined agenda-setting theory, as initial correlational studies gave way to more empirically sophisticated designs that enabled clearer causal links and stronger conceptualizations (McCombs & Valenzuela, 2020).

Researchers now agree that the media not only tell us what is important in a general way, but they also provide ways of thinking about specific issues by the signs, symbols, terms, and sources they use to define the issue in the first place. This perspective—that the media do not simply tell us what to think *about*, but also what to think—has been broadly referred to as framing (similar to issue framing described above, but at the aggregate level). In this view, public problems are social constructions (Borah, 2011). That is, groups, institutions, and advocates are in competition to identify problems, move them onto the public agenda, and define them, in competition across spatial contexts and over time (Druckman, 2022). This view suggests that the media's agenda-setting function is not independent but is in fact shaped by various community groups, institutions, and advocates, which has implications for those in public health who seek to use the media to raise public salience and awareness of specific problems. For example, although there is considerable evidence that immigration policy is a determinant of health, little is known about the mechanisms through which such policy shapes health processes and outcomes, such as health behaviors and care seeking. Guided by theories of agenda setting and issue framing, Trinidad Young and colleagues focused on one potential mechanism—news coverage of US immigration policy—by conducting a content analysis of such coverage during the 2010s. They found that most coverage focused on exclusionary immigration policies at the federal level, despite a marked increase in integration policies in recent years, with immigrants tending to be framed either negatively as criminals or positively as part of families (Young et al., 2021). By understanding these patterns in news coverage, advocates may be positioned to agitate for reporting that better reflects the current state of immigration policy and, in turn, bolster public support for policies that center on immigrant health and health equity.

Communication researchers increasingly consider the role of *priming* alongside agenda-setting and framing effects (Scheufele & Tewksbury, 2006). With roots in cognitive social psychology, priming refers to the activation of certain emotions, thoughts, or ideas that are embedded in our minds—specifically, in associative networks, or mental models that link together nodes, which represent concepts (Ewoldsen & Rhodes, 2020). In psychology, an associative network that is activated can affect how subsequent concepts are evaluated; applied to communication research, media content can activate relevant networks, and this activation can have behavioral consequences. In the immigration policy example from above, for example, news media coverage could prime stereotypes of immigrants that already exist within people's associative networks, and such activation could shape the way people think about immigration policy and, ultimately, whether they support efforts to advance immigrant health, with implications for political agenda-setting at the societal level.

Cultivation

By the 1960s, television had replaced radio as the new medium of the day, and its presence in homes across the US raised concerns about its impact, especially the effects of televised violence on children. In 1968, George Gerbner was appointed by President Johnson's National Commission on the Causes and Prevention of Violence to study the content of television programs. Thus began Gerbner's long-running Cultural Indicators project, which assessed both the prevalence and nature of violence portrayals ("message system analysis") and whether exposure to such portrayals might shape people's perceptions of the world ("cultivation analysis"). The theory of *cultivation* emerged from this research program, positing that habitual television exposure shapes people's beliefs about the nature of the world (Gerbner et al., 1980), and that the heavier that exposure, the more likely a person is to subscribe to television's version of social reality (Gerbner et al., 2002). One of the project's most compelling findings was that heavy television viewing was associated with an overestimation of crime and violence—or, put another way, the belief that the world was a mean and dangerous place ("mean world syndrome") (Gerbner et al. 1980).

Fundamentally, cultivation is a theory about dominant media rather than about television, specifically. It suggests that the messages (or, in Gerbner's terms, the message systems) to which we are exposed—repetitively, cumulatively, over the long term—shape our perceptions of social reality. Thus, cultivation is no less relevant today, despite the differences between the current media ecosystem and the one that existed when cultivation research began. That said, recent research has focused less on generalized television media exposure than content- or genre-specific exposure. For example, studies have linked local television news viewing in particular with fatalistic beliefs about cancer prevention (see, e.g., Niederdeppe et al., 2010). From a public health perspective, cultivation theory underscores the notion that health messages, both planned and unplanned, can operate as a set and offer a prevailing view of the world. A media campaign about a given health behavior therefore does not operate in a vacuum, but as part of a complex message ecosystem.

Communication and Health Equity

There are two primary strands of media effects research that foreground issues of health equity. The first is research on communication inequalities, which has historical roots in the knowledge gap hypothesis; the second is research on communicating about health inequity.

Conventional wisdom once held that persistent social problems could be resolved through public education alone. Yet, with the work of Tichenor, Donohue, and Olien in the 1970s, it became clear that knowledge and information are unequally distributed across population groups. Referring to this observation as the *knowledge gap hypothesis*, they proposed that an increasing flow of information into a social system (from a media campaign, for example) would be more likely to benefit groups of higher socioeconomic status (SES) than those of lower SES (Tichenor et al., 1970). In other words, increasing the information available in the system would only exacerbate existing differences in knowledge between these groups. The disturbing implication of this research was that media campaigns would actually perpetuate inequities. This implication is also at the core of the related theory in public health that posits that social conditions are a "fundamental cause" of disease because better social conditions convey resources (including access to health information, but also power, money, access to care, and other advantages) that contribute to better health (Link & Phelan, 1995).

The knowledge gap hypothesis was one of the first theoretical perspectives in the media effects tradition to draw attention to the role of the social environment in shaping media influence (Viswanath & Finnegan, 1996)—and it attracted the attention of scholars and policymakers alike. For instance, Viswanath's early research applied the knowledge gap hypothesis in the health context (Viswanath et al., 1991), but ultimately he broadened the concept to include inequalities across other communication dimensions. And so emerged a body of research that systematically documents a broad range of *communication inequalities*, defined as (1) differences among social groups in the generation, manipulation, and distribution of information at the institutional level, and (2) differences among social groups in their ability to access, process, retain, and act on information at the individual level (Viswanath et al., 2022). Communication inequalities at the institutional level have been observed among organizations. For example, consider the marketing and promotional budgets of the tobacco industry ($8.2 billion in 2019 in the United States alone; CDC, 2021) and food and beverage industry (estimated at $1.8 billion in the United States in 2009 in marketing to children and adolescents; FTC, 2012), and contrast these to the limited communication capacity of community-based organizations working to prevent tobacco use or promote healthy eating among youth. At the individual level, studies show the pervasiveness of communication inequalities across several dimensions, including information access and processing (e.g., Lin et al., 2014), information avoidance (e.g., McCloud et al., 2013), and differential effects of communication interventions (e.g., Lee et al., 2022). Unfortunately, such inequalities have become more pronounced during the COVID-19 pandemic (Viswanath et al., 2020).

A second strand of research on communication and health equity builds upon this work by considering how communication can be leveraged to alleviate health inequities. Specifically, research in this space has focused on how strategic communication can (1) raise public awareness of health inequities (which remains low, particularly for disparities by race and income; Gollust et al., 2022), (2) shape perceptions that such inequities are serious and should be addressed, (3) influence beliefs about who or what is responsible for such inequities, (4) promote support for policies that could reduce inequities, and (5) mobilize key stakeholders and groups to advocate for social change (Niederdeppe et al., 2013). For example, in the recent study noted in the above discussion about narratives, Niederdeppe et al. (2021) tested several evidence-based strategies to generate public support for investments in early childhood education, finding that policy narratives—"short stories with a setting, characters, and a plot that unfolds over time and offers a policy solution to a social problem" (p. 1088)—may be a promising message strategy, particularly for persuading people who are inclined to oppose such policies.

Applications

This section illustrates how the key theories described above can be applied to pressing health issues, both in the United States (Application 1) and globally (Application 2). Both examples describe empirical research that demonstrates the importance of selected theories in an applied health communication context.

Application 1: COVID-19 Vaccine Uptake in the United States in 2021

After all the early COVID-related health and political communication issues in 2020, as described at the beginning of this chapter, the first coronavirus vaccine for people 16 years of age and older became available on December 11, 2020 under an emergency use authorization from the Food and Drug Administration. The vaccine was first available only to healthcare professionals and other groups deemed essential, and subsequently to groups defined by characteristics such as age and risk, following guidance from the CDC (Dooling et al., 2021). By April 19, 2021, once there was sufficient vaccine supply, all adults across all states became eligible.

Survey evidence almost immediately demonstrated significant differences between different groups in COVID-19 vaccine uptake, which can be explained by several of the communication theories described above. First, national surveys, such as the Kaiser Family Foundation (KFF) COVID-19 Vaccine Monitor, continually demonstrated that Republicans expressed more concerns about the vaccine and lower intentions to get vaccinated; ultimately, far fewer Republicans (54%) than Democrats (86%) reported receiving at least one dose of the vaccine by July 2021 (Kirzinger et al., 2021). These significant nationwide political patterns were increasingly evident even at the community level as well (Kates et al., 2022). Since then, many studies have sought to understand these links between political partisanship, ideology, and coronavirus vaccination behavior—and the role of communication in producing the observed polarization in vaccine beliefs (e.g., Gadarian et al., 2022; Viswanath et al., 2021). For instance, one study tested the effects of various media frames (issue frames) about COVID-19 vaccines and found that a message that emphasized social norms (describing others' willingness to get the vaccine) increased vaccine intentions, whereas a message that aimed to politicize the vaccine (emphasizing President Trump's pressure on the FDA to approve a vaccine quickly) reduced vaccine intentions; the authors observed no moderation by partisanship (Palm et al., 2021). Another study tested the effects of explicit partisan cues versus scientific cues in messaging about vaccines (Golos et al., 2022); the concept of motivated reasoning would suggest that the partisan cues should produce politically polarized responses. In fact, the authors observed a wide gap in vaccine intentions by respondents' partisanship, with the scientific cue particularly effective at increasing vaccine intentions, especially among Democrats (Golos et al., 2022). These findings illuminate the importance of information processing theories, showing that partisanship is a significant predisposition that can shape responses to health messaging.

Another major difference that emerged early in vaccine-related survey data involved concerns about vaccines expressed by people of color. For instance, in February 2021, 34% of Black adults said they would "wait and see" about the vaccine, compared to only 18% of White adults who expressed this hesitant perspective (Hamel et al., 2021). These differences are likely related to historical and contemporary distrust of the healthcare system and the structural racism that these systems reinforce (Momplaisir et al., 2021). Later that year, differences in reported intentions translated into racial differences in vaccine uptake. By July 2021, 70% of White adults had received at least one dose, compared to 65% of Black adults and 61% of Hispanic adults. Although the vaccine was available for free and there was abundant media attention to vaccines, in both news media and campaign PSAs, a communication inequality perspective helps understand in part why these disparities emerged (see, e.g., Viswanath et al., 2020).

Communication inequalities point to the importance of group differences in the ability to act on information (such as availability of free vaccines), which includes the ability to take time off from work to get the vaccine or recover from side effects, as well as to access vaccine sites (by locating these close to where communities of color live and work). They also point to relevant structural factors at play, including a lack of prioritization and outreach in geographic areas with social vulnerability, and the use of age-based allocation schemes that tended to promote earlier vaccination among older White adults (Hughes et al., 2021; Wrigley-Field et al., 2021).

Application 2: Tobacco Imagery in Popular Entertainment Media in India

For more than two decades, researchers have studied whether exposure to portrayals of tobacco use in entertainment media, particularly movies, influences tobacco uptake among youth. This work has arguably produced one of the most robust literatures documenting the influence of media on health. In its 2008 monograph on media and tobacco use, the US National Cancer Institute drew a bold conclusion: "The total weight of the evidence from cross-sectional, longitudinal, and experimental studies, combined with the high theoretical plausibility from the perspective of social influences [sic], indicates a causal relationship between exposure to movie smoking depictions and youth smoking initiation" (Davis et al., 2008, p. 19). This finding was later echoed by the US Surgeon General's report (2012) on preventing tobacco use among youth and young adults.

Research on tobacco imagery in entertainment media has been conducted both in and outside the United States, and it has been especially important as the tobacco epidemic has shifted from developed to developing countries. One country that has confronted the challenge of such portrayals is India, with its thriving Bollywood movie industry and prevalent tobacco use (nearly 267 million Indian tobacco users aged 15+, as of 2016–2017; WHO, 2022). Early observational research showed findings similar to those observed in the United States and elsewhere. Compared with low-exposure adolescents, adolescents with high exposure to tobacco use in popular Bollywood movies were significantly more likely to report ever using tobacco, adjusting for potential covariates (Arora et al., 2012). Given the popularity of Bollywood movie stars, the authors argued that actors' behavior in films could influence youth. This argument is consistent with two underlying theoretical explanations offered in previous research (Davis et al., 2008): (1) positive portrayals of tobacco use, or a risk behavior shown in the absence of negative consequences, could be persuasive from a modeling perspective (as described in Social Cognitive Theory; see Chapter 9); and (2) frequent tobacco portrayals could lead to the perception that tobacco use is prevalent (as suggested by theories of descriptive normative influence).

More recent longitudinal research among Indian youth did not find evidence of lagged, or subsequent, associations with smoking uptake (Kulkarni et al., 2021), and researchers suggested that this could be due to the presence of on-screen health warnings. Due at least in part to communication research evidence, the 2003 Indian tobacco-free film rules (which were updated in 2012) indicated that any film with tobacco imagery must include a 20-second audiovisual health warning in the beginning and middle of the film, as well as visual health warnings displayed on screen while tobacco products or use appear. Unfortunately, content analytic research suggests that such warnings are not strictly enforced, and tobacco imagery remains prevalent in films in India (Kulkarni et al., 2020). Research should continue to monitor and evaluate whether any reductions in tobacco imagery contribute to decreased tobacco use among youth. Implementation challenges notwithstanding, the fact that Indian law requires strategic health messaging in the face of movie smoking portrayals provides a compelling illustration of how planned and unplanned applications of communication for health often compete for audience attention (see Figure 17.1).

Discussion and Conclusions

Like every discipline, communication and, specifically, media effects research, has struggled with unresolved challenges. First, the term "effects" in media effects signals fundamental causality, and yet demonstrating causality is no easy task. Many researchers use randomized controlled experiments to test for message effects (e.g., Bigman, 2014; Hall et al., 2018), and these studies provide important insights into how messages shape short-term attitudes and intentions. However, these methods are harder to use to assess effects on longer-term outcomes like behavior change. This methodological challenge is particularly true in when evaluating health communication campaigns, the most successful of which are large, naturally occurring programs that do not constrain people's exposure to campaign messages—and so, by definition, cannot be assessed via a rigid randomized trial design (Hornik, 2002). Thus, researchers aiming to evaluate media campaigns need to use alternative designs that respect the way communication actually flows through social systems, while still limiting threats to validity and maximizing the potential for causal inference (e.g., true and constructed cohort studies, time series designs; Hornik, 2002). Such designs do not enable the same causal claims as trials, but they can get close while still allowing identification of campaign-driven health behavior change.

There are also ongoing challenges in measuring key constructs. Perhaps most salient is the question of how best to capture media exposure—an important construct, as it is often the central independent variable in media effects and health communication research. After all, if someone is not exposed to media content, whether directly or indirectly, then they cannot be influenced by it. Measuring media exposure is becoming increasingly complex given the ever-growing number and breadth of information sources to which the public is exposed, from social media to digital advertising to streaming TV services. Over the years there have been several syntheses of and validity studies on measuring media exposure, including a special issue of *Communication Methods and Measures* dedicated to this topic in 2016 (De Vreese & Neijens, 2016). Such work has summarized the breadth of measures available, their strengths and limitations, and their applications. It has also provided evidence of measures that perform best against a set of validity criteria (e.g., nomological validity, discriminant validity). Also, these reviews have laid out directions for future research on measure development.

Finally, there is the pressing challenge of developing an evidence base for effective communication interventions to address phenomena such as conflicting scientific information in the media, mis/disinformation, and politicization of health and science issues—issues that predated but also became more urgent with COVID-19. The extant evidence for such interventions is stronger in some areas than others. For instance, there has been considerable work on strategies to mitigate and even prevent the adverse consequences of exposure to mis/disinformation, much (though certainly not all) of it spurred by the COVID-19 pandemic (see, for example, van der Linden, 2022). In contrast, little is known about how best to limit the now well-documented undesirable effects of exposure to conflicting health information, including worrisome downstream carryover (or spillover) effects of such information on people's receptivity to unrelated health messages for which there is scientific consensus (e.g., fruit and vegetable consumption, physical activity) (Nagler et al., 2021). And although there is some initial evidence that forewarning messages could guard or "inoculate" against the negative effects of exposure to politicized information (Fowler et al., 2022), research in this space is nascent.

Summary

Communication theories and approaches described in this chapter underscore how critical it is for both researchers and practitioners to consider the broader media ecosystem—including multiple information sources, channels, and messages—in trying to understand the effects of planned and unplanned communication on health behavior and its antecedents. The COVID-19 experience has illuminated longstanding features of the media environment that have important implications for health and health behavior change, including fragmented information sources, proliferation of messengers, media distrust, polarization, and spread of misinformation. Communication science, with its strong theoretical grounding and empirical support, can help relevant stakeholders (including researchers, program planners, and communication practitioners) to make predictions and evaluations of the effects of health messaging on public perceptions and behaviors. Attention to this body of science can assist in targeting resources to more effectively use communication to improve the public's health and advance health equity.

References

Arora, M., Mathur, N., Gupta, V. K., Nazar, G. P., Reddy, K. S., & Sargent, J. D. (2012). Tobacco use in Bollywood movies, tobacco promotional activities and their association with tobacco use among Indian adolescents. *Tobacco Control, 21*(5), 482–487.

Baker, P., & Karni, A. (2020). "Trump accuses media and Democrats of exaggerating coronavirus threat." *The New York Times.*

Bandura, A. (1986). *Social foundations of thought and action.* Englewood Cliffs, NJ: Prentice Hall.

Barry, C. L., Brescoll, V. L., & Gollust, S. E. (2013). Framing childhood obesity: How individualizing the problem affects public support for prevention. *Political Psychology, 34*(3), 327–349.

Berelson, B. (1948). Communications and public opinion. In W. Schramm (Ed.), *Communications in modern society* (pp. 167–185). Urbana, IL: University of Illinois Press.

Bigman, C. A. (2014). Social comparison framing in health news and its effect on perceptions of group risk. *Health Communication, 29*(3), 267–280.

Borah, P. (2011). Conceptual issues in framing theory: A systematic examination of a decade's literature. *Journal of Communication, 61*(2), 246–263.

Braddock, K. & Dillard, J. P. (2016). Meta-analytic evidence for the persuasive effect of narratives on beliefs, attitudes, intentions, and behaviors. *Communication Monographs, 83*(4), 446–467.

Brehm, J. W. (1966). *A theory of psychological reactance.* New York: Wiley.

CDC. (2021). Tobacco industry marketing. https://www.cdc.gov/tobacco/data_statistics/fact_sheets/tobacco_industry/marketing/index.htm

Chaiken, S., Liberman, A., & Eagly, A. (1989). Heuristic and systematic information processing within and beyond the persuasion context. In J. S. Uleman & J. A. Bargh (Eds.), *Unintended thought* (pp. 212–252). New York: Guilford Press.

Davis, R. M. (Ed.) Gilpin, E., Loken, B., Viswanath, K., & Wakefield, M. (2008). *The role of the media in promoting and reducing tobacco use* (No. 19). US Department of Health and Human Services, National Institutes of Health, National Cancer Institute Tobacco Control Monograph Series.

De Vreese, C. H., & Neijens, P. (2016). Measuring media exposure in a changing communications environment. *Communication Methods and Measures, 10*(2–3), 69–80.

Dhawan, D., Bekalu, M., Pinnamaneni, R., McCloud, R., & Viswanath, K. (2021). COVID-19 news and misinformation: Do they matter for public health prevention? *Journal of Health Communication, 26*(11), 799–808.

Dillard, J. P., & Shen, L. (2013). *The Sage handbook of persuasion.* Thousand Oaks, CA: Sage.

Dillard, J. P., & Shen, L. J. (2005). On the nature of reactance and its role in persuasive health communication. *Communication Monographs, 72*(2), 144–168.

Dooling, K., Marin, M., Wallace, M., McClung, N., Chamberland, M., Lee, G. M., Talbot, H. K., Romero, J. R., & Oliver, S. E. (2021). The Advisory Committee on Immunization Practices' updated interim recommendation for allocation of COVID-19 vaccine—United States, December 2020. *Morbidity and Mortality Weekly Report, 69*(51–52), 1657.

Druckman, J. N. (2022). A framework for the study of persuasion. *Annual Review of Political Science, 25*, 65–88.

Entman, R. (1993). Framing: Toward clarification of a fractured paradigm. *Journal of Communication, 34*(4), 51–58.

Ewoldsen, D. R., & Rhodes, N. (2020). Media priming and accessibility In M. B. Oliver, A. A. Raney, J. Bryant (Eds.), *Media Effects: Advances in Theory and Research* (pp. 83–99). New York: Routledge.

Fishbein, M., & Yzer, M. C. (2003). Using theory to design effective health behavior interventions. *Communication Theory, 13*(2), 164–183.

Fowler, E. F., Nagler, R. H., Banka, D., & Gollust, S. E. (2022). Effects of politicized media coverage: Experimental evidence from the HPV vaccine and COVID-19. *Progress in Molecular Biology and Translational Science, 188*, 101–134.

FTC. (2012). A review of food marketing to children and adolescents: Follow-up report. https://www.ftc.gov/sites/default/files/documents/reports/review-food-marketing-children-and-adolescents-follow-report/121221foodmarketingreport.pdf

Gadarian, S. K., Goodman, S. W., & Pepinsky, T. B. (2022). *Pandemic politics*. Princeton, NJ: Princeton University Press.

Gerbner, G., Gross, L., Morgan, M., & Signorielli, N. (1980). The "mainstreaming" of America: Violence profile number 11. *Journal of Communication, 30*(3), 10–29.

Gerbner, G., Gross, L., Morgan, M., Signorielli, N., & Shanahan, J. (2002). Growing up with television: Cultivation processes. *Media Effects: Advances in Theory and Research, 2*(1), 43–67.

Gollust, S. E., Barry, C. L., & Niederdeppe, J. (2017). Partisan responses to public health messages: Motivated reasoning and sugary drink taxes. *Journal of Health Politics, Policy and Law, 42*(6), 1005–1037.

Gollust, S. E., Fowler, E. F., Vogel R. I., Rothman A. J., Yzer M., & Nagler, R. H. (2022). Americans' perceptions of health disparities over the first year of the COVID-19 pandemic: Results from three nationally-representative surveys. *Preventive Medicine, 162*, 107–135.

Gollust, S. E., Nagler, R. H., & Fowler, E. F. (2020). The emergence of COVID-19 in the US: A public health and political communication crisis. *Journal of Health Politics, Policy and Law, 45*(6), 967–981.

Golos, A. M., Hopkins, D. J., Bhanot, S. P., & Buttenheim, A. M. (2022). Partisanship, messaging, and the COVID-19 vaccine: Evidence from survey experiments. *American Journal of Health Promotion, 36*(4), 602–611.

Gottfried, J., & Liedke, J. (2021). *Artisan divides in media trust widen, driven by a decline among Republicans*. Pew Research Center. https://www.pewresearch.org/fact-tank/2021/08/30/partisan-divides-in-media-trust-widen-driven-by-a-decline-among-republicans/

Green, M. C., & Brock, T. C. (2000). The role of transportation in the persuasiveness of public narratives. *Journal of Personality and Social Psychology, 79*(5), 701–721.

Hall, M. G., Sheeran, P., Noar, S. M., Boynton, M. H., Ribisl, K. M., Parada Jr, H., Johnson, H., & Brewer, N. T. (2018). Negative affect, message reactance and perceived risk: How do pictorial cigarette pack warnings change quit intentions? *Tobacco Control, 27*(e2), e136–e142.

Hamel, L., Sparks, G., & Brodie, M. (2021). KFF COVID-19 Vaccine Monitor: February 2021. https://www.kff.org/coronavirus-covid-19/poll-finding/kff-covid-19-vaccine-monitor-february-2021/

Hinyard, L. J., & Kreuter, M. W. (2007). Using narrative communication as a tool for health behavior change: a conceptual, theoretical, and empirical overview. *Health Education & Behavior, 34*(5), 777–792.

Hornik, R. (2002). *Public health communication: Evidence for behavior change*. New York: Routledge.

Hughes, M. M., Wang, A., Grossman, Pun E., Whiteman, A., Deng, L., Hallisey, E., Sharpe, D., Ussery E. N., Stokley, S., Musial, T., Weller, D. L., Murthy, B. P., Reynolds, L., Gibbs-Scharf, L., Harris, L., Ritchey, M. D., & Toblin, R. L. (2021). County-level COVID-19 vaccination coverage and social vulnerability—United States, December 14, 2020–March 1, 2021. *Morbidity and Mortality Weekly Report, 70*(12), 431.

Kates, J., Tolbert, J., & Rouw, A. (2022). The Red/Blue divide in COVID-19 vaccination rates continues: An update. https://www.kff.org/policy-watch/the-red-blue-divide-in-covid-19-vaccination-rates-continues-an-update/

Kennedy, B., Tyson, A., & Funk, C. (2022). Americans' trust in scientists, other groups declines. https://www.pewresearch.org/science/2022/02/15/americans-trust-in-scientists-other-groups-declines/

Kirzinger, A., Sparks, G., Hamel, L., Lopes, L., Kearney, A., Stokes, M., & Brodie, M. (2021). KFF COVID-19 Vaccine Monitor: July 2021. https://www.kff.org/coronavirus-covid-19/poll-finding/kff-covid-19-vaccine-monitor-july-2021/

Kosicki, G. M. (1993). Problems and opportunities in agenda-setting research. *Journal of Communication, 43*(2), 100–127.

Kulkarni, M. M., Kamath, A., Kamath, V. G., Lewis, S., Bogdanovica, I., Bains, M., Cromwell, J., Fogarty, A., Arora, M., Nazar, G. P., Ballal, K., Naik, A. K., Bhagawath, R., & Britton, J. (2021). Prospective cohort study of exposure to tobacco imagery in popular films and smoking uptake among children in southern India. *PLoS One, 16*(8), e0253593.

Kulkarni, M. M., Kamath, V. G., Cranwell, J., Britton, J., Nazar, G. P., Arora, M., Ballal, K., & Kamath, A. (2020). Assessment of tobacco imagery and compliance with tobacco-free rules in popular Indian films. *Tobacco Control, 29*(1), 119–121.

Lazarsfeld, P. F., Berelson, B., & Gaudet, H. (1968). *The people's choice*. New York: Columbia University Press.

Lee, E. W., McCloud, R. F., & Viswanath, K. (2022). Designing effective eHealth interventions for underserved groups: Five lessons from a decade of eHealth intervention design and deployment. *Journal of Medical Internet Research, 24*(1), e25419.

Lin, L., Jung, M., McCloud, R. F., & Viswanath, K. (2014). Media use and communication inequalities in a public health emergency: A case study of 2009–2010 pandemic influenza A virus subtype H1N1. *Public Health Reports, 129*(6 Suppl4), 49–60.

Link, B., & Phelan, J. (1995). Social conditions as fundamental causes of disease. *Journal of Health and Social Behavior, 35*(Extra Issue), 80–94.

Lippmann, W. (1922). *Public opinion.* New York: Free Press.

McCloud, R. F., Jung, M., Gray, S. W., & Viswanath, K. (2013). Class, race and ethnicity and information avoidance among cancer survivors. *British Journal of Cancer, 108*(10), 1949–1956.

McCombs, M., & Shaw, D. (1972). The agenda setting function of the mass media. *Public Opinion Quarterly, 36,* 176–187.

McCombs, M., & Valenzuela, S. (2020). *Setting the agenda: Mass media and public opinion.* Hoboken, NJ: John Wiley & Sons.

Momplaisir, F., Haynes, N., Nkwihoreze, H., Nelson, M., Werner, R. M., & Jemmott, J. (2021). Understanding drivers of coronavirus disease 2019 vaccine hesitancy among blacks. *Clinical Infectious Diseases, 73*(10), 1784–1789.

Nagler, R. H., Fowler, E. F., & Gollust, S. E. (2017). Women's awareness of and responses to messages about breast cancer overdiagnosis and overtreatment: Results from a 2016 national survey. *Medical Care, 55*(10), 879.

Nagler, R. H., Vogel, R. I., Gollust, S. E., Rothman, A. J., Fowler, E. F., & Yzer, M. C. (2020). Public perceptions of conflicting information surrounding COVID-19: Results from a nationally representative survey of US adults. *PLoS One, 15*(10), e0240776.

Nagler, R. H., Vogel, R. I., Gollust, S. E., Yzer, M. C., & Rothman, A. J. (2021). Effects of prior exposure to conflicting health information on responses to subsequent unrelated health messages: Results from a population-based longitudinal experiment. *Annals of Behavioral Medicine, 56*(5), 498–511.

Niederdeppe, J., Bigman, C. A., Gonzales, A. L., & Gollust, S. E. (2013). Communication about health disparities in the mass media. *Journal of Communication, 63*(1), 8–30.

Niederdeppe, J., Bu, Q. L., Borah, P., Kindig, D. A., & Robert, S. A. (2008). Message design strategies to raise public awareness about social determinants of health and population health disparities. *Milbank Quarterly, 86*(3), 481–513.

Niederdeppe, J., Fowler, E., Goldstein, K., & Pribble, J. (2010). Does local television news coverage cultivate fatalistic beliefs about cancer prevention? *Journal of Communication, 60*(2), 230–253.

Niederdeppe, J., Roh, S., & Shapiro, M. A. (2015). Acknowledging individual responsibility while emphasizing social determinants in narratives to promote obesity-reducing public policy: A randomized experiment. *PLoS One, 10*(2), e0117565.

Niederdeppe, J., Winett, L. B., Xu, Y., Fowler, E. F., & Gollust, S. E. (2021). Evidence-based message strategies to increase public support for state investment in early childhood education: Results from a longitudinal panel experiment. *Milbank Quarterly, 99*(4), 1088–1131.

Palm, R., Bolsen, T., & Kingsland, J. T. (2021). The effect of frames on COVID-19 vaccine resistance. *Frontiers in Political Science, 3,* 41.

Petty, R. E., & Cacioppo, J. T. (Eds.) (1986). The elaboration likelihood model of persuasion. *Communication and persuasion* (pp. 1–24). New York: Springer.

Rothman, A. J., Bartels, R. D., Wlaschin J., & Salovey, P. (2006). The strategic use of gain- and loss-framed messages to promote healthy behavior: How theory can inform practice. *Journal of Communication, 56*(s1), S202–S220.

Scheufele, D. A., & Tewksbury, D. (2006). Framing, agenda setting, and priming: The evolution of three media effects models. *Journal of Communication, 57*(1), 9–20.

Shen, F. Y., & Edwards, H. H. (2005). Economic individualism, humanitarianism, and welfare reform: A value-based account of framing effects. *Journal of Communication, 55*(4), 795–809.

Southwell, B. G. (2013). *Social networks and popular understanding of science and health: Sharing disparities.* Baltimore: Johns Hopkins University Press.

Stroud, N. J. (2011). *Niche news: The politics of news choice.* New York: Oxford University Press.

Surgeon General's Report. (2012). *Preventing tobacco use among youth and young adults: A report of the surgeon general.* Washington, DC: US Government Printing Office.

Taber, C. S., & Lodge, M. (2006). Motivated skepticism in the evaluation of political beliefs. *American Journal of Political Science, 50*(3), 755–769.

Tichenor, P. J., Donohue, G. A., & Olien, C. N. (1970). Mass media flow and differential growth in knowledge. *Public Opinion Quarterly, 34*(2), 159–170.

Tversky, A., & Kahneman, D. (1981). The framing of decisions and the psychology of choice. *Science, 211*(4481), 453–458.

van der Linden, S. (2022). Misinformation: susceptibility, spread, and interventions to immunize the public. *Nature Medicine, 28*(3), 1–8.

Viswanath, K., Bekalu, M., Dhawan, D., Pinnamaneni, R., Lang, J., & McLoud, R. (2021). Individual and social determinants of COVID-19 vaccine uptake. *BMC Public Health, 21*(1), 1–10.

Viswanath, K., & Finnegan Jr, J. R. (1996). The knowledge gap hypothesis: Twenty-five years later. *Annals of the International Communication Association, 19*(1), 187–228.

Viswanath, K., Finnegan Jr, J. R., Hannan, P. J., & Luepker, R. V. (1991). Health and knowledge gaps: Some lessons from the Minnesota Heart Health Program. *American Behavioral Scientist, 34*(6), 712–726.

Viswanath, K., Lee, E. W., & Pinnamaneni, R. (2020). We need the lens of equity in COVID-19 communication. *Health Communication, 35*(14), 1743–1746.

Viswanath, K., McCloud, R. F., & Bekalu, M. A. (2022). Section 7: Communication, health and equity: structural influences. In T. L. Thompson & N. G. Harrington. (Eds.) *Routledge handbook of health communication* (pp. 426–440). New York: Routledge.

Vraga, E. K., & Jacobsen, K. H. (2020). Strategies for effective health communication during the coronavirus pandemic and future emerging infectious disease events. *World Medical & Health Policy, 12*(3), 233–241.

WHO. (2022). Tobacco. https://www.who.int/india/health-topics/tobacco

Wrigley-Field, E., Kiang, M. V., Riley, A. R., Barbieri, M., Chen, Y.-H., Duchowny, K. A., Matthay, E. C., Van Riper, D., Jegathesan, K., Bibbins-Domingo, K., & Leider J. P. (2021). Geographically targeted COVID-19 vaccination is more equitable and averts more deaths than age-based thresholds alone. *Science Advances, 7*(40), eabj2099.

Xu, Z., Lin, C. A., Laffidy, M., & Fowks, L. (2022). Perpetuating health disparities of minority groups: The role of US Newspapers in the COVID-19 pandemic. *Race and Social Problems, 14*(4), 1–12.

Young, D. G., Rasheed, H., Bleakley, A., & Langbaum, J. B. (2022). The politics of mask-wearing: Political preferences, reactance, and conflict aversion during COVID. *Social Science & Medicine, 298*, 114836.

Young, M. E., Sarnoff, H., Lang, D., & Ramírez, A. S. (2021). Coverage and framing of immigration policy in US Newspapers. *Milbank Quarterly, 100*(1): 78–101.

Yzer, M., Rhodes, K., Nagler, R. H., & Joseph, A. (2021). Effects of culturally tailored smoking prevention and cessation messages on urban American Indian youth. *Preventive Medicine Reports, 24*, 101540.

PART FIVE

USING THEORY IN RESEARCH AND PRACTICE

CHAPTER 18

INTRODUCTION TO USING THEORY IN RESEARCH AND PRACTICE

The Editors

This chapter provides highlights from each chapter in the section, discusses emerging developments and challenges, and comments on the state of the art in the use of theory in health behavior research and practice. Using theory thoughtfully and appropriately is not simple, but it should be rewarding. This discussion aims to provoke thought and debate and stimulate further reading, rather than to provide definitive answers or prescriptions for the field.

Preceding sections of the book show that theories often are complementary, and that some fit within broader models. Generally, theories can be used most effectively if they are integrated within a comprehensive planning framework. Such a framework assigns a central role to research as an input to determine the situation and needs of the population to be served, resources available, and the progress and effectiveness of the program at various stages. Part Five gives specific examples of how theories can be combined for greater impact.

Theory-Based Planning Models

In Chapter 19, María Fernández and co-authors describe two well-developed planning models, PRECEDE-PROCEED and Intervention Mapping (IM), that can be used to integrate and apply diverse theoretical frameworks. Both models take comprehensive approaches that begin with assessing the problem and population and continue to evaluate, based on a theoretically informed logic model. They illustrate the ways behavior change theories can be applied and incorporated into a systematic planning process and note the challenges of applying the models. Similar to some theories discussed in earlier chapters, using these planning models can be demanding and laborious for practitioners and community groups. But when mastered, they can lead to effective, appropriate health behavior change programs.

While health behavior theories are critical tools, they do not substitute for adequate planning and research. However, theories help in interpreting problem situations and in planning feasible, promising interventions and appropriate program evaluations. Theories aid in articulating assumptions behind intervention strategies and can be useful in pinpointing intermediate steps that should be assessed in evaluations.

Health Behavior: Theory, Research, and Practice, Sixth Edition. Edited by Karen Glanz, Barbara K. Rimer, and K. Viswanath.
© 2024 John Wiley & Sons, Inc. Published 2024 by John Wiley & Sons, Inc.
Companion website: www.wiley.com/go/glanz/healthbehavior6e

The PRECEDE/PROCEED Model centers on the systematic application of theory and previous research to assess local needs, priorities, circumstances, and resources (Green & Kreuter, 1991). Concepts of priority, changeability, and community preferences should be considered, along with analytical and empirical findings about health behavior determinants. For example, health experts concerned with effecting distribution of safe drinking water must understand how people in communities think about water sources and what beliefs might be amenable to change. These ideas are also consistent with concepts presented in earlier chapters on community engagement, implementation, and dissemination.

Fernández and colleagues also review IM, a framework for developing theory- and evidence-based multilevel health behavior/education programs, and illustrate how IM has been applied. IM can help guide program planners toward explicit specification of how to use both theory and empirical findings to develop effective health behavior interventions.

Behavioral Economics

In Chapter 20, Jessica Cohen and Harsha Thirumurthy provide the rationale for key constructs of, and applications of, behavioral economics to health improvement programs. The foundations of behavioral economics lie in classical economics and expected utility theory, blended with a grounding in theories and evidence from psychology and sociology. While not a theory, behavioral economics provides important tools and constructs to understand human behavior. Behavioral economics has received growing attention in recent years, with applications in several fields in which anticipated costs and benefits play a central role: labor markets, wage policies, savings and retirement, and organizational behavior (National Academies of Science, Engineering & Medicine, 2023). Its application to health behavior, health policy, and health care use is emerging rapidly, as described in Chapter 20.

Behavioral economics aims to increase the explanatory power of economics by grounding it in psychological and social foundations. It uses insights from cognitive psychology, sociology, and decision analysis. Behavioral economics recognizes that people make decision errors in weighing the costs and benefits of their actions, and that message framing can influence how people react to persuasive communications. Key implications from behavioral economics for health behavior change suggest that incentives can improve health behaviors, and the way incentives are delivered can matter more than the amount of incentives. This idea, also consistent with Applied Behavior Analysis and Social Cognitive Theory (Chapter 9), has been used in health behavior intervention research by the authors and others with substantial success.

In Chapter 20, Cohen and Thirumurthy report on successful studies that increased uptake of HIV testing and reduced inappropriate opioid prescribing. Both applications illustrate how concepts from behavioral economics can be effective when they are incorporated into patient-facing and provider-facing health care structures. These approaches can be sustained over time and have been shown to be cost-effective and to save lives by reducing fatal overdoses.

Social Marketing

In Chapter 21, Storey and colleagues review the purpose, key components, and methods of social marketing. They illustrate the application of social marketing in two health communication programs: a project in Kenya that supports adoption of behaviors and access to products and services to improve health; and a project in Indonesia that sought to expand the availability of various contraceptive methods and to increase the use of longer-acting methods when appropriate for not having any more children or spacing the next birth.

Social marketing is a process that promotes desired voluntary behaviors among members of a target market, by offering attractive benefits and/or reducing barriers associated with healthful choices. It involves the adaptation of commercial marketing technologies to promote socially desirable goals. In Chapter 21, Storey, Kumoji, Rareiwa, and Wahyuningrum take a fresh look at Social Marketing. They emphasize how social marketing can be applied within a strategic health communication framework and link key theories of health communication and health behavior to the effective practice of social marketing.

Success with social marketing is most likely when marketers accurately determine the perceptions, needs, and wants of target markets and satisfy them through the design, communication, pricing, and delivery of appropriate, competitive, and visible offerings. The process is consumer-driven, not only expert-driven. This orientation is consistent with principles of community organization, and its product development approach parallels the innovation development process of diffusion theory. At the same time, it shares an economic perspective with behavioral economics, a field of inquiry that relates individual behaviors to economic variables (Bickel and Vuchinich, 2000, Chapter 20). Both social marketing and behavioral economics are adapted from an economic or market-based foundation: social marketing uses some principles from commercial marketing, whereas behavioral economics builds on classic economic theory.

As with the PRECEDE/PROCEED Model and IM, social marketing provides a framework to identify what drives and maintains behavior and behavior change. It also requires identification of potential intermediaries, channels of distribution and communication, and actual and potential competitors. As the authors indicate, theories of health behavior can guide the analytical process in social marketing and aid in the formulation of intervention strategies and materials. They explicitly illustrate four theories that contribute to social marketing approaches: Theory of Planned Behavior, Extended Parallel Processing Model, Social Cognitive Theory, and diffusion of innovations. Because of the focus on understanding consumers (or target audiences), social marketing models are robust for use in diverse and unique populations, including disadvantaged groups and ethnic minorities, and in many countries. In fact, it is often thought that social marketing programs tend to be inherently culturally sensitive because they follow a consumer-oriented process. In social marketing, it is always important to identify and fulfill demand—that is, to "start where the people are."

Social Media

Chapter 22 by Bekalu and Viswanath is new for this edition, focusing on the burgeoning use of social media and health. The authors discuss evidence for associations between social media use, health behaviors, and health, and describe examples of interventions for smoking cessation and COVID-19 mitigation that use social media to improve health and health behavior.

Social media is a broadly defined communication channel and process, not a specific theory or organized approach to developing interventions or messages. It straddles several theoretical frameworks presented earlier in the book, including media effects theories, social networks, and social support. Bekalu and Viswanath zero in on two issues: (1) social media use as a behavior and how it affects mental and physical health outcomes, and (2) the role and effects of social media platforms and networks as channels for health interventions.

The latter issue, use of social media to deliver health behavior interventions, is most directly tied to the other chapters' emphasis on use of theory in research and practice. Such strategies are a type of "digital strategy," which has become increasingly widely used, and often use theoretical foundations (Ajie & Chapman-Novakofski, 2014; Swindle et al., 2022). Key questions in considering social-media-based interventions are whether they attract the intended audience (Heckman et al., 2021) and whether they are effective when disseminated beyond initial efficacy testing.

Cross-Cutting Propositions About Using Theory

We offer some key cross-cutting propositions to readers to put the use of health behavior theory in perspective. These ideas are germane to the review and discussion of the chapters in this section and throughout this book.

1. We should not confuse *using* or *applying* theory with testing theory or developing theory. They are fundamentally different activities with their own distinct, although complementary, methodologies.
2. Testing efficacy or effectiveness of theory-based interventions does not constitute testing a theory or theories per se.
3. It is likely that the strongest interventions will be built from multiple theories. The most replicable and transparent interventions will be built in a way that the contributions of each theory can be understood.
4. When combining theories, it is important to clearly think through the unique contribution of different theories to the combined model. If this is not done carefully or well, the "new" combined approach may be redundant, overlapping, and hard to interpret in the context of established theories.
5. Rigorous tests of theory-based interventions, including measurement and analyses of mediators and moderators, are the building blocks of the evidence base in health behavior.

6. Theory use, testing, and development will be enhanced by use of shared instruments and reporting. The more we can build on past efforts, the more we are likely to advance the public's health. We recommend adaptations of the protocol concept used in clinical research so that it is much more transparent and accessible to understand what measures were used to accompany particular theories and how theory is turned into interventions. Good examples can be found in the literature (Glanz et al., 2005; Harte et al., 2022) but more are needed, and intervention researchers should publish protocol papers more routinely.

7. Theory, research, and practice are part of a continuum for understanding the determinants of behaviors, testing strategies for change, and implementing effective interventions (see Chapters 16 and 19).

8. There is as much to learn from failure as there is to learn from success. Researchers and practitioners who develop and test theory-based interventions should publish their findings when they are negative *and* when they are positive.

9. There is no substitute for knowing the audience. This applies to the conduct of fundamental research to understand determinants of health behavior as much as it applies to developing health promotion programs for specific individuals, groups, and communities. Participatory research (Chapter 15) and program design improve the odds of success.

The authors of the next four chapters in Part Five describe tools, strategies, models, and issues for applying theories. This section of *Health Behavior: Theory, Research and Practice* tackles the complexity of health behavior and health promotion at multiple levels. A basic theme is that if intervention strategies are based on a carefully researched understanding of the determinants of behavior and environments, and if systematic approaches to tailoring, targeting, implementation, and evaluation are used, the chances are good that programs will be effective. And if they are not, then there should be good information about why an intervention did not work. Understanding past failure is critical to future success.

Moving Forward

After becoming familiar with some contemporary theories of health behavior, the challenge is to use them within a comprehensive planning process. They should be aligned with cultural and geographical circumstances and designed using technology that aligns with what is revealed during the planning steps. Researchers and practitioners can increase the odds of success by examining health and behavior at multiple levels, as articulated in ecological models (Chapter 3).

At its simplest, an ecological perspective emphasizes two main options: change people, and/or change the environment. The most powerful approaches will use both options together. Activities most directly tied to changing *people* are derived from individual-level theories like Health Belief Model, Transtheoretical Model of Change, and Reasoned Action Approach. In contrast, activities aimed at changing the *environment* draw on community-level theories. In between are Social Cognitive Theory, social support, and social networks. Each of these focuses on reciprocal relations among persons or between individuals and their environments.

Theoretical frameworks are guides in the pursuit of successful efforts, maximizing flexibility and helping apply abstract concepts of theory in ways that are most useful in diverse work settings and situations. Knowledge of theory and comprehensive planning systems offers a great deal. Other key elements of effective programs are a good program-to-audience match; accessible and practical information; active learning and involvement; and skill building, practice, and reinforcement. Strong interventions will often but not always be built on theory, but theory alone cannot lead to effective interventions. Theory helps one ask the right questions, and effective planning enables you to zero in on these elements in relation to a specific problem. Still, theory must be turned into effective interventions, and these must be applied with fidelity and evaluated well. A lot happens between theory and behavior change. Effective use of theory for practice and research requires practice but can yield important dividends in efforts to enhance the health of individuals and populations. In the end, we should ask ourselves whether our work has made a difference. Developing better theories is a means to that end.

The modern field of health behavior dates back only about 80 years, and progress has accelerated most rapidly in the past 30 years. As the chapters in this book have shown, many of the early ideas of social and behavioral theorists serve as solid foundations for our work today. To accelerate progress, we should stand on the shoulders of the pioneers in the field, equip ourselves to be explorers, address today's problems with new tools, and anticipate the challenges of the future.

References

Ajie, W. N., & Chapman-Novakofski, K. M. (2014). Impact of computer-mediated, obesity-related nutrition education interventions for adolescents: A systematic review. *Journal of Adolescent Health, 54*(6), 631–645.

Bickel, W. K., & Vuchinich, R. E. (Eds.). (2000). *Reframing health behavior change with behavioral economics.* Mahwah, NJ: Lawrence Erlbaum Associates.

Glanz, K., Steffen, A., Elliott, T., & O'Riordan, D. (2005). Diffusion of an effective skin cancer prevention program: Design, theoretical foundations, and first-year implementation. *Health Psychology, 24*(5), 477–487.

Green, L. W., & Kreuter, M. W. (1991). *Health promotion planning: An educational and environmental approach.* Mountain View, CA: Mayfield.

Harte, R., Norton, L., Whitehouse, C., Lorincz, I., Jones, D., Gerald, N., Estrada, I. Sabini, C., Mitra, N., Long, J., Cappella, J., Glanz, K., Volpp, K. G., & Kangovi, S. (2022). Design of a randomized controlled trial of digital health and community health worker support for diabetes management among low-income patients. *Contemporary Clinical Trials Communications, 5*, 100878.

Heckman, C. J., Riley, M., Khavjou, O., Ohman-Strickland, P., Manne, S. L., Yaroch, A. L., Bhurosy, T., Coups, E. J., & Glanz, K. (2021). Cost, reach, enrollment, and representativeness of recruitment efforts for an online Skin Cancer Risk Reduction Intervention Trial for young adults. *Translational Behavioral Medicine, 11*(10), 1875–1884.

National Academies of Sciences, Engineering, and Medicine. (2023). *Behavioral economics: Policy impact and future directions.* Washington, DC: The National Academies Press. https://doi.org/10.17226/26874.

Swindle, T., Poosala, A. B., Zeng, N., Børsheim, E., Andres, A., & Bellows, L. L. (2022). Digital intervention strategies for increasing physical activity among preschoolers: Systematic review. *Journal of Medical Internet Research, 24*(1), e28230.

CHAPTER 19

PLANNING MODELS FOR THEORY-BASED HEALTH PROMOTION INTERVENTIONS

María E. Fernández
Christine Markham
Patricia Dolan Mullen
Melissa Peskin
Shari Esquenazi-Karonika

KEY POINTS

This chapter describes two different frameworks (models) that can guide systematic development of theory- and evidence-based health promotion programs: PRECEDE-PROCEED (Green & Kreuter, 1991, 2005, 2022) and Intervention Mapping (Bartholomew et al., 2016).

The chapter presents:

- An overview of the two planning models, PRECEDE-PROCEED and Intervention Mapping, and the major steps in each model.

- Description of how these models can be used to integrate theory and evidence into program planning and evaluation.

- Case examples that describe the process of applying PRECEDE-PROCEED and Intervention Mapping.

- Adaptation of evidence-based interventions and planning implementation strategies using Intervention Mapping.

Vignette

Angela, a recent MPH graduate and new employee at the city health department, has been charged with planning a program to increase HPV vaccination in the city as a key strategy to reduce incidence and mortality from cervical and other HPV-related cancers. Reviews of vaccination records indicate that the city's rates are below the state average for HPV vaccination initiation and for completion of the vaccination series.

Angela forms a team to plan a health promotion program and holds a meeting with stakeholders that includes healthcare providers and community members. The group immediately starts suggesting ways to address the problem. "We need to scare parents into vaccinating their children," said a teacher. "They don't get that they are putting their kids at risk if they don't vaccinate them." Another planning group member said, "The most important thing is access. I bet people aren't getting their kids vaccinated because they cannot find a place where they can get the vaccine for free."

Angela reflects on her academic training on theories and frameworks in health promotion, to better understand the reasons parents may not be vaccinating their children against HPV. She thinks about the Health Belief Model and wonders whether perceived risk is a factor, or perhaps perceived severity. She also remembers reading about how the beliefs about outcomes (that the vaccine will work) could also influence behavior. Surely, it is important to use theory in planning, but how? Angela realizes she needs a way to organize the discussions, her knowledge about theory, and information from the published literature to create a plan (or map) on how to get from the problem to the solution. She decides to use Intervention Mapping to plan the program.

Health Behavior: Theory, Research, and Practice, Sixth Edition. Edited by Karen Glanz, Barbara K. Rimer, and K. Viswanath.
© 2024 John Wiley & Sons, Inc. Published 2024 by John Wiley & Sons, Inc.
Companion website: www.wiley.com/go/glanz/healthbehavior6e

Introduction

Planning frameworks and models guide program planners in the design of interventions to improve health and quality of life. They provide a series of steps and processes that help planners organize theory, evidence, and new data to inform program planning. These frameworks are particularly relevant in (1) helping planners apply health behavior and organizational theories to improve their understanding of the environmental and behavioral factors that influence health problems; and (2) designing interventions to address them.

We use the terms "framework" and "model" interchangeably throughout this chapter to mean a structure that elicits a hypothesized set of relationships among constructs and one or more behavior(s) or environmental factor(s) leading to health outcomes, and a set of processes to follow in the development of a health behavior or health promotion intervention.

Unlike *theories*, planning *frameworks* do not consist of a set of testable constructs and propositions that describe the relations between these constructs. A planning model is a scaffold or structure that provides an overview, or outline, of categories or concepts (Crosby & Noar, 2011); and often the steps to create, adapt, and evaluate interventions. Thus, while planning models often help incorporate and organize constructs of various theories, they are typically broader than individual theories, and they guide how theories should be applied to create change. They also help practitioners organize empirical evidence about the influences on health behavior and environment. The purpose of a planning framework, then, is to guide planners in identifying the full range of constructs that may be relevant for changing one or more behavior(s) and outcomes, describing the mechanisms through which change is likely to occur, and guiding the design of intervention components and materials.

A benefit of using planning models in intervention design is that they do not dictate the exact theory that should be used but instead, provide guidance about what types of theories *can be* used, and *when* and *how* to use theory. They can enable the use of constructs that are not explicitly theory-based (Glanz & Bishop, 2010; Hilliard et al., 2018) but can inform the planning process, providing guidance on several decisions in the intervention development process.

Using Planning Models to Apply Health Behavior Theory

Public health professionals and researchers interested in developing, implementing, and evaluating *interventions* approach the use of theory in fundamentally different ways from that of researchers generating new or testing existing *theories*. In intervention development, the primary goal is to diagnose problems and create programs that influence health outcomes rather than theory-testing (Bartholomew & Mullen, 2011); therefore, intervention developers often apply multiple theories and draw on empirical evidence and new research.

PRECEDE-PROCEED and Intervention Mapping

PRECEDE-PROCEED and IM are among the most widely used planning frameworks across an array of health behaviors, populations, and settings and have been used by people with varying levels of training (Bartholomew et al., 2016; Green et al., 2022). Both emphasize an ecological perspective and community engagement throughout the planning and implementation processes (Green et al., 2022). PRECEDE-PROCEED, with a longer history, follows a linear approach, emphasizing behavioral science theories to identify *predisposing, enabling, and reinforcing* factors that influence health behaviors. IM is an iterative six-step planning process that integrates multiple theories and models to design a multilevel intervention (behavioral, organizational, environmental). It places strong emphasis on understanding determinants of behavior, choosing theory-based methods to create change and developing interventions and implementation strategies based on theory, evidence, and new data.

PRECEDE-PROCEED Model

PRECEDE-PROCEED has been a cornerstone of health promotion practice for more than fifty years and has been used for planning health promotion interventions globally with more than 1600 published works describing its use as of August 2023 (http://www.lgreen.net). Developed in the 1970s, PRECEDE-PROCEED began to influence the health education field by describing an outcome-focused approach to planning that incorporates three categories of factors that influence behavior and, ultimately health problems: predisposing, reinforcing, and enabling factors. Of particular importance is the model's ecological approach to planning, which considers the relationships between individuals and their environments and incorporates multiple levels of influence on health and quality of life, including genetic, behavioral, social, and environmental factors (Bronfenbrenner, 1979; Marmot, 2000) (see Chapter 3). This model helps planners map these influences and recognize how they can influence health (Green et al., 2022).

The model emphasizes involvement of community members, particularly those directly affected by health problems and those who will be most influenced by programs or policy changes. This approach recognizes that community members' knowledge, experience, and insights concerning their health and quality of life, the behavioral and environmental conditions affecting them, and that their predisposing, reinforcing, and enabling influences, are critical to effective program planning. Community members, including potential intervention implementers and participants, help ensure that the intervention is locally relevant, and develop capacity in intervention development and evaluation.

PRECEDE-PROCEED has eight phases: four planning phases, one implementation/process evaluation phase, and three evaluation phases (Green et al., 2022). The first three phases help develop a logic model (theory) of the problem, starting with an assessment of quality of life and associated health problems that contribute to decreases in quality of life. Recognizing health, social conditions, and quality of life as closely intertwined and mutually influencing, the model leads planners through an analysis of the causes of health problems at multiple ecological levels and helps planners focus on determinants of health-related behaviors and environments. The latter phases of the PRECEDE-PROCEED framework are the PROCEED phases, which focus on the implementation, evaluation, and maintenance of health interventions (Figure 19.1) (Table 19.1).

Phase 1: Social Assessment: Quality of Life

Planners using this model identify the social conditions and their interpretations by community members, professionals, and organizational leaders and staff, and connect these understandings with potential health program strategies to

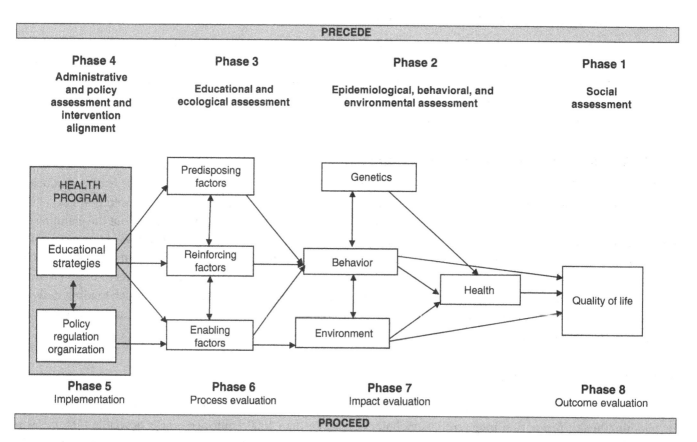

Figure 19.1 PRECEDE-PROCEED Planning Model
Source: Gielen et al., in Glanz et al. (2008)

Table 19.1   PRECEDE-PROCEED Model as a Structure for Using Theories and Constructs

Examples Theories and Principles by Ecological Level	Phase 1 Social Assessment	Phase 2 Epidemiological, Behavioral, and Environmental Assessments	Phase 3 Educational and Ecological Assessment	Phase 4 Administrative and Policy Assessment and Intervention Alignment
Community-Level	X	X	X	X
Participation and Relevance, e.g., Stakeholder Theory, Theories of Power, Coalition Theories	X	X	X	X
		X		X
Community Assessment, e.g., Systems Theories, Social Capital, and Community Capacity				
Intervention, e.g., Community Organization, Community Mobilization, Organizational Change, Diffusion of Innovation				
Interpersonal-Level		X	X	X
Social Cognitive Theory		X	X	
Adult Learning			X	
Interpersonal Communication			X	
Social Networks, and Social Support				
Individual-Level		X	X	
Social Cognitive Theory		X	X	
Theories of Self-Regulation			X	
Goal Setting and Planning			X	
Health Belief Model			X	
Transtheoretical Model of Behavior Change (Stages of Change)				
Theory of Reasoned Action				
Theory of Planned Behavior				
Information Processing				

accommodate diverse values and needs. The model recognizes that health, social conditions, and quality of life are closely intertwined and mutually influencing.

Planners can use a variety of sources to better understand quality of life concerns. These include surveys measuring unemployment/underemployment rates, poverty, transportation, pain, mental well-being, and health-related quality of life. A combination of methods can be used: interviews, focus groups, concept mapping, and citizen scientist projects (Rowbotham et al., 2023).

Several theoretical approaches to community engagement (see Chapter 15) and perspectives on community structure, needs and assets can be helpful at this phase, including systems theories (Foster-Fishman et al., 2007; McKnight & Kretzmann, 2012); theories regarding social networks (Valente & Pitts, 2017); and constructs of social capital and community capacity (Green et al., 2022; Springer & Evans, 2016). Other theories, for example, stakeholder theories (Kok et al., 2015) and coalition theories (Butterfoss & Kegler, 2009) can guide community engagement. Additional objectives for this phase are to articulate the rationale for selecting priority problems, and, ultimately, to use the documentation and rationale as variables in the evaluation of the resulting program.

Phase 2: Epidemiological Assessment I: Population Health

This phase involves a comprehensive examination of the health issues within a priority population. The aim is to understand the current health status, identify health determinants, and recognize the factors that contribute to the health problem. It includes data collection and analysis to provide a solid foundation for subsequent planning phases (Chapter 4 in Green et al., 2022).

An epidemiological analysis to identify and describe the health problem typically includes indicators such as mortality (death rates or years of potential life lost), morbidity (quality-adjusted life years or sick days), temporary or permanent disability (days lost from work or infertility), and cost (to communities, agencies, and health insurance providers). Examining data by subgroups (e.g., gender, socioeconomic status, age) can reveal differences and disparities associated with social determinants of health and help planners identify populations most in need.

In this phase, planners often use data from local, state, and national health surveys, disease registries, and medical claims databases; generally available electronically. Many websites provide extensive resources for both access and interpretation. Examples in the United States include the National Health Information Center at http://www.health.gov/nhic; the National Library of Medicine Databases and Electronic Resources at http://www.nlm.nih.gov/databases; the National Center for Health Statistics at http://www.cdc.gov/nchs; and the National Health Equity Atlas at https://nationalequityatlas.org.

Phase 2: Epidemiological Assessment II: Behavioral and Environmental Factors

In this phase, health planners carry out a *behavioral and environmental assessment* to identify what behaviors and environmental factors cause the health problem(s) and quality-of-life conditions. In the view of the model's authors, behavior can be thought of as occurring at three levels: (1) proximal behaviors, the direct actions or inactions of individuals or groups of individuals that are known to influence their own health or that of others who depend on them, e.g., their infants; (2) interpersonal behaviors, actions or inactions of others who have a direct impact on the social or physical environment of individuals at risk and thus influence their actions or inactions, e.g., parental policies regarding teen driving, and (3) distal behaviors, policy and enforcement actions, individually or collectively, on or by people acting in an organizational or policy environment (Chapter 5 in Green et al., 2022). The behavioral analysis describes what the at-risk group does that increases risk of experiencing the health problem. In the case of secondary and tertiary prevention, the analysis investigates what individuals do that increases the risk of disability or death from a health problem they already have. For example, lack of adherence to prescribed dietary, physical activity, and medication advice is a major barrier to the effective treatment of diabetes and can lead to the disease and increased disease burden (morbidity or mortality).

The *behavioral assessment* includes the following: (1) listing potential behavioral risks related to the health problem; (2) rating the importance and changeability of the behaviors; (3) choosing behavioral targets based on their dual ratings, and (4) specifying behavioral objectives. Typically, but not always, behaviors rated of greatest importance and changeability are selected as targets for action. In "d," behavioral objectives should include who is expected to change, the desired behavior or health practice to be achieved, how much change is to be achieved, and when the desired change is expected to occur.

The *environmental assessment* includes conditions in the social, physical, and biologic (including genetic) environments that influence the health problem directly or through its behavioral causes. In most analyses of health problems, the environment plays a significant and modifiable role in causing the problem either directly, such as exposure to lead-contaminated dust in lead poisoning, or indirectly through behavior and policies, such as lack of smoking bans in the workplace. In the case of genetics, a currently nonmodifiable factor may be quite important in understanding the health problem and identifying affected groups. Steps in the environmental analysis include selection of the most important and changeable environmental factors and specification of the environmental objective(s). In cases where environmental factors are too encompassing and complex for the scope of the project, PRECEDE-PROCEED authors recommend emphasizing additional social (organizational and economic) determinants that interact with behavior and are changeable by social action or policy change.

Several theories are useful when describing behavior and environment. For example, Social Cognitive Theory (SCT) (see Chapter 9) focuses on the reciprocal interaction of behavior and environment. Additionally, some theories are important for specifying the details of the behavior targeted for change. For example, Self-Regulation Theory (Vohs & Baumeister, 2016), theories of goal setting and planning (Latham & Arshoff, 2015), and the Transtheoretical Model of Behavior Change (Prochaska, 2013) (see Chapter 7) are theories that can help understand the steps people engage in to change behavior (see Table 19.1).

Phase 3: Educational and Ecological Assessment: Predisposing, Enabling, and Reinforcing Factors

This phase identifies and categorizes antecedents of behaviors and environmental conditions selected in the Phase 2 analysis as predisposing, enabling, and reinforcing. Predisposing factors refer to those factors that make individuals or communities more likely to engage in a particular health behavior or to have a particular health outcome. These factors are among the determinants that influence whether someone is inclined to adopt a certain behavior or make lifestyle choices that affect their health. Enabling factors facilitate changes in behavior and the environment—resources, social support, and skills. Reinforcing factors follow a behavior and provide the continuing reward or incentive for the action(s). (Fernandez et al., 2019).

These categories of factors all influence behavior and the environment directly or through their interactions. Once identified, selecting specific determinants to prioritize will depend not only on their importance and changeability but also on the resources and context available to address them. Additionally, the timing of the order in which these determinants are addressed can be informed by theory. For example, using the Transtheoretical Model (Chapter 7) would suggest that if the population or community does not have correct knowledge about the risk and behavior change needed or does not believe taking action will result in a positive outcome, then addressing predisposing factors should be the first priority.

Key constructs that address behavioral antecedents that can apply both to the at-risk group and to agents responsible for environmental conditions can be found in several theories/models, including: Health Belief Model (perceived severity and susceptibility, barriers and benefits, cues to action, and self-efficacy) (Chapter 5); Theory of Planned Behavior (attitudes, subjective norms, intention, and perceived behavioral control) (Chapter 6); and Social Cognitive Theory (self-efficacy, behavioral capability, and outcome expectations) (Chapter 9) (see Table 19.1).

Phase 4: Health Program and Policy Development I: Intervention Strategies

In this phase, the planner selects intervention strategies to address the program objectives. Planners: (1) match intervention strategies with the prioritized predisposing, enabling, and reinforcing factors and ecological level; (2) adapt prior interventions and community-preferred strategies that might have less evidence to support them, and if necessary, (3) patch those interventions to fill gaps in the evidence-based strategies by creating new intervention strategies and deriving specific strategies from more general "best practices"; (4) pool and blend intervention strategies into comprehensive programs, and (5) refine and test the full program (formative evaluation) to ensure its fit with the organization and community or population (Chapter 7 in Green et al., 2022).

Phase 4: Health Program and Policy Development II: Implementation Strategies

Here, planners work through concrete planning steps needed to implement the program—from adoption and initial implementation to full operation, program adjustment, and maintenance as well as program dissemination and scale-up. As Escoffery and Green put it: "Fundamentally, implementation challenges the notion that having a good idea or plan is enough." It asks, "How will that idea or plan express itself as action in the real world?" (Chapter 9 in Green et al., 2022). Thus, researchers are explicitly encouraged to contribute to an understanding of how interventions "work" in real-life situations.

Phases 5–8

Implementation planning starts by gathering data needed to develop a logic model, guiding selection and development of implementation tools. Such data can be sourced from manuals, a timeline, and a work plan that can be used for training and supervision as well as identification/development of the sources of data to monitor the program for process evaluation (Phase 5).

In the PROCEED Phases 5–8, the planner reaches back to the logic model of change, program objectives, program components, and the implementation plan to design data collection plans for evaluating the process (program monitoring), short and long-term outcomes, and economics. *Process evaluation* determines how well the program was implemented according to protocol. Short-term and intermediate evaluations assess "near-term" effects on predisposing, reinforcing, and enabling factors, as well as on behavioral and environmental factors. Finally, long-term outcome evaluation determines the effect of the program on health and quality of life indicators. Typically, the measurable objectives that are written in each phase of PRECEDE-PROCEED serve as milestones against which accomplishments are evaluated. Economic evaluation assesses the costs and consequences of one or more programs.

Applying the PRECEDE-PROCEED Model: Case Study

LISTEN UP (Locally Integrated Screening and Testing Ear aNd aUral Program) is an example of applying the PRECEDE-PROCEED model to develop and pilot test a pharmacy-based ear health service in two remote, rural communities in Australia. Details of the development process and results from a feasibility trial are reported elsewhere (Taylor et al., 2021, 2022).

The planning group used findings from a systematic review, an exploratory or scoping review, stakeholder surveys and interviews, and consultation with governing bodies and regulatory authorities, to inform needs assessment, intervention development, and implementation planning (Taylor et al., 2021). An advisory group, including governing bodies, regulatory authorities, and community organization representatives reviewed these data and provided ongoing consultation to ensure the LISTEN UP model fit the pharmacy and community.

Social Assessment and Epidemiological Assessment I

In Australia, one in six people experiences some form of hearing impairment, and 1.3 million people report preventable hearing loss (Australian Government Department of Health, 2022). Conductive hearing loss in Aboriginal and Torres Strait Islander peoples is a major public health problem, with rates as high as 90% in some remote communities (Macquarie University, 2022). In rural and remote areas, limited access to trained health professionals is a major barrier to universal ear health care. Findings from social and epidemiological assessments have shown that community pharmacists are well-positioned to provide expanded ear health services as they are often the only permanent health professional in these settings. Rural consumers, pharmacists, and health professionals ranked hearing tests as an important component of expanded pharmacy services and one that could be improved with adequate training and resources. The planning team set primary objectives for the six-month ear health feasibility study to improve rural consumer access to ear health care and determine pharmacists' level of preparedness and confidence to perform ear exams and make appropriate recommendations or referrals (Taylor et al., 2021).

Epidemiological Assessment II: Behavioral and Environmental Factors

Key behaviors of rural consumers included attending community pharmacies for ear complaints due to lengthy delays in obtaining doctors' appointments. Interviews with pharmacists indicated frequent provision of informal ear care services, including pain management options and referral recommendations, in some cases using otoscopy to examine patients' ears. Barriers included lack of time, space, and remuneration. Pharmacists also reported difficulty accessing health professionals, lack of permanent healthcare providers, and frequent staff turnover. Based on a literature review, survey, and interview findings, the planning group determined the following secondary objectives of the ear health strategy: (1) identify untreated ear conditions in rural communities; (2) improve collaboration between community pharmacy and general practitioner (GP) services; (3) provide targeted patient ear-health referrals to GP practice, and (4) support engagement of telehealth through the use of video-otoscopy and timely transfer of care (Taylor et al., 2021).

Educational and Ecological Assessment

Based on a literature review and discussions with stakeholders, rural pharmacists, and community leaders, the planning group determined that key *predisposing factors* included pharmacists' limited knowledge, skills, and equipment to diagnose or treat ear conditions appropriately. Consumer outcome expectations when presenting to community pharmacies with an ear complaint were either a product recommendation or referral to a GP or emergency department. Enabling factors included pharmacists' willingness to develop expanded practice models and their professional skills in ear-health care, and health providers' expectations that expanded pharmacy practice would improve healthcare for people living in rural and remote communities. Reinforcing factors included pharmacists' ability to retain equipment after completion of the feasibility study (Taylor et al., 2021, 2022).

Health Program and Policy Development I & II: Intervention and Implementation Strategies

The planning group consulted with two community pharmacists to assess the capacity of rural pharmacies to implement the intervention. Both pharmacies reported adequate personnel, time, and space for the project. The primary capital expense was purchasing equipment.

The primary intervention was to train pharmacists in ear-health care. Ear, nose, and throat specialists were consulted on the otoscopy and tympanometry skills required for pharmacists to effectively conduct ear examinations. The planning group collaborated with a nationally credentialed training organization to develop 55 hours of online training and 16 hours of face-to-face workshops. Training included foundations of ear health, anatomy and physiology, theoretical and practical sessions on ear condition recognition and assessment, and otoscopy and tympanometry skill development. An advisory panel consisting of medical experts and policy makers confirmed that the training and expanded service model were appropriate, acceptable, and well-aligned with the current rural pharmacy landscape; and compliant with policy, regulation, and legal requirements (Taylor et al., 2021).

The planning group then developed the LISTEN UP protocol with an integrated direct referral pathway to local GP providers. Using the protocol, trained pharmacists provided otoscopy and tympanometry assessments on consumers presenting to the community pharmacy with ear complaints, and made recommendations including no treatment, pharmacy only products, or GP referral.

PROCEED Phases

In the PROCEED segment of the model, the planning group addressed implementation, process, and outcome evaluation and conducted a six-month feasibility trial February–July 2021. Two community pharmacies located in remote rural communities and a GP (primary care) practice in each community participated. Pharmacists collected data on ear complaints ($n = 23$) for eight weeks prior to the intervention period. To assess the feasibility and potential impact of the intervention, the planning group used a pre-intervention comparison group ($n = 55$). During this time, 23 ear complaints were presented to the pharmacy.

Extensive qualitative data were collected to assess consumer, pharmacist, and GP satisfaction. Competing priorities related to COVID-19 vaccinations limited pharmacists' time for ear health. Further, because the intervention was not remunerated, other competing, funded services were a higher priority. Despite implementation challenges, 90% (50/55) of consumers were highly satisfied with the service and said they would recommend it, citing convenience, improved confidence and appreciation of the knowledge gained about their ear complaint. Pharmacists were motivated to upskill and manage workflow to incorporate the service and expected both consumers and GPs to be more accepting of future expanded services as a result of LISTEN UP (Taylor et al., 2022). Overall, PRECEDE-PROCEED provided a comprehensive model to guide the design and implementation of an acceptable and accessible ear health service for rural and remote communities in Australia. However, sustainability will require ongoing funding to provide resources including additional pharmacists, equipment, and training.

Intervention Mapping

The IM framework for planning multilevel health promotion programs (Bartholomew et al., 2016; Fernandez et al., 2019) was built on the foundation of PRECEDE-PROCEED. IM adds detail to the processes of intervention development, implementation, and evaluation. IM defines determinants of behavioral and environmental change, identifies theory-based change methods to influence those determinants, and designs practical applications of those change methods that fit with the population and setting. IM has guided the development of health promotion programs for many different health problems (Millet et al., 2022; Ravicz et al., 2022) and has helped guide community-based participatory research (CBPR) in planning efforts (Guzman-Tordecilla et al., 2022).

Each step of IM comprises several tasks, and the completion of all steps creates a blueprint or "map" for designing, implementing, and evaluating an intervention. The process is intended to be iterative using several "core processes" across steps including brainstorming, conducting a literature review, applying theory, and gathering information and/or new data. (Bartholomew et al., 2016; Ruiter & Crutzen, 2020).

Step 1: Needs and Assets Assessment

This step consists of four tasks: (1) establish a planning group; (2) conduct a needs and assets assessment; (3) describe the context for the intervention (including the community, population, and setting); and (4) state the intervention goals. A product of Step 1 is the logic model *of the problem* (Bartholomew et al., 2016). The developers of IM use a modified version of PRECEDE-PROCEED in this step, combining predisposing and reinforcing factors into one category of "personal" determinants: those cognitive and emotional factors that lead to either behavior of the risk group or the behaviors of persons in the environment. Enabling factors, or the environmental conditions that make the behavior of the risk group either easier or more difficult, are included in the "environment" box of the logic model. Following a description of the health and quality of life problem, the behavioral and environmental factors influencing the problem, and the determinants causing the risk behaviors and detrimental environmental conditions, planners articulate program goals that would result in improvements in health and quality of life.

Step 2: Intervention Outcomes and Objectives

The guiding question for planners (in Step 2) is: "What needs to change to decrease or eliminate the health problem and the behavioral and environmental risks?" To create the Logic Model of Change, planners utilize theory and evidence to describe the targets of change for the intervention. This step includes four tasks: (1) state the desired behavioral and environmental outcomes; (2) specify the performance objectives for behavioral and environmental outcomes; (3) select determinants for behavioral and environmental outcomes; and (4) construct matrices of change objectives.

The IM Logic Model of Change depicts hypothesized causal pathways of how the intervention (its methods and practical applications of those methods) influences determinants and behavior of both the at-risk group and the environmental change agents, and, ultimately, how these changes lead to health and quality of life outcomes. In this step, planners decide what behavioral and environmental factors are associated most strongly with improvement in health outcomes (relevance), and which are most changeable.

Some theories help consider what behaviors should be the target(s) for change. For example, Social Cognitive Theory (SCT) emphasizes the interaction between a person and their social and physical environments and is congruent with the emphasis of this IM step on the importance of change in both the at-risk group and the environment (see Chapter 9). Other theories specify the detail of the behavior targeted for change. For example, Self-Regulation Theory (Vohs & Baumeister, 2016) and theories of goal setting and planning (Latham & Arshoff, 2015) guide planners to break behavior change into the processes of self-monitoring, goal setting, planning, performing, and evaluating strategies. When thinking about change in organizations, political entities, or communities, theories at a higher ecological level can be helpful. These include theories of social support (Chapter 10), social networks (Chapter 11), organizational change (Hussain et al., 2018) and community organization (Wallerstein et al., 2020).

The next task in this step is to use theory, evidence, and new data to understand the hypothesized determinants of the behavioral changes for the at-risk group and environmental agents. These determinants answer the question of *why* the person at-risk, or the environmental agent, would contribute to a change in behavior or the environment condition respectively.

A central activity of IM is to create a matrix of the *change objectives* that specify *who and what* should change. Change objectives are the intersection of the performance objectives and the determinants guided by the question, "What must change in the determinant to bring about the performance objective?" The answers to this question form the cells of the matrix and become the targets for change in an intervention. In the middle school example described in the next section, the planning team asked, "What must the intervention change in knowledge, skills, and self-efficacy for students to avoid peers and potential dating partners that engage in unhealthy relationship behaviors?" The matrices guide decisions about what theory-based change methods will likely influence change in determinants.

Step 3: Methods and Practical Applications

Step 3 consists of three tasks: (1) generate intervention ideas with the planning group; (2) choose theory and evidence-based change methods; and (3) select or design practical applications to deliver change methods. In this step, planners make decisions about theory-based change methods and how best to apply them, generating possible program themes and major program components. A theory-based change method is a defined process for how interventions can influence change in the determinants of behavior of individuals, groups, or social structures. Different methods influence different determinants. Some theories used to understand or predict a behavior may offer little or no guidance on how to change determinants related to the behavior; thus, other theories may be needed for this purpose. For example, the Health Belief Model (HBM) suggests the importance of perceived susceptibility in predicting action but offers little guidance about how to change this belief (see Chapter 5). SCT, on the other hand, offers specific methods for affecting change in determinants (see Chapter 9).

Parameters of methods describe the way they should be translated into a practical application such that the application preserves the conditions for effectiveness ("instructions" for effective use of a method). For example, "modeling" (a method) is effective only *if* it is (1) reinforced; and (2) when observers pay attention, have adequate self-efficacy and skills, identify with the model, and observe a coping model rather than a mastery model (Bartholomew et al., 2016).

Step 4: Intervention Design and Production

Step 4 consists of four tasks: (1) define the intervention's structure and reach; (2) plan intervention-related messages, materials, and activities; (3) produce intervention materials, activities, and protocols; and (4) pretest, refine, and finalize materials and activities. As planners produce the program's materials and protocols, they must recognize that theory-based methods (from Step 3) are likely to be a major foundation of an intervention's "active ingredients" or expected mechanism of action of the intervention. As planners determine messages, content, and delivery of the program, they must keep in mind the determinants, methods, parameters, and potential delivery. In this step, theory-derived change methods are operationalized and included in practical delivery strategies that are woven into a coherent program with a defined scope and sequence. The final delivered interventions will often comprise a multicomponent and multilevel program targeting change in both at-risk groups and environmental agents, with each part of the program requiring materials and messages.

Step 5: Implementation Mapping

In this step, planners focus on designing strategies to ensure program adoption, implementation, and sustainment. Step 5 includes five tasks: (1) conduct a needs and assets assessment and identify program implementers; (2) identify implementation performance objectives and determinants to create matrices of change objectives; (3) choose change methods and implementation strategies; (4) produce implementation protocols and materials; and (5) evaluate implementation outcomes. An implementation plan, including designated strategies to accelerate and improve program use, is essential to ensure that the program is delivered as planned (with fidelity) and that it reaches the populations of interest.

While this step has been integral to the process since IM was first described, it recently gained considerable attention within the implementation science community as "Implementation Mapping" because of its utility in providing a systematic approach to the design of implementation strategies (Fernandez et al., 2019). IM can be used both as part of the initial planning of an intervention (as Step 5 in the six-step planning process) or independently to plan strategies for improving adoption, implementation and/or maintenance of existing evidence-based interventions (Kang & Foster, 2022; Pérez Jolles et al., 2022).

In Step 5, planners use similar processes of considering needs and assets as described in Step 1, and develop performance objectives, and identify determinants (Step 2). The subjects performing the tasks in this step, however, are the program adopters, implementers, and maintainers. Working with potential adopters and implementers as core members of the planning group at the onset of a project can form the foundation for developing program components that directly affect implementation.

Step 6: Evaluation Plan

In Step 6 planners propose process and outcome evaluation methods. This step consists of six tasks: (1) Write effect and process evaluation questions; (2) Find indicators and measures for assessment; (3) Specify the evaluation design; (4) Complete the evaluation plan; (5) Pilot test the intervention and finalize the evaluation plan; and (6) Interpret/act on evaluation findings. The foundation for evaluating an IM-designed intervention is the products of earlier steps. The logic model of change and matrices for the intervention and its implementation suggest the constructs that could be measured, ranging from the ultimate effect on quality of life or health problems to near term effects to further right on the logic model (e.g., change in determinants). This will depend on the quality of the evidence already available. For example, since the effect of low birth weight on infant health and the contribution of maternal tobacco smoking to low birth weight is already known, the evaluator should focus on maternal smoking.

Process evaluation should always be conducted to confirm the extent to which the program was implemented with fidelity and reached the intended beneficiaries and environmental change agents, was received and acceptable. Ongoing or intermittent monitoring allows for learning about problems or gaps that allows for adjustment.

Applying the Intervention Mapping Framework

The following application illustrates how researchers used IM to develop a healthy relationship program for early adolescent youth that includes youth, parent, and school components.

Me & You: Building Healthy Relationships

Me & You: Building Healthy Relationships is an effective healthy relationship program for middle school students (Peskin et al., 2019). School-based programs are an efficient strategy to promote healthy relationship behaviors, which may lead to reduced bullying and teen dating violence (DV). Teen dating violence is a complex problem that affects many teens in the United States each year (CDC, 2023) and is influenced by multiple levels of the socio-ecological model (Chapter 3) (e.g., youth, family, and school staff). (Banyard et al., 2006; Foshee et al., 2011).

Step 1: Needs and Assets Assessment

The multidisciplinary planning team included behavioral scientists, epidemiologists, psychologists, and other public health professionals. They used several methods to gain input and ensure the program met the needs of the priority population (predominantly African American and Hispanic middle school students attending a large, urban school district in the south-central United States): (1) formation of an ethnically diverse 15-member teen advisory board (TAB); (2) focus groups with parents and teenagers from the priority population, and (3) school district presentations and meetings. All students attended middle schools with high participation in the free or reduced school lunch program, an indicator of low socio-economic status.

The planning group used theory (social cognitive theory, social ecological model) (Bandura, 1986; Sallis et al., 2008) and evidence to guide their needs assessment and complete the logic model of the problem. Because the priority population was middle school students, they identified unhealthy emotional, physical, and sexual relationship behaviors, from dating partners and peers, as target behaviors. Further, because they often share similar risk factors (Coker et al., 2014) and co-occur (Reeves & Orpinas, 2012; Ybarra et al., 2016), unhealthy relationship behaviors encompassed both perpetration and victimization.

As shown in Figure 19.2, the planning group's needs assessment revealed that youth exposed to DV experience multiple health problems, including increased risk of depression, suicidal ideation, anxiety, substance use, risky sexual behavior, and physical injury, and quality of life outcomes such as poor academic performance and poor life satisfaction and increased risk of future relationship difficulties, including adult intimate partner violence. Environmental factors,

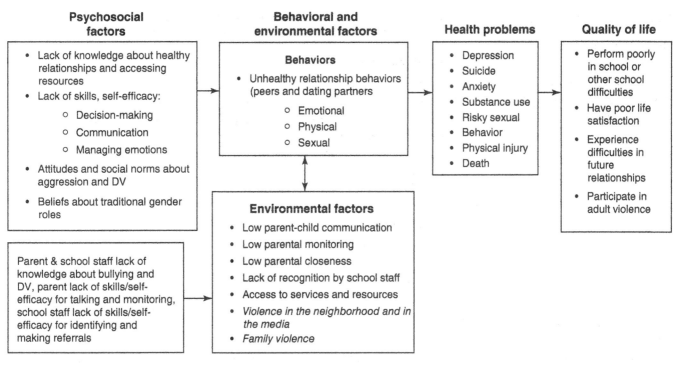

Psychosocial factors

- Lack of knowledge about healthy relationships and accessing resources
- Lack of skills, self-efficacy:
  - Decision-making
  - Communication
  - Managing emotions
- Attitudes and social norms about aggression and DV
- Beliefs about traditional gender roles

Parent & school staff lack of knowledge about bullying and DV, parent lack of skills/self-efficacy for talking and monitoring, school staff lack of skills/self-efficacy for identifying and making referrals

Behavioral and environmental factors

Behaviors

- Unhealthy relationship behaviors (peers and dating partners
  - Emotional
  - Physical
  - Sexual

Environmental factors

- Low parent-child communication
- Low parental monitoring
- Low parental closeness
- Lack of recognition by school staff
- Access to services and resources
- *Violence in the neighborhood and in the media*
- *Family violence*

Health problems

- Depression
- Suicide
- Anxiety
- Substance use
- Risky sexual
- Behavior
- Physical injury
- Death

Quality of life

- Perform poorly in school or other school difficulties
- Have poor life satisfaction
- Experience difficulties in future relationships
- Participate in adult violence

Figure 19.2 Logic Model of the Problem

such as low parental communication about healthy relationships, and low parental monitoring or closeness are associated with increased teen dating violence, and school staff often fail to recognize unhealthy peer or dating relationships or lack skills and perceive barriers toward identifying dating violence and referring youth to support staff. Finally, many psychosocial determinants such as knowledge, self-efficacy, attitudes, social norms and beliefs influence adolescent behavior. These findings emphasized the need for effective healthy relationship education for early adolescents.

In their asset assessment, the planning group recognized that schools would be an ideal setting for this intervention because youth spend most of their daytime hours in school. Additionally, the school district expressed an interest in their 6th graders participating in a healthy relationship curriculum as DV is prevalent among 6th graders (Orpinas et al., 2012; Orpinas et al., 2013). Based on data from previous programs, the planning group specified the following program goals:

1. After one year of the program, the percentage of students in the intervention group who report perpetrating any type of DV will be 8 percentage points lower than the percentage of students who do not receive the intervention.

2. After one year of the program, the percentage of students in the intervention group who report being victimized by any type of DV will be 8% points lower than the percentage of students who do not receive the intervention.

Step 2: Intervention Outcomes and Objectives

Working from the logic model of the problem, the team identified intervention outcomes to guide the development of the program's content and evaluation. Behavioral and environmental outcomes are included in Table 19.2 along with the detail of what specific behaviors students, parents, and school staff would have to perform to achieve these outcomes (performance objectives). The planning group then used social cognitive theory, social emotional learning, the social ecological model (Bandura, 1986; Sallis et al., 2008; Weissberg et al., 2015), their literature review, and data from the needs assessment to answer the question, "Why would a participant do a particular behavior?" The team then developed a matrix of change objectives for each behavior and environmental condition by asking "What needs to change related to this determinant to influence this performance objective?" For example, for Behavioral Objective 1 in Table 19.2: "What needs to change about self-efficacy regarding healthy relationships to evaluate one's own behavior in past and current peer and/or dating relationships?"

Table 19.2 Behavioral Outcomes, Environmental Outcomes, and Performance Objectives for *Me & You: Building Healthy Relationships* Program

Behavioral Outcome (BO) Students will:	Associated Performance Objectives
BO.1. Have healthy peer and dating relationships (i.e., that are free of emotional, physical, and sexual violence)	1. Evaluate their own behaviors within past and current peer and/or dating relationships.
	2. Evaluate peers' and/or dating partner's behaviors within past and current peer and/or dating relationships.
	3. Use effective communication strategies to foster healthy peer and dating relationships (e.g. conflict resolution, problem solving, and active consent).
	a. Use active consent (give and obtain) when engaging in sexual behaviors.
	4. Manage emotional responses (e.g. love, anger, anxiety, stress, depression, jealousy) to foster healthy peer and dating relationships.
	5. Avoid peers and potential dating partners that engage in unhealthy relationship behaviors.
	6. Avoid alcohol and drug use.
	7. Get out of unhealthy peer and/or dating relationships.
	8. Manage unhealthy peer and/or dating relationships that are unavoidable.
	9. Disclose abusive dating relationships (emotionally, physically, or sexually abusive either in-person and/or electronically).
	10. Access resources to help respond to current violent dating relationships and to prevent potential DV.

Environmental Outcomes (EO) Parents will:	
EO.1. Communicate with their child about healthy peer and dating relationships	1. Plan to discuss with their child how to have healthy peer and dating relationships (i.e., that are free of emotional, physical, and sexual violence).
	2. Create the appropriate times, locations, and activities to talk with their child about healthy peer and dating relationships.
	3. Use effective communication strategies when talking with their child (e.g., active listening, being nonjudgmental).
	4. Discuss with their child strategies for having healthy peer and dating relationships (e.g., conflict resolution, problem solving, effective communication).
	5. Discuss with their child strategies for managing their emotional responses appropriately (e.g., love, anger, anxiety, stress, depression, jealousy) in peer and dating relationships.
	6. Discuss strategies with their child for getting out of unhealthy peer and dating relationships.
	7. Discuss strategies with their child for avoiding peers and potential dating partners that engage in unhealthy relationship behaviors.
	8. Establish and discuss rules regarding how their child will spend time in friendship and dating activities (i.e., where, when, with whom) and use media (TV, internet, video games, music).
	9. Monitor adherence to the rules they establish with their child with respect to how they will spend time in friendship and dating activities (i.e., where, when, with whom) and use media (TV, internet, video games, music).
	10. Discuss with their child resources for avoiding and getting out of unhealthy relationship.

Environmental Outcomes (EO) School Staff will:	
EO.2. School staff (program facilitators, nurses, counselors, social workers, school leadership) will recognize DV among youth, respond appropriately, and refer to resources.	1. Use active listening when engaging with youth in discussions about their relationship experiences.
	2. Answer questions and concerns youth may have about relationships.
	3. Provide resources for youth.
	4. Maintain confidentiality standards with youth.
	5. Adhere to reporting laws.

Step 3: Methods and Practical Applications

After completing Step 2 tasks, the planning group selected potential theory-based methods shown to be effective for healthy relationships education (Foshee et al., 2004; Wolfe et al., 2009) and matched them to specific change objectives in the matrices. These methods included: active learning, group discussion, anticipated regret, chunking, modeling, scenario-based risk information, planning coping response, skills training with guided practice, resistance to social pressure, goal-setting, information about others' approval, and cultural similarity. The group then developed practical applications to operationalize these methods for the priority population and setting. Table 19.3 presents examples of methods and practical applications for 6th-grade students to develop healthy peer and dating relationships.

Table 19.3   Student Outcome: Partial Example Methods and Practical Applications

Behavioral Objective 1: Students will have healthy peer and dating relationships that are free of emotional, physical, and sexual violence

Knowledge		
Determinants and Change Objectives	**Method(s)**	**Application(s)**
Knowledge about the consequences of healthy and unhealthy peer and potential dating partner relationships	Discussion Anticipated regret	Group processing about role model stories related to the consequences of unhealthy relationships, and consequences of not having active consent
Knowledge related to the steps for managing emotions Knowledge related to the steps for having healthy relationships	Chunking	Using acronyms to describe the steps ("Relax, Rewind Replay"; "Select, Detect, Protect")
Knowledge of the characteristics of effective avoidance, refusal, and communication skills for fostering healthy relationships and/or avoiding unhealthy relationships	Modeling	Characters in stories demonstrate effective and ineffective refusal and communication skills

Skills and Self-Efficacy		
Skills and self-efficacy to identify and evaluate their behaviors in relationships	Scenario-based risk information	Students evaluate animated scenarios that demonstrate healthy and unhealthy relationships behaviors Assessment quizzes with remediation
Skills and self-efficacy for managing emotional responses Skills and self-efficacy for using effective communication skills to foster healthy relationships	Planning coping responses Guided practice	Students learn the "Relax, Rewind, Replay" paradigm to help them identify and manage emotional responses through animated role model scenarios
Skills and self-efficacy to use refusal/avoidance strategies to avoid peers and potential dating partners that engage in unhealthy relationships behaviors	Resistance to social pressure Modeling Goal setting	Facilitators demonstrate the skill and then the students do in-class and/or virtual online role-plays in which they practice the skill; Feedback is provided to the student Students set goals for their relationships on a private online "graffiti wall"

Perceived Norms		
Perceived norms that peers: • decide to have healthy relationships and do not tolerate violence in relationships • identify and evaluate behaviors within their relationships • manage emotional responses • use effective avoidance, refusal, and communication skills for fostering healthy relationships and/or avoiding unhealthy relationships	Discussion Information about others' approval Cultural similarity	Group processing and quizzes about role model stories related to the characteristics of healthy relationships, signs of unhealthy relationships, characteristics of active consent "Teens talk" (peer videos) on healthy friendships, pressures in relationships, dating relationships (what makes them healthy and unhealthy), strategies for managing emotions

Step 4: Intervention Design and Production

These practical applications (Step 3) were then grouped into distinct program components for students, parents, and school staff to create the scope (content) and sequence (lesson order) for *Me & You*. The *student component* consisted of thirteen 25-minute lessons, which included five group-based classroom lessons, five individual computer-only lessons, and three hybrid classroom-computer blended to provide opportunities for group and personalized learning and to discuss group norms. The *parent component* included two parent newsletters, and three parent-child take-home activities to encourage parent-child communication about healthy dating relationships. The *school staff component* was a two-day teacher training prior to curriculum implementation and a school newsletter that highlighted information about TDV and bullying and provided strategies for recognizing and referring related incidents.

The planning group purposefully chose the program theme, "*Me & You: Building Healthy Relationships (Me & You)*" as it related to developing skills to "build healthy relationships" rather than "preventing teen DV." Feedback from school staff and students suggested that the latter had a more negative connotation to parents. Further, this theme suggested that the skills learned in this program could be applied to other relationships as well, including those with peers, family members, and others.

Step 5: Implementation Mapping

Program planners faced three challenges regarding program adoption, implementation, and sustainability: (1) obtaining support at the school district and local school level for program adoption; (2) identifying and training teachers for program delivery, and (3) facilitating the sustainability of *Me and You* within a school district. In Step 5 as in Step 2, planners wrote behavioral outcomes and performance objectives for each. In addition, they identified relevant determinants, methods and practical applications, and implementation strategies to facilitate program adoption and sustainability.

Step 6: Evaluation Plan

Program planners can use the logic model of change to identify evaluation outcomes. Most often, the relationship between the behavioral and health and quality of life effects have been established previously, but determinants should be measured to verify whether the objectives selected in Steps 2 and 5, respectively, have been achieved (Bartholomew et al., 2016). Some of the effects of this program measured in a randomized controlled trial with urban middle school students included DV perpetration and victimization (behavioral outcomes) as well as norms for boy-against-girl violence and girl-against-boy violence, conflict-resolution skills, and attitudes about sexting (determinants) (Peskin et al., 2019). Students who received *Me and You* reported less favorable norms for boy-against-girl violence and girl-against-boy violence, greater constructive conflict-resolution skills, and more negative attitudes about sexting than did the comparison students (Peskin et al., 2019). The evaluation plan was derived directly from the previous steps of IM.

Summary

This chapter presented two models for developing theory-based health promotion interventions. Both frameworks have been used extensively in health promotion planning, with PRECEDE-PROCEED beginning in the late 1970's and IM beginning in the late 1990's. Both of these frameworks have been used across the globe in settings such as schools, communities, and workplaces, and have been used for planning multilevel interventions for many health topics. These frameworks take an ecological approach to planning and provide guidance for the use of theory both to understand health problems and to plan interventions that influence the determinants of those problems. Both also start with the important assumption that a diagnostic process should be undertaken before program components are selected. While the frameworks can be used in tandem, they are most often used independently and can guide planners to incorporate the use of theory, evidence, new data, and community engagement to make planning and implementation decisions.

Both planning frameworks underscore the importance of engaging the priority population and other stakeholders in collaborative planning to increase intervention ownership, relevance, and appeal (Bartholomew et al., 2016; Grembowski, 2016). The concept of the importance of co-creation of interventions with priority populations being true collaborative partners helps ensure that programs address community needs and contexts and increase the potential for sustainment over time (Hawe, 2015).

Both frameworks use logic models and graphic illustrations that depict the relationship between elements or components of interest. The logic models used in each framework are similar in some ways but also have several differences. They differ in how the determinants of behaviors and environmental conditions are categorized (predisposing, reinforcing, and enabling in PRECEDE-PROCEED vs. personal determinants in IM). Another difference is that in IM, the logic model includes a description of intervention methods and practical applications, and how they are proposed to influence the determinants of behavior and environmental conditions that drive health and quality of life.

Both IM and PRECEDE-PROCEED have been used to guide community-based work and are flexible enough to be useful tools for CBPR (Belansky et al., 2011). Because they do not specify or restrict which theories and constructs should be used to understand problems and create solutions, these frameworks are useful for a wide range of health problems and have been used broadly to address health disparities and problems in under-resourced communities worldwide (Bryant-Stephens et al., 2020). The frameworks also have been applied to influence detailed reporting of health promotion interventions (Bartholomew & Mullen, 2011), to understand theory-based change methods at the community level (Wallerstein et al., 2020), and to guide the adaptation of evidence-based interventions in new settings (Bartholomew et al., 2016).

References

Australian Government Department of Health. (2022). Ear health. https://www.health.gov.au/health-topics/ear- health

Bandura, A. (1986). *Social foundations of thought and action: A social cognitive theory.* Englewood Cliffs, NJ: Prentice-Hall.

Banyard, V. L., Cross, C., & Modecki, K. L. (2006). Interpersonal violence in adolescence: Ecological correlates of self-reported perpetration. *Journal of Interpersonal Violence, 21*(10), 1314–1332.

Bartholomew, L. K., & Mullen, P. D. (2011). Five roles for using theory and evidence in the design and testing of behavior change interventions. *Journal of Public Health Dentistry, 71*(Supp.1), S20–S33.

Bartholomew, L. K., Parcel, G. S., Kok, G., Gottlieb, N. H., & Fernandez, M. E. (2016). *Planning health promotion programs: An intervention mapping approach* (4th ed.). San Francisco, CA: Jossey-Bass.

Belansky, E. S., Cutforth, N., Chavez, R. A., Waters, E., & Bartlett-Horch, K. (2011). An adapted version of intervention mapping (AIM) is a tool for conducting community-based participatory research. *Health Promotion Practice, 12*(3), 440–455.

Bronfenbrenner, U. (1979). *The ecology of human development: Experiments by nature and design.* Cambridge, MA: Harvard University Press.

Bryant-Stephens, T., Kenyon, C., Apter, A. J., Wolk, C., Williams, Y. S., Localio, R., Toussaint, K., Hui, A., West, C,, Stewart, Y., McGinnis, S., Gutierrez, M., & Beidas, R. (2020). Creating a community-based comprehensive intervention to improve asthma control in a low-income, low-resourced community. *Journal of Asthma 57*(8), 820–828.

Butterfoss, F. D., & Kegler, M. C. (2009). The community coalition action theory. *Emerging Theories in Health Promotion Practice and Research, 2,* 237–276.

Centers for Disease Control and Prevention. (2023). YRBSS results. https://www.cdc.gov/healthyyouth/data/yrbs/results.htm

Coker, A. L., Clear, E. R., Garcia, L. S., Asaolu, I. O., Cook-Craig, P. G., Brancato, C. J., & Fisher, B. S. (2014). Dating violence victimization and perpetration rates among high school students. *Violence Against Women, 20*(10), 1220–1238.

Crosby, R., & Noar, S. M. (2011). What is a planning model? An introduction to precede-proceed. *Journal of Public Health Dentistry, 71,* S7–S15. https://doi.org/10.1111/j.1752-7325.2011.00235.x

Fernandez, M. E., Ruiter, R. A. C., Markham, C. M., & Kok, G. (2019). Intervention mapping: Theory- and evidence-based health promotion program planning: Perspective and examples. *Frontiers in Public Health, 7,* 209.

Foshee, V. A., Bauman, K. E., Ennett, S. T, Linder, G. F., Benefield, T., & Suchindran, C. (2004). Assessing the long-term effects of the Safe Dates program and a booster in preventing and reducing adolescent dating violence victimization and perpetration. *American Journal of Public Health, 94*(4), 619–24.

Foshee, V. A., Reyes, H. L., Ennett, S. T., Suchindran, C., Mathias, J. P., Karriker-Jaffe, K. J., Bauman, K. E., & Benefield, T. S. (2011). Risk and protective factors distinguishing profiles of adolescent peer and dating violence perpetration. *Journal of Adolescent Health, 48*(4), 344–350.

Foster-Fishman, P. G., Nowell, B., & Yang, H. (2007). Putting the system back into systems change: A framework for understanding and changing organizational and community systems. *American Journal of Community Psychology, 39*(3–4), 197–215.

Glanz, K., & Bishop, D. B. (2010). The role of behavioral science theory in development and implementation of public health interventions. *Annual Review of Public Health, 31*(1), 399–418.

Glanz, K., Rimer, B. K., Viswanath, K., (Eds.) (2008). *Health behavior and health education: theory, research, and practice* (4th ed.). San Francisco: Jossey-Bass.

Green, L. W., & Kreuter, M. W. (1991). *Health promotion planning: An educational and environmental approach.* Mountain View, CA: Mayfield.

Green, L. W., & Kreuter, M. W. (2005). *Health program planning: An educational and ecological approach* (4th ed.). Boston, MA: McGraw-Hill.

Green, L. W., & Kreuter, M. W. (2022). *Health promotion planning: An educational and ecological approach.* Mountain View, CA: Mayfield.

Green, L. W., Gielen, A. C., Ottoson, J. M., Peterson, D. V., & Kreuter, M. W. (2022). *Health program planning, implementation, and evaluation: Creating behavioral, environmental and policy change.* Baltimore: Johns Hopkins University Press.

Grembowski, D. (2016). *The practice of health program evaluation*. SAGE.

Guzman-Tordecilla, D. N., Lucumi, D. & Peña, M. (2022). Using an intervention mapping approach to develop a program for preventing high blood pressure in a marginalized Afro-Colombian population: A community-based participatory research. *Journal of Primary Prevention, 43*, 209–224. https://doi.org/10.1007/s10935-022-00668-1

Hawe, P. (2015). Lessons from complex interventions to improve health. *Annual Review of Public Health, 36*, 307–323.

Hilliard, M. E., Riekert, K. A., & Ockene, K. A. (2018). *The handbook of health behavior change* (5th ed.). Springer.

Hussain, S. T., Lei, S., Akram, T., Haider, M. J., Hussain, S. H., & Ali, M. (2018). Kurt Lewin's change model: A critical review of the role of leadership and employee involvement in organizational change. *Journal of Innovation & Knowledge, 3*(3), 123–127.

Kang, E., & Foster, E. R. (2022). Use of implementation mapping with community-based participatory research: Development of implementation strategies of a new goal setting and goal management intervention system. *Frontiers in Public Health, 10*, 834473.

Kok, G., Gottlieb, N. H., Peters, G. J. Y., Mullen, P. D., Parcel, G. S., Ruiter, R. A. C., Fernández, M. E., Markham, C., Bartholomew, L. K. (2015). A taxonomy of behavior change methods: An intervention mapping approach. *Health Psychology Review, 15*, 1–16.

Latham, G. P., & Arshoff, A. S. (2015). Planning: A mediator in goal-setting theory. In M. D. Mumford & M. Frese (Eds.), *The psychology of planning in organizations* (pp. 105–120). Routledge.

Macquarie University. (2022). Hearing health in Aboriginal & Torres Strait Islander peoples. https://www.mq.edu.au/__data/assets/pdf_file/0006/1076073/Indignous-Hearing-Health_Symposium-Proceedings-Final_MCMAHON.pdf

Marmot, M. (2000). Multilevel approaches to understanding social determinants In L. F. Berkman & I. Kawachi (Eds.). *Social Epidemiology* (pp. 349–367).

Mcknight, J. L. & Kretzmann, J. P. (2012). 10. Mapping community capacity. In M. Minkler (Ed.), *Community Organizing and Community Building for Health and Welfare* (pp. 171–186). Ithaca, NY: Rutgers University Press. https://doi.org/10.36019/9780813553146-012

Millet, N., McDermott, H. J., Moss, E. L., Edwardson, C. L., & Munir, F. (2022). Increasing physical activity levels following treatment for cervical cancer: An intervention mapping approach. *Journal of Cancer Survivorship, 16*, 650–658. https://doi.org/10.1007/s11764-021-01058-y

Orpinas, P., Nahapetyan, L., Song, X., McNicholas, C., & Reeves, P. M. (2012). Psychological dating violence perpetration and victimization: Trajectories from middle to high school. *Aggressive Behavior, 38*(6), 510–520.

Orpinas, P., Hsieh, H. L., Song, X., Holland, K., & Nahapetyan, L. (2013). Trajectories of physical dating violence from middle to high school: Association with relationship quality and acceptability of aggression. *Journal of Youth and Adolescence, 42*, 551–565.

Pérez Jolles, M., Fernández, M. E., Jacobs, G., De Leon, J., Myrick, L., & Aarons, G. A. (2022). Using implementation mapping to develop protocols supporting the implementation of a state policy on screening children for adverse childhood experiences in a system of health centers in inland Southern California. *Frontiers in Public Health, 10*, 876769.

Peskin, M. F., Markham, C. M., Shegog, R., Baumler, E. R., Addy, R. C., Temple. J. R., Hernandez, B., Cuccaro, P. M., Thiel, M. A., Gabay, E. K., & Tortolero Emery, S. (2019). Adolescent dating violence prevention program for early adolescents: The Me & You randomized controlled trial, 2014-15. *American Journal of Public Health, 109*(10), 1419–1428. https://doi.org/10.2105/AJPH.2019.305218

Prochaska, J. O. (2013). Transtheoretical model of behavior change. In M. D. Gellman & J. R. Turner (Eds.), *Encyclopedia of Behavioral Medicine* (pp. 997–2000). New York: Springer.

Ravicz, M., Muhongayire, B., Kamagaju, S., Klabbers, R. E., Faustin, Z., Kambugu, A., Bassett, I., & O'Laughlin, K. (2022). Using intervention mapping methodology to design an HIV linkage intervention in a refugee settlement in rural Uganda. *AIDS Care, 34*(4), 446–458.

Reeves, P. M., & Orpinas, P. (2012). Dating norms and dating violence among ninth graders in Northeast Georgia: Reports from student surveys and focus groups. *Journal of Interpersonal Violence, 27*(9), 1677–1698.

Rowbotham, S., Walker, P., Marks, L., Irving, M., Smith, B. J. and Laird, Y. (2023) Research Involvement and Engagement Building capacity for citizen science in health promotion: a collaborative knowledge mobilisation approach. *Research Involvement and Engagement, 9*, 36.

Ruiter, R. A. C., & Crutzen, R. (2020). Core processes: How to use evidence, theories, and research in planning behavior change interventions. *Frontiers in Public Health, 24*(8), 247.

Sallis, J. F., Owen, N., & Fisher, E. B. Ecologic models of health behavior. (2008). In K. Glanz, B. K. Rimer, & K. Viswanath (Eds.), *Health behavior and health education: Theory, research, and practice* (pp. 462–484). Jossey-Bass.

Springer, A.E. & Evans, A.E. (2016. Assessing environmental assets for health promotion program planning: A practical framework for health promotion practitioners. *Health Promotion Perspectives, 6*(3), 111–118.

Taylor, S., Cairns, A., & Glass, B. (2021). Developing an ear health intervention for rural community pharmacy: Application of the PRECEDE-PROCEED model. *International Journal of Environmental Research and Public Health, 18*, 6456. https://doi.org/10.3390/ijerph18126456

Taylor, S., Cairns, A., & Glass, B. D. (2022). Feasibility, accessibility and acceptability a pharmacist-led ear health intervention at rural community pharmacies (LISTEN UP): A mixed-methods study in Queensland, Australia. *BMJ Open, 12*, e057011.

Valente, T. W., & Pitts, S. R. (2017). An appraisal of social network theory and analysis as applied to public health: Challenges and opportunities. *Annual Review of Public Health, 38*, 103–118.

Vohs, K. D., & Baumeister, R. F. (Eds.). (2016). *Handbook of self-regulation: Research, theory, and applications.* Guilford Publications.

Wallerstein, N., Oetzel, J. G., Sanchez-Youngman, S., Boursaw, B., Dickson, E., Kastelic, S., Koegel, P., Lucero, J. E., Magarati, M., Ortiz, K., Parker, M., Peña, J., Richmond, A., & Duran, B. (2020). Engage for equity: A long-term study of community-based participatory research and community-engaged research practices and outcomes. *Health Education & Behavior, 47*(3), 380–390.

Weissberg, R. P., Durlak, J. A., Domitrovich, C. E., & Gullotta, T. P. (2015). *Social and emotional learning: Past, present, and future.* The Guilford Press.

Wolfe, D. A., Crooks, C., Jaffe, P., Chiodo, D., Hughes, R., Ellis, W., Stitt, L., & Donner, A. (2009). A school-based program to prevent adolescent dating violence: a cluster randomized trial. *Archives of Pediatrics & Adolescent Medicine, 163*, 692–699.

Ybarra, M. L., Espelage, D. L., Langhinrichsen-Rohling, J., Korchmaros, J. D., & Boyd, D. (2016). Lifetime prevalence rates and overlap of physical, psychological, and sexual dating abuse perpetration and victimization in a national sample of youth. *Archives of Sexual Behavior, 45*, 1083–1099.

CHAPTER 20

BEHAVIORAL ECONOMICS AND HEALTH

Jessica L. Cohen

Harsha Thirumurthy

KEY POINTS

- Behavioral economics can provide a better descriptive and predictive model of human behavior than previous economic models that assume fully rational behavior.

- The behavior of consumers, patients, healthcare providers, and other individuals often is shaped by biases in decision-making, reliance on mental shortcuts, and social forces.

- Behavioral economics principles can be useful for designing scalable interventions and subtle policy changes that result in better health outcomes.

Vignette

Early in the 21st century, malaria was the leading cause of child mortality in sub-Saharan Africa, and malaria deaths had been increasing since the early 1990s. A primary driver of this worrisome trend was the decreasing efficacy of the first-line treatment for malaria, chloroquine. Chloroquine-resistant strains of the malaria parasite had gained the advantage, and malaria illness became much more difficult and expensive to treat. But there was reason to be hopeful because new, highly effective antimalarial medications—Artemisinin Combination Therapies (ACTs)—had been developed, and there was strong commitment from agencies like the Global Fund to Fight AIDS, Tuberculosis and Malaria to heavily subsidize these medications so that they were widely available and affordable. These medications were sure to save lives. But along with the relief came worry: would the malaria parasite quickly gain resistance to ACTs too? Preserving the efficacy of ACTs for current and future malaria patients would require a major push to improve adherence to antimalarial medications.

Patient adherence to medications means that they fill the prescription, take the correct dosage at the right time, in the right way, and finish the full course of the medication for a prescribed period of time. Medication nonadherence undermines the efficacy of treatment for illnesses and, in some cases, can threaten the future efficacy of the treatment itself. Nonadherence to antimicrobials is a known driver of pathogen resistance to effective therapies, threatening our ability to effectively treat infections in the future (Murray et al., 2022).

Even though ACTs to treat malaria are only a three-day treatment course, more than 1/3 of patients are nonadherent (Cohen & Saran, 2018). To make sure that ACTs are truly curing patients' illnesses, the global health community and national malaria control programs have to ensure that the rollout of ACTs is accompanied by efforts to promote adherence. But what should policymakers do to increase adherence? The correct policy response hinges on having a good understanding of the reasons why people may not adhere to medications. For example, if policymakers assume that patients are not finishing their medication because they do not understand the proper way to take them, then training pharmacists and doctors to counsel patients more thoroughly on adherence is the right approach. On the other hand, if patients are nonadherent because they are forgetting to take their medication, then a different approach such as phone-based reminders is needed. And if the issue is that people feel fine after a while and stop taking the medications, then a more effective communication strategy about the continued importance of adherence will be useful.

Introduction

The problem of medication nonadherence in this chapter's opening vignette provides a helpful illustration of how behavioral economics insights can be useful—and how they differ from standard economic models of decision-making. It also illustrates why behavioral economics can usually offer a more intuitive lens through which to make sense of how and why people behave the way they do. If we have a more accurate understanding of behavioral drivers, policies and intervention approaches will be more effective and more cost-effective.

A traditional economic framework would conceptualize nonadherence as a patient's *choice*—patients who do not adhere choose to do so because that is the best decision for them based on the information they have, their preferences, and other factors (Cohen & Saran, 2018). Put simply, the patient would be weighing the expected benefits of adhering to the medication with the expected costs. For example, the main expected benefit of adherence is the guarantee of maximum health benefit from the medicine and the expected costs include things like side effects, the hassle of taking the medicine, etc. If this model is the right way of understanding adherence, then policy approaches could include things like providing patients with information regarding the benefits of adherence (e.g., on the bottle label) or formulating the drug so it has fewer side effects.

A behavioral economics lens of nonadherence would not necessarily assume patients are making the choice that is optimal for them or, even, that they are making a choice at all. For example, people may forget to take the medication, especially if their symptoms are mild and are thus not very salient or "top of mind." Indeed, ACTs tend to decrease patients' malaria symptoms quite quicky, with most of the symptom relief happening within the first day or two. Patients may be skipping the third day of the medication because they feel better and forget they need the pills. In this case, approaches to improving ACT adherence could focus on SMS reminder messages, e.g., text messages from the pharmacy or clinician's office (Volpp et al., 2017). Behavioral economics can help expand the lens with which we understand behavioral drivers of health decisions, allowing us to target the relevant behavioral barrier or barriers and design more effective policies and interventions.

Patient nonadherence is just one example of the ways individuals' decisions are instrumental in shaping health outcomes around the world. While environmental and structural factors are critically important in influencing population health, so are a wide variety of human behaviors ranging from individuals' decisions to use prevention services to healthcare providers' decisions to prescribe medications. Despite major biomedical advances in recent decades, behavioral factors often limit the overall effectiveness of those advances when it comes to improving population health. In the cases of cancer screening, childhood immunization, and pharmacologic management of chronic conditions, poor uptake, or adherence can pose major barriers to health improvement. Recent efforts to deploy COVID-19 vaccines around the world proved just how central human behavior is in controlling the spread of infectious diseases. Behavioral economics offers insights into health behavior and decision-making, from explanations for suboptimal engagement in healthy behavior to suggestions for policies and interventions that promote healthy behavior.

In this chapter, we describe several major ideas from behavioral economics and explain how they can be useful for explaining and influencing health behavior. We begin by summarizing the standard economic theory of human behavior and then contrasting it to behavioral economics theories. We then discuss key concepts in behavioral economics and summarize existing empirical evidence on how behavioral economics has been applied to health.

Theories of Human Behavior: From Standard Economics to Behavioral Economics

Standard Economic Theory

To understand human behavior and identify promising behavior change interventions, the discipline of economics has commonly relied on a model grounded in the assumption that individuals are rational, self-interested decision-makers who seek to maximize their "utility," or well-being. The model posits that three important factors influence our choices: (1) "preferences" that characterize our tastes and values, (2) relative prices associated with the various choices available, and (3) the constraints on available resources such as time or money. Preferences describe individuals' likes and dislikes, the extent to which they value the present relative to the future, and the degree of risk or uncertainty they are willing to tolerate—all of which can influence one's propensity to engage in certain health behaviors. Prices reflect the costs of purchasing health products and services. And finally, resource constraints usually refer to the amount of income available for procuring health products and services and time constraints that can influence health behaviors. We discuss each of these factors before explaining how behavioral economics theories represent a departure from this standard approach to understanding human behavior.

For many health behaviors, it is easy to see why individual preferences might be important. There may be substantial variation across individuals, e.g., in their liking for certain types of foods or for certain forms of exercise. Some individuals may place greater emphasis on the future costs or benefits stemming from their behaviors. As a result, they may be less likely to smoke cigarettes or more likely to take medications as prescribed. These temporal preferences are associated with both health behaviors and outcomes in several studies (Bradford et al., 2017; Thirumurthy et al., 2015). Preferences toward risk are other relevant decision-making factors. Heterogeneity in risk preferences and the association between risk preferences and risky health behaviors have been documented in many studies (Anderson & Mellor, 2008).

The propensity to use health services or engage in healthy behaviors can also be influenced through the provision of health information to people. This insight has motivated many public health campaigns that aim to raise awareness about the importance of healthy behaviors or the harms of unhealthy behaviors. Empirical evidence on the effects of information provision is mixed. Some studies have documented large impacts of one-time information provision. For example, a study in Kenya found that simply informing teenage girls about the risk of unsafe sex with older men who have a higher likelihood of being HIV-positive led to sexual behavior change and reduced pregnancy risk for the girls (Dupas, 2011). Larger-scale testing and applications of this approach to other types of behavior and in other countries have shown more muted effects, however. In the United States, researchers and policymakers have sought to influence food choices by providing caloric and other nutrition information on food items. Again, there is some evidence that this type of information can alter people's preferences and behavior (Shangguan et al., 2019; Wisdom et al., 2010), but nutrition labeling is not consistently effective across settings such as restaurants (Fernandes et al., 2016). These examples underscore the idea that, when designing public health interventions to promote healthy behavior, the provision of information alone may be insufficient.

Prices are the second fundamental determinant of health behavior in traditional economic models. Prices are highly relevant to understand health behavior and continue to shape health policy in important ways. A large literature has shown that prices of health products and services influence demand. The RAND health insurance experiment showed long ago that healthcare utilization is driven by the prices people face (Manning et al., 1987). In low-income countries, randomized trials have demonstrated that people's demands for life-saving health products and services are highly sensitive to prices even when prices are extremely low. One study from Kenya showed that demand for insecticide-treated mosquito nets to prevent malaria was extremely sensitive to small increases in price above zero (Cohen & Dupas, 2010), and another study from Zambia showed high price sensitivity for water-purification products (Ashraf et al., 2010). Similarly, a recent study in Zimbabwe found a 25% decline in demand for HIV self-tests among people offered self-tests for $0.50 instead of being offered them for free (Chang et al., 2019). A key lesson that emerges from these studies in low-income countries is that there is a compelling rationale for fully subsidizing healthcare products and services instead of charging user fees for them (Cohen, 2019). This is especially the case for health products and services associated with infectious diseases, where usage by one individual can influence health outcomes of other individuals.

In addition to public subsidies, two other policy measures also follow directly from the recognition that prices influence people's decisions. One is use of taxes to raise prices faced by individuals and thereby curb certain unhealthy behaviors. Another is use of financial incentives to increase benefits associated with certain health behavior and thereby promote those healthier behaviors. Taxes are a widely used policy measure not only for raising government revenue but also for changing human behavior (Chaloupka et al., 2011). Cigarette taxes are perhaps the most prominent example of taxes as a lever for behavior change in global health. Multiple studies have shown that taxes are an effective way to reduce smoking rates, particularly in combination with other measures such as information campaigns and reduced access to and restrictions on advertising (Davis 2008). More recently, in response to growing concern about rising obesity, some governments have begun to impose taxes on sugar-sweetened beverages. Studies from Mexico and individual cities in the United States have suggested that this is one way to reduce sugar-sweetened beverage consumption (Colchero et al., 2016; Silver et al., 2017; Roberto et al., 2019). Financial incentives (which we discuss in the next section in the context of present bias) have a clear and compelling rationale even in the standard model of decision-making. Just as subsidies lower the prices faced by consumers and thereby boost demand, incentives can offset various opportunity costs associated with seeking health services and bring down the full price faced by consumers.

Resources available to individuals are the third and final determinant of health behavior in standard economic models of decision-making. A core prediction of economic theory is that when all else is equal, individuals facing financial barriers or time constraints will be less able to access healthcare than those without such issues. This provides further motivation for interventions such as price subsidies or health insurance with limited cost-sharing (i.e., small deductible, copayments, or coinsurance); in recent years, there have been a number of efforts in low- or middle-income countries to expand access to health insurance. Another policy response to curb the effects of poverty on health has been the provision of unconditional cash transfers. Many countries have expanded unconditional cash transfer programs with the goal of both alleviating poverty and improving health outcomes (Pega et al., 2022). Later, in this chapter, we discuss additional ways in which poverty can influence health outcomes by summarizing recent research on the psychological consequences of poverty.

Historical Development of Behavioral Economics Theories

Behavioral economics has received increasing attention because of its conceptual appeal in describing and influencing human behavior. In addition, it has considerable potential to offer relatively low-cost and unobtrusive solutions to some of the most serious health problems around the world. Behavioral economics theories address some of the important limitations of standard economic theories of health behavior. For example, it is often not the case that people make fully rational decisions, that they are driven primarily by self-interest, or that they have stable preferences. Standard economic theories also ignore the fact that individuals' preferences and behaviors are strongly influenced by factors such as what those in one's social network are doing.

Over the past several decades, leaders in behavioral economics have described how people's decisions differ from standard economic models (see Table 20.1). While economists such as Herb Simon mapped out concepts of "bounded

Table 20.1 Standard Economic Theory Versus Behavioral Economics

Standard Economic Theory	Behavioral Economics
Core theory: expected utility maximization	Core theory: prospect theory
Assumes perfect rationality	Recognizes that people make decision errors
Starting point independent	Assessment depends on your starting point
Framing does not matter	Framing affects assessment even when utilities are the same
Stable preferences	Time inconsistent preferences
People discount the future at constant rates	People discount the near future to a greater degree and have time-inconsistent discounting
Interventions considered only when a person's actions adversely affect others (negative externalities)	Interventions considered when people will harm their future selves (internalities)
Regulations and policies generally geared to protecting people from the actions of others	Regulations and policies often geared to protecting people from themselves.

rationality" in the 1950s (Simon, 1955), and Maurice Allais in 1953 laid out the Allais Paradox (to a group of leading economists) (Allais, 1953) as a contradiction to standard expected utility maximization, the publication of Prospect Theory by Kahneman and Tversky (1979) is widely credited with being seminal in the development of behavioral economics. Prospect Theory provided an overarching conceptual framework to describe what Kahneman and Tversky and others had observed in a number of studies about human behaviors that could not be explained by expected utility theory. In essence, Prospect Theory has several important components that include: (1) how people feel about a set of possible outcomes depends on their starting point. This is the notion of reference-dependence in which decisionmakers evaluate outcomes as gains or losses depending on their starting point; (2) there is diminished sensitivity to both gains and losses, depending on the starting point; and (3) people exhibit *loss aversion* (the reduction in one's welfare due to a monetary loss is much stronger than the gain in welfare due to an equivalent gain) (Kahneman, 2011; Kahneman & Tversky, 1979). Another important implication of this theory is that people *over*-weight small probabilities (nonlinear probability weighting).

The importance of reference points is illustrated nicely by an example Kahneman gives in his book *Thinking Fast and Slow* (Kahneman, 2011). Consider two people who today each have $4 million. Standard models would consider them to have roughly equivalent utility of wealth. However, imagine that as of yesterday, one of the two had $1 million and the other had $7 million. Clearly, the person who had $1 million yesterday should be ecstatic today and the one who had $7 million yesterday would be despondent. Diminishing sensitivity to changes in wealth (or utility more broadly) is illustrated by this example: consider the utility of getting an extra $500 when your wealth is $1 million as opposed to if you have no money. The utility of this extra $500 is much greater if you have no (or very little) money than if you already have a lot.

A number of studies have shown that people have what Kahneman calls a "loss aversion ratio" in a range of 1.5–2.5; that is, people dislike losing more than they like winning (Novemsky & Kahneman, 2005). For example, when given a 50/50 chance of winning $150 or losing $100, most people would not voluntarily choose this gamble because the potential pain of losing $100 is greater than the joy of winning $150. Under standard expected utility maximization, it would be a "no-brainer" to take this gamble since the expected utility is 0.5(−$100) + 0.5 ($150) or $25.

Key Concepts in Behavioral Economics and Empirical Examples

The potential of behavioral economics for population health is that many of the same messages, incentives, and choice structures used so effectively to lure people into situations where they may be exploited or encouraged toward unhealthy behaviors can be redirected to attract them to healthier choices that can improve their long-term well-being (Table 20.2 provides an overview of several key concepts). Decision errors affect policymakers as well, with broader ramifications for the types of policies that are developed and adopted. In this section, we describe some of the key concepts from behavioral economics, including examples of decision errors and how they can be used to enhance the effectiveness of programs aimed at improving health behaviors.

Present Bias and Financial Incentives

Many health-related behaviors require us to make tradeoffs between present and future costs and benefits. Seeking preventive care, for example, requires incurring immediate time costs and potential economic costs in exchange for achieving better health in the future. For such behaviors, the *immediacy* of costs and benefits often influences decisions to a much greater extent than would be expected from the rational tendency to discount the future. When individuals engage in such *present-biased* decision-making, they may be less likely to engage in health behaviors that have large benefits—behaviors like quitting smoking, exercising, or using preventive services. Such decision-making also implies, however, that we may be able to guide individuals toward forward-looking, healthy behaviors by offering them immediate, salient rewards or lowering the immediate costs associated with engaging in those behaviors.

Present bias in decision-making motivates the widespread use of financial and nonfinancial incentives for healthy behaviors in many parts of the world. A study in rural India found that providing caregivers nonfinancial incentives worth approximately $1 per immunization (along with reliable services) led to significantly higher immunization rates (Banerjee et al., 2010). Another study in Malawi found that small financial incentives ranging from $0.20 to $3 led to

Table 20.2   Relevance of Selected Behavioral Economics Principles to Health

Concept	Definition	Relevance for Health	Suggested interventions and solutions	Citations
Present Bias	When making decisions, people place substantial weight on the immediate costs and benefits associated with those decisions rather than the future costs and benefits.	Smoking cessation Exercise Health insurance plan choice	Financial incentives	Halpern (2018) Abaluck and Gruber (2011) Patel (2016)
Decision Fatigue	Repeated decision-making results in decreased mental capacity and exhaustion which can diminish performance or hinder optimal decision-making.	Provider behaviors Vaccinations Chronic disease self-management	Clinical decision support systems Active choice interventions Checklists	Kawamoto (2005) Donato (2007)
Status Quo Bias/Defaults	People tend to prefer the status quo/default option when given multiple options.	Prescribing behavior Provider behavior	Changing default settings	Chiu (2018) Patel et al. (2014) Olson et al. (2015)
Availability Bias	People overestimate the probability of an event due to recent or salient examples of similar events in their memory. Correspondingly, people underestimate the probability of an event due to the lack of readily available examples.	Clinical decision making	Algorithms or standardization to help decision-making	Singh (2021) Sibbald (2013)
Social Norms	Implicit or explicit rules/standards of a group and a person's perception of those rules/standards inform their beliefs and behaviors.	Prescribing behavior HIV testing	Peer comparison feedback comparing prescribing rates Interventions to correct norms	Patel (2018) Tsai (2021)
Framing	Conveying the same message using different wording or presentation changes reception and resulting decisions.	COVID Vaccinations Preventative behaviors (cancer, smoking, exercise)	Loss-framed messages to reduce risk perception, benefit-target framing (society) Gain-framed messages	Gursoy et al. (2022) Gallagher and Updegraff (2012)
Limited Attention and Salience	Having a finite amount of attention and processing-capacity results in limited consideration of options.	Hand hygiene Vaccinations/screenings	Reminder posters Active choice	Grant and Hofmann (2011) Kim (2018)

higher HIV-testing uptake among adults (Thornton, 2008). Incentives to promote healthier behaviors have not always succeeded, however, and there are a number of lessons to be learned from these examples as well (Thirumurthy et al., 2019a). For example, incentives have generally been less effective in promoting repeated health behaviors like medication adherence (Thirumurthy et al., 2019b; Volpp et al., 2017), which often requires frequent, nearly daily pill-taking and therefore makes it harder to motivate with frequent incentives. For incentive interventions to succeed, it is important that payments be delivered as close in time as possible to the behaviors of interest. With new technologies that make it possible to monitor behaviors like medication adherence or physical activity, however, the potential for devising more effective incentive-based interventions is likely to grow. Alternative designs of incentives that leverage the power of lotteries or loss aversion can also help. For example, financial incentives framed as a loss were effective for achieving physical activity goals in one study conducted in the United States (Patel et al., 2016a).

Status Quo Bias and the Power of Defaults

In many realms of decision-making, people choose the option placed in front of them—the default option—instead of investing cognitive effort to choose a different option. This preference for the default option is typically referred to as *status quo bias*, and it explains many behaviors, such as loyalty to specific brands or meal choices at restaurants. Status quo bias can, however, lead to suboptimal health behaviors. For example, at a fast-food restaurant, many consumers may accept the standard side dishes that automatically come with a fast-food meal. The widespread preference for default options has several explanations. First, choosing an option other than the default requires cognitive effort, as one must spend time and decision-making "bandwidth" to survey other options and choose an alternative. Second, defaults may convey an implicit level of endorsement from person or organization who is offering the choices—those who are designing the choice environment. Finally, loss aversion may come into play if choosing options other than the default is seen as less desirable.

In many cases, the power of defaults can be used to steer people toward healthy behaviors. Opt-out screening programs for various diseases rely on status quo bias, as any given individual will be automatically screened or tested unless they proactively decline (Montoy et al., 2016). Physician prescribing behaviors also can be influenced by default settings. In one prominent study at a US health system, there was a 23% point increase in generic medication prescribing rates after an opt-out checkbox labeled "dispense as written" was added to the prescription screen in the electronic health record (if the checkbox was left unchecked, the generic-equivalent medication was prescribed) (Patel et al., 2016b). In several studies, default settings in the electronic health record (e.g., setting the default to 10 tablets instead of no default) either reduced the quantity of opioids prescribed by healthcare professionals or increased compliance with the default quantity of opioid medications (Delgado et al., 2018; Montoy et al., 2020).

Limited Attention and Salience

Another central insight from behavioral economics is that the human mind has limited capacity to attend to all the potentially relevant information and considerations in our lives. In making decisions, our cognitive bandwidth is limited. Most decisions involve some degree of uncertainty, e.g., uncertainty about the chances that a behavior will result in an outcome, uncertainty about all potential outcomes, and uncertainty about how we will feel about that outcome. The human mind is simply not designed to attend to all that information and find an optimal decision the way a computer is. Relatedly, we all have many competing priorities for our time and attention—multiple projects at work or school; families and friends to attend to; our health, nutrition, and wellbeing—and our attention is not always focused on the most important of those competing priorities. Rather, our limited attention is often focused on the priority that is most salient, most recent, or, in some other way, most likely to be at top of mind. Examples of limited attention in public health include medication nonadherence, insufficient take-up of influenza and COVID vaccinations, and inadequate handwashing and infection control among healthcare workers. Common interventions aimed at increasing the salience of targeted health behaviors in the context of limited attention are SMS reminders (Wagstaff et al., 2019), healthcare provider checklists (Boyd et al., 2017), and active choice frameworks (Keller et al., 2011).

Decision Fatigue

When we must make repeated cognitively effortful decisions, studies show that our mental capacity and the quality of our decision-making deteriorate. For example, healthcare providers see many patients back-to-back over the course of a day, with many visits involving the processing of extensive patient information, a diagnostic decision that must be made, and the creation of a course of action. Behavioral economics research has shown that provider decision making changes over the course of the day, with providers increasingly likely to act in ways that require less effort over time. For example, for providers to decline a prescription request for antibiotics or opioids from patients, providers must take time to counsel patients about why these medications may not be needed or may cause more harm than benefit. Research has shown that prescriptions for antibiotics and opioids increase over the course of a provider's shift during the day (Linder et al., 2014; Neprash & Barnett, 2019), as does the decision to refer a patient for physical therapy rather than surgery (Persson et al., 2019). Promising interventions to combat decision fatigue include clinical decision support systems and nudge reminders, or small changes that are easy and usually inexpensive to implement.

Framing Effects

A large literature in behavioral economics, marketing, and psychology has demonstrated the significant role of the framing of information and choices in decision-making (Levin et al., 1998). In standard economic theory, only the actual content of the information that is presented to people should make a difference in decision-making, but behavioral economics studies have repeatedly shown that the way in which the information is presented (wording that is used, presentational style, etc.) can matter as well. One prominent example is "loss-framed" versus "gain-framed" messages, where the former highlight the consequences of *not* choosing a particular behavior, and the latter highlight the benefits of choosing that behavior (Rothman & Salovey, 1997). Evidence suggests that gain-framed messages—such as the benefits of quitting smoking or getting vaccinated—are more likely to encourage preventive health behaviors than loss-framed messages—such as the consequences of continuing to smoke or not getting vaccinated (Gallagher & Updegraff, 2012). One can also change the framing using different time horizons (e.g., the daily vs. annual cost of a subscription), different denominators (e.g., per population vs. per population-at-risk) and different wording (e.g.,"95% fat-free" versus "5% fat").

Social Norms

Many people look to the actions of others to guide their own decisions and behaviors. In a wide range of domains in which we make choices, social norms—the standards for behavior within a particular community or social group—strongly influence behavior. This goes against some predictions from standard economic theory, which suggests that our decisions are driven mainly by private costs and benefits. Social norms theory makes an important distinction between *descriptive norms* (what we observe other people do) and *injunctive norms* (what others believe we *ought* to do) (Reid et al., 2010). (Also see Chapter 6 on Reasoned Action Approaches.) The power of social norms can be deployed strategically by governments and organizations that seek to encourage people to engage in certain behaviors. One prominent example comes from the United States, where social comparisons have been used to encourage households to conserve energy in their homes. When households received monthly "home energy reports" that featured personalized energy use feedback, comparisons of the household's recent energy use to that of 100 neighbors with similar house characteristics, as well as energy conservation tips, there were immediate declines in energy consumption (Allcott & Rogers, 2014). Even though there was some decline in consumers' energy conservation efforts as they became habituated to the monthly reports, long-term reductions in energy use due to the reports continued. Social comparisons have also been used to influence the behavior of healthcare providers. For example, in one study conducted in the United States, peer comparisons were found to be effective in reducing inappropriate antibiotic prescribing for acute respiratory tract infections (Meeker et al., 2016). Another study found that peer comparison feedback significantly reduced opioid prescription quantities at emergency departments and urgent care sites in the United States (Navathe et al., 2022).

Applications

Application 1: Promoting HIV Testing

The global response to the AIDS pandemic is now entering its fifth decade. In the past two decades especially, there has been remarkable progress against HIV/AIDS in many parts of the world. Deaths due to AIDS peaked in 2004 when about two million people died of AIDS-related illnesses worldwide. The number of deaths per year has since declined nearly 70%, with about 650,000 deaths in 2021 (UNAIDS, 2022). The number of people newly infected with HIV has also fallen substantially since the peak of 3.2 million new HIV infections in 1996. While there is a major need for further progress against HIV/AIDS—1.5 million people were newly infected with HIV in 2021—it can be illuminating to examine some of the ways in which principles from behavioral economics have informed the global response to HIV/AIDS.

Increasing awareness of HIV status has been a central priority in many countries around the world. For people living with HIV, getting tested can enable them to access treatment that not only improves their health and prolongs their life but also eliminates the risk of transmission. When coverage and uptake of HIV testing services are very low, the majority of people living with HIV will typically be unaware of their HIV status and will access HIV testing services only when they become very sick (usually with advanced HIV disease). Thus, it is remarkable that in the past two decades, the percentage of people living with HIV who are aware of their own status has risen in nearly every part of the world—from less than 10% in 2000 to 85% in 2021. How was this dramatic progress achieved? While many factors are undoubtedly important, strategies rooted in the behavioral economics principles discussed in this chapter—such as the use of defaults and role of present bias—have played an essential role.

In the standard way that HIV testing services are offered at most clinics and health facilities, clients must agree to an HIV test being performed after receiving pre-test counseling (an "opt-in" approach). In this case, informed consent is like the consent that is usually required for special tests (like liver biopsy) or surgical interventions in clinical settings. However, both experimental and nonexperimental studies have found that this standard approach to testing results in lower uptake of HIV testing than an "opt-out" approach in which clients must specifically decline the HIV testing after receiving basic pre-test counseling if they do not want the test to be performed. The opt-out approach represents a clear illustration of the power of default settings to influence choices. It is also like what typically occurs for clinical investigations involving some X-rays, blood tests, and other noninvasive procedures. Often, providers' recommendations lead to the HIV tests being performed unless a patient declines. Studies conducted in South Africa and the United States have shown that opt-out testing results in much higher testing uptake (Leon et al., 2010; Montoy et al., 2016). The opt-out approach was also found to be highly cost-effective (Wagner et al., 2020). Although much debate has occurred about whether health facilities should adopt opt-out or opt-in approaches, it is notable that opt-out testing has become very common in many health programs around the world—particularly during antenatal care, when HIV testing is central to preventing mother-to-child transmission of HIV.

There are other ways in which behavioral economics principles have been useful for motivating or explaining the approaches that countries have used to promote HIV testing. In the United States and any countries in sub-Saharan Africa, community-based delivery of HIV testing services has become common. These include testing offered by mobile clinics (e.g., mobile vans or temporary tents set up in communities) as well as home-based testing services. One reason why such approaches are effective in increasing testing coverage is that they significantly reduce the immediate costs (transport costs, time costs, hassle costs) associated with getting an HIV test (Chamie et al., 2021). Since present-biased decision-making suggests that immediate costs influence behavior, community-based delivery of services can boost uptake more than use of facility-based delivery of services.

Application 2: Curbing Inappropriate Opioid Prescribing

The opioid epidemic is among the most significant public health crises in American history, with over 500,000 fatal opioid overdoses occurring in the United States between 2010 and 2020 (Mattson et al., 2021). There is substantial variation in provider practice regarding opioid prescribing, and finding effective policy approaches to reducing opioid prescribing among providers has been a central feature of the effort to reduce the scope and toll of the opioid epidemic (Barnett et al., 2017).

Policy approaches to reducing unnecessary opioid prescribing based on traditional economics would likely focus on providers' information about the potential risks and benefits of opioid prescribing. Clinical training and continuing medical education aimed at improving knowledge regarding opioid prescribing guidelines and harmful effects of opioid prescribing is one such approach. Implicitly, this approach is premised on the problem of imperfect information—that is, providers are not aware of, or have inaccurate beliefs regarding, the likelihood of abuse when they prescribe opioids. Other policy approaches that use traditional economic frameworks as a starting point may target the providers' expected costs and benefits of prescribing opioids, e.g., by increasing the penalties for unnecessary prescribing or increasing reimbursement rates for alternative approaches to pain management.

Policy approaches to reducing unnecessary opioid prescribing may be more effective if they incorporate behavioral economics concepts such as limited attention, mental models, and social norms, than if they focus strictly on interventions that flow from rational decision making, such as information and incentives. For example, several studies have demonstrated that using defaults in electronic health records systems reduces opioid prescription rates. In one such study (Bachhuber et al., 2021), a randomized controlled trial evaluated the impact of lowering the default setting for the number of opioid pills prescribed in an electronic health records system. Thirty-six primary and emergency care centers in a New York health system were randomized to either a control arm or to a treatment arm in which the electronic health records system had a default setting of 10 tablets for patients receiving new opioid prescriptions. In the status quo (reflected in the control arm), the electronic health records system would present either a default of 30 tablets or no default at all. In all facilities, the number of tablets prescribed was fully modifiable—the only difference was the default setting. The researchers found that the introduction of a relatively low default opioid prescribing setting significantly reduced the number of opioid tablets prescribed. They also found no evidence that patients in the treatment arm returned to providers for more opioid prescription reorders (Bachhuber et al., 2021), which could have reduced some of the benefits of the initial reduction in prescribing. As noted above, defaults can have powerful impacts on decision-making due to the normal human tendency to stick with a status quo. This trial illuminates how default settings in electronic health records systems can have a substantial impact on healthcare provider decision-making.

In another example of how behavioral economics has been used in designing new approaches to opioid prescribing, Doctor and colleagues (Doctor et al., 2018) conducted a randomized controlled trial testing the impact of clinician notification regarding fatal overdoses among patients to whom they prescribed opioids. In the trial, clinicians who had written opioid prescriptions for a patient who subsequently experienced a fatal overdose were randomized into either a control arm or an arm that received a letter, signed by the Chief Deputy Medical Examiner, notifying them of the death. The letter also included information on the number of prescription drug deaths and on the state's prescription drug-monitoring program, and it outlined guidelines for safe prescribing. This intervention drew on several insights from behavioral economics. First, it drew on our tendency to overweight recent salient events in decision-making ("*availability bias*"; see Table 20.2), a tendency supported by several studies that found that recent adverse events experienced among a provider's patients can influence a provider's decision-making (Han et al., 2020; Ly, 2021; Wang et al., 2022). Second, it draws on our tendency to change behavior when we are being observed and believe that we may not be acting in compliance with peer norms (see Table 20.2). Knowing one's behavior is being observed could increase the amount of cognitive effort put into the decision regarding whether to prescribe or could simply shift behavior more toward social norms/averages. The study (Doctor et al., 2018) found that this intervention significantly reduces opioid prescribing relative to the comparison group.

Discussion and Conclusions

The field of behavioral economics has had an important impact on the study of health behavior and on the design of health policies and programs. "Nudge units" and "behavioral insights teams," designed to incorporate insights from behavioral economics into the design of public policies, have been formed within the governments of the United States, the United Kingdom, Australia, and many other countries. A recent study estimated that nearly 200 such units have been formed globally (DellaVigna & Linos, 2022). The UK Behavioral Insights team has developed the "Mindspace" (Messenger, Incentives, Norms, Defaults, Salience, Priming, Affect, Commitments, Ego) framework to help policymakers choose and apply nudge strategies to influence behavior (Matjasko et al., 2016). Nudge units have designed policies and strategies to tackle a wide range of health behaviors among both patients and providers, including antibiotic prescribing, smoking, and vaccination. The World Health Organization and United Nations also have formed behavioral insights teams, opening up the possibility for behavioral economics to contribute to global health policy and practice (Ghebreyesus, 2021).

Insights from behavioral economics increasingly are influencing the design of products and services in the private sector as well. For example, many employers offer incentive-based wellness programs to their employees that incorporate behavioral economic insights regarding the design of optimal incentives (e.g., cash payments for exercising or for quitting smoking) (Loewenstein et al., 2013). CVS Caremark has used behavioral economic findings to improve medication adherence (Girdish et al., 2017; Matlin et al., 2015). Finally, behavioral economic concepts such as pre-commitment, status quo bias, and salience all play an important role in the design of health-related digital applications such as StickK, Noom, and Beeminder.

Systematic reviews of research testing the effectiveness of behavioral economic nudges in health care generally point toward meaningful, yet often modest, impacts. Several reviews have found that clinician-directed nudges can increase compliance with clinical guidelines and motivate targeted behavior change (Last et al., 2021; Nwafor et al., 2021; Yoong et al., 2020). Although these studies generally have found that nudges can effectively guide desirable clinician behavior, important gaps in this research remain. First, certain types of nudge strategies for directing clinician behavior have been tested much more extensively than others. For example, interventions that use information framing (often in the form of peer comparison) and choice guiding (e.g., through assignment of default options) make up most nudge strategies (Last et al., 2021). Second, most of these studies take place in the United States and other high-income settings. Generating more evidence regarding the impact of behavioral economic strategies to improve healthcare-provider quality of care in low- and middle-income countries is an important priority. Third, many clinician-directed nudges have been tested over a short time frame and within a single setting (Last et al., 2021). While more evidence on the long-term effectiveness of incentives and behavioral nudges is needed, existing studies indicate that the effects of interventions typically decline after interventions are stopped (Harkins et al., 2017; Volpp et al., 2009). One study found that interventions designed by government nudge units and implemented "at scale" (impacting millions of people) have had a positive, significant impact on targeted behavior change, but that the effects are substantially smaller in magnitude than those found in academic studies often conducted at a smaller scale (DellaVigna & Linos, 2022).

Some critics of behavioral economics argue that its application to health policy can be paternalistic and potentially coercive. Using peoples' known cognitive biases and judgment errors to influence their choices may be seen as deceptive and restrictive of personal freedom. For example, we have already described how powerful the selection of a default option can be, with most people tending to use the default across a wide range of choices. But who gets to decide what the default should be, and how do we know it is "best"? Behavioral nudges have been tested in a number of highly consequential choice settings, including advance directives for end-of-life care (Halpern et al., 2013) and organ donation (Johnson & Goldstein, 2003). However, behavioral economists argue that nudges do not remove autonomy or restrict people's freedom of choice in any way and, in that sense, are "libertarian paternalism" (Thaler & Sunstein, 2009). They also argue that all choices are made in some kind of choice architecture—someone is setting a default or choosing how information is conveyed—so why not then choose the choice architecture that is likely to lead to the most desired outcome? Finally, they argue that behavioral economics is not attempting to change people's preferences but, rather, helping them overcome obstacles to achieving the behaviors they actually want to adopt.

Another criticism of behavioral economics is that behavioral nudges have often not translated into large impacts at scale (DellaVigna & Linos, 2022). One potential reason for this modest impact is because of the tendency for behavioral-economic-inspired interventions to be focused on individual-level choices ("i-frame" interventions) instead of changes to the overall system ("s-frame" interventions) in which individuals make these choices (Chater & Loewenstein, 2022). For example, a range of i-frame interventions have been tested to combat obesity—one of the most pressing public health concerns in the United States and elsewhere—including healthy eating (Arno & Thomas, 2016), weight-loss incentives (Li et al., 2021) and nudges to increase gym attendance (Milkman et al., 2021), with notable but varying effects that may fade over time (Chater & Loewenstein, 2022). While behavioral nudges that help people accomplish their desired diet and exercise habits may be an important part of addressing obesity, a focus on individual-level behavior change may be detracting from needed system-level changes, including regulation, taxation, increasing activity-friendly environments, and promoting smaller serving sizes. It is likely that public health problems will need to be addressed through a combination of i-frame and s-frame approaches, as research in one area informs the other.

The field of behavioral economics now has global influence, informing the design of policies, programs, and products in government, health systems, and the private sector. A major priority for behavioral economics is to strengthen the evidence base within low- and middle-income countries. Much research is needed to uncover how behavioral economics could help inform strategies to combat major illnesses like malaria in these settings, and to strengthen quality of healthcare in resource-strained health systems. Another critical priority for behavioral economics is research and evaluation focused on health equity. While behavioral economics has offered critical insights into improvements in healthcare utilization and quality, the implications of behavioral economic nudges for health equity rarely have been explored.

Summary

Whereas traditional economic theories justify seemingly poor decisions as reflections of some implied but hidden rational choice, behavioral economics sees our seemingly poor decisions as errors that can be corrected or even prevented. Many people have trouble dieting, exercising, and saving money and are prone to procrastination even when the cumulative consequences are severe. While many commercial enterprises exploit these decision errors, the potential of behavioral economics lies in the growing evidence that some of the same messages, incentives, and choice structures used so effectively to lure people into situations where they may be exploited can be redirected to attract them to healthier choices that improve their long-term well-being. The potential for using insights from behavioral economics to improve health behavior is substantial. In fact, in the past decade, many organizations, health systems, and even governments have begun to implement and test interventions that are motivated by behavioral economics. Ongoing efforts like these have substantial potential to improve health outcomes globally. At the same time, additional pathways and opportunities to improve health are also necessary because nudges and other behavioral economics interventions may be insufficient. For example, raising taxes on cigarettes and other unhealthy goods where it is in the public interest to consume less is a powerful economic policy tool. When these types of "structural" policies and measures are implemented alongside behavioral economics interventions, major improvements in population health are possible.

References

Abaluck, J. & Gruber, J. (2011). Choice inconsistencies among the elderly: evidence from plan choice in the medicare Part D program. *American Economic Review, 101*(4), 1180–1210. https://doi.org/10.1257/aer.101.4.1180

Allais, P. M. (1953). Le Comportement de L'Homme Rationnel Devant le Risque: Critique Des Postulats Et Axiomes de L'ecole Americaine. *Econometrica, 21*(4), 503–546.

Allcott, H., & Rogers, T. (2014). The short-run and long-run effects of behavioral interventions: Experimental evidence from energy conservation. *American Economic Review, 104*(10), 3003–3037. https://doi.org/10.1257/aer.104.10.3003

Anderson, L. R., & Mellor, J. M. (2008). Predicting health behaviors with an experimental measure of risk preference. *Journal of Health Economics, 27*(5), 1260–1274. https://doi.org/10.1016/j.jhealeco.2008.05.011

Arno, A., & Thomas, S. (2016). The efficacy of nudge theory strategies in influencing adult dietary behaviour: A systematic review and meta-analysis. *BMC Public Health, 16*, 676. https://doi.org/10.1186/s12889-016-3272-x

Ashraf, N., Berry, J., & Shapiro, J. M. (2010). Can higher prices stimulate product use? Evidence from a field experiment in Zambia. *American Economic Review, 100*(5), 2383–2413. https://doi.org/10.1257/aer.100.5.2383

Bachhuber, M. A., Nash, D., Southern, W. N., Heo, M., Berger, M., Schepis, M., Thakral, M., & Cunningham, C. O. (2021). Effect of changing electronic health record opioid analgesic dspense quantity defaults on the quantity prescribed: A cluster randomized clinical trial. *JAMA Network Open, 4*(4), e217481–e217481. https://doi.org/10.1001/jamanetworkopen.2021.7481

Banerjee, A. V., Duflo, E., Glennerster, R., & Kothari, D. (2010). Improving immunisation coverage in rural India: Clustered randomised controlled evaluation of immunisation campaigns with and without incentives. *BMJ, 340*, c2220. https://doi.org/10.1136/bmj.c2220

Barnett, M. L., Olenski, A. R., & Jena, A. B. (2017). Opioid-prescribing patterns of emergency physicians and risk of long-term use. *New England Journal of Medicine, 376*(7), 663–673. https://doi.org/10.1056/NEJMsa1610524

Boyd, J., Wu, G., & Stelfox, H. (2017). The impact of checklists on inpatient safety outcomes: A systematic review of randomized controlled trials. *Journal of Hospital Medicine, 12*(8), 675–682. https://doi.org/10.12788/jhm.2788

Bradford, D., Courtemanche, C., Heutel, G., McAlvanah, P., & Ruhm, C. (2017). Time preferences and consumer behavior. *Journal of Risk and Uncertainty, 55*(2), 119–145. https://doi.org/10.1007/s11166-018-9272-8

Chaloupka, F. J., Straif, K., & Leon, M. E. (2011). Effectiveness of tax and price policies in tobacco control. *Tobacco Control, 20*(3), 235–238. https://doi.org/10.1136/tc.2010.039982

Chamie, G., Napierala, S., Agot, K., & Thirumurthy, H. (2021). HIV testing approaches to reach the first UNAIDS 95% target in sub-Saharan Africa. *Lancet HIV, 8*(4), e225–e236. https://doi.org/10.1016/S2352-3018(21)00023-0

Chang, W., Matambanadzo, P., Takaruza, A., Hatzold, K., Cowan, F. M., Sibanda, E., & Thirumurthy, H. (2019). Effect of prices, distribution strategies, and marketing on demand for HIV self-testing in Zimbabwe: A randomized clinical trial. *JAMA Network Open, 2*(8), e199818. https://doi.org/10.1001/jamanetworkopen.2019.9818

Chater, N., & Loewenstein, G. F. (2022). The i-Frame and the s-Frame: How focusing on the individual-level solutions has led behavioral public policy astray. *SSRN Electronic Journal.* https://doi.org/10.2139/ssrn.4046264

Chiu, A. S., Jean, R. A., Hoag, J. R., Freedman-Weiss, M., Healy, J. M., & Pei, K. Y. (2018). Association of lowering default pill counts in electronic medical record systems with postoperative opioid prescribing. *JAMA Surgery, 153*(11), 1012–1019. https://doi.org/10.1001/jamasurg.2018.2083

Cohen, J. L. (2019). The enduring debate over cost sharing for essential public health tools. *JAMA Network Open, 2*(8), e199810–e199810. https://doi.org/10.1001/jamanetworkopen.2019.9810

Cohen, J., & Dupas, P. (2010). Free distribution or cost-sharing? Evidence from a randomized malaria prevention experiment*. *The Quarterly Journal of Economics, 125*(1), 1–45. https://doi.org/10.1162/qjec.2010.125.1.1

Cohen, J., & Saran, I. (2018). The impact of packaging and messaging on adherence to malaria treatment: Evidence from a randomized controlled trial in Uganda. *Journal of Development Economics, 134*, 68–95. https://doi.org/10.1016/j.jdeveco.2018.04.008

Colchero, M. A., Popkin, B. M., Rivera, J. A., & Ng, S. W. (2016). Beverage purchases from stores in Mexico under the excise tax on sugar sweetened beverages: observational study. *BMJ, 352*, h6704. https://doi.org/10.1136/bmj.h6704

Davis, R. M. (Ed.). (2008). *The role of the media in promoting and reducing tobacco use* (No. 19). US Department of Health and Human Services, National Institutes of Health, National Cancer Institute.

Delgado, M. K., Shofer, F. S., Patel, M. S., Halpern, S., Edwards, C., Meisel, Z. F., & Perrone, J. (2018). Association between electronic medical record implementation of default opioid prescription quantities and prescribing behavior in two emergency departments. *Journal of General Internal Medicine*, *33*(4), 409–411. https://doi.org/10.1007/s11606-017-4286-5

DellaVigna, S., & Linos, E. (2022). RCTs to scale: Comprehensive evidence From two nudge units. *Econometrica*, *90*(1), 81–116. https://doi.org/10.3982/ECTA18709

Doctor, J. N., Nguyen, A., Lev, R., Lucas, J., Knight, T., Zhao, H., & Menchine, M. (2018). Opioid prescribing decreases after learning of a patient's fatal overdose. *Science*, *361*(6402), 588–590. https://doi.org/10.1126/science.aat4595

Donato, A. A., Motz, L. M., Wilson, G., & Lloyd, B. J. (2007). Efficacy of multiple influenza vaccine delivery systems in a single facility. *Infection Control & Hospital Epidemiology*, *28*(2), 219–221. https://doi.org/10.1086/511797

Dupas, P. (2011). Do teenagers respond to HIV risk information? Evidence from a field experiment in Kenya. *American Economic Journal: Applied Economics*, *3*(1), 1–34. https://doi.org/10.1257/app.3.1.1

Fernandes, A. C., Oliveira, R. C., Proença, R. P. C., Curioni, C. C., Rodrigues, V. M., & Fiates, G. M. R. (2016). Influence of menu labeling on food choices in real-life settings: A systematic review. *Nutrition Reviews*, *74*(8), 534–548. https://doi.org/10.1093/nutrit/nuw013

Gallagher, K. M., & Updegraff, J. A. (2012). Health message framing effects on attitudes, intentions, and behavior: A meta-analytic review. *Annals of Behavioral Medicine*, *43*(1), 101–116. https://doi.org/10.1007/s12160-011-9308-7

Ghebreyesus, T. A. (2021). Using behavioural science for better health. *Bulletin of the World Health Organization*, *99*(11), 755–755. https://creativecommons.org/licenses/by/3.0/igo/. https://doi.org/10.2471/BLT.21.287387

Girdish, C., Shrank, W., Freytag, S., Chen, D., Gebhard, D., Bunton, A., Choudhry, N., & Polinski, J. (2017). The impact of a retail prescription synchronization program on medication adherence. *Journal of the American Pharmacists Association*, *57*(5), 579–584. e571. https://doi.org/10.1016/j.japh.2017.05.016

Grant, A. M. & Hofmann, D. A. (2011). It's not all about me:motivating hand hygiene among health care professionals by focusing on patients. *Psychological Science*, *22*(12), 1494–1499. https://doi.org/10.1177/0956797611419172

Gursoy, D., Ekinci, Y., Can, A. S., & Murray, J. C. (2022). Effectiveness of message framing in changing COVID-19 vaccination intentions: Moderating role of travel desire. *Tourism Management*, *90*, 104468.

Halpern, S. D., Loewenstein, G., Volpp, K. G., Cooney, E., Vranas, K., Quill, C. M., McKenzie, M. S., Harhay, M. O., Gabler, N. B., Silva, T., Arnold, R., Angus, D. C., & Bryce, C. (2013). Default options in advance directives influence how patients set goals for end-of-life care. *Health Affairs (Millwood)*, *32*(2), 408–417. https://doi.org/10.1377/hlthaff.2012.0895

Halpern, S. D., Harhay, M. O., Saulsgiver, K., Brophy, C., Troxel, A. B., & Volpp, K. G. (2018). A pragmatic trial of E-cigarettes, incentives, and drugs for smoking cessation. *New England Journal of Medicine*, *378*(24), 2302–2310. https://doi.org/10.1056/NEJMsa1715757

Han, D., Khadka, A., McConnell, M., & Cohen, J. (2020). Association of unexpected newborn deaths with changes in obstetric and neonatal process of care. *JAMA Network Open*, *3*(12), e2024589–e2024589. https://doi.org/10.1001/jamanetworkopen.2020.24589

Harkins, K. A., Kullgren, J. T., Bellamy, S. L., Karlawish, J., & Glanz, K. (2017). A trial of financial and social incentives to increase older adults' walking. *American Journal of Preventive Medicine*, *52*(5), e123–e130. https://doi.org/10.1016/j.amepre.2016.11.011

Johnson, E. J., & Goldstein, D. (2003). Medicine. Do defaults save lives? *Science*, *302*(5649), 1338–1339. https://doi.org/10.1126/science.1091721

Kahneman, D. (2011). *Thinking, fast and slow*. New York, NY: Farrar, Straus & Giroux.

Kahneman, D., & Tversky, A. (1979). Prospect theory: An analysis of decision under risk. *Econometrica*, *47*, 263–291.

Kawamoto, K., Houlihan, C. A., Balas, E. A., & Lobach, D. F. (2005). Improving clinical practice using clinical decision support systems: a systematic review of trials to identify features critical to success. *Bmj*, *330*(7494), 765. https://doi.org/10.1136/bmj.38398.500764.8F

Keller, P., Harlam, B., Loewenstein, G., & Volpp, K. (2011). Enhanced active choice: A new method to motivate behavior change. *Journal of Consumer Psychology*, *21*, 376–383. https://doi.org/10.1016/j.jcps.2011.06.003

Kim, R. H., Day, S. C., Small, D. S., Snider, C. K., Rareshide, C. A. L., & Patel, M. S. (2018). Variations in influenza vaccination by clinic appointment time and an active choice intervention in the electronic health record to increase influenza vaccination. *JAMA Network Open*, *1*(5), e181770–e181770. https://doi.org/10.1001/jamanetworkopen.2018.1770

Last, B. S., Buttenheim, A. M., Timon, C. E., Mitra, N., & Beidas, R. S. (2021). Systematic review of clinician-directed nudges in healthcare contexts. *BMJ Open*, *11*(7), e048801. https://doi.org/10.1136/bmjopen-2021-048801

Leon, N., Naidoo, P., Mathews, C., Lewin, S., & Lombard, C. (2010). The impact of provider-initiated (opt-out) HIV testing and counseling of patients with sexually transmitted infection in Cape Town, South Africa: A controlled trial. *Implementation Science*, *5*, 8. https://doi.org/10.1186/1748-5908-5-8

Levin, I. P., Schneider, S. L., & Gaeth, G. J. (1998). All frames are not created equal: A typology and critical analysis of framing effects. *Organizational Behavior and Human Decision Processes*, *76*(2), 149–188. https://doi.org/10.1006/obhd.1998.2804

Li, R., Zhang, Y., Cai, X., Luo, D., Zhou, W., Long, T., Zhang, H., Jiang, H., & Li, M. (2021). The nudge strategies for weight loss in adults with obesity and overweight: A systematic review and meta-analysis. *Health Policy*, *125*(12), 1527–1535. https://doi.org/10.1016/j.healthpol.2021.10.010

Linder, J. A., Doctor, J. N., Friedberg, M. W., Reyes Nieva, H., Birks, C., Meeker, D., & Fox, C. R. (2014). Time of day and the decision to prescribe antibiotics. *JAMA Internal Medicine*, *174*(12), 2029–2031. https://doi.org/10.1001/jamainternmed.2014.5225

Loewenstein, G., Asch, D. A., & Volpp, K. G. (2013). Behavioral economics holds potential to deliver better results for patients, insurers, and employers. *Health Affairs*, *32*(7), 1244–1250. https://doi.org/10.1377/hlthaff.2012.1163

Ly, D. P. (2021). The influence of the availability heuristic on physicians in the emergency department. *Annals of Emergency Medicine*, *78*(5), 650–657. https://doi.org/10.1016/j.annemergmed.2021.06.012

Manning, W. G., Newhouse, J. P., Duan, N., Keeler, E. B., & Leibowitz, A. (1987). Health insurance and the demand for medical care: Evidence from a randomized experiment. *The American Economic Review*, *77*(3), 251–277. http://www.jstor.org/stable/1804094

Matjasko, J. L., Cawley, J. H., Baker-Goering, M. M., & Yokum, D. V. (2016). Applying behavioral economics to public health policy: Illustrative examples and promising directions. *American Journal of Preventive Medicine*, *50*(5 Suppl. 1), S13–S19. https://doi.org/10.1016/j.amepre.2016.02.007

Matlin, O. S., Kymes, S. M., Averbukh, A., Choudhry, N. K., Brennan, T. A., Bunton, A., Ducharme, T. A., Simmons, P. D., & Shrank, W. H. (2015). Community pharmacy automatic refill program improves adherence to maintenance therapy and reduces wasted medication. *American Journal of Managed Care*, *21*(11), 785–791.

Mattson, C. L., Tanz, L. J., Quinn, K., Kariisa, M., Patel, P., & Davis, N. L. (2021). Trends and geographic patterns in drug and synthetic opioid overdose deaths—United States, 2013-2019. *Morbidity and Mortality Weekly Report (MMWR)*, *70*(6), 202–207. https://doi.org/10.15585/mmwr.mm7006a4

Meeker, D., Linder, J. A., Fox, C. R., Friedberg, M. W., Persell, S. D., Goldstein, N. J., Knight, T. K., Hay, J. W., & Doctor, J. N. (2016). Effect of behavioral interventions on Inappropriate antibiotic prescribing among primary care practices: A randomized clinical trial. *JAMA*, *315*(6), 562–570. https://doi.org/10.1001/jama.2016.0275

Milkman, K. L., Gromet, D., Ho, H., Kay, J. S., Lee, T. W., Pandiloski, P., Park, Y., Rai, A., Bazerman, M., Beshears, J., Bonacorsi, L., Camerer, C., Chang, E., Chapman, G., Cialdini, R., Dai, H., Eskreis-Winkler, L., Fishbach, A., Gross, J. J., Duckworth, A. L. (2021). Megastudies improve the impact of applied behavioural science. *Nature*, *600*(7889), 478–483. https://doi.org/10.1038/s41586-021-04128-4

Montoy, J. C., Dow, W. H., & Kaplan, B. C. (2016). Patient choice in opt-in, active choice, and opt-out HIV screening: Randomized clinical trial. *BMJj*, *532*, h6895. https://doi.org/10.1136/bmj.h6895

Montoy, J. C. C., Coralic, Z., Herring, A. A., Clattenburg, E. J., & Raven, M. C. (2020). Association of default electronic medical record settings with health care professional patterns of opioid prescribing in emergency departments: A randomized quality improvement study. *JAMA Internal Medicine*, *180*(4), 487–493. https://doi.org/10.1001/jamainternmed.2019.6544

Murray, C. J. L., Ikuta, K. S., Sharara, F., Swetschinski, L., Robles Aguilar, G., Gray, A., Han, C., Bisignano, C., Rao, P., Wool, E., Johnson, S. C., Browne, A. J., Chipeta, M. G., Fell, F., Hackett, S., Haines-Woodhouse, G., Kashef Hamadani, B. H., Kumaran, E. A. P., McManigal, B., Naghavi, M. (2022). Global burden of bacterial antimicrobial resistance in 2019: A systematic analysis. *The Lancet*, *399*(10325), 629–655. https://doi.org/10.1016/S0140-6736(21)02724-0

Navathe, A. S., Liao, J. M., Yan, X. S., Delgado, M. K., Isenberg, W. M., Landa, H. M., Bond, B. L., Small, D. S., Rareshide, C. A. L., Shen, Z., Pepe, R. S., Refai, F., Lei, V. J., Volpp, K. G., & Patel, M. S. (2022). The effect of clinician feedback interventions on opioid prescribing. *Health Affairs*, *41*(3), 424–433. https://doi.org/10.1377/hlthaff.2021.01407

Neprash, H. T., & Barnett, M. L. (2019). Association of primary care clinic appointment time with opioid prescribing. *JAMA Network Open*, *2*(8), e1910373–e1910373. https://doi.org/10.1001/jamanetworkopen.2019.10373

Novemsky, N., & Kahneman, D. (2005). The boundaries of loss aversion. *Journal of Marketing Research*, *42*, 119–128.

Nwafor, O., Singh, R., Collier, C., DeLeon, D., Osborne, J., & DeYoung, J. (2021). Effectiveness of nudges as a tool to promote adherence to guidelines in healthcare and their organizational implications: A systematic review. *Social Science & Medicine*, *286*, 114321. https://doi.org/10.1016/j.socscimed.2021.114321

Olson, J., Hollenbeak, C., Donaldson, K., Abendroth, T., & Castellani, W. (2015). Default settings of computerized physician order entry system order sets drive ordering habits. *Journal of Pathology Informatics*, *6*, 16.

Patel, M. S., Day, S., Small, D. S., Howell, J. T., Lautenbach, G. L., Nierman, E. H., & Volpp, K. G. (2014). Using default options within the electronic health record to increase the prescribing of generic-equivalent medications. *Annals of Internal Medicine*, *161*(10_Supplement), S44–S52. https://doi.org/10.7326/M13-3001

Patel, M. S., Asch, D. A., Rosin, R., Small, D. S., Bellamy, S. L., Heuer, J., Sproat, S., Hyson, C., Haff, N., Lee, S. M., Wesby, L., Hoffer, K., Shuttleworth, D., Taylor, D. H., Hilbert, V., Zhu, J., Yang, L., Wang, X., & Volpp, K. G. (2016a). Framing financial incentives to increase physical activity among overweight and obese adults: A randomized, controlled trial. *Annals of Internal Medicine*, *164*(6), 385–394. https://doi.org/10.7326/M15-1635

Patel, M. S., Day, S. C., Halpern, S. D., Hanson, C. W., Martinez, J. R., Honeywell, S., Jr., & Volpp, K. G. (2016b). Generic medication prescription rates after health system-wide redesign of default options within the electronic health record. *JAMA Internal Medicine*, *176*(6), 847–848. https://doi.org/10.1001/jamainternmed.2016.1691

Pega, F., Pabayo, R., Benny, C., Lee, E. Y., Lhachimi, S. K., & Liu, S. Y. (2022). Unconditional cash transfers for reducing poverty and vulnerabilities: Effect on use of health services and health outcomes in low- and middle-income countries. *Cochrane Database of Systematic Reviews*. https://doi.org/10.1002/14651858.CD011135.pub3

Persson, E., Barrafrem, K., Meunier, A., & Tinghög, G. (2019). The effect of decision fatigue on surgeons' clinical decision making. *Health Economics*, *28*(10), 1194–1203. https://doi.org/10.1002/hec.3933

Reid, A. E., Cialdini, R. B., & Aiken, L. S. (2010). Social norms and health behavior. *Handbook of Behavioral Medicine: Methods and Applications*, *3*, 263.

Roberto, C. A., Lawman, H. G., LeVasseur, M. T., Mitra, N., Peterhans, A., Herring, B., & Bleich, S. N. (2019). Association of a beverage tax on sugar-sweetened and artificially sweetened beverages with changes in beverage prices and sales at chain retailers in a large urban setting. *JAMA : The Journal of the American Medical Association*, *321*(18), 1799–1810. https://doi.org/10.1001/jama.2019.4249

Rothman, A. J., & Salovey, P. (1997). Shaping perceptions to motivate healthy behavior: The role of message framing. *Psychological Bulletin*, *121*(1), 3–19.

Shangguan, S., Afshin, A., Shulkin, M., Ma, W., Marsden, D., Smith, J., Saheb-Kashaf, M., Shi, P., Micha, R., Imamura, F., & Mozaffarian, D. (2019). A meta-analysis of food labeling effects on consumer diet behaviors and industry practices. *American Journal of Preventive Medicine*, *56*(2), 300–314.

Sibbald, M., de Bruin, A. B., Cavalcanti, R. B., & van Merrienboer, J. J. (2013). Do you have to re-examine to reconsider your diagnosis? Checklists and cardiac exam. *BMJ Quality & Safety*, *22*(4), 333–338. https://doi.org/10.1136/bmjqs-2012-001537

Silver, L. D., Ng, S. W., Ryan-Ibarra, S., Taillie, L. S., Induni, M., Miles, D. R., Poti, J. M., & Popkin, B. M. (2017). Changes in prices, sales, consumer spending, and beverage consumption one year after a tax on sugar-sweetened beverages in Berkeley, California, US: A before-and-after study. *PLoS Medicine*, *14*(4), e1002283. https://doi.org/10.1371/journal.pmed.1002283

Simon, H. A. (1955). A behavioral model of rational choice. *Quarterly Journal of Economics*, *69*, 99–118.

Singh, M. (2021). Heuristics in the delivery room. *Science*, *374*(6565), 324–329. https://doi.org/10.1126/science.abc9818

Thaler, R. H., & Sunstein, C. R. (2009). *Nudge: Improving decisions about health, wealth, and happiness*. (Rev. and expanded ed.). Penguin Books.

Thirumurthy, H., Hayashi, K., Linnemayr, S., Vreeman, R. C., Levin, I. P., Bangsberg, D. R., & Brewer, N. T. (2015). Time preferences predict mortality among HIV-infected adults receiving antiretroviral therapy in Kenya. *PLoS One*, *10*(12), e0145245. https://doi.org/10.1371/journal.pone.0145245

Thirumurthy, H., Asch, D. A., & Volpp, K. G. (2019a). The uncertain effect of financial incentives to improve health hehaviors. *JAMA*, *321*(15), 1451–1452. https://doi.org/10.1001/jama.2019.2560

Thirumurthy, H., Ndyabakira, A., Marson, K., Emperador, D., Kamya, M., Havlir, D., Kwarisiima, D., & Chamie, G. (2019b). Financial incentives for achieving and maintaining viral suppression among HIV-positive adults in Uganda: A randomised controlled trial. *Lancet HIV*, *6*(3), e155–e163. https://doi.org/10.1016/S2352-3018(18)30330-8

Thornton, R. (2008). The demand for, and impact of, learning HIV status. *American Economic Review*, *98*(5), 1829–1863.

Tsai, A. C., Kakuhikire, B., Perkins, J. M., Downey, J. M., Baguma, C., Satinsky, E. N., Gumisiriza, P., Kananura, J., & Bangsberg, D. R. (2021). Normative vs personal attitudes toward persons with HIV, and the mediating role of perceived HIV stigma in rural Uganda. *Journal of Global Health*, *11*, 04956. https://doi.org/10.7189/jogh.11.04056

UNAIDS. (2022). *In danger*. UNAIDS Global AIDS Update.

Volpp, K. G., Troxel, A. B., Pauly, M. V., Glick, H. A., Puig, A., Asch, D. A., Galvin, R., Zhu, J., Wan, F., DeGuzman, J., Corbett, E., Weiner, J., & Audrain-McGovern, J. (2009). A randomized, controlled trial of financial incentives for smoking cessation, *New England Journal of Medicine*, *360*(7), 699–709. https://doi.org/10.1056/NEJMsa0806819

Volpp, K. G., Troxel, A. B., Mehta, S. J., Norton, L., Zhu, J., Lim, R., Wang, W., Marcus, N., Terwiesch, C., Caldarella, K., Levin, T., Relish, M., Negin, N., Smith-McLallen, A., Snyder, R., Spettell, C. M., Drachman, B., Kolansky, D., & Asch, D. A. (2017). Effect of electronic reminders, financial incentives, and social support on outcomes after myocardial infarction: The HeartStrong randomized clinical trial. *JAMA Internal Medicine, 177*(8), 1093–1101. https://doi.org/10.1001/jamainternmed.2017.2449

Wagner, Z., Montoy, J. C. C., Drabo, E. F., & Dow, W. H. (2020). Incentives versus defaults: Cost-effectiveness of behavioral approaches for HIV screening. *AIDS and Behavior, 24*(2), 379–386. https://doi.org/10.1007/s10461-019-02425-8

Wagstaff, A., van Doorslaer, E., & Burger, R. (2019). SMS nudges as a tool to reduce tuberculosis treatment delay and pretreatment loss to follow-up. A randomized controlled trial. *PLoS One, 14*(6), e0218527. https://doi.org/10.1371/journal.pone.0218527

Wang, A. Z., Barnett, M. L., & Cohen, J. L. (2022). Changes in cancer screening rates following a new cancer diagnosis in a primary care patient panel. *JAMA Network Open, 5*(7), e2222131–e2222131. https://doi.org/10.1001/jamanetworkopen.2022.22131

Wisdom, J., Downs, J. S., & Loewenstein, G. (2010). Promoting healthy choices: Information versus convenience. *American Economic Journal: Applied Economics, 2*(2), 164–178. https://doi.org/10.1257/app.2.2.164

Yoong, S. L., Hall, A., Stacey, F., Grady, A., Sutherland, R., Wyse, R., Anderson, A., Nathan, N., & Wolfenden, L. (2020). Nudge strategies to improve healthcare providers' implementation of evidence-based guidelines, policies and practices: A systematic review of trials included within Cochrane systematic reviews. *Implementation Science, 15*(1), 50. https://doi.org/10.1186/s13012-020-01011-0

CHAPTER 21

SOCIAL MARKETING

J. Douglas Storey
Evelyn Kumoji
Fred Rariewa
Yunita Wahyuningrum

KEY POINTS

This chapter will:

- Define social marketing, its basic principles, and how they can be applied in strategic health communication.

- Link commonly used theories of health communication and health behavior to the effective practice of social marketing.

- Describe the uses of research in the formation, implementation, and evaluation stages of social marketing programs.

- Provide examples of international social marketing programs that illustrate how principles and processes of social marketing contribute to social change and behavior change.

Vignette

Meet Sara. Sara and her husband Adel live in a low-income neighborhood of a major city in the Global South. They have a son and a daughter, aged 5 and 2 years old. Like most of their neighbors, they struggle to make ends meet. They rely on small, local retail shops for family health supplies like hygiene products and basic pharmaceuticals. There is a government hospital a few miles away, but it is always crowded and seeing a health worker there takes more time than Sara can afford. She occasionally pays a close neighbor, who is a private midwife, for care and advice about her personal and family health needs. Sometimes she searches for answers on the internet using her cell phone but does not always find the information she needs.

Sara and Adel do not want any more children—at least for the next couple of years—but they are not sure about the best way to prevent another pregnancy. Condoms are available at the local retail shop and the midwife provides injectable contraceptives that work for a month at a time, but paying for that for the next three years or more would be challenging. Last week, Sara tried to talk to the local retail shop owner about alternatives to condoms, but he did not have any other over-the-counter options and got impatient when she asked too many questions. Sara does not know who to turn to for help with these important decisions.

Sara and Adel are facing challenges at multiple levels. The people they can turn to for help are not knowledgeable or prepared to help them make healthy choices, and in some cases, the commodities they need are not easily available. In the past, a typical health communication campaign to address these challenges would focus on what Sara and Adel needed to know to understand specific health issues like child health, birth spacing, and family planning (FP), and support them to make healthy choices. Other strategies might have focused on improving service-provider communication skills to teach clients about specific health issues and decisions. However, increased client knowledge or motivation, by itself, is unlikely to overcome the many challenges that prevent Sara and Adel from achieving what they want—a healthy, happy family, and good quality of life—even if they know how and want to.

Health Behavior: Theory, Research, and Practice, Sixth Edition. Edited by Karen Glanz, Barbara K. Rimer, and K. Viswanath.

With a comprehensive, well-designed social marketing program in place, Sara and Adel might see more salient messages in the media, around the community, or on her phone about contraceptive options for couples with small children. Her midwife would be more knowledgeable about the benefits of birth spacing and trained to help her choose a contraceptive that is right for her and Adel's stage of family life. The local retail shop owner would have a better stock of family health products, displayed in attractive and informative ways to appeal to customer needs and would be better prepared to answer Sara's questions and refer her to services that he cannot provide. Encouraged by activists from a local NGO, Sara and Adel could feel empowered to speak up at community meetings about their health needs. In response, local government leaders would potentially introduce subsidies to make certain health services and products more accessible and affordable for low-income households.

Introduction

Seventy years ago (1951–1952), the psychologist G.D. Wiebe famously asked, "Why can't you sell brotherhood like soap?" The notion that promoting universal goodwill and marketing a common cleaning product might be equated strains the imagination, but it has had enormous appeal and generated controversy ever since. What we now call social marketing—generally understood as the use of principles of commercial marketing to promote desirable social conditions—has evolved and grown in sophistication while informing efforts to create positive social and behavior change in all parts of the world and across nearly the full spectrum of issues reflected in the United Nations Sustainable Development Goals (United Nations, 2023). The field of public health, in particular, has been a major domain of social marketing research, theory development, and practice, and has produced compelling evidence of effectiveness in improving health outcomes on both large and small scales.

The translation of commercial marketing into social marketing approaches is complicated. Marketers of soap typically have much larger budgets than marketers of brotherhood, as well as much larger infrastructures dedicated primarily to the marketing function. They also are more often focused on selling specific brands (for example, Pedialyte™) rather than generating demand for a product category (e.g., oral rehydration products) or a class of behavior (e.g., treatment of diarrheal disease) that could be practiced in different ways. Like commercial marketing, social marketing also seeks to influence behavior, but with broader social implications, including shifts in attitudes, norms, and social priorities in ways that serve the public interest in addition to individual needs.

What distinguishes social marketing from other health promotion and health communication approaches? Why should one consider social marketing as a strategy for influencing positive health behaviors? How can principles of social marketing be used in the current media environment defined by rapidly spreading information and dominated by online and digital communication? The rest of this chapter will address these questions drawing examples from social marketing programs in non-US settings and two case studies from Kenya and Indonesia.

Definition of Social Marketing

Social marketing began to take shape in the late 1960s (Kotler & Levy, 1969). The term itself is usually attributed to Kotler and Zaltman (1971) who originally defined it as "a social influence technology involving the design, implementation and control of programs aimed at increasing the acceptability of a social idea or practice in one or more groups of target adopters" (Kotler & Roberto, 1989, p. 24). Some of the earliest applications of social marketing may have occurred in public health, specifically FP campaigns in India in the 1960s (Harvey, 1999). Since then, social marketing has evolved through extensive application and scholarship.

Andreasen's definition is one of the most concise and comprehensive: "Social marketing is the *application of commercial marketing technologies* to the analysis, planning, execution and evaluation of programs *designed to influence the voluntary behavior* of target audiences in order *to improve their personal welfare and that of their society*" (Andreasen, 1994, p. 11; emphasis added). These three highlighted aspects—the use of a commercial marketing perspective to influence voluntary behavior for individual and social good—lie at the heart of all social marketing efforts. The *focus* on outcomes that improve personal and social *welfare* is the primary feature that distinguishes social from commercial marketing.

To the features noted by Andreasen (1994, 2006), it is worth highlighting another one derived from Bagozzi (1974, 1978): the mutual fulfillment of self-interest through **voluntary exchange**. Voluntary exchange from a consumer's view means that the interaction with a marketer fulfills a felt need or desire, the perceived cost of which—in social, economic, psychological, and/or physical terms—does not outweigh the perceived gain. Voluntary exchange from a marketer's point of view primarily means providing a good or service that is in *their* best interest, often expressed in financial terms. In the case of social marketing, consumers and marketers presumably share the same goal, namely increasing benefits to all parties not just those in a position to pay for a product.

While debates over the definition of social marketing will continue, social marketing is now a well-developed area of scholarship and practice. Major international, regional, and national associations such as the International Social Marketing Association (https://isocialmarketing.org/), the European Social Marketing Association (https://european-socialmarketing.org/), and the Latin American Social Marketing Association (http://www.mercadeosocial.org/) serve networks of professionals and scholars. Expansion continues; the relatively new African Social Marketing Association held its first regional conference in 2023.

Basic Principles of Social Marketing

In this section, we describe four principles that have made social marketing popular and effective as a health promotion strategy: (1) focus on behavioral outcomes, (2) prioritize consumers' rather than marketers' benefits, (3) use audience segmentation, and (4) draw on a marketing perspective.

Focusing on behavior: In the past, "products" were defined broadly to include ideas (such as FP, protecting the environment), attitudes (such as preference for small family size, approval of recycling), availability of services (such as FP clinics, recycling centers) and behaviors (such as using hormonal contraceptives, recycling glass bottles). But Andreasen (1994, 2006) and others argue that the proper objective of social marketing is to influence behavior. It is not enough to promote the purchase of products or services; people must obtain *and* use them because usually it is use, rather than possession *per se*, that confers benefit. A condom marketing campaign would have to be judged unsuccessful if condoms were not used effectively and consistently as they were meant to be—to prevent disease and pregnancy. In other words, the focus on behavior is inextricably linked to the second principle, consumer benefit.

Prioritizing consumer benefits: A general dimension of communication campaigns—*locus of benefit* (Rogers & Storey, 1987)—refers to whether successful achievement of program objectives primarily benefits the program designers or the program audience. Compared to commercial marketing campaigns, social marketing campaigns primarily benefit members of the audience or society at large in the form of such outcomes as better health or a cleaner and more stable environment, although some have suggested that co-creation of value by marketers and consumers with common goals means benefits (and costs) are mutually shared (Lefebvre, 2012). Nevertheless, consumer or societal benefit is paramount.

Using audience segmentation: The principle of audience segmentation refers to the identification of relatively homogeneous subgroups and the development of marketing strategies customized to the characteristics of each subgroup. Different subgroups require different strategies because they value different benefits associated with a product, prioritize cost considerations differently, seek and obtain product information or social support for behavior change through different channels, and respond differently to some message formats or appeals than others. Segmentation strategies typically consider socioeconomic, cultural, geographical, psychographic, and age characteristics of an audience as well as patterns of use (such as high or low, frequent or infrequent, experienced or inexperienced) to identify clusters that respond or relate in similar ways to a product (see Warner, 2019; Wonneberger et al., 2020; Noar & Harrington, 2016 for examples of segmentation and cultural tailoring approaches).

Consider an adolescent reproductive health campaign focused on reducing teenage pregnancy. Within the age range of 14–18 years, some individuals are sexually active, and some are not. An audience segmentation strategy for teenage pregnancy prevention based on sexual activity status might focus on condom use for teens who are sexually active and abstinence or delay of sexual debut for teens who are not sexually active. Each product/behavior would have its own bundle of benefits, product and message placement, description of costs and benefits, and promotional strategy (perhaps using different types of role models) appropriate for each audience segment.

Maintaining a market perspective: Another principle of social marketing that sets it apart from other forms of persuasive communication is the concept of the market itself. First, a market perspective requires adoption of a *consumer orientation*; that is, markets revolve around consumer needs and desires and the ways in which decisions are made to satisfy those needs.

Second, the functioning of markets depends on the *circulation of information* about products that are available, what they cost, how they can be used, what benefits they provide, and where to obtain them. Third, promoted products always face *competition* for the consumer's attention and resources in a dynamic marketplace of ideas, priorities, and choices.

Some social marketing approaches refer to strategies addressing an *upstream* focus on infrastructural change (such as policy or regulatory requirements) or a *downstream* focus on individual change (such as knowledge, attitudes, or practices) (Andreasen, 2006). Often, upstream and downstream strategies need to be coordinated to change upstream structural conditions that pose downstream barriers to individual change.

The Role of Social Marketing Within a Strategic Communication Framework

In all societies, social marketing communication occurs within three principal domains: the social-political environment, health-service delivery systems, and among individuals within communities and households (Pollock & Storey, 2012; Storey et al., 2005; USAID, 2001). Communication within each of these domains combines to change audiences and institutions over time, making the environment more supportive of healthy practices, improving the performance of health services, and increasing the likelihood of preventive or protective health practices. To the extent that these changes are durable, improved health outcomes can be sustained. (For more discussion of multi-level thinking about health education and health behavior, see Chapter 3).

Within this larger framework, three approaches can be selected depending on needs and resources: *product-driven* approaches, *consumer- or demand-driven* approaches, and *market-driven* approaches.

Product-driven approaches: Product-driven approaches aim to increase the appeal of a product and differentiate it positively from alternatives. *Branding*, for example, identifies a product category and associates it with desirable attributes: *Under Armour* athletic gear, *Apple* iPhones, the *Google* search engine. Non-commercial "products" have brand identities, too: the *World Wildlife Federation* for environmental issues, *Amnesty International* for social justice issues, and the *truth FinishIt* brand (Evans et al., 2018) for tobacco cessation are examples of popular, internationally recognized brands of social activism. Branded products are then associated with a consistent bundle of promised benefits or ideas (such as quality, creativity, societal impact, truth). Consumers come to expect those attributes and return to or support those products again and again in anticipation of predictable outcomes.

A classic example of social marketing is Indonesia's highly successful national FP program, which in 1988 introduced the Blue Circle (*Lingkaran Biru*) as the brand image for products and services provided by urban, private sector doctors and midwives, then expanded it to cover a national range of products and services available everywhere (Mize & Robey, 2006; Piotrow et al., 1997). Eventually, the Blue Circle logo appeared in many forms: with the letters KB (*Keluarga Berencana* or FP); as signs indicating hospitals, clinics, pharmacies, and other facilities where contraceptives and services were available; on contraceptive product packaging; on posters, billboards, and televised PSAs promoting providers who offered value-added Blue Circle services; on car wheel covers; and as decoration on village gates to indicate the community's support for families choosing to practice FP. Even old automobile tires were painted blue and mounted on fence posts lining country roads. Almost non-stop national and local campaigns over more than 20 years, many of them featuring the Blue Circle, contributed to a rapid increase in contraceptive use from 23% of married women in 1977 to 58% in 2012 and a drop in the total fertility rate (TFR) from 5.6 to 2.6 average number of births in a woman's lifetime during the same period (BPS & ICF International, 2013). By the late 1990s, FP and small family size had become so engrained that even the economic crisis and political instability that Indonesia and much of Asia suffered from 1998 to 2002 had little effect on contraceptive use rates, even though commodities became more expensive and harder to obtain (Frankenberg et al., 2003; Storey & Schoemaker, 2006). It is important to note that social marketing's role was complemented and reinforced by other societal changes.

Consumer-driven approaches: Consumer-driven approaches aim at building demand for the product so that maintaining behavioral momentum shifts from the marketing organization to consumers. The Indonesian Blue Circle program illustrates this principle: during the economic crisis, markets responded to sustained demand for contraception, and people sought new sources of contraceptive supplies to continue protecting themselves from unwanted pregnancy. One strategy for achieving and sustaining consumer demand is to target social norms (Burchell et al., 2013). This approach is based on the theory that much behavior is influenced by perceptions about what is "typical" or socially acceptable and the perceived sanctions or rewards that result from deviating from or complying with those norms (Cislaghi & Heise, 2018; Yanovitsky & Rimal, 2006). Evoking thoughts of important reference groups or significant others (Ajzen, 1991), sometimes in a more general sense ("other teens your age") and sometimes in a very personalized way through group activities within peer networks can bring norms into focus and encourage compliance with them (see Chapter 11 on Social Networks).

Unfortunately, the misperception of norms is common. The perceived frequency of behavior (descriptive norm) is likely to be either underestimated when behaviors are less publicly visible, sensitive, taboo, or illegal (e.g. teenage sex or drug use) or overestimated for highly publicized behaviors (e.g., binge drinking in college campuses). But social-norms marketing can be used to inform people about the *actual* frequency of positive behaviors within groups they care about to create salient social pressure (injunctive norms), shift perceptions of relatively rare but dramatically visible negative behaviors, or introduce and promote new norms by spreading images of it in the mass media (Kincaid, 2004).

Market-driven approaches. An extension of consumer (or demand) driven approaches are market-driven ones that are positioned in relation to economic, commercial, or socio-structural forces. For example, a market-driven approach to responsible drinking must position its product (e.g., alcohol-free social interaction, or observing a "dry" January) as normative or as an attractive alternative to the commercial (e.g., seasonal) competition.

Sometimes, to counter unhealthy practices, a new brand can be introduced that reframes an old or customary behavior in a new way. For example, the *Saleema* campaign in Sudan (Evans et al., 2019; Johnson et al., 2018) aimed to encourage the abandonment of female genital mutilation (FGM), a widespread traditional practice reinforced by a variety of social and religious normative beliefs. The campaign created the character of Saleema, a young girl whose parents decided to abandon the practice of FGM because she was already "perfect, as God created her." Saleema dressed in bright colors (red, yellow, orange, and green) and clothing using those colors were featured in campaign materials including posters, television spots, and banners. People were encouraged to wear those colors as a way of expressing their support for abandonment and as a way of honoring God's work.

The Role of Theory and Research in Social Marketing

Social marketing is a strategic approach to social and behavior change that draws on behavioral theories to develop strategies and execute change.

The Use of Theory. Many of the health behavior theories discussed throughout this book can guide the planning and evaluation of social marketing programs. Some theories operate primarily at an individual level, while others focus more on interpersonal, group, or even structural levels. Key ideas and applications of four key theories often used in social marketing research and design are summarized in Table 21.1.

Theories offer insights into determinants of behavior which can be confirmed through formative research and published literature. For example, according to Diffusion of Innovations Theory (see Chapter 16), the adoption of a new behavior is more rapid if it (1) is perceived to have a *relative advantage* over current behavior, (2) is *compatible* with one's daily routine, priorities, and values, (3) seems *relatively easy* to adopt or practice, (4) can be *tried without great risk* before committing to it, and (5) can be *observed in action* to see what outcomes others experience before trying it oneself (Rogers, 2003). By examining the perceived characteristics of a product among potential consumers, marketers can design a message strategy to reinforce positive perceptions and change negative perceptions to increase the likelihood of acceptance and adoption.

Social marketers also use theories to segment audiences in meaningful ways. For example, the Extended Parallel Processing Model (EPPM) and its close relative, the Risk Perception Attitude Framework (elements of which appear in the Integrated Behavioral Model—see Chapter 6), describe the interaction between perceived threat and perceived efficacy, which influence information seeking or avoidance (Rimal & Real, 2003), and behavioral decision-making

Table 21.1 Applications of Major Theories and Research in Social Marketing

Theoretical framework	Applications of Framework		
	Identify Motives for Action	**Identify Message Strategies**	**Identify Target Audiences**
Extended Parallel Processing Model (EPPM) (Witte, 1994)	• To what extent is the health issue thought to pose a serious and personal threat (costs of inaction)? • To what extent are proposed actions perceived to be effective (response efficacy or benefit of action)? • How do people perceive their ability to enact the behavior (personal efficacy)?	• Create messages that increase understanding of the threat and explain or demonstrate how responses can effectively reduce the threat • Create messages that explain how to achieve the recommended response • Explain how to overcome barriers to recommended response	• Segment audiences into categories representing levels of perceived threat and efficacy
Reasoned Action/ Planned Behavior (Ajzen, 1991)	• What are the advantages (benefits) and disadvantages (costs), both personal and social, of a health behavior?	• Change beliefs about and evaluations of consequences (costs and benefits) of action • Change perceptions of subjective norms • Change motivations to comply with subjective norms	• Define primary audiences (those who would benefit from attitude change) • Define secondary audiences (significant others of those to be influenced)
Social Cognitive Theory (Bandura, 1986, 1997)	• What perceived personal and social incentives or reinforcements (benefits) affect learning and action? • What perceived personal and social barriers (costs) affect learning and action?	• Provide models of effective action that are appealing and compelling • Encourage rehearsal and trial of the behavior • Provide feedback and reinforcement for behavioral attempts • Provide incentives for performance of the proposed behavior	• Define primary audiences (those who would benefit from attitude change) • Define secondary audiences (potential role models and advocates)
Diffusion of Innovations (Rogers, 2003)	• How do members of the audience perceive the behavioral innovation? • What relative advantage (benefits) does it offer? • How complex or risky is it (costs)? • Can consequences (costs and benefits) of the behavior be observed? • Is the behavior compatible with current practices (costs)? • What social influences or networks exist in the environment that encourage or discourage the action (social costs and benefits)?	• Show and explain the benefits of the proposed action • Explain how to do it in simple terms • Show how new behavior fits with or grows out of current practices • Encourage those who already practice the behavior to advocate it to others	• Segment audience according to perceptions of the behavior • Target people who are key network members (opinion leaders)

(Witte, 1994). Splitting both the threat and efficacy dimensions into low and high categories can create a 2 × 2 typology of audience segments.

Various stage theories of behavior change, such as the Transtheoretical Model (Prochaska & DiClemente, 1992) (see Chapter 7), also can be used to identify segments of the overall audience who may be at different stages of change and to tailor messages accordingly: some are barely aware of a health issue and need to be alerted to it, while others are knowledgeable and capable of responding but lack motivation to act or to sustain healthy behavior over time.

Uses of Research. Research plays a role across all stages of health programs from design through implementation and evaluation (see also Chapter 19 on theory-based planning models). Because consumer decision-making and behavior are complex and situational, systematic research into the conditions and dynamics of targeted behaviors helps validate program planning decisions, increases the likelihood that programs will succeed and makes it possible to attribute change to specific aspects of the strategy.

During the design phase of a program, social-behavioral research helps planners determine the prevalence of the problem overall and among specific subaudiences; select audiences to target in order to achieve maximum individual and societal benefit; identify the unique communication needs, media habits, and preferences of the different audience segments; catalog the social, cultural, and structural/environmental factors that positively or negatively influence behavior and that may be amenable to change; and identify sources of personal influence over the behavior of audience members. Organizational research and environmental scans help identify organizations or social institutions that influence the intended audiences and might be engaged as partners to support the program and available resources. Concept testing and message pretesting are essential research steps in the design process that help planners explore and determine an optimum marketing mix and craft compelling messages.

During the implementation phase, monitoring or process evaluation provides answers to such questions as: Is the program being implemented as designed? Are activities and materials reaching the intended audience? Is the timing of activities and message distribution going as planned? Is the program beginning to have an impact? Does the program need adjustment and fine-tuning at mid-course? Sometimes, programs can take advantage of existing data collection systems or activities such as media reach data, health services statistics, and web analytics.

Finally, during the evaluation phase of the program, population-based social-behavioral and cost-effectiveness research helps determine how well a program met its objectives. It can explain why a program is effective (or not), including the effects of different activities or messages on different audience segments, determine the magnitude of change, and demonstrate what aspects of the program contributed to those changes. It can measure the cost of achieving specific outcomes or impacts and indicate which parts of the program should be continued or strengthened.

As an example of how compelling good research can be in the practice of social marketing, consider the concept of return on investment (ROI), or what a program can expect to gain for the resources expended to promote a product or behavior. Naturally, marketers wish to gain more than they spend, or at least to break even. In commercial settings the monetary cost of producing, promoting, and distributing a product or service must be more than offset by what consumers pay in exchange for it. Social marketing campaigns often are obliged to serve all audience members in need, not just those in a position to pay for a product, so they may offer products for free or at subsidized prices to increase social benefits. The social marketing organization and its donors may tolerate a financial loss (cost of commodities and distribution) if the social benefits to society (for example, lower birth rates or fewer HIV infections) are judged to offset those costs. However, those social benefits are rarely quantified in monetary terms. Increasingly, members of the donor community (USAID and the Bill and Melinda Gates Foundation, for example) are trying to get a better handle on how to calculate ROI.

Several studies have illustrated how to do this through cost-effectiveness analysis of HIV prevention communication campaigns in South Africa. Kincaid and Parker (2008) used data from a population-based survey that measured program exposure, preventive behaviors, and seroprevalence/HIV status to estimate that 701,495 HIV infections were *prevented* between 2000 and 2005 due to an increase in protective behaviors attributable to the campaign. Extrapolating from the average $8,000 lifetime cost of providing government subsidized anti-retroviral therapy to HIV-positive patients, they calculated that the $2.3 million national campaign would save the South African government $5.6 billion in health care costs over 20 years. A similar analysis estimated a $1.1 billion savings resulting from 132,066 infections averted due to condom use at first sex among youth (Kincaid et al., 2014). These are powerful arguments for investment in preventive health campaigns.

International Social Marketing Applications

In this section, we profile two health communication programs from a social marketing perspective: the TRANSFORM project in Kenya supporting communities to adopt behaviors and access products and services to improve health, livelihood, and overall wellbeing, and the Improving Contraceptive Method Mix (ICMM) project in Indonesia, which sought to expand the range of available contraceptive methods and increase the use of longer-acting methods for couples who wanted no more children or wanted to space their next birth for longer periods of time. We describe how each program reflects the four main principles of social marketing (focusing on behavior, benefiting consumers, maintaining a market perspective, and using audience segmentation) as well as how each used theory and research to guide decision-making.

Case Study #1: Kenya TRANSFORM Project (2018–2020)

Intervention Background

TRANSFORM (Transform, 2021) is a multi-country, joint partnership between Unilever, the United Kingdom's Foreign Commonwealth Development Office (FCDO), and EY (Ernst & Young Global Limited) established in 2015. This project uses a transformative marketing approach to increase the scale and sustainability of health behavior change related to nutrition, hygiene, and sanitation by expanding and strengthening market-based, social-enterprise initiatives, particularly those using digital strategies, and increasing access to quality products and services in low-and-middle-income countries in sub-Saharan Africa and South Asia. Social enterprises are businesses with societal and/or environmental objectives (Barone & Estevez, 2020).

In Kenya, TRANSFORM involves a digitally-based collaboration between public-sector donors and community-based, private-sector businesses that sell health products, but typically do not think of themselves as health promoters or educators. *UJoin*, a cellphone-friendly online platform, was designed to support small business *(duka)* owners—micro-retailers—in informal settlements of Nairobi (UJoin, 2020). *Duka* owners who chose to participate in *UJoin* could access business and financial courses, obtain online mentoring, take advantage of networking opportunities, and access health and product information related to products they stock (Cassanitti, 2020). *UJoin* also encouraged and supported *duka* owners to become a new category of public health educators for their customers.

Duka owners serve marginalized, low-income communities that often have less access to health information (see Chapter 17) and more constrained access to commercial resources than other community members. They are trusted community members and have longstanding relationships with their customers (Kimani et al., 2012). There are about 166,796 *duka* owners in Kenya (Mwiti, 2018), but 90% of them have no formal training in business operations, entrepreneurship (TechnoServ, 2020), or sales accounting (Waweru, 2018). Yet, 95% of Kenya consumers patronize *dukas* at one time or another, often for products related to critical health issues such as nutrition, hygiene, and sanitation. Helping *duka* owners become health advocates and health promoters helps strengthen their own business development and relationships with their consumer base.

To use *UJoin* digital technologies effectively, it was necessary to tailor strategies based on how *duka* owners vary in their attitudes and practices related to online resources. But prior to TRANSFORM, little was known about how *duka* owners perceived their potential role in health promotion, and how much interaction and communication they already had with customers about the health benefits of the commodities they sold. So, data were collected between 2019 and 2020 to understand the use of *UJoin* and its impact on *duka* operations and to refine the digital strategy. Although content on the *UJoin* platform ultimately reaches and benefits *duka* customers, this formative research focused primarily on *duka* owners themselves as an audience and as a networked community whose changes in behavior could transform the whole marketing system in Nairobi.

How TRANSFORM Reflects the Social Marketing Framework

Focus on behavior. Duka owners were encouraged to: (1) access and use *UJoin* to learn new technical business skills and network with each other; (2) discuss health information and health promotion with their peers; and (3) share health information and promote healthy behavior among their customers.

Focus on consumer benefit. UJoin was positioned to provide numerous benefits that could improve business performance of *duka* owners, including increased knowledge of health issues, health behaviors, and health products their shop addressed and strengthened entrepreneurial skills on such topics as accounting, sales, and customer relations. They also increased their ability to benefit consumers by sharing information with other *duka* owners, connecting with the mainstream health industry and thus gaining self-confidence as independent business owners.

Maintaining a market perspective. TRANSFORM identified unique features of health marketing ecosystem in Nairobi. For example, it recognized the underappreciated role and capacity of *duka* owners as frontline service providers and focused on them as an audience and key actors in a structural intervention, and tailored messaging to their situations. The program also sought to strengthen the entire health marketing infrastructure by improving access among the urban poor, an underserved but important consumer base.

Audience segmentation. Kenya TRANSFORM identified three distinct subgroups of *duka* owners requiring tailored message strategies:

• Endorsers. These *duka* owners were more likely to believe that use of *UJoin* was a norm in the *duka* community, they enjoyed discussing business with and learning from other *duka* owners, and they were confident they could discuss health issues with customers. Therefore, messaging for them encouraged networking with other *duka* owners, particularly about the use of *UJoin*.

- Skeptics, These *duka* owners believed that *UJoin* was supported by other *duka* owners but were less knowledgeable about it and the resources it provided and lacked confidence in their ability to communicate with customers about health-related matters. Therefore, messaging for them emphasized success stories from other *duka* owners about the use of *UJoin* and tips for communicating with customers to increase their business.

- Unengaged. While these *duka* owners appreciated *UJoin*, they were less likely to perceive participation as a norm among their peers. Nevertheless, they had generally positive attitudes toward business-related websites. Therefore, messaging for them emphasized the resources available through *UJoin* and encouragement to network with other *duka* owners, particularly Endorsers.

Use of Theory and Research

TRANSFORM supported quantitative research during the project design phase to understand *duka* owners' roles in providing health services and products in marginalized communities of Nairobi, and their use of digital to increase their entrepreneurial capacity. A survey collected data from over 800 male and female *duka* owners and the data were subjected to latent class analysis to identify the distinct audience segments described above (Kumoji et al., 2022). The survey also examined key theoretical constructs related to the intended behavior changes among *duka* owners.

Theoretical constructs from the Diffusion of Innovations framework were used to identify motivations to adopt *UJoin*; Social Learning Theory helped identify perceived self-efficacy and role modeling as keys to *duka* owner participation in *UJoin*; and the Theory of Reasoned Action was used to identify outcome expectancies and perceived community and business norms. Survey findings about perceived subjective norms and community support for use of *UJoin* among members of the *duka* community helped inform recommendations for how to encourage more uptake and use of *UJoin* resources.

In summary, The TRANSFORM project in Kenya and its use of the innovative online collaborative platform *UJoin*, illustrates a focused social marketing strategy that prioritized strengthening a relatively neglected segment of the health-services market, namely low-income urban communities in Nairobi and the micro-retailers that serve them. It provided new benefits to a particular class of social marketing actors—*duka* owners—bringing them closer to mainstream marketing resources, information, and services. It systematically studied and analyzed that population to identify important subgroups within it that had different needs for information and support and then tailored messaging to those different subgroups. And it drew inspiration from core theories of communication and behavior change to inform its research design, measured concepts, and strategies.

Case Study #2: Improving Contraceptive Method Mix in Indonesia (ICMM)

Intervention Background

The ICMM (2017) Project in Indonesia (2012–2016) was a transformative social marketing project aimed at improving informed choice of contraceptive methods among FP clients by altering existing health service policies and processes, budgeting and management, and improving capacity for and effectiveness of health communication and health promotion activities at regional and local levels in private and public sectors. A key priority of the project was to shift market emphasis on the use of short-term contraceptive methods (oral pills and injectable contraceptives) to address client demand for more diverse options, especially longer-term methods (IUDs and contraceptive implants) for clients who wanted to delay pregnancy for periods longer than one year.

ICMM was funded by the US Agency for International Development (USAID) and the Australian Department of Foreign Affairs and Trade (DFAT) and led by the Indonesia office of the Johns Hopkins Center for Communication Programs (CCP), the Directorate of Family Health at the Indonesian Ministry of Health (MOH), and the National Family Planning Coordination Board (BKKBN). ICMM was conducted in three districts in East Java province and three districts in West Nusa Tenggara province as demonstration sites.

In a mature national family planning program like Indonesia's, where contraceptive use is already relatively high, the emphasis tends to shift from increasing contraception in general to minimizing unintended pregnancies through consistent, effective use of contraceptives. Beginning in the early 2000s during the Asian economic crisis and a subsequent decentralization of most major government agencies and services, the mix of methods available and widely used in Indonesia changed. The overall rate of modern contraceptive use between 2012 and 2017 was about 57–58% of married women aged 15–49 (BPS & ORC Macro, 2017). But those women often had difficulty accessing a wide range of methods and finding the method they wanted. Although Indonesian couples are more likely to want to limit births rather than space them, most women use short-acting methods, primarily injectable contraceptives that must be administered every one to three months, depending on the type. Long-acting and reversible methods (LARCs) such as IUDs and hormonal implants are often not widely available. This lack of method choice often results in dissatisfaction with and discontinuation of a method or inconsistent or intermittent use of a method that increases the odds of unintended pregnancy. Meanwhile, the decentralization of government responsibility from the national to the provincial (state) level resulted in uneven institutional support for FP services especially at the district and village level because not all localities prioritized them equally.

ICMM was designed to transform the market for contraceptives by affecting upstream conditions: improving the supply chain of commodities (especially for LARCs), advocating for increased local prioritization of FP budgets and staffing, improving knowledge management in service delivery, increasing demand for longer-term methods, and improving the effectiveness of FP communication to increase the downstream range of options couples have and to help them choose and access contraceptives that best match their fertility intentions. This required a focus not just on the primary audience of FP clients, but on secondary audiences that could improve the enabling environment and facilitate clients' informed method choice.

How ICMM Reflects the Social Marketing Framework

Within the historical context of Indonesian social marketing of FP described above, some ways the ICMM approach reflected core principles of social marketing are summarized in Table 21.2. Specific behaviors were identified for both primary and secondary audiences, and specific benefits were identified for each of those audiences and prioritized actions that would inform motivational messaging. A marketing perspective was reflected in the use of an integrated whole-market approach that recognized multiple levels within the existing infrastructure, and audience segments were differentiated to allow targeted resource allocation, strategic focus, and messaging.

In addition to the core principles described in Table 21.2, ICMM used sophisticated theoretical frameworks and multiple complementary research and evaluation methods including: (1) behavioral modeling based on ideational (psychosocial) factors; (2) a pre-post evaluation design with treatment and comparison districts; (3) creation and monitoring of local working group activities in 1,400 villages; (4) documentary review and interviews with district and local officials about changes in policy, regulations, planning, and budgeting processes over the course of the project; (5) documentation of changes in budget allocations for district level and local FP program activities (staffing, communication materials production, health worker training, and outreach); (6) monitoring of commodity availability and supply chain improvements; and (7) use of a representative sample survey of over 26,000 married women of reproductive age in treatment and comparison districts to assess the effects of program exposure on ideational variables, changes in availability of preferred FP methods, and contraceptive method adoption decisions.

This integrated research and evaluation design produced compelling evidence of change in most of the major outcome variables and structural changes in the market associated with exposure to intervention activities and messaging (ICMM, 2017).

Overall, the ICMM project demonstrates the power of a full-market approach designed to address individual customer knowledge, attitudes, and behaviors, as well as the enabling political, structural, and funding environment that makes positive consumer behavior more likely. It illustrates how important building coalitions and partnerships can be in mobilizing resources and empowering communities to participate in their own pursuit of new opportunities and health improvement. Finally, it illustrates, like the TRANSFORM project in Kenya, the value of drawing on theoretical frameworks to guide research planning both before and after a project, to use data to inform strategic thinking and messaging, and then to carefully measure the effects of the intervention to learn from the experience, communicate that experience to donors and project partners, and plan for the future.

Table 21.2   Core Social Marketing Principles Reflected in the ICMM Project

Focus on Behavior	Actions Encouraged
Family Planning Clients	• Select and correctly use a contraceptive method consistent with fertility intentions (shorter-term methods or long-acting reversible methods) • Discuss appropriate method choice with health workers/midwives during service visits or outreach contact • Switch to long term methods whenever appropriate
Health Professionals	• Help clients make more informed method choices consistent with personal fertility intentions
Government Leaders	• Increase advocacy for improved contraceptive method mix • Become more client-oriented by prioritizing client needs • Increase advocacy for annual work plans, larger budgets, and improved supply chain management and monitoring and knowledge management among service providers.
Community Leaders	• Draft and secure approval for the necessary decrees and authorization documents that would allow local control over budgeting • Increase budgets and allocation of village development funds for family planning services and supplies

Focus on Consumer Benefit	Benefits Emphasized
Family Planning Clients	• Greater contraceptive security in terms of commodity supply • Increased satisfaction with the family planning method chosen • Reduced risk of unintended pregnancy
Health Professionals	• More political and material support for day-to-day family planning activities • Better access to information and commodities • Greater self-efficacy and job satisfaction
Regional and Local Civil Leaders	• Strengthened relationships and coordination throughout the health services bureaucracy • Increased access to funding and control over those resources • Stronger program coordination and access to resources • Improved status among constituents and community members who experience local program success
National Leaders in the MOH and BKKBN	• Opportunity to develop and test a new decentralized model of family planning social marketing with potential for national scale-up

Maintaining a Market Perspective	Aspects of an Integrated Whole-Market Approach
	• Working with national and regional policy and regulatory structures • Addressing commodity supply, chain-management systems, and knowledge management • Strengthening regional- and district-level service delivery staffing and processes • Increasing civil society (NGO) capacity for and involvement in healthcare delivery • Mobilizing local media and communication resources to promote informed method choices tailored to audience segments • Development of a comprehensive Advocacy Framework (see Figure 21.1) • Build commitment across multiple levels, stakeholder groups, and sectors (education, labor, health, women's empowerment, human resources) • Developing annual advocacy work plans, and implementing, evaluating, and refining the plans for the next annual cycle

Audience Segmentation	Segments Prioritized

	• Married couples
	  ○ Short-term spacers
	  ○ Long-term spacers
	• Health professionals
	• Government leaders (national, regional, and local)
	• Civic/community leaders (including faith groups, professional associations, and NGOs)

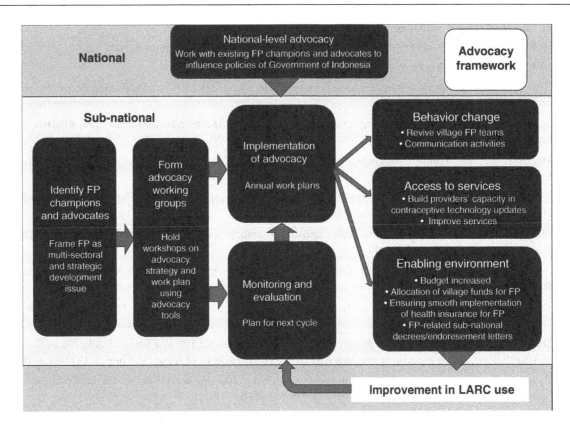

Figure 21.1 ICMM Family Planning (FP) Advocacy Framework
(*Source:* Adapted from ICMM, 2017)/Johns Hopkins University

Summary

This chapter has introduced the core principles and some examples of social marketing to improve health behavior and health outcomes. Social marketing is not—any more than other approaches described in this book—a panacea for overcoming public health challenges. Nevertheless, in its systematic approach to understanding audience characteristics and the market structure surrounding behavioral decisions, social marketing offers powerful guidelines for communication planning.

Social marketing draws attention to factors beyond the individual level toward ways that communication can affect—even transform—social conditions through policy change (think of fluoridation of water, iodization of salt, automotive safety regulations), legislation (such as mandatory seat belt use and bans against use of mobile phones while driving) and normative change (reduced HIV/AIDS stigma, abandonment of FGM), thereby facilitating the voluntary uptake of beneficial health behaviors. Even so, social marketing strategies necessarily work backward from the existing needs and conditions of consumers' lives to identify and reduce barriers and create structures that facilitate beneficial behavior. In both commercial and social marketing, it is sometimes necessary to build or create value, but in social marketing it is always important to identify and fulfill demand. Creating appealing messages about the product is important, but this must be done together with considerations of the cost-benefit ratio, where the exchange is likely to take place, what forces compete against the product for attention and resources, and how the entire social ecology of decision-making affects health choices and sustained health outcomes.

References

Ajzen, I. (1991). The theory of planned behavior. *Organizational Behavior and Human Decision Processes, 50*(2), 179–211.

Andreasen A. (1994). Social marketing: Definition and domain. *Journal of Public Policy & Marketing, 13*(1), 108–114.

Andreasen, A. (2006). *Social marketing in the 21st century.* Thousand Oaks, CA: Sage.

Bagozzi, R. P. (1974). Marketing as an organized behavioral system of exchange. *Journal of Marketing, 38*(4), 77–81.

Bagozzi, R. P. (1978), Marketing as exchange. *American Behavioral Scientist, 21*(4), 535–556.

Bandura, A. (1986). *Social foundations of thought and action: A social cognitive theory.* Prentice-Hall, Inc.

Bandura, A. (1997). *Self-efficacy: The exercise of control.* New York: W.H. Freeman.

Barone, A., & Estevez, E. (2020). *Business essentials: Social enterprise.* Investopedia. DOtdash Publishing. https://www.investopedia.com/terms/s/social-enterprise.asp

BPS & ICF International. (2013). *Indonesian demographic and health survey 2012.* Jakarta, Indonesia: BPS, BKKBN, Kemenkes, and ICF International.

BPS & ORC Macro. (2017). *Indonesian demographic and health survey.* Calverton, MD; Ministry of Health [Indonesia]: Macro International.

Burchell, K., Rettie, R., & Patel, K. (2013). Marketing social norms: Social marketing and the "social norm approach". *Journal of Consumer Behaviour, 12,* 1–9. https://doi.org/10.1002/cb.1395

Cassaniti, J. (2020). Influence networks relating to health knowledge among Nairobi's micro-retailers and their clients. *Electronic Journal of Knowledge Management, 18*(3), 302–324.

Cislaghi, B., & Heise, L. (2018). Theory and practice of social norms interventions: Eight common pitfalls. *Globalization and Health, 14*(1), 1–10.

Evans, W. E., Rath, J. M., Hair, E. C., Snider, J. W., Pitzer, L., Greenberg, M., Xiao, H., Cantrell, J., & Vallone, D. (2018). Effects of the truth FinishIt brand on tobacco outcomes. *Preventive Medicine Reports, 9,* 6–11. https://doi.org/10.1016/j.pmedr.2017.11.008

Evans, W. D., Donahue, C., Snider, J., Bedri, N., Elhussein, T. A., & Elamin, S. A. (2019). The Saleema initiative in Sudan to abandon female genital mutilation: Outcomes and dose response effects. *PLoS One, 14*(3), 1–14. https://doi.org/10.1371/journal.pone.0213380

Frankenberg, E., Sikoki, B., & Suriastini, W. (2003). Contraceptive use in a changing service environment: Evidence from Indonesia during the economic crisis. *Studies in Family Planning, 34*(2), 103–116.

Harvey, P. D. (1999). *Let every child be wanted: How social marketing in revolutionizing contraceptive use around the world.* Westport, CT: Auburn House.

ICMM (Improving Contraceptive Method Mix). (2017). Improving contraceptive method mix in East Java and West Nusa Tenggara, Indonesia. Final report: ICMM Associate Award, January 5, 2017. Baltimore, MD, Johns Hopkins Center for Communication Programs. https://drive.google.com/file/d/10qNrXnUwqrxZ0s1hIJ4mViPtVUSeuwtD/view

Johnson, A. C., Evans, W. D., Barrett, N., Badri, H., Abdalla, T., & Donahue, C. (2018). Qualitative evaluation of the Saleema campaign to eliminate female genital mutilation and cutting in Sudan. *Reproductive Health, 15*(1), 1–8. https://doi.org/10.1186/s12978-018-0470-2

Kimani, S. W., Kagira, E. K., Kendi, L., & Wawire, C. M. (2012). Shoppers perception of retail service quality: Supermarkets versus small convenience shops (Dukas) in Kenya. *Journal of Management and Strategy, 3*(1), 55. https://doi.org/10.5430/jms.v3n1p55. http://citeseerx.ist.psu.edu/viewdoc/download?doi=10.1.1.825

Kincaid, D. L. (2004). From innovation to social norm: Bounded normative influence. *Journal of Health Communication, 9*(1), 37–57.

Kincaid, D. L., & Parker, W. (2008). *National AIDS communication programs, HIV prevention behavior and HIV infections averted in South Africa, 2005.* Pretoria, South Africa. Johns Hopkins Health and Education in South Africa.

Kincaid, D. L., Babalola, S., & Figueroa, M.E. (2014). HIV communication programs, condom use at sexual debut, and HIV infections averted in South Africa, 2005. *Journal of Acquired Immune Deficiency Syndromes, 66*(3), S278–S284.

Kotler, P., & Levy, S.J. (1969). Broadening the concept of marketing. *Journal of Marketing, 33,* 10–15

Kotler, P. & Roberto, N. L. (1989). *Social marketing: Strategies for changing public behavior.* New York: Free Press.

Kotler, P., & Zaltman, G. (1971). Social marketing: An approach to planned social change. *Journal of Marketing, 35,* 3–12.

Kumoji, E., Oyenubi, O., Rhoades, A., Cassaniti, J., Rariewa, F., & Ohkubo, S. (2022). Understanding the audience for a digital capacity-building platform for micro-retailers in Nairobi, Kenya: A latent class segmentation analysis. *Social Marketing Quarterly, 28*(2): 147–268.

Lefebvre, R.C. (2012). Transformative social marketing: Co-creating the social marketing discipline and brand. *Journal of Social Marketing, 2*(2): 118–129.

Mize, L., & Robey, B. (2006). *A 35 Year commitment to family planning in Indonesia: BKKBN and USAID's Historic Partnership.* Baltimore, MD: Johns Hopkins Bloomberg School of Public Health/Center for Communication Programs.

Mwiti, L. (2018). *Family-owned dukas suffer major losses, closures in 2017.* The Standard. https://www.standardmedia.co.ke/financial-standard/article/2001290114/family-owned-dukas-suffer-major-lossesclosures-in-2017/

Noar, S. M., & Harrington, N. G. (2016). Tailored communications for health-related decision-making and behavior change. In M. A. Diefenbach, S. Miller-Halegoua, & D. J. Bowen (Eds.), *Handbook of health decision science* (pp. 251–263). New York, NY: Springer.

Piotrow, P. T., Kincaid, D. L., Rimon, J. G., & Rinehart, W. (1997). *Health communication: Lessons from family planning and reproductive health.* Westport, CT: Praeger.

Pollock, J. C., & Storey, J. D. (2012). Comparing health communication. In F. Esser, & T. Hanitzsch (Eds.), *Handbook of comparative communication research* (pp. 161–182). New York: Taylor & Francis.

Prochaska, J., & DiClemente, C. (1992). The transtheoretical approach. In J.C. Norcross, & M.R. Goldfield (Eds.), *Handbook of psychotherapy integration* (pp. 300–334). New York: Basic Books.

Rimal R., & Real, K. (2003). Perceived risk and efficacy beliefs as motivators of change: Use of the risk perception attitude (RPA) framework to understand health behaviors. *Human Communication Research, 29,* 370–399.

Rogers, E. M. (2003). *Diffusion of innovations* (5th ed.). New York: Free Press.

Rogers, E., & Storey, J. D. (1987). Communication campaigns. In C. Berger & S. Chaffee (Eds.), *Handbook of Communication Science* (pp. 814–846). Thousand Oaks, CA, Sage.

Storey, J.D., & Schoemaker, J. (2006). *Communication, normative influence and the sustainability of health behavior over time: A multilevel analysis of contraceptive use in Indonesia, 1997–2003* [Paper presentation]. Annual Conference of the International Communication Association, Dresden, Germany.

Storey, J. D., Figueroa, M. E., & Kincaid, D. L. (2005). *Health competence communication: A systems approach to sustainable preventive health. Technical report.* Baltimore, MD: Johns Hopkins Bloomberg School of Public Health/Center for Communication Programs.

TechnoServ (2020). Transforming communities through micro-retailers. https://www.technoserve.org/blog/smart-fixes-for-smart-shops-transforming-communities-through-micro-retailer/

Transform (2021). About transform. https://www.transform.global/Intro.aspx/

UJoin (2020). UJoin. *Every1mobile.* https://www.every1mobile.com/our-work/ujoin/

United Nations. (2023). *Sustainable Development Goals.* United Nations Department of Economic and Social Affairs (UNDESA), Division for Sustainable Development Goals (DSDG). New York: United Nations. https://sdgs.un.org/goals. Accessed 2 February 2023.

USAID (United States Agency for International Development). (2001). *Draft concept paper: Communication activity approval document.* Washington, DC: United States Agency for International Development, Office of Population and Reproductive Health.

Warner, L. A. (2019). Using homeowners' association membership to define audience segments for targeted local social marketing interventions: Implications from a statewide study. *Social Marketing Quarterly, 25*(4), 291–307.

Waweru, A. (2018). *Success on every corner: How mom-and-pop shops can drive growth in Africa.* TechnoServe: Business Fights Poverty. https://businessfightspoverty.org/articles/success-on-everycorner-how-mom-and-pop-shops-can-drive-growth-in-africa/

Witte, K. (1994). Fear control and danger control: A test of the Extended Parallel Processing Model (EPPM). *Communication Monographs, 61,* 113–134.

Wonneberger, A., Meijers, M. H. C., & Schuck, A. R. T. (2020). Shifting public engagement: How media coverage of climate change conferences affects climate change audience segments. *Public Understanding of Science, 29*(2), 176–193. https://doi.org/10.1177/096366251988647410.1177/1524500419882978

Yanovitsky, L., & Rimal, R. N. (2006). Communication and normative influence: An introduction to the special issue. *Communication Theory, 16*(1), 1–6.

CHAPTER 22

SOCIAL MEDIA AND HEALTH

Mesfin A. Bekalu
K. Viswanath

KEY POINTS

This chapter will:

- Propose an overarching definition of social media and discuss challenges in conceptualizing, defining, and measuring social media use related to health.

- Discuss evidence for associations between social media use, health behaviors, and health.

- Review and provide examples of interventions that use social media to improve health and health behavior.

Vignette

Mary is 45, working for a marketing company, busy with her career, raising a family, and taking care of her parents. She is active in her community and volunteers her time at her children's school with little time for herself. In her last routine mammogram, a growth was found in her breast, and she was diagnosed with early-stage breast cancer. Suddenly she had multiple decisions to make about which medical procedures to undergo. And the decision making would be made under stressful conditions, including a lack of time and information. She had a great medical team and outstanding support from her colleagues, family, and friends. Still, she wanted information from others with similar experiences. She joined a social media group for women with breast cancer. Initially, she just followed others and learned from them. Over time, however, she became active—posting questions and seeking answers—and she was gratified to hear from others who were going through similar experiences. Her social media "friends" helped her through emotional ups and downs, giving her tips, ideas, and support. Mary found the group so helpful that she began sharing her own experience and offering support to others. Being part of the group helped her navigate one of the most frightening experiences of her life. While there are many in-person support groups in her community, the social media group allowed her to seek and get support any time of the day or night from people all over the world. It helped her cope, navigate, and thrive despite her condition.

This chapter addresses the role of social media in health and health behavior, drawing on systematic reviews and recently published studies. We will discuss the literature on social media use and health under two broad categories. One focuses on social media use as a behavior and investigates how it affects health outcomes. A second category examines the role and effects of social media platforms and networks as channels for health interventions.

Health Behavior: Theory, Research, and Practice, Sixth Edition. Edited by Karen Glanz, Barbara K. Rimer, and K. Viswanath.
© 2024 John Wiley & Sons, Inc. Published 2024 by John Wiley & Sons, Inc.
Companion website: www.wiley.com/go/glanz/healthbehavior6e

Introduction

There are many definitions of "social media." Key elements of definitions include one or more of these features of different social media platforms: (1) interactions, communications, and conversations among family or friends or members of aligned affinity or geographic communities; (2) curation and sharing content; (3) expression of opinions; and/or (4) shopping. Table 22.1 describes the main categories of social media, a definition of each category, and examples of platforms in each category.

Why are Social Media Important?

There are three main reasons why social media are important and relevant to public health issues and health behavior. First, the penetration of social media is broad and deep. There are more than 4.7 billion social media users worldwide, and the average social media user visits or uses 7.4 different social media platforms every month (DataReportal, 2023). Social media use has become an important digital activity in the lives of people across age groups and geographies. Second, as face-to-face social interactions have diminished across societies, social media networks complement and, in some cases, substitute for decreasing face-to-face social interactions and may even affect health-related outcomes (Bekalu et al., 2021), though the empirical evidence is somewhat mixed (Rumas et al., 2021). During the COVID-19 pandemic, in-person interactions decreased, and social media use increased. In 2020, the average time US users spent on social media was 65 minutes daily, compared to 55 minutes in prior years (Tankovska, 2021). Third, social media are being used increasingly as tools and channels for health promotion and disease prevention interventions, such as in smoking cessation (Naslund et al., 2017), HIV and sexual health (Cao et al., 2017), cancer patient support, and physical activity and dietary behaviors (Goodyear et al., 2021; Günther et al., 2021).

How Users Engage with Social Media Platforms and Content

Users' engagement with social media platforms and content can be studied along three dimensions: user activity, communication partners, and content.

User Activity

Researchers have categorized users' activities into passive versus active use and examined the differential effects on health outcomes. Active use refers to the production and sharing of social media content (Verduyn et al., 2015, 2017).

Table 22.1   Broad Categories of Social Media

Social Media Category	Main Features and Functions	Examples
Social Networks	• Mainly used to connect with friends, family, professional colleagues, and brands • Provide platform for personal, human-to-human interactions	Facebook, Twitter, LinkedIn
Media Sharing Networks	• Used mainly for sharing images and videos	Instagram, Snapchat, YouTube
Discussion Forums	• Often used by communities and special interest groups to pose questions and share information about a variety of topics	Reddit, Quora, Digg
Bookmarking and Content Curation Networks	• Used for searching, sharing, and curating content and media	Pinterest, Flipboard
Consumer Review Networks	• Used for obtaining and sharing reviews of products and services	Yelp, Zomato, TripAdvisor
Blogging and Publishing Networks	• Enable users (mostly authors) to publish articles, opinions, or product reviews • Enable direct participation and interaction between readers and host blogger or other blog participants	WordPress, Tumblr, Medium
Social Shopping Networks	• Help users follow different brands, share interesting things, and make purchases • Enable businesses to create brand awareness, boost engagement, and sell products	Polyvore, Etsy, Fancy
Interest-Based Networks	• Enable users to connect with other people who have the same sorts of hobbies or interests	Goodreads, Houzz, Last.fm

Passive use refers to content consumption (e.g., browsing newsfeeds and one's own or others' profiles). Most studies of user engagement have examined the differential effects of users' passive versus active use of social media platforms. In a longitudinal study, for example, Frison and Eggermont found differential effects of Facebook use on adolescents' well-being depending on whether use was "active" or "passive" (Frison & Eggermont, 2020). In their study, active Facebook use (engaging in exchanges with other users) was associated with positive outcomes, but passive Facebook use (viewing others' posts and profiles without engaging in exchanges) sometimes resulted in less healthy strategies for coping with stress. Notably, although the active versus passive dichotomy has been studied to explain differential effects of social media use on coping and health, the validity of the dichotomy has been questioned. Users' engagement on social media might be captured more accurately on a continuum rather than as completely active or completely passive.

Uses and Gratifications Theory, which posits that media users are active agents who choose and use media to fulfill specific, personally salient needs (Katz et al., 1974), has often been used to describe social media use. The most common motives include seeking information, experiencing positive feelings, maintaining relationships, establishing new relationships, obtaining social recognition, building social connections, and expressing oneself (Pertegal et al., 2019). However, little research has examined the relationship between motives for social media use and health (Yang et al., 2021). The motives that have been associated with health outcomes include relationship formation, relationship maintenance, entertainment/passing time/fun, and escapism (Yang et al., 2021). Recent studies also have shown the role of fear of missing out (FOMO) as an important psychological drive for general and problematic use of social media (Balta et al., 2020; Beyens et al., 2016; Yang et al., 2021). For example, Beyens et al. (2016) showed that increased FOMO was associated with increased stress related to Facebook use.

Communication Partners

Social media interactions with close associates are generally related to positive psychosocial well-being (Burke & Kraut, 2016; Yang et al., 2021) while "friending," "following," or interacting with strangers sometimes are related to lower self-esteem and poorer social adjustment and life satisfaction among young adults in college (Eşkisu et al., 2017; Yang & Lee, 2020). One Instagram study found that people tended to compare themselves less favorably and reported more depressive symptoms when they followed a higher percentage of strangers (Lup et al., 2015). Another study (Lin & Utz, 2015) found that individuals experienced greater happiness after reviewing a positive post from a close friend. These findings should be taken as examples, not definitive findings, because of the variable design features and quality of the studies.

Content

Content of feeds and posts on social media is another dimension of engagement. For example, social media are often used to spread misinformation and disinformation. Health *misinformation* is defined as "any health-related claim of fact that is false, based on current scientific consensus" (Chou et al., 2020). Health *disinformation* is defined as deliberate distortion or misrepresentation of health-related information to support the sender's political or economic interests. In the context of COVID, this flow of information was characterized by WHO as an *infodemic*, that is, a great amount of information including false or misleading information on the pandemic. There is some support for the idea that misinformation can promote vaccine hesitancy (Borges Do Nascimento et al., 2022).

Social Media Use and Health Inequities

Inequalities in social media use follow some of the same patterns as differences in the use of mass media more generally. Differences in access to, engagement with, processing of and ability to act upon health information, or *communication inequalities*, are pervasive among population groups of different socioeconomic status (SES) and residence (Bekalu et al., 2016; Viswanath et al., 2021). While differences in access to and use of mass media have declined steadily, some differences persist in use of all types of communication media, with higher income groups using more cable and satellite television, Internet, newspapers, and media that require recurring fees (Viswanath et al., 2012; Whitacre et al., 2015). More educated and higher-income groups have more access to these information resources compared with lower SES groups. Income, education, and ethnicity are also associated with discrepancies in "going online" for health information and may influence active seeking of health information.

Differences in social media use between other groups also occur, though such differences may or may not constitute inequalities. For example, according to recent data in the U.S., social media use differs by age, with 84% of those between 18 and 29 years reporting the use of at least one social media platform compared to 45% of those 65 years and older (Pew Research Center, 2021). There are also notable differences by income, education, and residence, with over 75% of those earning $75,000 or higher, with college education, and with urban residence, respectively, reporting using at least one social media platform compared to 64–69% of those earning less than $30,000, with high school or less education, and rural residence (Pew Research Center, 2021). Such differences are parallel to more general health inequities (Lee & Viswanath, 2020; Viswanath et al., 2020, 2021).

A study of a nationally representative sample of American adults found that the association of social media use with social well-being and self-rated health (SRH) also varied across population subgroups (Bekalu et al., 2019). While the benefits seem to be generally higher among younger, better educated, and white racial/ethnic groups, harms seem to be higher among older, less educated, and minority racial/ethnic groups (Bekalu et al., 2019).

Inequalities in social media use also may magnify differences found in population health surveillance. When social media are used to monitor incidence and/or prevalence of physical and mental health conditions in populations (Merchant et al., 2019), this may complement and enhance traditional surveillance systems. But it may also exacerbate the impact of "data absenteeism," where data from disadvantaged groups are not represented or are underrepresented in health studies (Lee & Viswanath, 2020; Viswanath et al., 2022). Thus, the age-, income-, education- and residence-based differences in use of social media may contribute to data absenteeism if social media is used for public health surveillance.

Effects of Social Media on Health

The impact of social media use on health and health behavior is a topic of growing interest. To date, the research on both positive and negative impacts of social media on health and behavior is mixed and inconclusive. Figure 22.1 presents a framework of pathways through which social media, as one element of the complex information ecosystem, can influence health (physical, mental, and social) and health behaviors. As the framework shows, individuals could be exposed to social media and several other information sources at multiple levels: interpersonal, organizational, and mass media (Also see Chapters 3, 9, and 11). Exposure to these sources could be from naturally occurring communication processes and/or from planned communications and interventions. Effects of exposure to information sources should be seen against the backdrop of demographic characteristics and social factors. As indicated by the bidirectional vertical arrows in the figure, there can be mutual influence between routine/unplanned and planned communication processes, and individuals could be exposed to complementary or contradictory information from both processes. The framework also depicts the bidirectional nature of relationships between social media and background factors and health outcomes, as indicated by the two-headed horizontal arrows.

This framework illustrates factors that have been used in research to examine effects of social media on health and behavior. Researchers have studied social media use for a range of health behaviors, including smoking, alcohol use, diet, and sleep. Several studies have examined these questions in youth and college students; the findings are intriguing but also have important methodological limitations. A study using longitudinal data from a nationally representative sample of American youth found that watching and posting tobacco-related content on social media were associated with greater tobacco use among youth nationwide (Pérez et al., 2022). Similarly, in another study, it was reported that for adolescents, greater social media use and heavier exposure to advertisements and e-cigarette content in social media were associated with greater risk for e-cigarette use (Vogel et al., 2021). Further, exposure to peers' alcohol-related content on social media during the initial six weeks of college was found to predict alcohol consumption six months later (Boyle et al., 2016). A systematic review of literature on the link between social media use and dietary behaviors among children and adolescents found that greater social media use was associated with skipping breakfast, increased intake of unhealthy snacks and sugar-sweetened beverages, and lower fruit and vegetable intake, in both short-term experimental exposure studies and large cross-sectional surveys (Sina et al., 2022). However, the experiments were limited by single outcome measures, and the cross-sectional surveys cannot discern causal relationships.

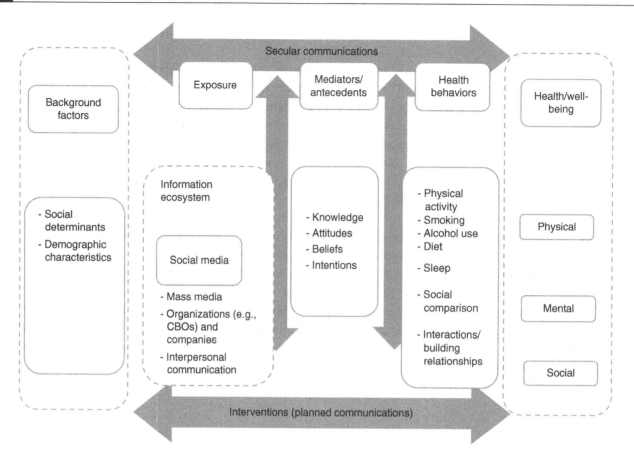

Figure 22.1 Social Media and Health in the Broader Ecosystem of Information, Behavior, and Health

In a survey among a sample of Midwestern university students in the U.S., Lee and colleagues found positive correlations of social media use with higher levels of C-reactive protein (a marker of chronic inflammation), more somatic symptoms, and more visits to doctors or health centers for an illness (Lee et al., 2022). The survey could not discern whether the health issues were causes of high social media use or effects, or whether they were both a result of some other factor(s).

One concern about the harmful effects of social media is articulated by the *displacement hypothesis*—that social media may displace health-promoting behaviors, such as physical activities and adequate sleep. A study drawing data from a nationally representative longitudinal sample of 12,866 young people ages 13 years to 16 years in England found that very frequent social media use increased in both boys and girls as they got older. The study also showed that mental health problems were related to cyberbullying and displacement of sleep or (to a small degree) less physical activity among girls (Viner et al., 2019). The negative effects from frequent use of social media were found only among girls in this study, suggesting the moderating role of gender (Viner et al., 2019). Thus, the picture is complicated when studying how social media are associated with mental health and social well-being outcomes.

A meta-analysis examining the association of different dimensions of social media use found that depressive symptoms were significantly, but weakly, associated with time spent using social media and intensity of social media use. However, the association of depressive symptoms to <u>problematic</u> social media use (e.g., social media use in combination with addictive symptoms) was moderate and significantly higher than for time spent or intensity of use (Cunningham et al., 2021). Another recent systematic review reported that different dimensions of social media use (time spent, type of activity, investment, and addiction) were correlated with depression, anxiety, and psychological distress (Keles et al., 2019) while also noting caveats due to methodological limitations such as of cross-sectional design, sampling, and measures.

The question of whether and how social media use impacts health itself has also garnered attention from the public and policy makers alike. Important questions are whether social media could be categorically bad or good for health, and whether there is sufficient evidence supporting any policy intervention. As shown by Figure 22.1, the effects of social media on physical health and well-being (emotional and social well-being) should be seen within the complex information ecosystem. Causal relationships are complex and often bi-directional (various health conditions leading to problematic use of social media).

A narrative review of trends in studies of social media and well-being by Kross and colleagues indicated that several experiments in recent years have found small, negative effects of social media use on well-being (Kross et al., 2021). They acknowledge that well-being is a complex construct, and that increasing evidence suggests that social media can either enhance or diminish health (physical, mental, and social), depending on how people use them (Kross et al., 2021). This notion is supported by data from a survey of nationally representative American adults that found routine use of social media and emotional connection with social media had divergent associations with social well-being, positive mental health, and self-rated health (Bekalu et al., 2019). Routine use of social media was associated positively with all three types of well-being; while emotional connection to social media was associated negatively with all the three outcomes. This is consistent with the above-noted Cunningham meta-analysis that found negative impacts of problematic social media use.

In summary, the literature on the impact of social media on health is mixed and inconclusive. The notion that "social media" is a singular phenomenon and can have good or bad effects on health is overly reductionist and simplistic, and more nuanced analyses need to be interpreted within their specific contexts. A recent field experiment in the United Kingdom on the effects of social media hiatus (short breaks from social media commonly known as "digital detoxing") on well-being did not find any positive effects (Przybylski et al., 2021). In addition, while a systematic review of reviews found that misinformation can negatively affect mental health (Borges Do Nascimento et al., 2022), eight of 31 reviews in that study also reported *positive* health outcomes, some finding that several social media platforms generated significantly improved knowledge and awareness, higher compliance with health recommendations, and more positive health-related behaviors among users of social media compared to other conventional information dissemination tools.

Methodology and Measurement in Research on Social Media and Health

Almost every review of the literature on the use and effects of social media on health raises methodological and measurement challenges (Kross et al., 2021; Orben, 2020; Valkenburg, 2022). Early research dating back to 2005 through 2010s mainly used self-report and cross-sectional methods, and studies did not examine the effects of social media on health over time (Kross et al., 2021). While there has been an increase in the number of longitudinal and experimental studies, researchers have argued that a need remains for research that allows for study of within-person associations of social media use with health (Valkenburg, 2022). While most studies that examined the effects of social media use on health have used conventional methods (e.g., cross-sectional, longitudinal, and/or experimental), some studies about use of social media platforms for public health surveillance (tracking and predicting diseases) have employed additional, innovative methods such as data mining and natural language processing (Merchant et al., 2019). Because social media-based surveillance systems can have many limitations and challenges, including noise, demographic bias, privacy issues, etc., the best methods may be hybrid studies that supplement traditional surveillance data with data from search queries, social media posts, and crowdsourcing (Aiello et al., 2020; Gupta & Katarya, 2020). These innovative methods have also been used to investigate social media as a tool or platform for health interventions.

Measurement approaches that can account for the complex nature of users' social media experiences are also still needed. Research should distinguish between measuring the amount of use, type of use (e.g., active versus passive), extent of users' engagement (e.g., emotional connection), valence of experience (positive versus negative), type of platform used, and the type of content consumed. Moreover, according to a recent systematic review, most studies (about 80%) do not use any theories (Bekalu et al., 2023). More theory-based studies would enhance our understanding of the mechanisms and conditions that characterize the effects of social media use on health behavior and health outcomes.

Health Behavior Interventions that Use Social Media

A growing body of research is investigating the use of social media as a channel for health promotion and/or disease prevention interventions. Social media can be harnessed for health behavior change interventions in many ways, including the provision of information, support networks, and skills that reinforce positive behaviors. Unlike conventional mass media, too, social media can be used to target and engage specific population groups and individuals. Social media technologies can provide platforms for interactivity whereby each audience member can react to the message source. Social media communications can also be either synchronous or asynchronous, providing audiences with the opportunity to interact with the message anytime and anywhere. Beyond disseminating health information, moreover, social media can provide interventionists with virtual social networks to support health behavior change (Chapter 11). Virtual social networks can be naturally occurring or created as part of an intervention.

Overall, reviews of the literature offer sufficient evidence for the effectiveness of social media interventions aiming at changing a range of health behaviors related to both infectious and non-infectious (non-communicable) diseases, including numerous published trials and several systematic reviews and meta-analyses on the effectiveness of social media interventions to change health behaviors and promote well-being. A recent Cochrane review that combined data for a variety of outcomes, for example, concluded that social media interventions may increase physical activity and improve well-being (Petkovic et al., 2021). Also, in a systematic review on theory-based social media interventions to address vaccine hesitancy, Li and colleagues found that the Health Belief Model (Chapter 5) was the most frequently deployed theory, and that most interventions used tools such as educational posts, dialogue-based groups, interactive websites, and personal reminders (Li et al., 2022). The review also found evidence that theory-based interventions triggered positive behavior changes more than atheoretical interventions, supporting the efficacy of theory-based interventions delivered through social media.

The causal mechanisms through which social media interventions lead to changes in health behaviors, such as increased physical activity, could be related to cognitive effects of exposure to targeted health messages and/or the social influence, social norms, and social support from a virtual social network. A randomized controlled trial investigating whether promotional messaging or peer networks on social media can increase physical activity found that social influence from anonymous online peers was more successful than promotional messages for improving physical activity (Zhang et al., 2015). Also, a recent review examining the behavior change techniques used in social media interventions for promoting healthy behaviors in adults found that interactive techniques such as "liking," "retweeting," "smiling," "congratulating," and "badging" were common techniques used in social media interventions to encourage healthful behaviors (Simeon et al., 2020).

Social Media Interventions and Health Inequities

It has been argued that the goal of public health communication interventions should include bridging communication gaps in health outcomes between population subgroups (Bekalu, 2014). However, communication inequalities sometimes play a key role in exacerbating health disparities (Bekalu et al., 2017; Viswanath et al., 2021). A systematic review that examined the effectiveness of social media interventions for health behavior change found that social media interventions had a significant, moderate-sized, positive effect on behavior change among populations experiencing health inequities despite significant heterogeneity across studies (Vereen et al., 2021). According to this review, social media interventions may be a promising intervention approach to encourage behavior change and mitigate health inequities.

Social media may also be useful to address global inequalities in health and health-related outcomes. Since social media use is increasing globally, in general, and in low- and middle-income countries (LMICs), in particular (Poushter et al., 2018), it is important to investigate whether these technologies can be effective tools for public health interventions. A systematic review of studies that examined the effectiveness of social media-based interventions for health behavior change in LMICs found most studies showed that social media interventions were effective. Also, several social media interventions for HIV/AIDS prevention have been shown to be effective in promoting HIV testing among men who have sex with men (MSM) in both high- and middle-income countries (Cao et al., 2017). However, some studies of the effectiveness of social media interventions did not quantify the level of social media engagement or use a theory or a conceptual model of behavior change, thus limiting the interpretation of those studies (Seiler et al., 2022).

Applications of Social Media for Health Behavior Interventions

Two examples illustrate how social media has been used for health behavior interventions.

Break-it-Off (BIO) Smoking Cessation Campaign

Break-it-Off (BIO) is an innovative, multicomponent, web-based, and social media approach to smoking cessation (Baskerville et al., 2016). The campaign, developed and implemented by the Canadian Cancer Society, was aimed at young adult smokers aged 19–29 in six provinces across Canada to engage them in smoking cessation through use of a website and social media. BIO used a "break-up" metaphor, comparing quitting smoking with ending a romantic relationship, to provide support and encourage young smokers to "break up" with their smoking addiction.

The intervention guided users through the challenging stages of ending an unhealthy relationship with smoking: getting it over with, staying split up, and moving on with life. Users could also learn through the website about established quit methods, such as telephone counseling, nicotine patches, and nicotine gum. They could upload a video of their "break-up with smoking" experience as well as announce their break-up status to friends via Facebook.

BIO was evaluated using a quasi-experimental design with baseline and three-month follow-up data from smokers exposed to BIO ($n = 102$ at follow-up) and a comparison group of Smokers' Helpline (SHL) users ($n = 136$ at follow-up). Findings demonstrated that the campaign resulted in reaching a wide swath of young adults and led to significantly higher quit attempts and quit rates compared with SHL users alone.

The success of this intervention may be attributed to social influence, social norms, and social support delivered through virtual social networks. For example, when smokers posted videos about their "break-up" experiences and/or announced their break-ups, they exerted a form of social influence that encouraged others in the network to follow suit. As elaborated in Social Cognitive Theory (see Chapter 9), individuals learn by observing the behaviors of others (modeling) and that learning can occur intentionally or unintentionally (Bandura, 2001, p. 271).

Facebook Advertising Campaign on COVID-19 Mitigation Measures

In November 2020, the number of COVID-19 cases was rapidly increasing across the United States, and, owing to concerns that holiday travel would exacerbate the problem, the Centers for Disease Control and Prevention recommended that people stay home for the Thanksgiving and Christmas holidays. In this context, researchers (Breza et al., 2021) ran a large, clustered, randomized controlled trial with Facebook users in randomly selected zip codes in the United States. The purpose of the study was to identify whether short videos delivered through Facebook would influence population-level holiday travel and, in turn, cause a decline in COVID-19 cases after the holidays.

Researchers worked with physicians and nurses before Thanksgiving and Christmas to record 20-second videos to encourage people to stay home for the holidays. They then disseminated the videos as sponsored content (ads) to Facebook subscribers in randomly selected zip codes in 820 counties in 13 states. Over 11 million people (35% of users in the targeted regions) received at least one ad before Thanksgiving, and over 23 million people (66% of users in targeted regions) received at least one video before Christmas. On average, each user reached by the campaign received 2.6 videos at Thanksgiving and 3.5 at Christmas.

The primary COVID-related outcome was COVID-19 infections recorded at the zip code level in the two-week period starting five days after the holiday. Infections declined by 3.5% in intervention compared to control zip codes. Researchers concluded that social media messages recorded by health professionals before the winter holidays in the United States led to a significant reduction in holiday travel and subsequent COVID-19 infections.

This study seems to have exploited a unique characteristic or capacity of social media: targeting and engaging people in specific regions and/or population groups. This distinctive ability distinguishes social media from conventional mass media such as television where messages are usually pushed out to largely undifferentiated mass audiences.

Future Directions

In a relatively short time, social media have become ubiquitous and have transformed the way people interact. This rapid change has led to concerns about their effects on health, especially the health of youth and adolescents. A close look at the literature reveals a large, though scattered, body of research that has examined the effects of social media use on a range of health-related outcomes over the past decade. However, the evidence is mixed and inconclusive, and low-quality research methods reduce the strength of any conclusions from these studies.

There are helpful, harmful, and benign ways of interacting with social media technologies; accordingly, there are positive, negative, and neutral effects of social media on health. Preoccupation with negative effects may lead to societal "moral panics" as was the case with mass media, in general, and television, in particular, several decades ago (Walsh, 2020). A limited understanding of both the negative and positive effects of these platforms on population health may misplace research agenda and public policies. We must understand not only how social media use could become addictive and harmful but also the ways and conditions in which these ubiquitous platforms can be leveraged to redress the lack of in-person social interactions and thereby improve population health.

Future research should consider individual and social factors that moderate and mediate the effects of social media use on health outcomes. Moreover, there is a need to go beyond time-based predictors (investigating the effects of time spent on social media) to content-based predictors (type of content, including its valence, consumed on social media) (Valkenburg, 2022). Most studies on the effects of social media use on health lump a range of different types of social media platforms or search for aggregate effects (Bekalu et al., 2022; Kross et al., 2021). Because different social media platforms have different features and affordances (properties or environments that permit social action), a more precise picture of the associations between social media platforms and health might be obtained from studying individual platforms.

Researchers have called for a "causal effect heterogeneity" approach to the study of social media use and health (Valkenburg, 2022). Instead of relying on average associations derived from heterogeneous populations of social media users who differ in how they select and respond to social media, we need causal effect models that enable us to better understand why and how individuals differ in their responses to social media use.

Given the usefulness of theory to guide researchers in their search to understand why and how social media use influences health and well-being, the limited presence of theory in the social media literature is a concern as well. Theories can be useful to inform research design, develop measures, and interpret findings. Atheoretical studies sometimes fail to give attention to the underlying processes and mechanisms that might explain why social media use may lead to harmful or beneficial outcomes.

References

Aiello, A. E., Renson, A., & Zivich, P. N. (2020). Social media- and internet-based disease surveillance for public health. *Annual Review of Public Health, 41*, 101–118.

Balta, S., Emirtekin, E., Kircaburun, K., & Griffiths, M. D. (2020). Neuroticism, trait fear of missing out, and phubbing: The mediating role of state fear of missing out and problematic Instagram use. *International Journal of Mental Health and Addiction, 18*, 628–639. https://doi.org/10.1007/s11469-018-9959-8.

Bandura, A. (2001). Social cognitive theory of mass communication. *Media Psychology, 3*, 265–299.

Baskerville, N. B., Azagba, S., Norman, C., McKeown, K., & Brown, K. S. (2016). Effect of a digital social media campaign on young adult smoking cessation. *Nicotine and Tobacco Research, 18*(3), 351–360. https://doi.org/10.1093/ntr/ntv119.

Bekalu, M. A. (2014). Communication inequalities and health disparities. *Information Development, 30*(2), 189–191.

Bekalu, M. A., Eggermont, S., & Viswanath, K. (2016). HIV/AIDS communication inequalities and associated cognitive and affective outcomes: A call for a socioecological approach to AIDS communication in Sub-Saharan Africa. *Health Communication, 32*(6), 685–694. https://doi.org/10.1080/10410236.2016.1167999.

Bekalu, M. A., Eggermont, S., & Viswanath, K. V. (2017). HIV/AIDS communication inequalities and associated cognitive and affective outcomes: A call for a socioecological approach to AIDS communication in Sub-Saharan Africa. *Health Communication, 32*(6), 685–694. https://doi.org/10.1080/10410236.2016.1167999.

Bekalu, M. A., Sato, T., & Viswanath, K. (2022). Social media use and well-being: Systematic review. Working Paper.

Bekalu, M. A., McCloud, R. F., Minsky, S., & Viswanath, K. (2021). Association of social participation, perception of neighborhood social cohesion, and social media use with happiness: Evidence of trade-off (JCOP-20-277). *Journal of Community Psychology, 49*(2), 432–446. https://doi.org/10.1002/jcop.22469.

Bekalu, M. A., McCloud, R. F., & Viswanath, K. (2019). Association of social media use with social well-being, positive mental health, and self-rated health: Disentangling routine use from emotional connection to use. *Health Education and Behavior, 46*(2), 69–80. https://doi.org/10.1177/1090198119863768.

Bekalu, M. A., Sato, T., & Viswanath, K. (2023). Conceptualizing and measuring social media use in health and well-being studies: Systematic review. *Journal of Medical Internet Research, 25*, e43191. https://doi.org/10.2196/43191.

Beyens, I., Frison, E., & Eggermont, S. (2016). "I don't want to miss a thing": Adolescents' fear of missing out and its relationship to adolescents' social needs, Facebook use, and Facebook related stress. *Computers in Human Behavior, 64*, 1–8.

Borges Do Nascimento, I. J., Beatriz Pizarro, A., Almeida, J., Azzopardi-Muscat, N., André Gonçalves, M., Björklund, M., & Novillo-Ortiz, D. (2022). Infodemics and health misinformation: A systematic review of reviews. *Bulletin of the World Health Organization, 100*(9), 544–561. https://doi.org/10.2471/BLT.21.287654.

Boyle, S. C., LaBrie, J. W., Froidevaux, N. M., & Witkovic, Y. D. (2016). Different digital paths to the keg? How exposure to peers' alcohol-related social media content influences drinking among male and female first-year college students. *Addictive Behaviors, 57*, 21–29. https://doi.org/10.1016/j.addbeh.2016.01.011.

Breza, E., Stanford, F. C., Alsan, M., Alsan, B., Banerjee, A., Chandrasekhar, A. G., Eichmeyer, S., Glushko, T., Goldsmith-Pinkham, P., Holland, K., Hoppe, E., Karnani, M., Liegl, S., Loisel, T., Ogbu-Nwobodo, L., Olken, B. A., Torres, C., Vautrey, P. L., Warner, E. T., Wootton, S., & Duflo, E. (2021). Effects of a large-scale social media advertising campaign on holiday travel and COVID-19 infections: a cluster randomized controlled trial. *Nature Medicine, 27*(9), 1622–1628. https://doi.org/10.1038/s41591-021-01487-3.

Burke, M., & Kraut, R. E. (2016). The relationship between Facebook use and well-being depends on communication type and tie strength. *Journal of Computer-Mediated Communication, 21*(4), 265–281. https://doi.org/10.1111/jcc4.12162.

Cao, B., Gupta, S., Wang, J., Hightow-Weidman, L. B., Muessig, K. E., Tang, W., Pan, S., Pendse, R., & Tucker, J. D. (2017). Social media interventions to promote HIV testing, linkage, adherence, and retention: Systematic review and meta-analysis. *Journal of Medical Internet Research, 19*(11), e394. https://doi.org/10.2196/jmir.7997.

Chou, S. W. Y., Gaysynsky, A., & Cappella, J. N. (2020). Where we go from here: Health misinformation on social media. *American Journal of Public Health, 110*(S3), S273–S275. https://doi.org/10.2105/AJPH.2020.305905.

Cunningham, S., Hudson, C. C., & Harkness, K. (2021). Social media and depression symptoms: A meta-analysis. *Research on Child and Adolescent Psychopathology, 49*(2), 241–253. https://doi.org/10.1007/s10802-020-00715-7.

DataReportal. (2023). Global social media statistics. https://datareportal.com/social-media-users

Eşkisu, M., Hoşoğlu, R., & Rasmussen, K. (2017). An investigation of the relationship between Facebook usage, Big Five, self-esteem and narcissism. *Computers in Human Behavior, 69*. https://doi.org/10.1016/j.chb.2016.12.036.

Frison, E., & Eggermont, S. (2020). Toward an integrated and differential approach to the relationships between loneliness, different types of Facebook use, and adolescents' depressed mood. *Communication Research, 47*(5), 701–728.

Goodyear, V. A., Wood, G., Skinner, B., & Thompson, J. L. (2021). The effect of social media interventions on physical activity and dietary behaviours in young people and adults: A systematic review. *International Journal of Behavioral Nutrition and Physical Activity, 18*(1), 1–18.

Günther, L., Schleberger, S., & Pischke, C. R. (2021). Effectiveness of social media-based interventions for the promotion of physical activity: Scoping review. *International Journal of Environmental Research and Public Health, 18*(24), 13018. https://doi.org/10.3390/ijerph182413018.

Gupta, A., & Katarya, R. (2020). Social media based surveillance systems for healthcare using machine learning: A systematic review. *Journal of Biomedical Informatics, 108*. https://doi.org/10.1016/j.jbi.2020.103500.

Katz, E., Blumler, J.G., & Gurevitch, M. (1974). Utilization of mass communication by the individual. In J.G. Blumler and E. Katz (Eds.), *The uses of mass communications: Current perspectives on gratifications research* (pp. 19–31). Beverly Hills: Sage Communications.

Keles, B., McCrae, N., & Grealish, A. (2019). A systematic review: The influence of social media on depression, anxiety and psychological distress in adolescents. *International Journal of Adolescence and Youth, 25*(1), 79–93. https://doi.org/10.1080/02673843.2019.1590851.

Kross, E., Verduyn, P., Sheppes, G., Costello, C. K., Jonides, J., & Ybarra, O. (2021). Social media and well-being: Pitfalls, progress, and next steps. *Trends in Cognitive Sciences, 25*(1), 55–66.

Lee, D. S., Jiang, T., Crocker, J., & Way, B. M. (2022). Social media use and its link to physical health indicators. *Cyberpsychology, Behavior, and Social Networking, 25*(2), 87–93.

Lee, E. W. J., & Viswanath, K. (2020). Big data in context: Addressing the twin perils of data absenteeism and chauvinism in the context of health disparities research. *Journal of Medical Internet Research, 22*(1), e16377. https://doi.org/10.2196/16377.

Li, L., Wood, C. E., & Kostkova, P. (2022). Vaccine hesitancy and behavior change theory-based social media interventions: A systematic review. *Translational Behavioral Medicine, 12*(2), 243–272.

Lin, R., & Utz, S. (2015). The emotional responses of browsing Facebook: Happiness, envy, and the role of tie strength. *Computers in Human Behavior, 52*, 29–38. https://doi.org/10.1016/j.chb.2015.04.064.

Lup, K., Trub, L., & Rosenthal, L. (2015). Instagram# instasad?: Exploring associations among Instagram use, depressive symptoms, negative social comparison, and strangers followed. *Cyberpsychology, Behavior, and Social Networking, 18*(5), 247–252.

Merchant, R. M., Asch, D. A., Crutchley, P., Ungar, L. H., Guntuku, S. C., Eichstaedt, J. C., Hill, S., Padrez, K., Smith, R. J., & Schwartz, H. A. (2019). Evaluating the predictability of medical conditions from social media posts. *PLoS One, 14*(6), e0215476. https://doi.org/10.1371/journal.pone.0215476.

Naslund, J. A., Kim, S. J., Aschbrenner, K. A., McCulloch, L. J., Brunette, M. F., Dallery, J., Bartels, S. J., & Marsch, L. A. (2017). Systematic review of social media interventions for smoking cessation. *Addictive Behaviors, 73*, 81–93. https://doi.org/10.1016/j.addbeh.2017.05.002.

Orben, A. (2020). Teenagers, screens and social media: A narrative review of reviews and key studies. *Social Psychiatry and Psychiatric Epidemiology, 55*(4), 407–414. https://doi.org/10.1007/s00127-019-01825-4.

Pérez, A., Spells, C. E., Bluestein, M. A., Harrell, M. B., & Hébert, E. T. (2022). The longitudinal impact of seeing and posting tobacco-related social media on tobacco use behaviors among youth (aged 12–17): Findings from the 2014–2016 Population Assessment of Tobacco and Health (PATH) Study. *Tobacco Use Insights, 15*, 1179173X221087554.

Pertegal, M. Á., Oliva, A., & Rodríguez-Meirinhos, A. (2019). Development and validation of the Scale of Motives for Using Social Networking Sites (SMU-SNS) for adolescents and youths. *PLoS One, 14*(12), e0225781. https://doi.org/10.1371/journal.pone.0225781.

Petkovic, J., Duench, S., Trawin, J., Dewidar, O., Pardo Pardo, J., Simeon, R., DesMeules, M., Gagnon, D., Hatcher Roberts, J., Hossain, A., Pottie, K., Rader, T., Tugwell, P., Yoganathan, M., Presseau, J., & Welch, V. (2021). Behavioural interventions delivered through interactive social media for health behaviour change, health outcomes, and health equity in the adult population. *Cochrane Database of Systematic Reviews*, (5), CD012932.

Pew Research Center. (2021). Social media fact sheet. https://www.pewresearch.org/internet/fact-sheet/social-media/?menuItem=d102dcb7-e8a1-42cd-a04e-ee442f81505a.

Poushter, J., Bishop, C., & Chwe, H. (2018). Social media use continues to rise in developing countries but plateaus across developed ones. *Pew Research Center, 22*, 2–19.

Przybylski, A. K., Nguyen, T. V. T., Law, W., & Weinstein, N. (2021). Does taking a short break from social media have a positive effect on well-being? Evidence from three preregistered field experiments. *Journal of Technology in Behavioral Science, 6*, 507–514.

Rumas, R., Shamblaw, A. L., Jagtap, S., & Best, M. W. (2021). Predictors and consequences of loneliness during the COVID-19 pandemic. *Psychiatry Research, 300*, 113934.

Seiler, J., Libby, T. E., Jackson, E., Lingappa, J., & Evans, W. (2022). Social media–based interventions for health behavior change in low- and middle-income countries: Systematic review. *Journal of Medical Internet Research, 24*(4), e31889. https://doi.org/10.2196/31889.

Simeon, R., Dewidar, O., Trawin, J., Duench, S., Manson, H., Pardo, J. P., Petkovic, J., Roberts, J. H., Tugwell, P., Yoganathan, M., Presseau, J., & Welch, V. (2020). Behavior change techniques included in reports of social media interventions for promoting health behaviors in adults: Content analysis within a systematic review. *Journal of Medical Internet Research, 22*(6), e16002. https://doi.org/10.2196/16002.

Sina, E., Boakye, D., Christianson, L., Ahrens, W., & Hebestreit, A. (2022). Social media and children's and adolescents' diets: A systematic review of the underlying social and physiological mechanisms. *Advances in Nutrition, 13*(3), 913–937.

Tankovska, H. (2021). Social media use during COVID-19 worldwide—statistics & facts. Statista. https://www.statista.com/topics/7863/social-media-use-during-coronavirus-covid-19-worldwide.

Valkenburg, P. M. (2022). Social media use and well-being: What we know and what we need to know. *Current Opinion in Psychology, 45*, 101294.

Verduyn, P., Lee, D. S., Park, J., Shablack, H., Orvell, A., Bayer, J., Ybarra, O., Jonides, J., & Kross, E. (2015). Passive Facebook usage undermines affective well-being: Experimental and longitudinal evidence. *Journal of Experimental Psychology. General, 144*(2), 480–488. https://doi.org/10.1037/xge0000057.

Verduyn, P., Ybarra, O., Résibois, M., Jonides, J., & Kross, E. (2017). Do social network sites enhance or undermine subjective well-being? A critical review. *Social Issues and Policy Review, 11*(1), 274–302. https://doi.org/10.1111/sipr.12033.

Vereen, R. N., Kurtzman, R., & Noar, S. M. (2021). Are social media interventions for health behavior change efficacious among populations with health disparities?: A meta-analytic review. *Health Communication, 38*(1), 133–140. https://doi.org/10.1080/10410236.2021.1937830.

Viner, R. M., Aswathikutty-Gireesh, A., Stiglic, N., Hudson, L. D., Goddings, A.-L., Ward, J. L., & Nicholls, D. E. (2019). Roles of cyberbullying, sleep, and physical activity in mediating the effects of social media use on mental health and wellbeing among young people in England: A secondary analysis of longitudinal data. *Lancet Child and Adolescent Health, 3*(10), 685–696. https://doi.org/10.1016/s2352-4642(19)30186-5.

Viswanath, K., Lee, E. W. J., & Pinnamaneni, R. (2020). We need the lens of equity in COVID-19 communication. *Health Communication, 35*(14), 1743–1746. https://doi.org/10.1080/10410236.2020.1837445.

Viswanath, K., McCloud, R. F., & Bekalu, M. A. (2021). Communication, health, and equity: structural influences. In T. L. Thompson & N. G. Harrington (Eds.), *The Routledge handbook of health communication* (pp. 426–440). New York: Routledge.

Viswanath, K., McCloud, R. F., Lee, E. W. J., & Bekalu, M. (2022). Measuring what matters: Data absenteeism, science communication, and the perpetuation of inequities. *The Annals of the American Academy of Political and Social Science, 700*(1), 208–219.

Viswanath, K., Nagler, R. H., Bigman-Galimore, C. A., McCauley, M. P., Jung, M., & Ramanadhan, S. (2012). The communications revolution and health inequalities in the 21st century: Implications for cancer control. *Cancer Epidemiology, Biomarkers and Prevention, 21*(10), 1701–1708. https://doi.org/10.1158/1055-9965.EPI-12-0852.

Vogel, E. A., Ramo, D. E., Rubinstein, M. L., Delucchi, K. L., Darrow, S. M., Costello, C., & Prochaska, J. J. (2021). Effects of social media on adolescents' willingness and intention to use e-cigarettes: An experimental investigation. *Nicotine and Tobacco Research, 23*(4), 694–701.

Walsh, J. P. (2020). Social media and moral panics: Assessing the effects of technological change on societal reaction. *International Journal of Cultural Studies, 23*(6), 840–859. https://doi.org/10.1177/1367877920912257.

Whitacre, B., Strover, S., & Gallardo, R. (2015). How much does broadband infrastructure matter? Decomposing the metro-non-metro adoption gap with the help of the National Broadband Map. *Government Information Quarterly, 32*(3), 261–269.

Yang, C., & Lee, Y. (2020). Interactants and activities on Facebook, Instagram, and Twitter: Associations between social media use and social adjustment to college. *Applied Developmental Science, 24*(1), 1–17. https://doi.org/10.1080/10888691.2018.1440233.

Yang, C. C., Holden, S. M., & Ariati, J. (2021). Social media and psychological well-being among youth: The multidimensional model of social media use. *Clinical Child and Family Psychology Review, 24*(3), 631–650. https://doi.org/10.1007/s10567-021-00359-z.

Zhang, J., Brackbill, D., Yang, S., & Centola, D. (2015). Efficacy and causal mechanism of an online social media intervention to increase physical activity: Results of a randomized controlled trial. *Preventive Medicine Reports, 2*, 651–657. https://doi.org/10.1016/j.pmedr.2015.08.005.

NAME INDEX

A

Abaluck, J., 263
Abraham, C., 16, 46, 48
Abrams, D. B., 83
Ackermann, R. T., 210
Adams, T. B., 80
Adjoian, T., 179
Adler, N. E., 6, 7
Ahmed, T. F., 51
Ahmed, W., 140
Aiello, A. E., 293
Ailshire, J. A., 122
Airhihenbuwa, C. O., 177
Ajie, W. N., 237
Ajzen, I., 12, 40, 41, 57–61, 63, 64, 69, 278, 279
Albarracin, D., 64, 69
Albertín, P., 127
Albright, C. L., 84
Alegria, A. A., 162
Alexander, C., 147
Al-Hasan, A., 51
Allais, P. M., 262
Allcott, H., 265
Allem, J. P., 145
Allen, A. M., 160
Allen, M., 209, 211
Allicock, M., 207
Al-Metwali, B. Z., 51
Alvarez-Galvez, J., 145
Amarel, D., 125
Amaro, H., 69
American Cancer Society, 207
American Institute of Stress, 157
American Psychological Association, 154, 156, 157, 160
Anderson, L. R., 260
Anderson, N. W., 175
Andreasen A., 275–277
Antonucci, T. C., 126
Arevalo, S., 179
Arias, E., 176
Armitage, C. J., 69
Arno, A., 268
Arora, M., 226
Arshoff, A. S., 244, 248
Artiga, S., 174
Asare, M., 110
Ashraf, N., 260
Aspinwall, L. G., 121
Atkins, L., 16
Auchincloss, A. H., 30

Averett, S. L., 106
Aveyard, P., 80, 83
Ayers, J. W., 145
Aziz, Z., 210

B

Babbie, E., 12, 13
Bachhuber, M. A., 266, 267
Bagozzi, R. P., 275
Bagramian, R. A., 32
Bailey, Z. D., 162, 169–171, 174, 177
Baker, P., 217
Balas, E. A., 201
Balestrieri, S. G., 73
Balta, S., 290
Bandura, A., 47, 58, 63, 76, 99, 101–106, 111, 112, 221, 250, 251, 279, 295
Banerjee, A. V., 262
Banik, R., 51
Banyard, V. L., 250
Barker, R. G., 24
Barnett, M. L., 264, 266
Barnett, N. P., 80
Barone, A., 281
Barrington-Trimis, J. L., 147
Barry, C. L., 222
Barth, J., 119, 123
Bartholomew, L. K., 11, 240, 247–249, 254, 255
Baskerville, N. B., 295
Basu, A., 105
Batavia, C., 162
Batis, C., 32
Baumann, A. A., 201, 211
Baumeister, R. F., 244, 248
Becker, M. H., 45, 48, 58
Bekalu, M. A., 237, 288–291, 293, 294, 296
Belansky, E. S., 254
Bell, D. A., 126, 177
Benitez, T. J., 84
Bennett, T. L., 125
Benowitz, N. L., 109
Benson, H., 158, 161
Benvenuti, M., 129
Berelson, B., 223
Berg, M. B., 51
Berjot, S., 161
Berkley-Patton, J. Y., 184, 192
Berkman, L. F., 117, 120, 123
Berkowitz, A. D., 95
Bernard, C., 154

Health Behavior: Theory, Research, and Practice, Sixth Edition. Edited by Karen Glanz,
Barbara K. Rimer, and K. Viswanath.
© 2024 John Wiley & Sons, Inc. Published 2024 by John Wiley & Sons, Inc.
Companion website: www.wiley.com/go/glanz/healthbehavior6e

SUBJECT INDEX

Health Behavior: Theory, Research, and Practice, Sixth Edition. Edited by Karen Glanz,
Barbara K. Rimer, and K. Viswanath.
© 2024 John Wiley & Sons, Inc. Published 2024 by John Wiley & Sons, Inc.
Companion website: www.wiley.com/go/glanz/healthbehavior6e